MacDonald's Atlas of

Procedures in Neonatology

Sixth Edition

MacDonald's Atlas of
Procedures in Neonatology

Sixth Edition

JAYASHREE RAMASETHU, MBBS, DCH, MD, FAAP

Professor of Clinical Pediatrics
Georgetown University Medical Center
Medical Director, Neonatal Intensive Care Unit
Associate Program Director, Neonatal Perinatal Medicine Fellowship Program
Division of Neonatal Perinatal Medicine
MedStar Georgetown University Hospital
Washington, DC

SUNA SEO, MD, MSc, FAAP

Assistant Professor of Clinical Pediatrics
Georgetown University Medical Center
Washington, DC

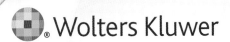

Philadelphia • Baltimore • New York • London
Buenos Aires • Hong Kong • Sydney • Tokyo

Acquisitions Editor: Robin Najar
Development Editor: Ashley Fischer
Editorial Coordinator: Emily Buccieri
Production Project Manager: David Saltzberg
Design Coordinator: Holly Reid McLaughlin
Senior Manufacturing Manager: Beth Welsh
Prepress Vendor: Aptara, Inc.

6th edition

9 8 7 6 5 4 3 2 1

Printed in China (or the United States of America)

978-1-4963-9425-5
Library of Congress Cataloging-in-Publication Data
available upon request

Library of Congress Control Number: 2019911905

shop.lww.com

*This book is dedicated to the newborn infants in our care
and to their parents who place their trust in us.*

Contributors

M. Kabir Abubakar, MD
Professor, Clinical Pediatrics
Georgetown University Medical Center
Attending Neonatologist/Director, Neonatal ECMO Program
Department of Pediatrics, Division of Neonatal Perinatal
    Medicine
MedStar Georgetown University Hospital
Washington, DC

Anne Ades, MD, MSEd
Professor, Clinical Pediatrics
University of Pennsylvania Perelman School of Medicine
Director, Neonatal Education
Department of Pediatrics, Division of Neonatology
Children's Hospital of Philadelphia
Philadelphia, Pennsylvania

Edward S. Ahn, MD
Professor, Neurosurgery and Pediatrics
Department of Neurologic Surgery
Mayo Clinic College of Medicine
Rochester, Minnesota

Hany Aly, MD, MSHS
Professor, Pediatrics
Case Western Reserve Lerner College of Medicine
Chairman, Department of Neonatology
Cleveland Clinic
Cleveland, Ohio

June Amling, MSN, RN, CNS, CWON, CCRN
Advanced Practice Nurse, Wound Team
Department of Plastic Surgery
Children's National Health System
Washington, DC

Jacob V. Aranda, MD, PhD, FRCPC, FAAP
Professor of Pediatrics and Ophthalmology and Director of
    Neonatology
Department of Pediatrics and Ophthalmology
State University of New York Downstate Medical Center
Brooklyn, New York

David Askenazi, MD, MSPH
Professor, Pediatrics, Nephrology
University of Alabama at Birmingham
Birmingham, Alabama

Stephen B. Baker, MD, DDS, FACS
Professor and Program Director
Department of Plastic Surgery
MedStar Georgetown University Hospital
Washington, DC

Megan E. Beck, MD
General Surgery Resident Physician
MedStar Georgetown University Hospital/Washington
    Hospital Center
Washington, DC

Alan Benheim, MD
Assistant Professor, Pediatrics
Virginia Commonwealth University School of Medicine
Richmond, Virginia
Pediatric Cardiology
Inova Children's Hospital
Fairfax, Virginia

Catherine M. Brown, MSN, RN, RNC-NIC
Staff Development Specialist II
Neonatal Intensive Care Unit
Virginia Hospital Center
Arlington, VA

Johanna M. Calo, MD
Assistant Professor of Pediatrics
Attending Neonatologist
Department of Pediatrics
State University of New York Downstate Medical Center
Brooklyn, New York

Joshua Casaos, BS
Johns Hopkins University School of Medicine
Division of Pediatric Neurosurgery
Baltimore, MD

Maura C. Caufield, MD
Dermatology
Colorado Center for Dermatology and Skin Surgery
Centennial, Colorado

A. Alfred Chahine, MD
Associate Professor, Surgery and Pediatrics
Department of Surgery
The George Washington University School of Medicine
Attending Surgeon
Children's National Health System
Washington, DC

Ela Chakkarapani, FRCPCH, MD
Consultant Senior Lecturer, Neonatology
St. Michael's Hospital
Translational Health Sciences
Bristol Medical School
Southwell street
Bristol, United Kingdom

Ha-Young Choi, MD
Assistant Professor, Pediatrics
Georgetown University Medical Center
Attending Neonatologist
Department of Pediatrics, Division of Neonatal Perinatal
    Medicine
MedStar Georgetown University Hospital
Washington, DC

Christine M. Clark, MD
Resident Physician, Otolaryngology
Department of Otolaryngology/Head and Neck Surgery
MedStar Georgetown University Hospital
Washington, DC

Marko Culjat, MD, PhD, FAAP
Neonatal Perinatal Medicine Fellow, Division of Neonatal
    Perinatal Medicine
MedStar Georgetown University Hospital
Washington, DC

Linda D'Angelo, BSN, RN-Retired
WOCN
Department of Nursing Georgetown University Hospital
    Washington, DC, USA

Peter A. Dargaville, MBBS, FRACP, MD
Professorial Research Fellow, Neonatology
Menzies Institute for Medical Research
University of Tasmania
Staff Specialist
Neonatal and Paediatric Intensive Care Unit
Royal Hobart Hospital
Hobart, Australia

Amber M. Dave, MD, FAAP
Neonatal-Perinatal Medicine Fellow
Division of Neonatal-Perinatal Medicine
MedStar Georgetown University Hospital
Washington, DC

Linda S. de Vries, MD, PhD
Em. Professor, Neonatal Neurology
University Medical Center Utrecht
Utrecht, the Netherlands

William F. Deegan III, MD
Pediatric Retina Surgeon
Virginia Hospital Center
Arlington, VA

Cynthia M. C. DeKlotz, MD
Assistant Professor of Clinical Medicine and Pediatrics
Georgetown University Medical Center
Pediatric and Adult Dermatologist
MedStar Washington Hospital Center/Georgetown
    University Hospital
Washington, DC

Catherine E. Demirel, PhD
Audiologist and Newborn Hearing Screening Coordinator
Department of Otolaryngology
MedStar Georgetown University Hospital
Washington, DC

Daniel R. Dirnberger, MD, FAAP
Medical Director of Neonatology
Nemours/Alfred I. duPont Hospital for Children
Wilmington, Delaware

Caitlin Drumm, MD
Assistant Professor
Department of Pediatrics
Uniformed Services University of the Health Sciences
Bethesda, Maryland
Attending Neonatologist
Department of Pediatrics
Brooke Army Medical Center
Fort Sam Houston, Texas

Jennifer A. Dunbar, MD
Associate Professor, Ophthalmology
Loma Linda University School of Medicine
Vice Chair for Clinical Affairs
Loma Linda Eye Institute
Loma Linda University Medical Center
Loma Linda, California

Debra A. Erickson-Owens, CNM, PhD
Associate Professor, Nursing
University of Rhode Island
Kingston, Rhode Island
Research Scientist, Pediatrics
Women & Infants Hospital
Providence, Rhode Island

Jane Germano, DO
Neonatologist
Department of Pediatrics and Neonatology
MedStar Washington Hospital Center
Washington, DC

Dorothy P. Goodman, BSN, RN, CWOCN
Wound, Ostomy and Continence Nurse
MedStar Georgetown University Hospital
Washington, DC

Allison M. Greenleaf, MSN, CPNP
Certified Pediatric Nurse Practitioner
Department of Pediatrics, Division of Neonatal Perinatal
    Medicine
MedStar Georgetown University Hospital
Washington, DC

Ashish O. Gupta, MD
Assistant Professor, Clinical Pediatrics
Sidney Kimmel Medical College
Thomas Jefferson University
Philadelphia, Pennsylvania
Attending Neonatologist
Nemours/Alfred I. DuPont Hospital for Children
Wilmington, Delaware

Earl H. Harley, Jr., MD
Professor, Otolaryngology
MedStar Georgetown University Hospital
Washington, DC

Traci Henderson, RPh
Clinical Pharmacist, Nephrology
Children's of Alabama
Birmingham, Alabama

Sarah A. Holzman, MD
Urology Chief Resident
MedStar Georgetown University Hospital
Washington, DC

Daryl Ingram, RN, BSN, CDN
Acute Dialysis Coordinator
Children's of Alabama
Birmingham, Alabama

Rajiv R. Iyer, MD
Department of Neurosurgery Johns Hopkins University
    School of Medicine
Division of Pediatric Neurosurgery
Neurosurgery Resident
The Johns Hopkins Hospital Baltimore, MD USA

Cyril Jacquot, MD, PhD
Associate Medical Director for Blood Donor Center
Divisions of Laboratory Medicine and Hematology
Children's National Health System
Assistant Professor, Pediatrics and Pathology
George Washington University School of Medicine
    and Health Sciences
Washington, DC

Kara Johnson, BSN, RN, WOC-RN, WCC
Senior Quality Outcomes Coordinator
Department of Nursing Science, Professional Practice, &
    Quality Outcomes
Children's National Health System
Washington, DC

Lindsay C. Johnston, MD, MEd
Associate Professor, Pediatrics
Yale School of Medicine
Attending Neonatologist, Pediatrics
Yale-New Haven Children's Hospital
New Haven, Connecticut

Karen Kamholz, MD, MPH
Associate Professor, Clinical Pediatrics
Georgetown University Medical Center
Program Director, Neonatal-Perinatal Medicine
    Fellowship Program
Department of Pediatrics, Division of Neonatal Perinatal
    Medicine
MedStar Georgetown University Hospital
Washington, DC

Anup C. Katheria, MD
Associate Professor, Pediatrics
Loma Linda School of Medicine
Loma Linda, California
Neonatology
Sharp Mary Birch Hospital for Women & Newborns
San Diego, California

Suhasini Kaushal, MD
Assistant Professor, Pediatrics
Department of Pediatrics; Division of Neonatal Perinatal
    Medicine
Georgetown University Medical Center
Attending Physician
Division of Neonatal Perinatal Medicine
MedStar Georgetown University Hospital
Washington, DC

Bavana Ketha, MD
Resident
Department of Surgery
MedStar Georgetown University Hospital
Washington, DC

Chahira Kozma, MD
Professor, Clinical Pediatrics
Georgetown University Medical Center
Washington, DC

Aaron J. Krill, MD
Assistant Professor
Department of Surgery
George Washington University
Pediatric Urologist
Children's National Medical Center
Washington, DC

Margaret Mary Kuczkowski, MSN, CRNP
Intermediate Care Nurse Practitioner
Neonatal Intensive Care Unit
MedStar Georgetown University Hospital
Washington, DC

Neha Kumbhat, MD, MS Epi
Clinical Neonatology Fellow, Neonatology/Pediatrics
Lucile Packard Children's Hospital
Stanford University School of Medicine
Palo Alto, California

Stephanie S. Lee, MD
Division of Newborn Medicine
St. Louis Children's Hospital
Washington University School of Medicine
St. Louis, Missouri

Lara M. Leijser, MD, MSc, PhD
Assistant Professor
Department of Pediatrics, Section of Neonatology
Cumming School of Medicine, University of Calgary
Alberta Health Services
Pediatrician/Neonatologist
Calgary, Canada

Naomi L. C. Luban, MD
Vice Chair of Academic Affairs
Medical Director of the Office of Human Subjects
    Protection
Children's National Health System
Professor, Pediatrics and Pathology
George Washington University School of Medicine and
    Health Sciences
Washington, DC

Mirjana Lulic-Botica, Pharm D, BCPS
Neonatal Clinical Pharmacy Specialist
Hutzel Women's Hospital, Detroit Medical Center
Detroit, Michigan

Louis Marmon, MD, PhD
Professor of Surgery and Pediatrics
George Washington University School of Medicine
Department of Surgery
Division of General and Thoracic Surgery
Children's National Medical Center
Washington, DC

Kathryn M. Maselli, MD
Surgical Resident
Department of Surgery
MedStar Georgetown University Hospital
Washington, DC

Harley Mason, MBBS, DCH
Paediatric Registrar Department of Paediatrics
Women's and Children's Services Royal Hobart Hospital
Tasmania, Australia

Amit M. Mathur, MBBS, MD, MRCP (UK)
Professor, Pediatrics
St. Louis University School of Medicine/SSM-Cardinal
    Glennon Children's Hospital
St. Louis, Missouri

Judith S. Mercer, PhD, FACNM
Advent Professor, Pediatrics
Brown University Alpent School of Medicine
Providence, Rhode Island
Consultant
Neonatal Research Institute
Sharp Mary Birch Hospital for Women & Newborns
San Diego, California

Gregory J. Milmoe, MD
Associate Professor, Otolaryngology/Head and Neck Surgery
Georgetown University Medical Center
Attending
Department of Otolaryngology/Head and Neck Surgery
MedStar Georgetown University Hospital
Washington, DC

Yunchuan Delores Mo, MD, MSc
Associate Medical Director for Blood Bank
Divisions of Laboratory Medicine and Hematology
Children's National Health System
Assistant Professor, Pediatrics and Pathology
George Washington University School of Medicine and
    Health Sciences
Washington, DC

Mohamed A. Mohamed, MD, MS, MPH
Professor of Pediatrics and Global Health
Director, Newborn Services Division
The George Washington University School of Medicine
Washington, DC

Aaron Mohanty, MCN
Associate Professor
Division of Neurosurgery, Department of Surgery
University of Texas Medical Branch
Galveston, Texas

Vincent Mortellaro, MD
Assistant Professor
Department of Surgery
University of Alabama at Birmingham
Birmingham, Alabama

Robert J. Musselman, DDS, MSD
Professor, Pediatric Dentistry
LSUHSC School of Dentistry
New Orleans, Louisiana

John North, MD
Neonatologist, Pediatrics
Neonatology/Inova Children's Hospital
Falls church, Virginia

Kimberly K. Patterson, DDS, MS
Assistant Professor, Graduate Program Director
Pediatric Dentistry
Medical University of South Carolina
Charleston, South Carolina

Jayashree Ramasethu, MBBS, DCH, MD, FAAP
Professor, Clinical Pediatrics
Georgetown University Medical Center
Medical Director, Neonatal Intensive Care Unit
Associate Program Director, Neonatal Perinatal Medicine
    Fellowship Program
Division of Neonatal Perinatal Medicine
MedStar Georgetown University Hospital
Washington, DC

Jolie Ramesar, MD, FAAP
Department of Pediatrics
Valley Children's Healthcare
Madera, CA

Anoop Rao, MD, MS
Instructor, Neonatology/Pediatrics
Stanford University School of Medicine
Stanford, California

Mary E. Revenis, MD
Associate Professor, Pediatrics
The George Washington University School of Medicine
    and the Health Sciences
Attending Neonatologist
Department of Neonatology
Children's National Medical Center
Washington, DC

Lisa M. Rimsza, MD
Professor and Consultant
Department of Laboratory Medicine and Pathology
Mayo Clinic
Scottsdale, Arizona

Priyanshi Ritwik, BDS, MS
Associate Professor, Pediatric Dentistry
LSUHSC School of Dentistry
New Orleans, Louisiana

Angela Rivera, RN
Staff Nurse
Neonatal Intensive Care Unit
MedStar Georgetown University Hospital
Washington, DC

Anne S. Roberts, MD
Department of General Surgery
Mid-Atlantic Permanente Medical Group
McLean, Virginia
Attending Surgeon
Virginia Hospital Center
Arlington, VA

Reem Saadeh-Haddad, MD
Associate Professor
Georgetown University Medical Center
Department of Pediatrics
MedStar Georgetown University Hospital
Washington, DC

Maame Efua S. Sampah, MD, PhD
Resident
Department of Surgery
Medstar Georgetown University Hospital
Washington, DC

Thomas T. Sato, MD
Professor, Surgery and Pediatric Surgery
Senior Associate Dean, Surgery
Medical College of Wisconsin
CEO
Children's Specialty Group
Children's Hospital of Wisconsin
Milwaukee, Wisconsin

Matthew A. Saxonhouse, MD
Associate Professor
Department of Pediatrics, Division of Neonatology
Levine Children's Hospital at Atrium Health
Charlotte, North Carolina

Melissa Scala, MD
Clinical Assistant Professor, Pediatrics
Lucile Packard Children's Hospital/Stanford University
Palo Alto, California

Kelly A. Scriven, MD
Resident Physician, Otolaryngology
Department of Otolaryngology/Head and Neck Surgery
Georgetown University Hospital
Washington, DC

Suna Seo, MD, MD, MSc, FAAP
Assistant Professor, Clinical Pediatrics
Georgetown University Medical Center
Washington, DC

Kara Short, MSN, CRNP
Pediatric Nurse Practitioner
Department of Pediatric Nephrology
Children's of Alabama
Birmingham, Alabama

Lamia Soghier, MD, MEd, FAAP
Associate Professor of Pediatrics
George Washington University School of Medicine and
    Health Sciences
Medical Unit Director of the Neonatal Intensive Care Unit
Children's National Health System
Washington, DC

Martha C. Sola-Visner, MD
Associate Professor, Pediatrics
Department of Pediatrics, Division of Newborn Medicine
Boston Children's Hospital/Harvard Medical School
Boston, Massachusetts

Ganesh Srinivasan, MD
Director, Neonatal-Perinatal Medicine Subspecialty
    Residency Program
Section of Neonatal-Perinatal Medicine
University of Manitoba
Winnipeg, Canada

Nathalie El Ters, MD
Instructor, Pediatrics
Washington University School of Medicine
St. Louis Children's Hospital
St. Louis, Missouri

Marianne Thoresen, MD, PhD
Professor, Neonatal Neuroscience
Bristol Medical School, University of Bristol
Honorary Consultant Neonatologist
St. Michael's Hospital
Bristol, United Kingdom

Manuel B. Torres, MD
Assistant Professor of Surgery and Pediatrics
Department of Surgery and Pediatrics
George Washington University School of Medicine and
    Health Sciences
Attending Pediatric Surgeon
Department of Surgery
Children's National Medical Center and MedStar
    Georgetown University Hospital
Washington, DC

Victoria Tutag-Lehr, BS Pharm, PharmD
Professor, Department of Pharmacy Practice
Clinical Pharmacy Specialist-Pediatric Pain
Eugene Applebaum College of Pharmacy and Health
    Sciences
Wayne State University
Detroit, Michigan

Gloria B. Valencia, MD, FAAP
Professor of Pediatrics and Medical Director of Newborn
    Intensive Care Unit
Department of Pediatrics
State University of New York Downstate Medical Center
Brooklyn, New York

Aimee Vaughn, BS, MSN, RNC-NIC
QI and Patient Safety Coordinator
MedStar Georgetown University Hospital
Washington, DC

Jessica S. Wang, MD
Plastic Surgery Resident
Department of Plastic and Reconstructive Surgery
MedStar Georgetown University Hospital
Washington, DC

Jennifer L. Webb, MD, MSCE
Medical Director of Therapeutic Apheresis
Division of Hematology
Children's National Health System
Assistant Professor, Pediatrics
George Washington University School of Medicine and
    Health Sciences
Washington, DC

Laura Welch, BSN, RN-BC, CPN, WOC-RN, WCC
Professional Practice Specialist
Department of Nursing
Children's National Health System
Washington, DC

Tung T. Wynn, MD
Assistant Professor, Pediatrics
Department of Pediatrics, Division of Pediatric
    Hematology/Oncology
University of Florida Shand's Children's Hospital
Gainesville, Florida

Video Contributors

The editors and contributors gratefully acknowledge the past video contributions of the following individuals:

Hany Aly, MD

Alan Benheim, MD, FACC, FAAP

John North, MD

Khodayar Rais-Bahrami, MD, FAAP

Jayashree Ramasethu, MBBS, DCH, MD, FAAP

Mary E. Revenis, MD

Lamia Soghier, MD, FAAP

Alfonso Vargas, III, MD

Illustration Contributors

The editors and contributors gratefully acknowledge the past illustration contributions of the following individuals:

Judy Guenther

Virginia Schoonover

Marko Culjat

Foreword

But chieflye the anatomye
Ye oughte to understand;
If ye will cure well anye thinge,
That ye doe take in hande......
—John Halle (1529–1568)

In the United Kingdom, where I completed my training in pediatrics in the early 1970s, pediatrics was not officially accredited as a medical specialty worthy of equal status with surgery and internal medicine until 1996, when the Royal College of Pediatrics and Child Health (RCPCH) received its Royal Charter. Neonatology subsequently emerged from the shadows as a key subspecialty of pediatrics, and academic neonatologists in the United Kingdom can now become free-standing professors of neonatology.

I received my training in neonatology in the United States, where the American Academy of Pediatrics (AAP) was founded in 1930. Despite this head start, neonatology was not formally accredited as a pediatric subspecialty by the AAP until 1975. The first Sub-Board examination in Neonatal-Perinatal Medicine was offered in the same year. Of course, in both countries, those interested in neonatal medicine had been building a substantial core curriculum and body of research for decades prior to subspecialty accreditation. Subsequent advances provided the opportunity for more vigorous physiologic support and monitoring during procedures, but also new side effects and potential complications.

Published in 1983, the first edition of the "*Atlas of Procedures in Neonatology*" was born out of the recognition that the body of procedures playing a critical role in neonatal intensive care was growing rapidly and that the neonatology trainee too frequently learned how to perform these procedures by observing a more senior trainee who had learned the same way. The literature on performance, complications, and outcome of individual procedures was widely scattered, difficult to access, and often deficient in anatomic detail and patient numbers.

The "Atlas" was designed to meet the need for a comprehensive resource providing a step-by-step evidence-based approach to each procedure, with emphasis on anatomy, physiology, and prevention of complications. When germane, alternative methodology and discussion of controversial points were also included. Over the years it has been truly gratifying to witness the evolution of this book into a trusted and frequently dog-eared reference found in neonatal intensive care units all over the world.

Key to the success of the "Atlas" is that it is written and edited by practitioners who actively engage in performing the procedures. I can now enjoy my retirement, happy in the knowledge that Drs Jayashree Ramasethu and Suna Seo have assumed the care and feeding of the "Atlas" and have produced an outstanding sixth edition!

Mhairi G. MacDonald, MBChB, DCH, FRCP(E), FAAP, FRCPCH
Professor Emeritus of Pediatrics
George Washington School of Medicine and Health Sciences
Washington, DC

Preface

In theory there is no difference between theory and practice. In practice there is.
　　　　　　　　　　　　　　　　　　　—Yogi Berra

The *Atlas of Procedures in Neonatology* was published first in 1983, and since then there have been four additional editions, each edition elucidating both common and uncommon procedures performed in newborn infants, with updated information and new techniques. With an enormous amount of information available on the Internet, is another edition of this book still warranted? We maintain that the "Atlas" remains a valuable resource for practicing clinicians with its emphasis on correct techniques, precautions, and potential complications, all in one handy, technology-independent source.

Dr. Mhairi MacDonald was an editor of the "Atlas" from the 1st edition through the 5th edition. She shepherded the "Atlas" over 30 years, ensuring it was current and accurate. Dr. MacDonald has retired from editing this book, and we have assumed this major responsibility. It is only fitting that the 6th edition is now named *MacDonald's Atlas of Procedures in Neonatology.*

In the past 50 years, since the specialty of Neonatology was formally recognized, we have focused on technology and techniques to help smaller and younger babies survive. In industrialized nations, we have probably reached the limits of neonatal viability at about 350 to 400 g birth weight and 22 weeks of gestation, although few survive at these extremes and even fewer survive intact. More recently, with the increasing recognition of the large numbers of preterm births and high neonatal mortality and morbidity in low and middle income countries, the emphasis has shifted to improving survival of all newborns around the world (Every Newborn Action Plan, WHO 2014). There is increasing focus on delivering babies in health care facilities, and a recognized need to improve neonatal care in such facilities.

The training of providers in neonatal procedures remains a vital part of neonatal care in special and intensive care units in industrialized nations as well as in low and middle income countries. Placement of an intravenous catheter in a preterm infant or drawing of a blood sample from an arterial stick may seem like minor procedures but they are performed innumerable times in busy units. Flawless execution of these common procedures saves time, supplies, and equipment and decreases stress on the infant and caregiver. Too often we have used the "see one, do one, teach one" model of learning, with the risk of missing important training due to lack of opportunity. Advances in respiratory care have reduced the incidence of pneumothorax in infants receiving intensive care and yet, when this complication arises, it is an emergency that requires immediate treatment with needle aspiration or placement of a chest tube. Many physicians lack the expertise to perform these procedures owing to lack of exposure and experience.

In order to circumvent this situation, simulation training has become the cornerstone for education in neonatal procedures. Although increasingly sophisticated high-fidelity models have been developed, many are unaffordable for programs around the world. In this edition, we include a chapter on how to make low-cost models for neonatal procedures using materials found in local hardware and toy stores. We have used these models successfully in training workshops at national and international meetings, and encourage the development of such models to improve knowledge and skills in neonatal health care providers around the world. We have added a section on checklists for common procedures that could be used for training purposes, so that critical steps of procedures are not missed.

In the "see one, do one, teach one" model, there is a potential risk of passing on less-than-ideal practices through generations of learners. Examples include the routine administration of calcium gluconate during exchange transfusions and the use of "prophylactic aggressive" phototherapy. In this edition of the "Atlas," as in previous editions, we have tried to find the best possible evidence for practices, and have discussed controversies where relevant. Some changes may be small, but we believe that small incremental changes in practice may lead to major improvements in neonatal care and advance the field of neonatology.

This edition of the "Atlas" also includes several new chapters. Delayed cord clamping was endorsed by the World Health Organization in 2007; its importance in preterm infants is being increasingly recognized and adopted into routine clinical practice. Amplitude-integrated EEG monitoring has become the standard of care in several neonatal intensive care units. Minimally invasive surfactant therapy is finding increased application. Ventriculoperitoneal shunts and their complications are not uncommon problems in the neonatal intensive care unit. A chapter has been devoted to wound care, a necessary skill to counteract the unfortunate complications of surgery or invasive procedures or sometimes to deal with congenital skin conditions that are similar to open wounds.

This text is bundled with a VitalSource eBook. Several chapters have accompanying videos that are also available with your access to the eBook. Instructions for activating your eBook are located on the inside front cover of the text.

The "Atlas" covers topics from capillary blood sampling to complex procedures like extracorporeal membrane oxygenation (ECMO) cannulation, and renal replacement therapy. We trust that these procedures will be performed by those who have the necessary training and qualifications. No textbook can replace the knowledge acquired by observation, simulation, and practice. We hope that the "Atlas" will be a valuable resource to all those who care for newborn infants, in special care nurseries and neonatal intensive care units around the world.

Practice isn't the thing you do once you're good. It's the thing you do that makes you good   —*Malcolm Gladwell*

Jayashree Ramasethu, MBBS, DCH, MD, FAAP

Suna Seo, MD, MSc, FAAP

Preface to the First Edition

The rapid advances in neonatology in the last 15 years have brought with them a welter of special procedures. The tiny, premature, and the critically ill term neonate is attached to a tangle of intravenous lines, tubes, and monitoring leads. As a result, more and more procedures are done at the bedside in the intensive-care nursery, rather than in a procedure room or operating room. With these technical advances has come the opportunity for more vigorous physiologic support and monitoring. With them also has come a whole new gamut of side effects and complications. The old dictum to leave the fragile premature undisturbed is largely ignored. It is therefore the responsibility of those who care for sick newborns to understand the complications as well as the benefits of new procedures and to make systematic observations of their impact on both morbidity and mortality. Unfortunately, the literature on outcome and complications of procedures is widely scattered and difficult to access. Manuals that give directions for neonatal procedures are generally deficient in illustrations giving anatomic detail and are often cursory.

We are offering *Atlas of Procedures in Neonatology* to meet some of these needs. A step-by-step, practical approach is taken, with telegraphic prose and outline form. Drawings and photographs are used to illustrate anatomic landmarks and details of the procedures. In several instances, more than one alternative procedure is presented. Discussion of controversial points is included, and copious literature citations are provided to lead the interested reader to source material. A uniform order of presentation has been adhered to wherever appropriate. Thus, most chapters include indications, contraindications, precautions, equipment, technique, and complications, in that order.

The scope of procedures covered includes nearly all those that can be performed at the bedside in an intensive-care nursery. Some are within the traditional province of the neonatologist or even the pediatric house officer. Others, such as gastrostomy and tracheostomy, require skills of a qualified surgeon. Responsibility for procedures such as placement of chest tubes and performance of vascular cutdowns will vary from nursery to nursery. However, some details of surgical technique are supplied for even the most invasive procedures to promote their understanding by those who are responsible for sick neonates. We hope this will help neonatologists to be more knowledgeable partners in caring for babies and will not be interpreted as a license to perform procedures by those who are not adequately qualified.

The book is organized into major parts (e.g., "Vascular Access," "Tube Placement," "Respiratory Care"), each of which contains several chapters. Most chapters are relatively self-contained and can be referred to when approaching a particular task. However, Part I, "Preparation and Support," is basic to all procedures. Occasional cross-referencing has been used to avoid repetitions of the same text material. References appear at the end of each part.

Many persons have contributed to the preparation of this atlas, and we are grateful to them all. Some are listed under Acknowledgments, and others have contributed anonymously out of their generosity and good will. A special thanks is due to Bill Burgower, who first thought of making such an atlas and who has been gracious in his support throughout this project.

If this atlas proves useful to some who care for sick newborns, our efforts will have been well repaid. Neonatology is a taxing field: strenuous, demanding, confusing, heartbreaking, rewarding, stimulating, scientific, personal, philosophical, cooperative, logical, illogical, and always changing. The procedures described in this atlas will eventually be replaced by others, hopefully more effective and less noxious. In the meantime, perhaps the care of some babies will be assisted.

Mary Ann Fletcher, MD

Mhairi G. MacDonald, MBChB, FRCP(E), DCH

Gordon B. Avery, MD, PhD

Acknowledgments

We would like to acknowledge the hard work of all the authors who contributed to this book, and thank all those who took photographs and sent us useful figures and x-rays. We understand the time commitment required to make this happen in the middle of busy schedules.

We would also like to thank the staff from Wolters Kluwer, Emily Buccieri, Ashley Fischer, and Robin Najar for their patience and flexibility in dealing with delays, and to Anamika Singh of Aptara for her help in coordinating the production of the book.

Contents

Section V   Vascular Access

Section VI   Respiratory Care

Section VII   Tube Placement and Care

Section VIII   Transfusions

SECTION IX Miscellaneous Procedures

Preparation and Support

Educational Principles of Simulation-Based Procedural Training

Ganesh Srinivasan

The Need

The traditional see one, do one, teach one, *and hope not to harm one* Halstedian model of graduated responsibility for acquisition of procedural skills has been termed "education by random opportunity." Rationing of work hours during residency training, the increasing breadth of technical skills required in neonatology, and the limited opportunity to acquire competence in the context of safety and time provide us with both a challenge and an opportunity to revisit traditional training and embrace innovative learning strategies.

The educational strategies best suited to address acquisition of procedural skills include didactic, audiovisual, simulated experiences and supervised clinical experiences with coaching and feedback.

Simulation enables repeated procedural exposure in a safe environment without compromising patient safety, that is, see a lot, simulate and train a lot, teach and assist a lot, *and harm none* (1–10). Although animal and other models have been used to teach and practice procedures used in neonates for the past 4 decades (**Fig. 1.1A–E** and **Table 1.1**) (3,8), the role of simulation-based training has made a paradigm shift in the past 20 years to an educational experience that helps address the need for integrated acquisition of technical skills, behavioral skills (including ability to work as part of a team), and cognitive skills—factors where deficits identified and not corrected may lead to adverse outcomes. The Neonatal Resuscitation Program™ has embraced simulation-based resuscitation training methodology to teach and evaluate competence in neonatal resuscitation (12). The recent advances and availability of virtual reality and augmented reality in addition to high fidelity simulators hold promise in advancing our goal of improving safety and quality for all while performing procedures. This chapter serves as a general overview of the current underlying educational principles of simulation-based training in neonatology (13–18).

Definition

Modern-day simulation is an immersive instructional strategy that is used to replace or amplify real experiences with guided experiences that evoke or replicate substantial aspects of the real world in a fully interactive manner.

The Theory of Simulation-Based Learning

Bloom's Taxonomy

According to Bloom's taxonomy of learning (**Fig. 1.2**), knowledge and comprehension are the simplest levels of learning. Simulation, when used with the goal of improving practice, can allow the learner to move from knowledge or comprehension to application, analysis, and synthesis, which are better indicators of competence.

Adult Learners

1. Are self-directed and self-regulated in their learning
2. Are predominantly intrinsically motivated to learn
3. Have previous knowledge and experience that are an increasing resource for learning
4. Through this previous experience, they form mental models that guide their behavior
5. Use analogical reasoning in learning and practice

The process of having an experience (concrete experience), reflecting on the experience (reflective observation),

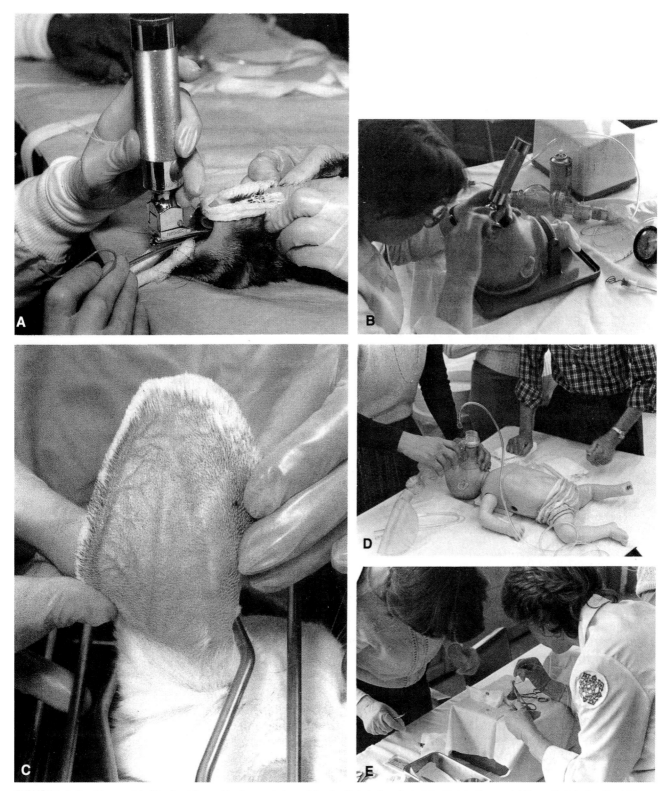

FIGURE 1.1 Teaching models (**A**) a ferret is used to demonstrate endotracheal intubation. **B:** An infant intubation model (Resusci Intubation Model, Laerdal Medical, Armonk, NY) is used to practice endotracheal intubation. A viewing port in the back of the head allows demonstration of anatomic relationships. **C:** A rabbit's ear has been shaved to demonstrate vessels for intravenous placement. **D:** A resuscitation model (Resusci Baby, Laerdal Medical) is used to practice bag and mask ventilation. **E:** An umbilical cord is used to practice catheter insertion. The cord is placed in an infant feeding bottle, filled with normal saline, and supported inside a cardboard box. The end of the cord projects through a cut nipple. (Reprinted with permission from MacDonald MG, Seshia MMK. *Neonatology: Pathophysiology and Management of the Newborn.* 4th ed. Philadelphia, PA: JB Lippincott; 1994.)

TABLE 1.1 Teaching Models Used to Teach Procedures

Manikin (Small Dolls with Soft Vinyl Skin)
To teach tracheotomy care:
    Create a hole in the doll's neck with a sharp instrument—a corkscrew works well.
    Insert a size 1 or size 0 tracheotomy tube.
    Tie the ties, and use as a model to teach proper suctioning and skin care techniques.
To teach umbilical catheter management:
    Puncture the doll's anterior abdomen using a 16-gauge Medicut needle.
    Insert needle through the doll's front and back, then remove.
    Thread an umbilical catheter through from front to back.
    Insert blunt needles onto catheter at both ends. An IV bag containing water tinted with red food coloring can be attached to the posterior end of the catheter to simulate blood.
To teach technique for drawing samples for blood gases:
    Insert a three-way stopcock into the umbilical catheter anteriorly and attach IV bag and tubing.
This system also can be used to teach arterial and venous blood pressure monitoring by transducer.
    To simulate arterial pressure, wrap a blood pressure cuff around the partially filled IV bag and inflate to 60–70 torr.
    For a venous line, inflate to 5–10 torr.

Resusci Head[a]
The model head used for endotracheal intubation can be modified to teach orogastric and nasogastric feeding by attaching a reservoir to the esophageal opening.

Rabbits
To teach placement of chest tube:
    Anesthetize a rabbit weighing approximately 2 kg using xylazine, 8.8 mg/kg IM. Wait 10 min, then administer ketamine HCl, 50 mg/kg IM.
    Place the rabbit on its back and shave or clip the chest hair as closely as possible. Use a commercial depilatory to remove remaining hair.
    Restrain the rabbit's fore- and hindpaws securely.
    Surgically drape the rabbit.
    Place electrodes on the chest wall for attachment to a cardiorespiratory monitor. Changes in ECG tracing due to the pneumothorax can then be demonstrated.
    Insert chest tube.

Weanling Kittens
To teach endotracheal intubation:
    Use kittens weighing 1–1.5 kg.
    Withhold food 8 h before intubation; however, allow water intake.
    Give ketamine HCl 20 mg/kg IM.
    Wait 10 min for full effect of ketamine HCl.
Examine larynx after every four or five attempts at intubation. If the laryngeal area is traumatized, allow 7–10 d for recovery.

Ferrets
To teach endotracheal intubation
    Withhold food 8 h before intubation; however, allow water intake.
    Give ketamine HCl, 5 mg/kg IM, and acepromazine maleate, 0.55 mg/kg IM, and allow to take effect.
    Maintain anesthesia with 40% of original dose IM as needed. If necessary, control sneezing with 0.5 mg/kg IM of diphenhydramine.
    Apply bland ophthalmic ointment to eyes to prevent desiccation.
Examine larynx for signs of trauma, as for kittens, and allow recovery between training sessions. Evidence of trauma was noted in 100% of ferrets after 10 intubations.

Placenta and Cord
To teach insertion of IV infusion lines and umbilical vessel catheters[b]:
    Preserve placenta and cord by freezing in individual containers.
    Allow 3–4 h for thawing before use.
    Use vessels on the fetal surface of the placenta to demonstrate insertion of peripheral IV needles and cannulae. Blood drawing also can be demonstrated.
    Cut a 15-cm length of cord to demonstrate the anatomy of the umbilical stump and the technique for arterial and venous catheterization. The cord may be placed in an infant's feeding bottle that contains saline. One end of the cord then protrudes through a suitably cut nipple and can be pulled out of the bottle for each attempt at the procedure.

[a]Laerdal Medical, Armonk, NY.
[b]Use of this model is not recommended unless HIV and hepatitis B virus status of source is known.
Reprinted with permission from Avery GB, MacDonald MG, Seshia MMK. *Avery's Neonatology: Pathophysiology and Management of the Newborn.* 4th ed. Philadelphia, PA: Lippincott Williams & Wilkins; 1994.

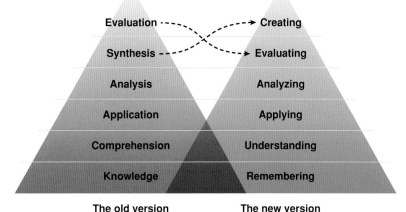

FIGURE 1.2 The older and newer versions of Bloom's taxonomy in the cognitive domain. (Reprinted with permission from Timby BK. *Fundamental Nursing Skills and Concepts.* 11th ed. Philadelphia, PA: Wolters Kluwer; 2016:109.)

developing mental models (abstract conceptualization), and testing that mental model (active experimentation) is based on Kolb's experiential learning cycle (**Fig. 1.3**).

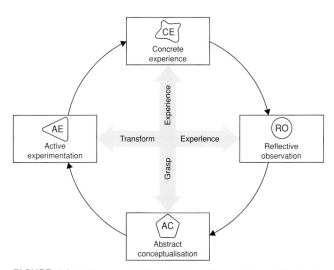

FIGURE 1.3 Kolb's experiential cycle forms the basis for adult simulation-based education. (From Kolb A, Kolb D, Experience Based Learning Systems. *Australian Educational Leader.* 2018;40(3):8–14. https://learning-fromexperience.com/downloads/research-library/eight-important-things-to-know-about-the-experiential-learning-cycle.pdf. Accessed July 11, 2019.)

Kolb's Experiential Learning Cycle

1. **Concrete experience (feeling):** Simulations provide concrete experiences that stress the learner, causing a significant change of body state to foster meaningful reflection of learner identified knowledge gaps.
2. **Reflective observation (watching):** Debriefing provides the opportunity for learners to reflect on the simulation and their performance. The learner observes before making a judgment and seeks optimal comprehension by viewing the experience from different perspectives. The educators can facilitate the process

by providing an objective view of the learner's performance.
3. **Abstract conceptualization (thinking):** Is the logical analysis of ideas and acting on intellectual understanding of a situation by the learner, and helps provide the educator with the opportunity to clarify the same. This results in a new mental model and understanding.
4. **Active experimentation (doing):** This new mental model and understanding, developed by the learner, requires immediate testing by active experimentation, in order to imprint new knowledge and effect long-term changes in practice.
5. Depending on the situation or environment, the learner may enter the learning style at any point and will best learn the new task if they practice all four modes in Kolb's cycle.

For example, *learning to place a radial arterial line:*

Reflective observation: Thinking about placing a radial line and watching another person place a line
Abstract conceptualization: Understanding the theory, indications and contraindications, hand washing and safety, and having a clear grasp of the concept
Concrete experience: Receiving practical tips and techniques from an expert
Active experience: Getting the opportunity and attempting to place a line under supervision

Procedural Skill Learning

Sawyer et al. have built on Kovacs psychomotor learning theory paradigm of *Learn, See, Practice and Do* and suggested a pedagogical framework incorporating two additional steps *Prove and Maintain* for the learner (19–22) (**Fig. 1.4**).

1. *Learn* the procedure and acquire requisite cognitive knowledge
2. *See* the procedure performed by instructor or preceptor
3. *Practice* the procedure with emphasis on error free deliberate practice and distributed practice

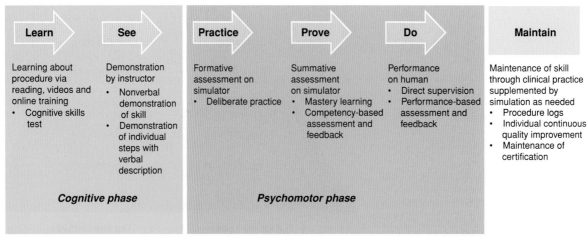

FIGURE 1.4 The progression of the development of expertise in procedural skills using Simpson's and Harrow's taxonomy of psychomotor skill development correlated with the Dreyfus and Dreyfus lexicon of medical skill acquisition. (Reprinted with permission from Sawyer T, White M, Zaveri P, et al. Learn, see, practice, prove, do, maintain: An evidence-based pedagogical framework for procedural skill training in medicine. *Acad Med.* 2015;90(8):1025–1033.)

4. *Prove:* Simulation-based mastery learning with evaluation and feedback
5. *Do:* Perform procedure on patient with direct supervision with real-time assessment and feedback
6. *Maintain:* Correct for "de-skilling" over time

Procedural Skills acquisition which includes the mental and motor activities required to execute a manual task progresses through a five stage continuum of *Guided response, Mechanism, Complex overt response, Adaptation, and Originating* (Fig. 1.5).

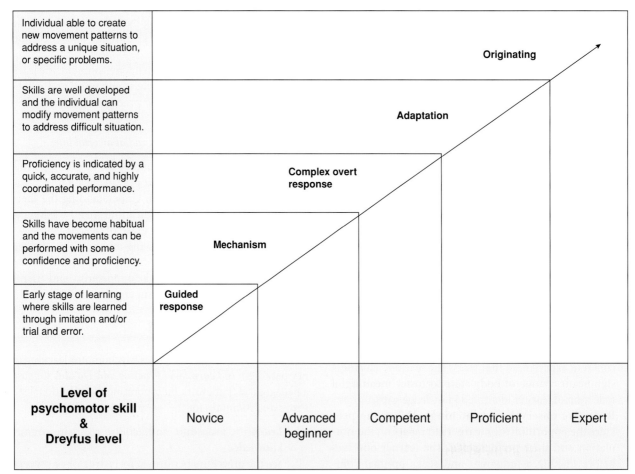

FIGURE 1.5 A proposed pedagogical framework for procedural skill training in medicine. (Reprinted with permission from Sawyer T, White M, Zaveri P, et al. Learn, see, practice, prove, do, maintain: An evidence-based pedagogical framework for procedural skill training in medicine. *Acad Med.* 2015;90(8):1025–1033.)

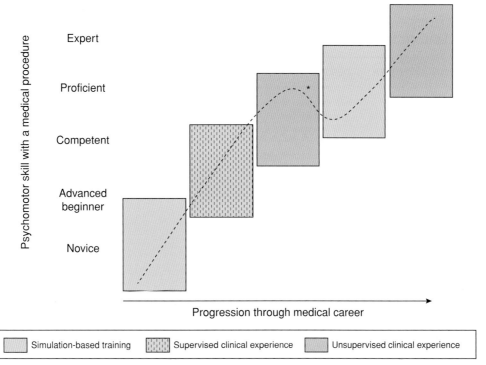

FIGURE 1.6 The theoretical interplay of simulation and clinical experience in procedural skill development and maintenance. The *dashed line* represents skill development and maintenance over time. The *asterisk* (*) indicates a clinical hiatus, or long break in clinical practice. (Reprinted with permission from Sawyer T, White M, Zaveri P, et al. Learn, see, practice, prove, do, maintain: An evidence-based pedagogical framework for procedural skill training in medicine. *Acad Med*. 2015;90(8):1025–1033.)

Competency-Based Medical Education and Simulation

An Entrustable Professional Activity is a key task of a discipline that an individual can be trusted to perform in a given health care context, once sufficient competence has been demonstrated. With the transition to competency-based medical education the interplay between simulation-based procedural training and supervised clinical experience is essential for achievement of competence and leading to mastery (**Fig. 1.6**).

SIMULATION-BASED TRAINING

Simulation-based training is pertinent to and can be incorporated into all aspects of procedural skills training.

The key components of simulation-based training include:

A. Identifying and Elucidating the Learning Objectives Specifically Amenable to Simulation

Clarity of planned learning objectives is integral to planning a useful simulation.

B. Pre-Practice Activities in Preparation for Simulation

1. Didactic training sessions
2. Pre-reading material
3. Audiovisual aids such as training videos and modules

C. Choosing the Optimal Simulator (Tables 1.1 to 1.3)

1. High-fidelity simulators
2. Low-fidelity simulators (see Chapter 2)
3. Procedural trainers (see Chapter 2)
4. Miscellaneous special training simulators
5. Augmented reality and Virtual reality devices and software

D. A Defined Simulation Environment

1. At a clinical learning and simulation facility
2. At the hospital or patient care facility
3. Adjacent to site where patient care is to be provided, and just before performing the procedure on the patient ("just-in-place and just-in-time training")
4. Tele-simulation using appropriate audiovisual tele-communication equipment for outreach training

TABLE 1.2 **Commercially Available Neonatal Task Training Simulators: Focused on Single Skills and Permit Learners to Practice in Isolation**

NAME	MANUFACTURER	DESCRIPTION	SIMULATOR
Baby Stap	Laerdal	Reproduction of a neonatal infant positioned for the practice of lumbar puncture techniques.	Photo by courtesy of Laerdal Medical.
Baby Umbi	Laerdal	Female newborn infant reproduction designed for the practice of umbilical catheterization.	Photo by courtesy of Laerdal Medical.
Laerdal Intraosseous Trainer	Laerdal	The Laerdal Intraosseous Trainer is designed for training in infant intraosseous infusion techniques.	Photo by courtesy of Laerdal Medical.
Infant IV Leg	Laerdal	The infant IV Leg is designed for training extremity venipuncture procedures and IV fluid administration in the superficial veins of the foot.	Photo by courtesy of Laerdal Medical.

TABLE 1.2 Commercially Available Neonatal Task Training Simulators: Focused on Single Skills and Permit Learners to Practice in Isolation (*Continued*)

NAME	MANUFACTURER	DESCRIPTION	SIMULATOR
Laerdal Infant Airway Management Trainer	Laerdal	Realistic anatomy of the tongue, oropharynx, epiglottis, larynx, vocal cords, and trachea	 Photo by courtesy of Laerdal Medical.
Neonatal Echo-cardiography Trainer	Echocom https://www. echocom.de/	Training simulator for echocardiography in neonates	 Photo by courtesy of Laerdal Medical.
Ultrasound Neonatal Head Phantom	Kyoto Kagaku Co., Ltd. https://www. kyotokagaku. com/products/ detail03/us-14. html		 US-14a normal US-14b abnormal

TABLE 1.3 Commercially Available Neonatal Simulators (High, Medium, and Low Fidelity)

NEONATAL SIMULATOR	MANUFACTURER	CAPABILITIES
NeoNatalie™ Photo by courtesy of Laerdal Medical.	Laerdal *https://www.laerdal.com/ca/products/simulation-training/obstetrics-pediatrics/*	■ The NeoNatalie™ simulator was developed to help train birth attendants in low resource countries through such programs as "Helping Babies Breathe" ■ Designed to facilitate effective learning of essential newborn care and neonatal resuscitation ■ Realistic size and appearance, natural weight and feel when filled with lukewarm water. Assessment of heart activity: Pulse beats felt through umbilicus. Lung ventilation: When the airway is correctly opened, the lungs can be ventilated with BVM. Chest compression: When correctly given are signaled by an audible click *Low to Medium Fidelity*
Newborn Anne™ Photo by courtesy of Laerdal Medical.	Laerdal	■ Newborn Anne accurately represents a full term (40 weeks), 50th percentile newborn female, measuring 21 in and weighing 7 lb ■ Airway features: Positioning the newborn to simulate opening the airway via head tilt, chin lift or jaw thrust, PPV (BVM, T-Piece resuscitator, or anesthesia bag), ET tube intubation, LMA insertion, OG tube insertion, stomach distension (when ET is misplaced), suctioning of the nares, nasopharynx, oropharynx, esophagus, and the lungs via an ET tube, meconium module for suction removal ■ Breathing features: Bilateral and unilateral chest rise and fall with mechanical ventilation. Pneumothorax—Needle thoracentesis left mid axillary ■ Cardiac features: Manual chest compression at appropriate depth and force ■ Circulation features: Manual umbilical pulse, vascular access, umbilical vein/artery access via patent umbilicus, IO access in left and right lower leg, tibial tuberosity and medial malleolus ■ Other features: Full articulation *Medium Fidelity*
Nita Newborn™ Photo by courtesy of Laerdal Medical.	Laerdal	■ The Nita Newborn is a model of a 4 lb, 16 in newborn female with realistic landmarks and articulation for vascular access procedures ■ Nose and mouth openings allow placement* of nasal cannulas, endotracheal tubes, nasotracheal tubes, and feeding tubes ■ Standard venipuncture in various sites facilitating blood withdrawal and fluid infusion, median, basilic and axillary sites in both arms, saphenous and popliteal veins in right leg, external jugular and temporal veins, PICC line insertion, securing, dressing and maintenance and umbilical catheterization *Nita Newborn does not have intubation capabilities *Low to Medium Fidelity*

TABLE 1.3 Commercially Available Neonatal Simulators (High, Medium, and Low Fidelity) (*Continued*)

NEONATAL SIMULATOR	MANUFACTURER	CAPABILITIES
SimNewB® Photo by courtesy of Laerdal Medical.	Laerdal	■ SimNewB is a newborn tetherless simulator co-created with the AAP, designed to help improve neonatal resuscitation and to meet the specific learning objectives of neonatal resuscitation protocols ■ Airway: Anatomically accurate, realistic airway. Lung recruitment maneuver, oral and nasal ET tube insertion, LMA insertion, positive-pressure ventilation, right mainstem intubation, suctioning, variable lung resistance, gastric tube insertion ■ Breathing/Respirations: Spontaneous breathing, with variable rate; bilateral and unilateral chest rise and fall with mechanical ventilation, normal and abnormal breath sounds, simulated oxygen saturation. Breathing complications: Pneumothorax, unilateral chest movement/breath sounds with mechanical ventilation. Unilateral needle thoracentesis located mid-axillary. ■ Cardiovascular system: Extensive ECG library, simulated ECG monitoring via 3-lead monitor ■ Vascular access: Patent, cuttable umbilicus with venous and arterial access for bolus or infusion, simulated blood flashback upon cannulation, bilateral IO access ■ Other features: Rotating (selectable) pupils with normal, blown and constricted pupils moving limbs: limp, tone, spontaneous motion and seizure, SimStore Scenarios include 7th edition NRP curricula ■ Circulation: Heart sounds, palpable umbilical pulse, bilateral brachial pulse, central cyanosis ■ Sounds: Vocal: grunt, breathing, crying, hiccups and others, Lung: Normal, stridor, pneumonia and others. Heart: Normal, diastolic murmur, systolic murmur and others. ■ Debriefing: Web-camera recording (SessionViewer PC), Debrief event log *High Fidelity*
Premature Anne Photo by courtesy of Laerdal Medical.	Laerdal	■ Premature Anne™ is a realistically proportioned 25-week preterm manikin developed in collaboration with AAP ■ Airway features: Anatomically accurate, realistic airway, ET tube insertion, Sellick maneuver, PPV, right mainstem intubation, suctioning, OG/NG tube insertion ■ Breathing features: Bilateral and unilateral chest rise and fall with mechanical ventilation ■ Breathing complications: Unilateral chest movement (right mainstem intubation) with mechanical ventilation ■ Cardiac: Realistic compressions ■ Vascular access: Patent, umbilicus that can be cut with venous and arterial access for bolus or infusion, simulated blood flashback upon cannulation of umbilical vein, peripheral IV access (dry ports only) ■ Sounds: Auscultation of lung sounds during ventilation *Medium to High Fidelity*

(continued)

TABLE 1.3 Commercially Available Neonatal Simulators (High, Medium, and Low Fidelity) (*Continued*)

NEONATAL SIMULATOR	MANUFACTURER	CAPABILITIES
Premature Anne with SimPad PLUS Photo by courtesy of Laerdal Medical.	Laerdal	■ Premature Anne, when paired with SimPad PLUS, helps place learners in scenarios that simulate real-life experiences. ■ All Premature Anne features plus breathing features, cyanosis, heart sounds and vocal sounds. ■ The AAP Premature Anne Pack consists of the Premature Anne simulator and a SimPad PLUS handheld remote with 8 pre-programmed scenarios written by the AAP and supports the NRP™ *High Fidelity*
Gaumard – Newborn HAL®S3010—Wireless and Tetherless, Full-Term Newborn Patient Simulator 	Gaumard *https://www.gaumard.com/products/pediatric-neonatal*	■ 40-week tether less newborn with breathing, pulses, color and vital signs that are responsive to hypoxic events and interventions; includes trending, crying, convulsions, oral and nasal intubation, airway sounds and extra tablet PC for control *High Fidelity*
Gaumard – SUPER TORY®S2220—Wireless and Tetherless, Advanced Full-Term Newborn Patient Simulator	Gaumard	■ Full-term newborn, weight: 8 lb, length: 21 in, tetherless, fully responsive during transport, wireless control at distances up to 300 ft (100 m) RF / 33 ft (10 m) Bluetooth, internal rechargeable battery provides up to 8 hours of operation. NOELLE® Fetus-Newborn wireless link capability, Tablet PC preloaded with UNI® (Gaumard's unified simulator control software), OMNI®2 tablet ready ■ Smooth and supple full-body skin with seamless trunk and limb joints. Programmable movement: blinking, mouth open and close, arm and leg flexion and extension, realistic joint articulation: neck, shoulder, elbow, hip, and knee, forearm pronation and supination. ■ Lifelike umbilicus and post cord detachment navel, palpable bony landmarks.

TABLE 1.3 Commercially Available Neonatal Simulators (High, Medium, and Low Fidelity) (*Continued*)

NEONATAL SIMULATOR	MANUFACTURER	CAPABILITIES
		■ **Airway:** Anatomically accurate oral cavity and airway, nasotracheal/orotracheal intubation (ETT, LMA), head tilt, chin lift, jaw thrust, NG/OG tube placement, BVM ventilation, neck hyperextension and flexion airway obstruction with event capture and logging, intubation depth detection and software event log. ■ **Breathing:** Spontaneous, continuous breathing, variable respiratory rates and inspiratory/expiratory ratios, programmable unilateral chest rise and fall, unilateral lung sounds synchronized with respiratory rate, programmable retractions, "see-saw" breathing, MV support, A/C, SIMV, CPAP, PCV, PSV, NIPPV, dynamic airway and lung controls, variable lung compliance, bilateral bronchi resistance, programmable respiratory efforts for weaning/liberation, unilateral chest rise with right mainstem intubation (automatic detection and logging), real-time ventilation feedback, bilateral, midaxillary pneumothorax sites support needle decompression and chest tube insertion, pneumothorax sites feature palpable bony landmarks, realistic skin for cutting and suturing, bleeding, tactile pleural pop, and fluid drain, visible chest rise during BVM ventilation, $EtCO_2$ monitoring using real sensors and monitoring devices. ■ **Circulatory:** Visible cyanosis, jaundice, paleness, and redness with variable intensities, manual capillary refill time assessment on the left foot (automatic detection and logging). ■ **Palpable pulses:** Brachial, femoral, and umbilical, pulse palpation event detection and logging, blood pressure dependent pulses, blood pressure monitoring using real NIBP cuff, audible Korotkoff sounds, preductal (right hand) and postductal (right foot) SpO_2 monitoring using real devices ■ **Cardiac:** Library of ECG rhythms with customizable beat variations, ECG monitoring using real devices, ECG-derived respiration monitoring (EDR), eCPR™ real-time quality feedback and reporting-time to CPR, compression depth/rate, compression interruptions, ventilation rate, excessive ventilation, CPR voice coach, chest compression depth sensor, defibrillate, cardiovert, and pace using real devices and energy, effective chest compressions generate palpable femoral pulses and ECG activity; healthy and abnormal heart sounds, virtual pacing and defibrillation ■ **Vascular access:** IV cannulation: bolus, infusion, and sampling-hand, scalp, umbilicus, umbilical catheterization (UVC/UAC): continuous infusion and sampling, bilateral IO tibial infusion ■ **Neurologic:** Crying/grunting with visible mouth movement, blinking eyes, seizures/convulsions, programmable muscle tone: active, reduced, and limp; programmable fontanel: depressed, normal, and bulging ■ **Gastrointestinal:** Programmable abdominal distension, urinary catheterization with return, normal and abnormal bowel sounds *Very High Fidelity*

(continued)

TABLE 1.3 Commercially Available Neonatal Simulators (High, Medium, and Low Fidelity) (*Continued*)

NEONATAL SIMULATOR	MANUFACTURER	CAPABILITIES
Gaumard – Newborn TORY® S2210—Wireless and Tetherless, Full-Term Newborn Patient Simulator 	Gaumard	■ 40-week term newborn, weight 2.7 kg, length 52.7 cm. Tetherless and wireless mobility: Tetherless and fully responsive even while being transported, Wireless control at distances of up to 300 ft, internal rechargeable battery provides up to 4 hours of tetherless operation. NOELLE® Fetus-Newborn wireless link. UNI® Unified Simulator Control Software, Virtual patient option, and other options depend on package. ■ Smooth and supple full-body skin, seamless trunk and limb joints, realistic joint articulation: neck, shoulder, elbow, hip, and knee, forearm pronation and supination, lifelike umbilicus, palpable landmarks including ribs and xiphoid process. Pneumatic and fluid reservoirs housed inside the body, airway, breathing, cardiac, vascular access, digestive and additional clinical features similar to but slightly less advanced as the S2220 version. *Very High Fidelity*
Gaumard – Premie HAL® S2209—Wireless and Tetherless, 30-Week Premature Neonate Patient Simulator 	Gaumard	■ The Premie HAL® S2209 is a lifelike, wireless and tetherless 30-week preterm patient simulator designed to facilitate the training of residents and health care professionals in the areas of preterm airway management, resuscitation, stabilization, transport, and intensive care *High Fidelity*

TABLE 1.3 Commercially Available Neonatal Simulators (High, Medium, and Low Fidelity) (*Continued*)

NEONATAL SIMULATOR	MANUFACTURER	CAPABILITIES
Gaumard – CODE BLUE® III Newborn S300.110— Advanced Life Support Newborn Patient Simulator	Gaumard	■ The Code Blue III Newborn offers simulation-based resuscitation learning, including programmable models for hypoxic events. The included OMNI 2 controller is a touchscreen interface *High Fidelity*
Gaumard – PEDI® Blue Newborn S320.101—Full-Term Newborn Patient Simulator with OMNI® 2	Gaumard	■ PEDI® Blue with OMNI® 2 is a full-term neonate patient simulator designed to aid in the training of neonatal nursing care and resuscitation skills. PEDI® Blue includes the OMNI® 2 control tablet, which features CPR feedback, virtual patient monitor support, and debriefing tools, in one package. The S320.101.250 Newborn HAL body adds a higher fidelity airway and limb articulation to the S320.100.250 model features *High Fidelity*

(*continued*)

TABLE 1.3 Commercially Available Neonatal Simulators (High, Medium, and Low Fidelity) (*Continued*)

NEONATAL SIMULATOR	MANUFACTURER	CAPABILITIES
Gaumard – PEDI® Blue Newborn S320.100—Full-Term Newborn Patient Simulator with OMNI® 2	Gaumard	■ The S320.100 PEDI® Blue neonatal manikin is a neonate newborn simulator which changes cyanosis color based upon an initial pre-selected condition and measures the effectiveness of CPR, airway ventilation and chest compression. The simulator has all the conventional features found in airway management trainers. Optional accessories include an intraosseous leg and an injection training arm *Medium Fidelity*
Gaumard – Newborn PEDI® S109—Full-Term Newborn Skills Trainer	Gaumard	■ Full-term neonate of average size and weight: 8 lb 19.5 in, smooth, full-body skin, available in light, medium, and dark skin tones, realistic resistance and range of joint articulation including flexible spine, detachable umbilical cord, palpable lumbar landmarks for proper needle insertion ■ Airway: Anatomically accurate oral cavity and airway: including gums, tongue, epiglottis, glottis, and vocal cords, practice endotracheal intubation with standard adjuncts, placement of supraglottic airway devices, Sellick maneuver, PPV via BVM, nasopharyngeal, or oropharyngeal intubation ■ Respiratory: Visible chest rise with positive-pressure ventilation, chest tube insertion ■ Cardiac: Realistic resistance for chest compressions and recoil, palpable pulses generated with manual pressure bulb: fontanelle, umbilical, brachial, and femoral ■ Vascular access: IV cannulation: bolus infusion, and sampling (hand, scalp, umbilicus), umbilical catheterization (UVC/UAC): access, continuous infusion, and sampling ■ Bilateral heel stick with blood draw, lumbar puncture, catheterization, infusion, and sampling, anterolateral thigh intramuscular injection, bilateral intraosseous tibial infusion ■ Gastrointestinal: NG/OG tube placement, feeding and suction through gastric tubes, ileostomy, colostomy, and suprapubic stomas for ostomy care and drainage exercises, interchangeable male and female genitalia, urinary catheterization with fluid return *Medium Fidelity*

TABLE 1.3 Commercially Available Neonatal Simulators (High, Medium, and Low Fidelity) (*Continued*)

NEONATAL SIMULATOR	MANUFACTURER	CAPABILITIES
Gaumard – Premie HAL®- S108.100—24-Week Preterm Newborn Skills Trainer	Gaumard	■ 24-week preterm neonate, length: 31.75 cm, weight: 600 g ■ Airway: Lifelike, anatomically accurate oral cavity and airway, lifelike gums and appropriately sized tongue, endotracheal intubation, Sellick maneuver, nose and oral cavity suction ■ Breathing: True-to-life lung compliance, visible chest rise following recommended flow, PIP, and PEEP values, supports standard positive pressure ventilation devices including BVM, CPAP, and mechanical ventilators ■ Cardiac: Pulses (manual)—brachial, femoral, umbilical, fontanelle, realistic chest recoil during CPR ■ Vascular access: IV cannulation—hand, scalp, UVC/UAC infusion and sampling, PICC line placement, navel insert ■ Gastrointestinal: Gastric distension, patent esophagus, NG/OG, intubation, gastric suction, and feeding *Medium Fidelity*
Gaumard – Premie™ Blue S108—Premature Newborn Patient Simulator with OMNI® 2	Gaumard	■ 28-week articulating preterm neonate ■ Omni 2® wireless tablet controller with interactive resuscitation tools ■ Realistic airway with tongue, vocal cords, trachea, and esophagus for airway management exercises, Realistic internal organs for CPR performance, simulate "heelstick" maneuver for capillary blood sample, BVM or CPR exercises, oral and nasal intubation, simulate suction procedures, bilateral lung expansion with realistic chest rise, peripheral and central cyanosis as well as healthy skin tone, use monitor to select rates of improvement and deterioration, pulse umbilicus using squeeze bulb, practice placement of umbilical lines practice intraosseous access, practice injection, and intravenous techniques *Medium to High Fidelity*

(continued)

TABLE 1.3 Commercially Available Neonatal Simulators (High, Medium, and Low Fidelity) (*Continued*)

NEONATAL SIMULATOR	MANUFACTURER	CAPABILITIES
Gaumard – Newborn S107—Multipurpose, Full-Term Patient Simulator	Gaumard	■ External stoma sites with internal tanks, oral, nasal, and digital intubation, suction, right/left mainstem bronchi, place NG/OG tubes, BVM with realistic chest rise, chest compression, umbilical catheterization, IO infusion, IV arm with variable palpable pulses *Low to Medium Fidelity*
Gaumard – Newborn PEDI® S105—Nursing Skills Patient Simulator		■ Full-body, full-term infant, built-in OMNI® 2 wireless connectivity, OMNI® 2—wireless tablet interface ■ Realistic airway with tongue, vocal cords, trachea, and esophagus for airway management exercises, oral or nasal intubation plus suctioning ■ eCPR™—Real-time CPR quality metrics with performance reporting, compression depth and rate, ventilation rate, excessive ventilation, no-flow time, CPR: Realistic internal organs and anatomical landmarks for CPR hand placement, realistic bilateral lung expansion with BVM ■ IV access on right arm and lower left leg, umbilical catheterization and infusion, IO access and infusion, articulating head, arms, legs cycles, palpable pulses: right brachial, radial, femoral, popliteal, and umbilical (manual bulb) *Medium Fidelity*

TABLE 1.3 Commercially Available Neonatal Simulators (High, Medium, and Low Fidelity) (*Continued*)

NEONATAL SIMULATOR	MANUFACTURER	CAPABILITIES
Gaumard – CPR Newborn S104—Patient Simulator with OMNI®	Gaumard	■ Includes all features of Susie Simon® S103 ■ Soft, lifelike faceskin with molded hair, fully articulating head and jaw with tongue, SAFE CPR™ individual disposable airways, arterial pulse point, IO access, and femoral venous site with OMNI® *Not intubatable *Low to Medium Fidelity*
Gaumard – SUSIE SIMON® S104—Newborn CPR Simulator	Gaumard	■ Includes all features of Susie Simon® S101 ■ Soft, lifelike faceskin with molded hair, fully articulating head and jaw with tongue, SAFE CPR™ individual disposable airways, arterial pulse points plus IO access and femoral venous site *Not intubatable *Low to Medium Fidelity*
Susie Simon® S101—Newborn CPR Patient Simulator	Gaumard	■ Soft, lifelike faceskin with molded hair, fully articulating head and jaw with tongue, SAFE CPR™ individual disposable airways, arterial pulse points *Not intubatable *Low to Medium Fidelity*

(continued)

TABLE 1.3 Commercially Available Neonatal Simulators (High, Medium, and Low Fidelity) (*Continued*)

NEONATAL SIMULATOR	MANUFACTURER	CAPABILITIES
Gaumard – SUSIE SIMON® S100—Nursing Care Newborn Patient Simulator	Gaumard	■ Soft and flexible faceskin, self-molded hair, realistic eyes, NG, simulated ear canal, arms and legs rotate within the torso body, soft hands, feet, fingers, and toes for heel stick and finger prick technique, soft upper body skin over torso for "babylike" feel, bathing and bandaging activity, intramuscular injection in upper thigh, interchangeable genitalia, urethral passage and bladder catheterization, enema administration *Not intubatable
Paul- 27 week premie	SIMCharacters GmbH	■ Preterm baby born in 27 + 3 weeks of gestation, highly realistic external anatomy including real hair. ■ Weight: 1,000 g, length: 35 cm. ■ Completely wireless product with 1.5 hours of battery use ■ Pathologic breathing patterns (nasal flaring, paradoxical respiration, substernal retractions, and grunting), highly realistic upper airway ideal for practicing endotracheal intubation and special neonatologic care strategies (MIST, INSURE), mechanical ventilation using bag-mask and Perivent® systems, automatic tube position detection during intubation, physiologic and pathologic lung parameters for machine-assisted ventilation, cyanosis and hyperoxia ■ Palpable pulse on the umbilical cord and all four limbs, sensors to detect the correct position and depth of an umbilical venous catheter (UVC), auscultatory respiratory, heart, and intestinal noises *Very High Fidelity*
Airway Paul	SIMCharacters GmbH	■ Slightly simplified version of Paul ■ Designed to provide a *High Fidelity*

TABLE 1.3 Commercially Available Neonatal Simulators (High, Medium, and Low Fidelity) (*Continued*)

NEONATAL SIMULATOR	MANUFACTURER	CAPABILITIES
C.H.A.R.L.I.E. Nursing Essentials and C.H.A.R.L.I.E. Nursing Med-Surg (LF0142103U and LF0142104U) LF01421U	Nasco Healthcare	■ LF01421U C.H.A.R.L.I.E. NRP Neonate—IV, IO, oral and nasal airway, CPR ■ 101-102200U SimVS Essentials—vitals cart, monitor, and tablet; BP cuff, pulse ox; thermometer; and glucometer *Medium to High Fidelity* ■ LF01421U C.H.A.R.L.I.E. NRP Neonate—IV, IO, oral and nasal airway, CPR ■ 101-102200U SimVS Essentials—vitals cart and monitor, BP cuff, pulse ox, thermometer ■ 800-102107U SimVS Larger SimVS Control Tablet; multifunction tablet that can present any one of the following presentations: hospital monitor, AED, ECG, defibrillator; nursing scenario set with hard copy. *Medium Fidelity*
ALS Infant Nursing Essentials and ALS Infant Nursing Med-Surg (101-09003U and 101-09004U) 101-090U	Nasco Healthcare	■ 101-090U ALS Full Body Infant, IO legs, ALS airway LMA, Sellick's maneuver, NG tube placement, IV sites, CPR capable, manual pulse points ■ 101-102200U SimVS Essentials—vitals cart, monitor, and tablet; BP cuff, pulse ox; thermometer *Medium Fidelity* ■ 101-090U ALS Full Body Infant, IO legs, ALS airway LMA, Sellick's maneuver, NG tube placement, IV sites, CPR capable, manual pulse points ■ 101-102200U SimVS Essentials—vitals cart and monitor, BP cuff, pulse ox, thermometer ■ 800-102107U SimVS Larger SimVS Control Tablet; multifunction tablet that can present any one of the following presentations: hospital monitor, AED, ECG, defibrillator; nursing scenario set with hard copy *Medium Fidelity*

(*continued*)

TABLE 1.3 Commercially Available Neonatal Simulators (High, Medium, and Low Fidelity) (*Continued*)

NEONATAL SIMULATOR	MANUFACTURER	CAPABILITIES
Micro-Preemie Nursing Essentials and Micro-Preemie Nursing Med-Surg (LF0128003U and LF0128004U) 	Nasco Healthcare	■ LF01280U Micro-Preemie—NRP neonate, IV, oral and nasal airway, CPR ■ 101-102200U SimVS Essentials—vitals cart, monitor, and control tablet; BP cuff; pulse ox; thermometer; and glucometer *Low to Medium Fidelity* ■ LF01280U Micro-Preemie—NRP neonate, IV, oral and nasal airway, CPR ■ 101-102200U SimVS Essentials—vitals cart and monitor, BP cuff, pulse ox, thermometer, glucometer ■ 800-102107U SimVS Larger SimVS Control Tablet; multifunction tablet that can present any one of the following presentations: hospital monitor, AED, ECG, defibrillator; nursing scenario set with hard copy
CAE Luna Base Photos by Lyudmil Iliev, provided courtesy of CAE Healthcare.	CAE Healthcare	■ Wireless and tetherless infant simulator ■ Mannequin: Newborn to 1 month, 21 in, 7 lb, interchangeable gender, bleeding via externally connected IV ■ Respiratory: Anatomically correct airway, oral endotracheal intubation, nasal endotracheal intubation, right mainstem intubation, laryngeal mask placement, oropharyngeal airway insertion, pre-made tracheostomy site, manual chest excursion, asymmetrical chest excursion, oral and nasopharyngeal suctioning ■ Neuro: Manual tristate pupils, manual adjustable fontanelle ■ Digestive and urinary: Feeding tube placement, distended abdomen, urinary catheterization with fluid return
CAE Lunabase Continued Photos by Lyudmil Iliev, provided courtesy of CAE Healthcare.	CAE Healthcare	■ Circulatory: Chest compressions, IO access, IM injections, peripheral venous access via cephalic vein, lateral marginal, foot vein, temporal vein, central venous access via umbilicus, SQ injections, peripheral arterial catheter placement, subclavian catheter placement ■ Musculoskeletal: Localized skin tones, Articulations—elbow, shoulder, hip, knee, neck, jaw, removable umbilical cord supporting cut-down *High Fidelity*

TABLE 1.3 Commercially Available Neonatal Simulators (High, Medium, and Low Fidelity) *(Continued)*

NEONATAL SIMULATOR	MANUFACTURER	CAPABILITIES
CAE Luna Live Photos by Lyudmil Iliev, provided courtesy of CAE Healthcare.	CAE Healthcare	▪ All CAE Luna base features and: Mannequin: internal battery, wireless facilitator control ▪ Respiratory: Lung sound auscultation, pneumothorax decompression, chest tube placement ▪ Digestive and urinary: Bowel sound auscultation ▪ Circulatory: Bilateral brachial pulses, variable pulse strength, library of cardiac rhythms, Commercial ECG device compatible, heart sound auscultation, chest compression metrics ▪ Options: SymDefib, commercial defibrillator compatible, physiologic model ▪ Other: Facilitator control software, emulated patient monitor software *High Fidelity*
CAE Luna Advanced Photos by Lyudmil Iliev, provided courtesy of CAE Healthcare.	CAE Healthcare	▪ All of CAE Luna Base and Live model features and: Respiratory: Laryngospasm, spontaneous breathing, variable respiratory rate and breathing patterns, detection of ventilated air, pneumothorax, decompression detection, substernal retractions, mechanical ventilation support ▪ Neuro: Seizures ▪ Circulatory: Femoral pulse, umbilical pulse ▪ Musculoskeletal: Circumoral cyanosis ▪ Options: External lung *Very High Fidelity*

BVM, bag-valve-mask ventilation; LMA, laryngeal mask airway; PICC, percutaneous intravenous central catheter; AAP, American Academy of Pediatrics; OG, orogastric; NG, nasogastric; IV, intravenous; IO, intraosseous; MV, mechanical ventilation; CPR, cardio pulmonary resuscitation; ET, endotracheal.

E. Pre-Scenario Briefing

1. Ensure confidentiality and respectfulness.
2. Acquaint participants with the capabilities of the simulator.
3. Clarify simulator strengths and weaknesses.
4. Enter into the "fiction contract": The learner agrees to suspend judgment of realism for any given simulation, in exchange for the promise of learning new knowledge and skills. (This helps to keep the focus on the learning objectives.)
5. Discuss the root of the scenarios.

F. Running the Appropriately Realistic, Challenging, and Well-Designed Scenario

1. Rehearse in advance
2. Thoughtful use of actor confederates and props to simulate realism
3. Choose the appropriate start, optimal duration, and finish
4. Achieve an optimal alert and activated state in the participants

G. Recording and Identifying the Knowledge and Performance Gaps of the Participants During the Scenario

1. Focused observation and recording
2. Use of checklists and global rating scales
3. Use of competency assessment tools
4. Use of video

H. Post-Scenario Debriefing

Post-scenario debriefing is the heart of the simulation:

1. Debriefing may focus on actions or both frames (internal images of reality) and actions and help trainees make sense of, learn from, and apply simulation experience to change frames of thought and resulting actions. The goal is to provide objective evaluative feedback.
2. The good judgment approach to debriefing, as advocated by the Center for Medical Simulation at Harvard, consists of four phases:
   a. **Preview phase:** Helps focus the debriefing content
   b. **Reactions phase:** Clears the air and sets the stage for discussion of feelings and facts

   c. **Understanding phase:** Promotes understanding of learner's performance, and explores the basis for learner's actions, using advocacy and enquiry
   d. **Summary phase:** Distills lessons learned for future use; what worked well, what should be changed

I. Evaluation of the Simulation Session

Each simulation session should be evaluated for its effectiveness in achieving its stated objectives.

1. Obtain an objective evaluation of the session from the participants and review of the same by the facilitators.
2. A post session debriefing of the facilitators is also strongly recommended for evaluating success and for future planning of effective simulation sessions.

Acknowledgements to:

The authors gratefully acknowledge the past contributions of Dr. Mhairi Macdonald and Dr. Jenny Rudolph.

References

1. Anderson JM, Warren JB. Using simulation to enhance the acquisition and retention of clinical skills in neonatology. *Semin Perinatol.* 2011;35:59–67.
2. Arafeh JM. Simulation-based training: the future of competency? *J Perinat Neonatal Nurs.* 2011;25:171.
3. Ballard HO, Shook LA, Locono J, et al. Novel animal model for teaching chest tube placement. *J Ky Med Assoc.* 2009;107:219–221.
4. Cates LA. Simulation training: a multidisciplinary approach. *Adv Neonatal Care.* 2011;11:95–100.
5. Cates LA, Wilson D. Acquisition and maintenance of competencies through simulation for neonatal nurse practitioners: beyond the basics. *Adv Neonatal Care.* 2011;11:321–327.
6. Gaba DM. The future vision of simulation in health care. *Qual Saf Health Care.* 2004;13(Suppl 1):i2–i10.
7. Halamek LP. The simulated delivery-room environment as the future modality for acquiring and maintaining skills in fetal and neonatal resuscitation. *Semin Fetal Neonatal Med.* 2008;13:448–453.
8. Halamek LP, Kaegi DM, Gaba DM, et al. Time for a new paradigm in pediatric medical education: teaching neonatal resuscitation in a simulated delivery room environment. *Pediatrics.* 2000;106:E45.
9. MacDonald MG, Johnson B. Perinatal outreach education. In: Avery GB, Fletcher MA, Macdonald MG, eds. *Neonatology: Pathophysiology and Management of the Newborn.* 4th ed. Philadelphia, PA: JB Lippincott Co.; 1994:32.
10. Kattwinkel J, Perlman JM, Aziz K, et al. Neonatal resuscitation: 2010 American Heart Association Guidelines for Cardiopulmonary Resuscitation and Emergency Cardiovascular Care. *Pediatrics.* 2010;126:c1400–c1413.

11. Murphy AA, Halamek LP. Educational perspectives. *NeoReviews*. 2005;6:e489.

12. Rudolph JW, Simon R, Dufresne RL, et al. There's no such thing as "nonjudgmental" debriefing: a theory and method for debriefing with good judgment. *Simul Healthc*. 2006;1:49–55.

13. Ericsson KA. Deliberate practice and the acquisition and maintenance of expert performance in medicine and related domains. *Acad Med*. 2004;79(10 Suppl):S70–S81.

14. Institute of Medicine. *To Err is Human: Building a Safer Health System*. Washington, DC: National Academies Press; 2000.

15. Clark DR. (2012). Kolb's learning styles and experiential learning model. Updated July 13, 2011. http://nwlink.com/~donclark/hrd/styles/kolb.html. Accessed April 23, 2012.

16. Rodgers DL. High-fidelity patient simulation: a descriptive white paper report. http://sim-strategies.com/downloads/Simulation%20White%20Paper2.pdf. Accessed April 23, 2012.

17. Sawyer T, White M, Zaveri P, et al. Learn, see, practice, prove, do, maintain: an evidence-based pedagogical framework for procedural skill training in medicine. *Acad Med*. 2015;90(8):1025–1033.

18. Sawyer T, Gray MM. Procedural training and assessment of competency utilizing simulation. *Semin Perinatol*. 2016;40(7):438–446.

19. Johnston L, Sawyer T, Nishisaki A, et al. Neonatal Intubation Competency Assessment Tool: Development and Validation. *Acad Pediatr*. 2019;19(2):157–164.

20. Griswold-Theodorson S, Ponnuru S, Dong C, et al. Beyond the simulation laboratory: a realist synthesis review of clinical outcomes of simulation-based mastery learning. *Acad Med*. 2015;90(11):1553–1560.

21. Manthey D, Fitch M. Stages of competency for medical procedures. *Clin Teach*. 2012;9(5):317–319.

22. Institute for Medical Simulation Comprehensive Instructor Workshop and Graduate Course material Copyright, all pages, Center for Medical Simulation, 2004–2011. Also personal communication JW Rudolph.

CHAPTER

2

Making Low-Cost Simulation Models for Neonatal Procedures

Jayashree Ramasethu, Suna Seo, and Ashish O. Gupta

Simulation training has become the cornerstone of procedural training in neonatal intensive care (1). The use of animal models such as anesthetized kittens, rabbits, ferrets, and chickens has fallen out of favor for ethical and logistic concerns (2–5). Increasingly sophisticated high-fidelity simulation models have been developed, but they are often expensive and unaffordable. Additionally, it is not clear that high-fidelity models offer major advantages in procedural training when compared to low-fidelity models (6).

In this chapter we describe how to make relatively inexpensive models for vital neonatal procedures, using materials that are easily available. These models have been used in training boot camps for Neonatal Perinatal Fellows and in Procedure Workshops at National Conferences. Other low-cost simulation models have been described in the literature for umbilical catheterization and for circumcision (7,8). There are quality commercial models available for neonatal intubation and lumbar puncture, procedures for which low-cost simulation models are urgently required.

Simulation training is most effective in temporal proximity to the time when the skills are likely to be used and frequent refresher training should be considered to prevent skills decay (9–11). The use of check lists (see Appendix A) to monitor and document compliance with all steps of the procedures is encouraged for competency training. Repeated training improves technique and reduces number of overall attempts (11). Team-based training to improve team work and communication, particularly for emergency scenarios, is vital to improve performance in real-life situations (12,13).

A. Equipment (Additional Model-Specific Equipment Is Listed for Each Model)

1. Polyurethane/vinyl or silicone baby dolls, 8 to 20″ long, with hollow torsos

2. Craft knife—hobby/exacto or box cutter
3. Scissors
4. Thick shelf liner (e.g., Nonadhesive Grip Premium Liner, Con-Tact Brand, Kittrich Corporation, La Mirada, CA)
5. Vinyl or latex gloves—skin colored
6. Food coloring—red and yellow
7. Duct tape or similar strong tape
8. Water
9. Permanent marker

B. Chest Tube Model (14)

This model may be used for thoracocentesis and chest tube placement simulations.

1. Equipment (in addition to the equipment listed in A):
   a. Electrical cable wire (14 gauge)
   b. Styrofoam pieces
   c. Inflated sandwich bags or bubble wrap with large bubbles
2. Procedure
   a. Cut away the anterior chest and abdominal wall of the doll (**Fig. 2.1**)
   b. Construct the clavicles and rib cage using 14-gauge electrical wire and tape (**Fig. 2.2**)
   c. Place styrofoam block in the middle of the rib cage to create two pleural cavities, and place inflated sandwich bags inside each cavity to simulate pneumothorax (**Fig. 2.3**)
   d. Wrap chest model with thick shelf liner (simulates muscle layer) (**Fig. 2.3**)
   e. Place inside chest cavity of hollow doll (**Fig. 2.4**)
   f. Ensure that ribs can be counted and that intercostal spaces may be palpated

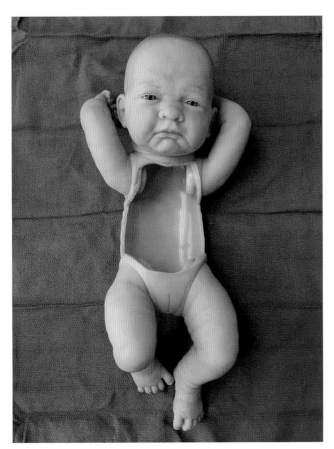

FIGURE 2.1 Doll with anterior chest and abdominal wall cut away.

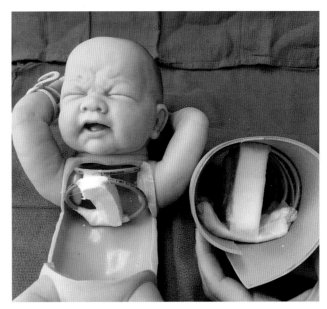

FIGURE 2.3 Chest tube model. Rib cage with styrofoam block to divide space into two pleural cavities, whole then covered with thick shelf liner to simulate chest wall/muscle.

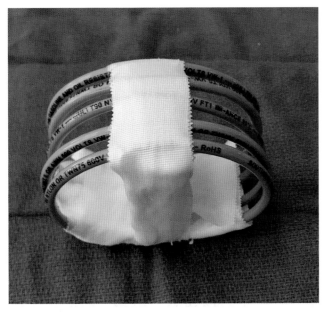

FIGURE 2.2 Chest tube model. Clavicles and rib cage constructed with electrical wire and tape.

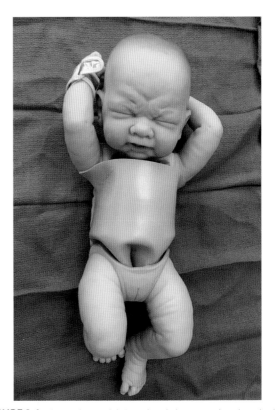

FIGURE 2.4 Chest tube model. Completed rib cage is placed inside chest cavity of doll.

g. Cover entire chest with cut and stretched skin colored glove or similar material (simulates skin) and mark nipples using permanent marker at 4th intercostal space (**Fig. 2.5**)

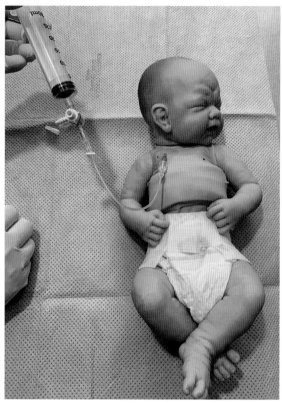

FIGURE 2.5 Chest tube model. Demonstration of needle thoracocentesis from 2nd right intercostal space in completed model (the sterile drapes have been removed to show the needle and landmarks).

C. Umbilical Catheter Model

This model may be used for umbilical artery and venous catheter placement as well as for exchange transfusion simulations.

1. Equipment (in addition to the equipment listed in A):
   a. Latex or silicone baby bottle nipple
   b. 1 to 2 in of silicone tubing with two narrow channels simulating umbilical arteries and one wider channel simulating umbilical vein (**Fig. 2.6**)
   c. Empty IV fluid bag or bottle—fill with water and red food coloring to simulate blood
   d. Clear plastic tubing to connect simulated umbilicus to IV fluid bag or bottle—appropriate length 24 to 36 inches
   e. Arterial clamp or similar clamp to regulate "blood" flow from IV fluid bag to bottle
2. Procedure
   a. Cut small opening at umbilical area in the doll's abdomen (**Fig. 2.6**). Cut a larger opening in the lumbosacral area of the doll (**Fig. 2.7**)

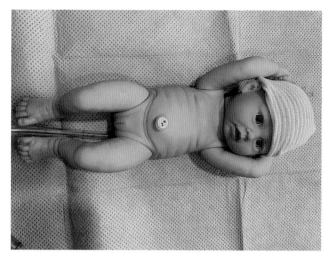

FIGURE 2.6 UAC/UVC model. Front view of doll showing simulated umbilicus.

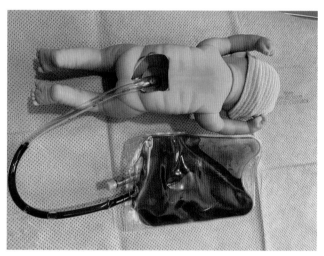

FIGURE 2.7 UAC/UVC model. Rear view of doll showing silicone tubing inserted into nipple which has been placed into umbilicus from within the abdominal cavity.

b. Cut tip of baby bottle nipple. Insert silicone tubing into the nipple
c. Attach one end of clear plastic tubing over the silicone tubing and the other end into the IV fluid bag/bottle. Place clamp on tubing to prevent "blood" from leaking (**Fig. 2.7**)
d. Insert the nipple/silicone tubing ensemble from the lumbosacral area into the umbilical area; ensure it fits snugly (**Fig. 2.8**)
e. Release the clamp to allow blood to flow into the tubing and up to the "umbilicus." Close clamp to prevent further blood flow until use during the procedure
f. During the simulation, the supervisor may regulate the blood flow, using the clamp

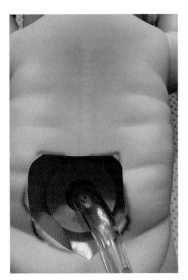

FIGURE 2.8 UAC/UVC model. Clear tubing connects silicon umbilicus to the blood bag.

D. Pericardiocentesis Model

1. Equipment (in addition to the equipment listed in A)
   a. Bulb and tubing from old sphygmomanometer
   b. Soft foam or cloth

2. Procedure
   a. Cut away anterior abdominal wall from doll, keeping the chest wall to simulate the rib margins and sternum. Make another small opening in the left "suprascapular" region of the doll (**Fig. 2.9A,B**)
   b. Mix yellow food coloring with water to make pale yellow fluid to simulate a transudate or parenteral alimentation fluid, which are the most common causes of pericardial effusion in babies in the NICU (see Chapter 42). Fill sphygmomanometer bulb and tubing with this fluid and clamp shut
   c. Place sphygmomanometer bulb into chest cavity; thread connecting tubing into the hole in the left suprascapular region of the doll (**Fig. 2.9A,B**)
   d. Place soft foam or cloth into the abdominal cavity to fill the remaining space and secure the sphygmomanometer bulb in place
   e. Cover chest and abdomen with thick shelf liner; secure shelf liner with tape or velcro over the back
   f. On palpation, the abdomen should feel soft and one should be able to feel the rib margins and the xiphisternal area
   g. Using a permanent marker, approximate and draw the nipples on the chest

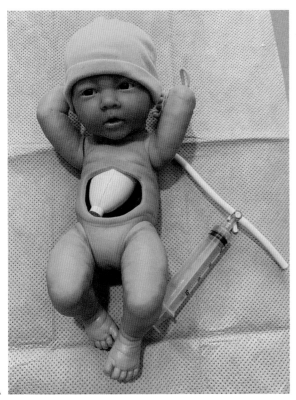

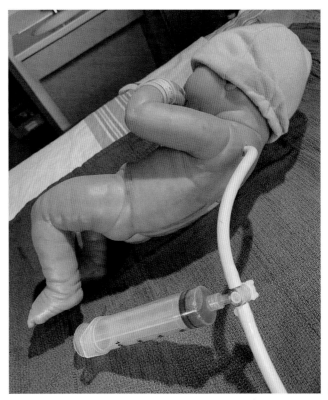

A   B

FIGURE 2.9 A: Pericardiocentesis model. Doll with anterior abdominal wall cut away and sphygmomanometer bulb inserted into chest. Note that the lower rib margin and xiphisternum are clearly defined. **B:** Pericardiocentesis model. Hole in the left suprascapular area through which the tube attached to the sphygmomanometer is threaded.

h. **Figure 2.10** demonstrates the xiphisternal approach to pericardiocentesis (see Chapter 42). The cannula pierces the sphygmomanometer bulb and pale yellow fluid may be aspirated. Once the cannula is removed, the thick rubber material of the bulb reseals easily, preventing leaking and allowing repeated use

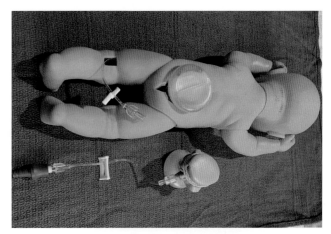

FIGURE 2.11 Suprapubic bladder aspiration model. Opening in sacral area of doll accommodates plastic bottle with yellow fluid simulating urine. Note plastic bottle cut to size, covered with shelf liner, with IV extension tubing attached.

e. Place bottle through the sacral opening in the doll, so the end covered with shelf liner abuts the abdominal wall (**Fig. 2.11**). Ensure that the bottle sits below the umbilicus. The lower edge of the bottle can be palpated to simulate the pubic symphysis

f. **Figure 2.12** shows the procedure of suprapubic aspiration. The butterfly needle pierces the suprapubic

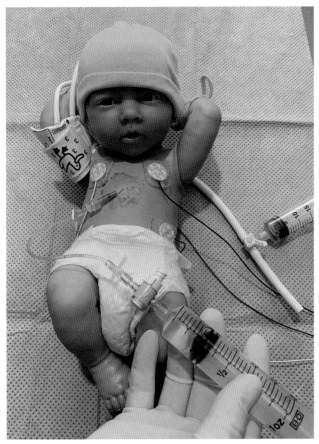

FIGURE 2.10 Pericardiocentesis model. Demonstration of pericardiocentesis on the completed model (the sterile drapes have been removed to show the needle and landmarks).

E. Suprapubic Bladder Aspiration Model

1. Equipment (in addition to the equipment listed in A)
   a. Small plastic bottle about 2 in tall (the depth of the doll's abdomen). A plastic bottle may be cut to size to fit
   b. IV extension set
   c. Rubber bands
2. Procedure
   a. Cover open end of plastic bottle with thick shelf liner using rubber bands (**Fig. 2.11**)
   b. Drill hole in side of bottle with sharp implement, and insert end of IV extension tubing
   c. Mix yellow food coloring with water to simulate urine; fill bottle (almost fully) with this fluid.
   d. Cut an opening in the sacral area of the doll

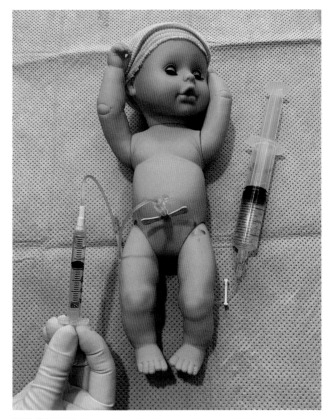

FIGURE 2.12 Suprapubic bladder aspiration model. Demonstration of suprapubic bladder aspiration in completed model. The sterile drapes have been removed to show the needle and landmarks.

skin and yellow fluid (urine) may be aspirated from the bottle under the surface

g. The IV extension tubing can be used to refill the bottle so the level of fluid remains high for repeated procedures

References

1. Sawyer T, Gray MM. Procedural training and assessment of competency utilizing simulation. *Semin Perinatol.* 2016; 40(7):438–446.

2. Hourihane JO, Crawshaw PA, Hall MA. Neonatal chest drain insertion—an animal model. *Arch Dis Child Fetal Neonatal Ed.* 1995;72(2):F123–F124.

3. Ballard HO, Shook LA, Iocono J, et al. Novel animal model for teaching chest tube placement. *J Ky Med Assoc.* 2009; 107(6):219–221.

4. Kircher SS, Murray LE, Julian ML. Minimizing trauma to the upper airway: a ferret model of neonatal intubation. *J Am Assoc Lab Anim Sci.* 2009;48:780–784.

5. Wadman M. Medical schools swap pigs for plastic. *Nature.* 2008; 453(7192):140–141.

6. Finan E, Bismilla Z, Whyte HE, et al. High-fidelity simulator technology may not be superior to traditional low-fidelity equipment for neonatal resuscitation training. *J Perinatol.* 2012;32(4):287–292.

7. Sawyer T, Gray M, Hendrickson M, et al. A real human umbilical cord simulator model for emergency umbilical venous catheter placement training. *Cureus.* 2018;10(11):e3544.

8. Roca P, Alvarado C, Stausmire JM, et al. Effectiveness of a simulated training model for procedural skill demonstration in neonatal circumcision. *Simul Healthc.* 2012;7(6): 362–373.

9. Thomas SM, Burch W, Kuehnle SE, et al. Simulation training for pediatric residents on central venous catheter placement: a pilot study. *Pediatr Crit Care Med.* 2013;14(9):e416–e423.

10. Andreatta PB, Dooley-Hash SL, Klotz JJ, et al. Retention curves for pediatric and neonatal intubation skills after simulation-based training. *Pediatr Emerg Care.* 2016;32(2): 71–76.

11. Kessler D, Pusic M, Chang TP, et al. Impact of just in time and just in place simulation on intern success with infant lumbar puncture. *Pediatrics.* 2015;135:e1237–e1246.

12. Reed DJW, Hermelin RL, Kennedy CS, et al. Interdisciplinary onsite team-based simulation training in the neonatal intensive care unit: a pilot report. *J Perinatol.* 2017;37(4):461–464.

13. Wetzel EA, Lang TR, Pendergrass TL, et al. Identification of latent safety threats using high-fidelity simulation-based training with multidisciplinary neonatology teams. *Jt Comm J Qual Patient Saf.* 2013;39(6):268–273.

14. Gupta AO, Ramasethu J. An innovative nonanimal simulation trainer for chest tube insertion in neonates. *Pediatrics.* 2014; 134(3):e798–e805.

CHAPTER

3

Informed Consent for Procedures

Karen Kamholz

In its "Hospital Interpretive Guidelines for Informed Consent," the United States Department of Health and Human Services, Centers for Medicare and Medicaid Services (CMS), regulates that a patient or a patient's surrogate "has the right to make informed decisions regarding his or her care" (1). Informed consent, in its most ideal form, is a collaborative process whereby a clinician informs a patient or patient's representative about a treatment or procedure including its indications, potential risks, anticipated benefits, possible alternatives, and expected outcome without the treatment; and further provides the opportunity for the decision maker to ask questions (2,3). The practice of informed consent should empower a patient or patient's representative to make a thoughtful assessment about whether to proceed with or refuse a treatment or procedure. A complete informed consent process encompasses not only the disclosure of information, but also an assessment of the decision maker's understanding of this information as well as his/her capacity for making medical decisions (4).

Purpose of Informed Consent

Informed consent serves three intersecting objectives:

1. protecting the legal rights of the individual
2. promoting the ethical practice in medicine
3. fulfilling the administrative demand on hospitals to ensure adequate informed consent (4)

Legally, informed consent provides patients protection from assault and battery. The 1914 case of Schloendorff v. Society of New York Hospital inaugurated the modern legal precept in America of consent, determining that a patient has a "right to determine what shall be done with his body" (5). In the 1950s, courts determined that physicians must disclose all pertinent facts needed for a patient to make an informed decision—the so-called "reasonable physician" standard. In the 1970s, the concept of the "reasonable person" standard arose, stating that the information disclosed

should be that which a reasonable person would want to know (5). According to this standard, patients or their surrogates should have all of the information they need to compare treatment options and make decisions based on their personal values, goals, and preferences (6).

Ethical principles of informed consent center on respect for patient autonomy, ensuring that individuals have "the capacity to live life according to [their] own reasons and motives" (2). By this precept, patients or their representatives will use the information that they receive to make informed, rational, autonomous decisions. While the nature of the risks, benefits, and alternative therapies discussed is at the discretion of, and based on the judgment of, the clinician obtaining the consent, enough detail should be provided to allow for the patient or the patient's representative to make an informed decision (5). The American Academy of Pediatrics (AAP) notes that, in certain instances, the discussion of provider-specific data or clinician experience is also warranted (2). With an ethical focus, experts have proposed that a more appropriate ideal for the informed consent process is a "shared decision-making" model in which providers make recommendations based on collaborative communication and an understanding of the family's goals and values (2). The administrative aspects of informed consent center on compliance, including the development of policies surrounding patient consent for treatment or procedures as well as the documentation of an adequate informed consent process.

What Are the Requirements for Informed Consent?

In addition to a signed consent form, there are four required components to an acceptable informed consent process:

1. Communication of adequate information allowing for an informed decision including details of the proposed procedure or treatment and the probability of success.

2. Assessment of the decision maker's understanding of the information conveyed.
3. Appraisal of the patient's or patient representative's capacity for appropriate decision making.
4. Assurance that the consent that is provided is voluntary (2).

Who May Obtain Consent

Little is written about who should be responsible for obtaining informed consent from a patient or a surrogate decision maker. Some institutions require that only the individual performing the procedure may obtain the consent (7). Others have suggested that individuals who are capable of performing a procedure should be able to obtain consent for that procedure, as they would be most likely to understand the potential risks and their frequency, as well as the anticipated benefits of a procedure. Additionally, those responsible for acquiring consents should have training to familiarize them with the specific requirements of the informed consent process (8). In practice, however, it is often trainees with relatively little hands-on experience who are tasked with obtaining consents for specific procedures from patients or their representatives (9).

Types of Informed Consent

There are a variety of approaches to obtaining informed consent for procedures for patients being cared for in the intensive care unit (ICU).

Informed consent can be:

- procedure specific for planned procedures
- bundled with one consent covering several procedures commonly performed in the ICU setting
- universal to cover all procedures performed during an ICU admission or a hospitalization

Weiss et al. surveyed many different types of adult ICUs about their consent practices for 16 procedures commonly performed in the ICU setting. They found that in the majority of ICUs, practitioners obtained procedure-specific consents. Only about 20% of ICUs had bundled procedure consents. About 25% acquired an overall consent for ICU admission, though some of these also asked for procedure-specific consents (10). Davis et al. explored the use of bundled consents covering 8 procedures frequently required in adult ICUs. They demonstrated a 70% increase in the frequency with which consent was documented prior to the procedure being performed. In both groups, the majority of consents were provided by patient surrogates rather than by the patients themselves. No decline was seen in comprehension of the procedure indications or risks with the bundled consent form (11). Other studies have shown increased family satisfaction following the introduction of a bundled consent form that

was presented and signed at a family meeting within the first 2 days of an ICU admission (12).

In a recent survey of informed consent practices in neonatal ICUs and pediatric ICUs, 70% of respondents reported using procedure-specific written consents. This was also the method respondents deemed most likely to satisfy all of the criteria for adequate informed consent (13). To date, however, studies of interventions to improve informed consent practices in NICUs are lacking.

What Is Required on a Procedure-Specific Informed Consent Form?

According to the CMS, a consent form must be completed prior to a procedure or treatment and in accordance with hospital guidelines as well as state and national laws (14). At a minimum, informed consent forms must include:

- Hospital or facility name
- Procedure to be performed
- Clinician responsible for performing the procedure
- A declaration that the procedure or treatment including the risks, benefits, and alternative therapies was explained to the patient or the patient's legal representative
- Signature of the patient or patient's representative
- Date and time of completion of the consent form

CMS suggests that a well-designed informed consent form could also include:

- The name of the clinician obtaining the consent
- A witness signature, including date and time
- Specific risks discussed
- As appropriate, a statement that other clinicians including trainees might be involved
- As appropriate, a statement that nonphysician practitioners with appropriate hospital privileges might be involved

While informed consent forms should promote the ideals of providing adequate information to assist patients or their representatives in making educated medical decisions, unfortunately in practice, this occurs infrequently. The forms are more often viewed as an administrative requirement rather than as documentation of a collaborative process of shared decision making. Studies suggest that few consent forms contain all of the required components for informed consent. Many are deficient in describing the rationale, specific benefits and serious risks, or outcome probabilities of the procedure (5,15,16). The intended purposes of the forms were more often for obtaining treatment authorization and protecting from liability, rather than assisting patients in decision making (15). Other concerns include the advanced education and language skills often required to understand forms and the short amount of time allocated for patients to consider the form (6). Each of these concerns may be amplified in the NICU setting. Parents who are confronted with laundry lists of potential procedural complications, unaccompanied by the likelihood of these risks occurring or a qualification of which risks are common and which are rare, may perceive the neonatologist and hospital as caring more about avoiding liability than providing a realistic assessment of the benefits and risks of a procedure. Such a form may do little more than paralyze parents with fear and indecision.

How "Informed" Is Informed Consent?

In practice, the informed consent process is often suboptimal. The information conveyed during the informed consent process must be adequate for a patient or patient's representative to make an informed decision, yet often the information provided does not achieve this goal (7,8). As Hall et al. note, "patients remember little of the information disclosed during the informed consent process and . . . their level of comprehension is often overestimated" (5). Studies suggest that informed consent standards are rarely met and that a majority of patients may believe that their consent gives "doctors control over what happened" (5,17). Achieving adequate informed consent is likely to be even more difficult in the ICU setting given the acute nature of the patient's illness. Patients and their representatives often feel vulnerable and stressed. Procedural consent is often done just prior to the procedure itself, which can leave patients feeling pressured to sign (7). Furthermore, in certain cases, language or cultural barriers can add an additional layer of complexity. In these cases, providers should engage medical translation services, rather than using family members as interpreters (18). Since patients or their representatives cannot meaningfully participate in medical decision making unless they are able to comprehend the risks, benefits, and alternatives of the treatments proposed, addressing each of these issues is crucial (7).

Several studies have examined a variety of techniques that overall improved decision makers' informed consent experience (2,6,8,19,20). These interventions range from patient information sheets to interactive computer programs or other audio/visual interventions, and from promoting extended discussions to employing teach-back techniques where clinicians have patients repeat key elements of a discussion to demonstrate understanding (8,19). Spatz et al. note that when decision aids were used, patients "had greater knowledge of the evidence, felt more clear about what mattered to them, had more accurate expectations about the risks and benefits, and participated more in the decision-making process" (6). These techniques added an average of less than 4 minutes, and often much less, to the consent process (19,20). Studies leading to these findings prompted the AAP to recommend that clinicians use multimedia presentations, repeat back, and increased time during informed consent discussion with patients or their representatives (2). In summary, the use of patient decision aids is recommended since they can "provide balanced, evidence-based information about treatment options" (6).

Special Issues Related to Informed Consent in the Context of Neonates

There are obviously special issues when it comes to obtaining informed consent for procedures in the neonatal ICU, as a surrogate must become the decision maker for the infant. In most cases, parents will serve as the patient's representative. They, in turn, are obligated to make caring decisions that are, based on their judgment, in the best interest of their child, giving consideration to the child's social, emotional, and health care needs within the framework of their family values and beliefs. The assumption is that parents understand their child better than others and will therefore serve as the best advocates for their child, minimizing risks while maximizing benefits (2). Cooke describes this responsibility as "informed parental permission" rather than informed consent (8). Parents of a critically ill neonate must also have adequate capacity to be able to provide proper informed consent. The AAP policy on informed consent notes that sometimes "parental distress presents a challenge for good informed decision-making" (2).

Another special condition that complicates informed consent in neonatology is when parents of an infant are not legally married. In certain jurisdictions, fathers who are not married to mothers are not able to provide consents or they cannot legally sign consent forms until after the infant's birth certificate is completed (8). It is important to know the laws in the region in which the care is being provided, especially since it is not infrequent that mothers are under the influence of medications or experience complications following delivery and are not able to provide informed consent for their infants in the immediate postpartum period (4). If a mother is unable, and a father is not permitted, to provide consent, only a legal guardian or a court may fill this role (8).

Another circumstance unique to pediatrics occurs when the mother of an infant is a minor herself. All US states recognize minor parents as the decision makers for their children, though it is suggested that these teenagers involve a parent or other trusted adult when they are faced with more difficult decisions (2). Furthermore, while minor parents have the right to make decisions for their children, unless they have been legally declared to be emancipated minors, the parents of these adolescents continue to be responsible for the health care decisions affecting their teenage children.

Consent Refusals

The AAP policy statement on informed consent notes that "clinicians have both a moral obligation and a legal responsibility to question and, if necessary, to contest surrogate and/or patient medical decisions that put the patient at significant risk of serious harm." There is a harm threshold below which parental decisions will not be tolerated, and parental autonomy becomes limited, since the state also has a responsibility to safeguard individuals who are unable to care for or protect themselves (4). Through a doctrine known as *parens patriae*, the state can challenge parental authority if child's well-being is at risk and assume court-ordered guardianship of the child (2,21).

Parents will sometimes have religious beliefs leading to the refusal of certain medical treatments, for example, when a mother who is a Jehovah's Witness has an extremely premature baby in need of a blood transfusion. The AAP policy on informed consent states that "children deserve effective medical treatment regardless of parental religious beliefs when such treatment is not overly burdensome and is likely to prevent substantial harm, serious disability, or death" (2). In addition to the state's obligation to protect the child, the rationale for refusing to withhold life-saving treatments for a child on religious grounds is that the child might not choose to accept these same religious doctrines in the future. As a result, the courts can assume temporary guardianship of the child and can consent to the needed treatment on their behalf. Providers can also ask the courts for temporary protective custody in situations in which a parent or guardian is intoxicated or otherwise impaired such that they are not able to provide informed consent for a period of time.

Emergency Procedures

It is not infrequent that procedures performed in the NICU are emergent in nature and informed consent is not required in situations that are imminently life threatening or in the treatment of serious conditions (8,21). AAP policy states that medical stabilization and treatment should never be withheld or delayed when reasonable efforts to contact a parent or guardian have been attempted and urgent interventions to prevent imminent and significant harm are necessary (2,18). Such situations include life- or limb-threatening conditions, severe pain, fractures, infections, and other conditions associated with possible significant impairment or dysfunction without urgent treatment. In these cases, the provider is acting in the best interest of the child and providing the emergency care as desired by reasonable persons under an "implied consent" (18). Documentation is important in these situations and should note both the emergent nature of the procedure as well as any attempts that were made to contact a parent or guardian. After initial stabilization, however, consent should be obtained prior to the provision of additional nonemergent treatments (18).

Summary

The informed consent process can be an effective method for building alliances with patients and their advocates, allowing providers to discuss goals of care, provide education, assess understanding, and build a shared model of decision making. Using educational materials, procedure-specific consent

forms, and a systematic approach facilitates this process. Proper education and training for all clinicians and trainees involved in the consent process is also essential. Finally, further research into methods of improving the informed consent process, especially in ICU settings, and in neonatology in particular, will benefit providers, patients, and families.

References

1. Centers for Medicare and Medicaid Services, Department of Health and Human Services. 42 CFR 482.13(b)(2). Condition of participation: Patient's rights [71 FR 71426, Dec. 8, 2006, as amended at 75 FR 70844, Nov. 19, 2010; 77 FR 29074, May 16, 2012].
2. Katz AL, Webb SA; Committee on Bioethics. Informed consent in decision-making in pediatric practice [technical report]. *Pediatrics*. 2016;138(2):e20161485.
3. The Joint Commission. Informed consent: More than getting a signature. *Quick Safety!* 2016;(21). https://www.jointcommission.org/assets/1/23/Quick_Safety_Issue_Twenty-One_February_2016.pdf. Accessed January 16, 2018.
4. Committee on Bioethics. Informed consent in decision-making in pediatric practice [policy statement]. *Pediatrics*. 2016;138(2):e20161484.
5. Hall DE, Prochazka AV, Fink AS. Informed consent for clinical treatment. *CMAJ*. 2012;184(5):533–540.
6. Spatz ES, Krumholz HM, Moulton BW. The new era of informed consent: getting to a reasonable-patient standard through shared decision making. *JAMA*. 2016;315(19):2063–2064.
7. Schenker Y, Meisel A. Informed consent in clinical care: practical considerations in the effort to achieve ethical goals. *JAMA*. 2011;305(11):1130–1131.
8. Cooke RW. Good practice in consent. *Semin Fetal Neonatal Med*. 2005;10(1):63–71.
9. Arnolds M, Feltman D. Are trainees prepared to obtain informed consent for bedside procedures in the ICU? Results from a nationwide survey of neonatology and pediatric critical care fellowship directors. E-PAS, Abstract/Poster number: 1484.700. Toronto, Canada; 2018.
10. Weiss EM, Kohn R, Madden V, et al. Procedure-specific consent is the norm in United States intensive care units. *Intensive Care Med*. 2016;42(10):1637–1638.
11. Davis N, Pohlman A, Gehlbach B, et al. Improving the Process of Informed Consent in the Critically Ill. *JAMA*. 2003;289(15):1963–1968.
12. Dhillon A, Tardini F, Bittner E, et al. Benefit of using a "bundled" consent for intensive care unit procedures as part of an early family meeting. *J Crit Care*. 2014;29(6):919–922.
13. Arnolds M, Feltman D. How informed consent for procedures is obtained in neonatal and pediatric ICUs: a nationwide survey. E-PAS, Abstract/Poster number: 3800.2. Toronto, Canada; 2018.
14. Centers for Medicare and Medicaid Services, Department of Health and Human Services. 42 CFR 482.24(c)(2)(i)(B)(v). Condition of participation: medical record services [51 FR 22042, June 17, 1986, as amended at 71 FR 68694, Nov. 27, 2006; 72 FR 66933, Nov. 27, 2007; 77 FR 29074, May 16, 2012].

15. Bottrell MM, Alpert H, Fischbach RL, et al. Hospital informed consent for procedure forms: facilitating quality patient-physician interaction. *Arch Surg*. 2000;135(1):26–33.

16. Bellieni CV, Coradeschi C, Curcio MR, et al. Consents or waivers of responsibility? Parents' information in NICU. *Minerva Pediatr*. 2018. doi: 10.23736/S0026-4946.18.05084-3.

17. Akkad A, Jackson C, Kenyon S, et al. Patients' perceptions of written consent: questionnaire study. *BMJ*. 2006;333(7567): 528.

18. Committee on Pediatric Emergency Medicine and Committee on Bioethics. Consent for emergency medical services for children and adolescents. *Pediatrics*. 2011;128(2):427–433.

19. Schenker Y, Fernandez A, Sudore R, et al. Interventions to improve patient comprehension in informed medical and surgical procedures: a systematic review. *Med Decis Making*. 2011;31(1):151–173.

20. Kinnersley P, Phillips K, Savage K, et al. Interventions to promote informed consent for patients undergoing surgical and other invasive healthcare procedures. *Cochrane Database Syst Rev*. 2013;(7):CD009445.

21. Courtney B, Hodge JG Jr; Task Force for Pediatric Emergency Mass Critical Care. Legal considerations during pediatric emergency mass critical care events. *Pediatr Crit Care Med*. 2011;12(6 Suppl):S152–S156.

4

Maintenance of Thermal Homeostasis

Anoop Rao and Melissa Scala

A. Definitions

1. Homeostasis: Fundamental mechanism whereby living things regulate their internal environment within tolerable limits, thus keeping a dynamic equilibrium and maintaining a stable, constant condition. From the Greek *homeo* (same, like) and *stasis* (stable state) (1).
2. Normal body temperature: The core body temperature is maintained by the term infant within the range of 36.5° to 37.5°C, and the skin temperature, from 0.5° to 1°C lower (2).
3. Neutral thermal environment: The range of ambient temperature required for the infant (for each gestational age and weight) to keep a normal body temperature and a minimal basal metabolic rate. In practice, it is the ambient temperature at which the core temperature of the infant at rest is between 36.5°C and 37. 5°C and the core and mean skin temperatures are changing less than 0.2°C/hr and 0.3°C/hr, respectively **(Table 4.1)** (3,4).
4. Thermoregulation: Mechanisms by which the infant tries to balance heat production and heat loss to accommodate the thermal environment (3–5).
5. Cold stress: The infant senses heat loss as a stress and responds with increased heat production and peripheral vasoconstriction, with centralization of circulation, in an effort to maintain the core temperature (6).
6. Hypothermia: Heat losses exceed heat production, dropping the infant's temperature below the normal range of 36.5° to 37.5°C (97.7° to 99.5°F) (7). Hypothermia can be a sign of sepsis.
   a. Mild hypothermia (cold stress): 36° to 36.4°C (96.8° to 97.5°F)
   b. Moderate hypothermia: 32° to 35.9°C (89.6° to 96.6°F)
   c. Severe hypothermia: Below 32°C (89.6°F)
7. Hyperthermia: An increase in the infant's temperature to above 37.5°C (99.5°F) due to a warm environment. Hyperthermia is less common than hypothermia but is equally dangerous. Clinically, it may be difficult to distinguish hyperthermia from fever (infectious origin); therefore, always consider both causes in any increase in temperature (7).

B. Background

1. Mechanisms of heat loss (8)
   a. Evaporation: Evaporation is the loss of body heat due to a moisture concentration differential between the infant's skin and surrounding air environment. For example, evaporation of amniotic fluid from the newborn skin.
   b. Conduction: The transfer of heat between two objects in contact, from the warmer to the cooler object. For example, an infant placed on a cold weighing scale.
   c. Convection: The transfer of heat by air currents that move across the exposed skin of the newborn. For example, an infant exposed to low temperature in the operating room.
   d. Radiation: The transfer of heat from the infant to another colder object, even if there is no contact between the two. After the first week of life, radiation becomes the most important route of heat loss in premature infants. For example, cold objects in the room transfer heat away from the infant.
2. **Effects of hypothermia**
   a. Hypothermia may have severe consequences in newborn infants and may even lead to arrhythmias and death (9,10)
   b. Peripheral vasoconstriction: Acrocyanosis, pallor, and coldness to touch
   c. Respiratory distress, apnea, and bradycardia (11,12)
   d. Depletion of caloric reserves and hypoglycemia, causing a shift to anaerobic metabolism and lactic acid production (13,14)

TABLE 4.1 Neutral Thermal Environmental Temperatures

AGE AND WEIGHT	RANGE OF TEMPERATURE (°C)	AGE AND WEIGHT	RANGE OF TEMPERATURE (°C)
0–6 hrs		**72–96 hrs**	
<1,200 g	34.0–35.4	<1,200 g	34.0–35.0
1,200–1,500 g	33.9–34.4	1,200–1,500 g	33.0–34.0
1,501–2,500 g	32.8–33.8	1,501–2,500 g	31.1–33.2
>2,500 g (and >36 wks)	32.0–33.8	>2,500 g (and >36 wks)	29.8–32.8
6–12 hrs		**4–12 days**	
<1,200 g	34.0–35.4	<1,500 g	33.0–34.0
1,200–1,500 g	33.5–34.4	1,501–2,500 g	31.0–33.2
1,501–2,500 g	32.2–33.8	>2,500 g (and >36 wks)	
>2,500 g (and >36 wks)	31.4–33.8	4–5 days	29.5–32.6
12–24 hrs		5–6 days	29.4–32.3
<1,200 g	34.0–35.4	6–8 days	29.0–32.2
1,200–1,500 g	33.3–34.3	8–10 days	29.0–31.8
1,501–2,500 g	31.8–33.8	10–12 days	29.0–31.4
>2,500 g (and >36 wks)	31.0–33.7	**12–14 days**	
24–36 hrs		<1,500 g	32.0–34.0
<1,200 g	34.0–35.0	1,501–2,500 g	31.0–33.2
1,200–1,500 g	33.1–34.2	>2,500 g (and >36 wks)	29.0–30.8
1,501–2,500 g	31.6–33.6	**2–3 wks**	
>2,500 g (and >36 wks)	30.7–33.5	<1,500 g	32.2–34.0
36–48 hrs		1,501–2,500 g	30.5–33.0
<1,200 g	34.0–35.0	**3–4 wks**	
1,200–1,500 g	33.0–34.1	<1,500 g	31.6–33.6
1,501–2,500 g	31.4–33.5	1,501–2,500 g	30.0–32.7
>2,500 g (and >36 wks)	30.5–33.3	**4–5 wks**	
48–72 hrs		<1,500 g	31.2–33.0
<1,200 g	34.0–35.0	1,501–2,500 g	29.5–32.2
1,200–1,500 g	33.0–34.0	**5–6 wks**	
1,501–2,500 g	31.2–33.4	<1,500 g	30.6–32.3
>2,500 g (and >36 wks)	30.1–33.2	1,501–2,500 g	29.0–31.8

For their table, Scopes and Ahmed had the walls of the incubator 1° to 2°C warmer than the ambient air temperatures. Generally speaking, the smaller infants in each weight group require a temperature in the higher portion of the temperature range. Within each time range, the younger the infant, the higher the temperature that is required.

Adapted from Scopes J, Ahmed I. Range of critical temperatures in sick and newborn babies. *Arch Dis Child*. 1966;41:417–419.

e. Increased oxygen consumption and metabolic demands result in metabolic acidosis—a strong pulmonary vasoconstrictor inducing hypoxemia and central cyanosis (15–17)

f. Mobilization of norepinephrine, TSH, T_4, and free fatty acids: Norepinephrine release promotes pulmonary hypertension and pulmonary ventilation–perfusion mismatch (18)

g. Decreased cardiac output, increased systemic vascular resistance, and decreased intestinal and cerebral blood flow (10)

h. Decreased number, activation, and aggregation of platelets (10)

i. Impaired neutrophil release and function (10)

j. Poor weight gain with chronic hypothermia (19)

k. Controlled hypothermia has a neuroprotective effect in term and near-term infants with moderate to severe hypoxic ischemic encephalopathy (20)

3. **Effects of hyperthermia or overheating** (7)

a. Peripheral vasodilatation: The skin is hot, the extremities are red, and the face is flushed. Diaphoresis present in full-term infants. Skin temperature is higher than core temperature.

b. Apnea, tachypnea.

c. Tachycardia and hypotension.

d. The infant assumes a spread-eagle posture.

e. Hyperactivity and irritability: The infant becomes restless and cries, then feeds poorly, with lethargy and hypotonia.

f. If hyperthermia is severe, shock, seizures, and coma may occur.

g. If the increase in temperature is due to hypermetabolism (infection), paleness, vasoconstriction, cool extremities, and a core temperature higher than skin temperature may be noted.

h. Hyperthermia is associated with adverse neurodevelopmental outcome in infants with hypoxic ischemic encephalopathy (21,22).

4. Factors affecting heat loss

a. Infant

(1) Large surface area relative to body mass

(2) Relatively large head with highly vascular fontanelle

(3) Skin maturation/thickness, epidermal barrier functionally mature at 32 to 34 weeks. Transepidermal water loss may be 10 to 15 times greater in preterm infants ≤25 weeks' gestation (2)

(4) Decreased stores of subcutaneous fat and brown adipose tissue in more premature infants (5)

(5) Inability to signal discomfort or trigger heat production (shivering) (5)

b. Environment (23)

(1) Physical contact with cold or warm objects (conduction)

(2) Radiant heat loss or gain from proximity to hot or cold objects (radiation)

(3) Wet or exposed body surfaces (evaporation). This is the main cause of heat loss in the first 30 minutes of life

(4) Air currents in nursery or in incubator fan (convection)

(5) Excessive or insufficient coverings or clothing

c. Other factors

(1) Metabolic demands of disease: Asphyxia, respiratory distress, sepsis (10)

(2) Pharmacologic agents (e.g., vasodilating drugs, maternal analgesics, and unwarmed IV infusions) (10)

(3) Medical stability of infant prior to procedure

(4) Thermogenic response matures with increase in postconception age (23)

C. Indications

1. Maintenance of thermal homeostasis is necessary in all infants at all times.

2. Particular attention should be paid when the neonate is in the delivery room, is very premature, or is undergoing diagnostic or therapeutic procedures.

D. Equipment, Techniques, and Complications

1. **Prevention of heat loss in the delivery room**

a. Warm environment (see **Table 4.1**), room temperature >25°C; place infant on a radiant warmer, dry the skin with a prewarmed towel, and then remove any wet towels immediately (7,13,24)

b. Use occlusive plastic blankets/bags **(Fig. 4.1)** (2,9,25).

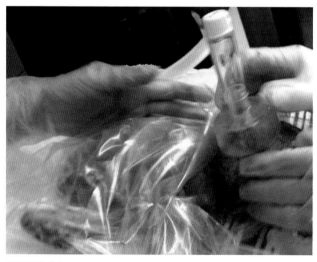

FIGURE 4.1 Extremely low–birth-weight preterm newborn wrapped in occlusive polyethylene sheet during resuscitation.

Polyethylene bags (20 cm × 50 cm) prevent evaporative heat loss in infants <29 weeks' gestation. Their diathermancy allows transmission of radiant heat to the infant. Immediately after delivery, open the bag under the radiant warmer; wrap the wet infant's body from the shoulders down, and dry only the head. Place hat on head. Remove the wrap after the infant has been stable in the neonatal intensive care unit (NICU), in a humidified environment, for 1 hour.

(1) Environment: Maintains temperature and reduces insensible water loss (IWL) by 25% (24,25)

(2) Access: Allows neonatal resuscitation (secure airway, intubation, and chest compressions), but vascular access is limited

(3) Asepsis: Limited by access

(4) Precautions: Record core temperature every 5 to 10 minutes until infant is stable

(5) Complications: Hyperthermia, skin maceration, risk of infection

c. Hats (2,9,26)

(1) Stockinette caps are not effective in reducing heat loss in term infants in the delivery room; there is insufficient evidence in preterm infants.

(2) Woolen hats may reduce or prevent heat loss in term infants in the delivery room.

2. **Prevention of heat loss in the NICU**

a. **Rigid plastic heat shields** (heat shielding)

(1) Environment: Reduces IWL by 25% (27)

(2) Access: Very limited

(3) Asepsis: Limited by access

(4) Precautions: Avoid direct skin contact

(5) Complications: Hyperthermia, skin maceration, risk of infection

b. **Heat lamp:** As an extra heat source (28)

(1) Environment: Increased IWL.

(2) Access: Limited by other equipment used (open incubator, bassinette walls).

(3) Asepsis: May be affected by limited access.

(4) Precautions: Record temperature every 5 to 10 minutes or use a continuous monitor. To avoid burns, do not place oily substances on infant's skin. Avoid heating incubator thermometer; apply manual temperature control (33° to 35°C) when using an open incubator. Keep infant approximately 60 to 90 cm from lamp bulb, and cover infant's eyes and genitals to protect from the light.

(5) Complications: Cooling or overheating of isolette due to failure to detach the thermistor from infant; dehydration.

c. **Warming mattress:** Extra heat source, for transport or radiology procedures (e.g., MRI). Effective in preventing and treating hypothermia in very-low-birth-weight infants (<1,500 g) in the delivery room (2,9,24). Some new incubators incorporate a warmed mattress in their design with the goal of minimizing infant temperature fluctuations during infant care times or procedures (e.g., Baby Leo incubator, Draeger, www.draeger.com).

(1) Environment: Heating through conduction; reduces heat requirements and IWL

(a) Heated water-filled mattress (keep at 37°C)

(b) Exothermic crystallization of sodium acetate mattress (TransWarmer Infant Transport Mattress, Prism Technologies, San Antonio, Texas) with a postactivation temperature of 39°C ± 1°C

(2) Access: Limited only by other equipment used

(3) Asepsis: Limited only by other equipment used

(4) Precautions: Record temperature every 10 to 20 minutes or use an infant servocontrol (ISC) continuous monitor

(5) Complications: Hypothermia, hyperthermia, burns

3. **Mechanical devices to maintain temperature**

a. **Thermal resistor (thermistor):** A probe placed on the anterior abdominal wall or on the back avoiding the interscapular area. Use a servocontrol incubator/radiant warmer to keep infant's temperature between 36.5°C and 36.8°C (28,29).

b. **Convection-warmed incubator (Fig. 4.2):** Ideal for maintaining neutral thermal environment and providing additional humidity for low-birth-weight or preterm infants.

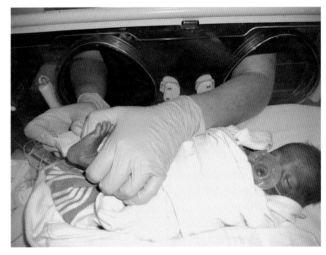

FIGURE 4.2 All aspects of homeostasis are maintained during a procedure by use of incubator portholes, swaddling, comfortable position, and sucrose/analgesia pacifier.

(1) Environment: Creates a microclimate for each infant. The incubator may be servocontrolled by the baby's skin or air temperature; temperature can also be set manually. Double plastic walls, insulated mattress, and forced-heated/humidified air minimize IWL and maintain temperature.

(2) Incubator temperature control is initially regulated by servocontrol (ISC) with baby's skin temperature being maintained between 36.5°C and 36.8°C. Once the baby's clinical condition has stabilized, umbilical catheters have been removed, incubator and baby's temperatures have remained stable, and the baby is clothed or swaddled; after several days or weeks based on the gestational age, the incubator may be set to air temperature. The incubator air temperature is generally set at the temperature the baby was using under ISC in the previous 24 hours, within the parameters of the neutral thermal environment (see **Table 4.1**).

(3) Humidity: Increases in humidity may decrease heat transfer via transdermal water loss and decrease metabolic demand (30). For infants over 30 to 32 weeks, the skin is thought to be mature enough that this mechanism of heat loss is negligible (4). For more preterm infants, changes in relative humidity by 20% may increase or decrease thermoneutral temperature by 1.5° to 1.9°C (31). A range of protocols exist for humidity targets and weaning but most recommend high humidity for infants born less than 28 to 30 weeks' gestation (ranging from 70% to 80%) with initiation of weaning by 7 days of life (32,33). Discontinuation of humidity may occur at 2 weeks of age or may be continued until 32 weeks CGA with a gradual wean. Decision to prolong weaning should consider the risk of delayed skin maturation and infection risk with longer periods of humidity (34,35).

(4) Access: Impeded by portholes, especially when working with assistants. Improved with new incubators/warmers to allow better access (e.g., Giraffe OmniBed neonatal care station [GE Medical Systems, Waukesha, Wisconsin]).

(5) Asepsis: Difficult to maintain wide sterile field and infant position.

(6) Precautions: Take infant's temperature before and after procedures. Use ISC and ensure that thermistor remains in place. Add an extra heat source (heat lamp) for unstable infants or stressful procedures. Clinical deterioration may require lifting the protective shield.

(7) Complications: Hyperthermia, hypothermia, unexpected break of aseptic field.

c. Radiant warmer bed: For unstable infants (28).
(1) Environment: Increases IWL by 50% in small preterm infants.
(2) Access: Unimpeded access to infants receiving intensive care.
(3) Asepsis: Ability to maintain infant position and wide sterile field; also allows assistants to participate.

(4) Precautions: Keep infant 80 to 90 cm from radiant heat. For premature infants, heat shielding must be added. Increase fluid infusions. Record temperature every 5 to 10 minutes or use a continuous monitor. To avoid burns, do not place oily substances on infant's skin.
(5) Complications: Hyperthermia and dehydration.

E. Resource-Limited Settings

1. The World Health Organization (WHO) Standard recommends measures to prevent hypothermia. These include warm delivery rooms, immediate drying, skin-to-skin contact, early breast-feeding, postponed bathing and weighing, appropriate clothing and bedding, and warm transportation and resuscitation (7).
2. Despite following these guidelines, in resource-limited settings, nearly half of low-birth-weight babies and two of five normal-birth-weight infants were hypothermic (36).
3. Hypothermia is a major cause of neonatal mortality (37).
4. The Neonatal Resuscitation Program and the International Liaison Committee on Resuscitation consensus statement recommends the use of a plastic wrap in addition to standard techniques in the delivery room for very–low-birth-weight infants (13).
5. Plastic bags, costing approximately 3 cents each, have been proven to reduce hypothermia (38).
6. Kangaroo mother care is a method of care for low-birth-weight babies that involves early, prolonged, and continuous skin-to-skin contact with a caregiver and exclusive and frequent breast-feeding. This form of care is known to stabilize the body temperature, promote breast-feeding, and prevent infection (39).

F. Special Circumstances/Considerations

1. Remember that very–low-birth-weight preterm infants and infants during the immediate newborn adaptation period are more vulnerable to hypothermia and IWL. This risk remains present for the first 2 to 4 weeks according to gestational age at birth.
   a. Regulate room temperature to one optimal for infant (28° to 30°C) (7).
   b. Prewarm all heating units, including radiant warmers and incubators.
2. For transport outside of the NICU, use a heated, battery-operated transport double-walled incubator.
   a. Plug incubator into wall outlet during procedure to allow battery to charge.
   b. Be aware that anesthesia may inhibit the infant's thermoregulatory capabilities.

3. Warm and humidify all anesthetic and respiratory gases to body temperature.

4. Gastroschisis/omphalocele: These abdominal wall defects increase the risk of heat loss, fluid imbalance, and visceral damage. The infant may be placed in a "bowel bag" from the torso down, or the entire abdomen may be wrapped in clean, clear plastic wrap. Avoid using saline soaked gauze, which may increase evaporative heat loss. Avoid visceral ischemia by keeping intestines directly above the abdominal wall defect or keep the infant in right lateral decubitus position (40).

5. Neural tube defects: Keep the infant in the prone position, cover the lesion with sterile nonadhesive dressing to minimize insensible water losses, and prevent hypothermia (41).

References

1. *Stedman's Electronic Medical Dictionary. Version 7.0.* Emerald Group Publishing; 2008.
2. Bissinger RL, Annibale DJ. Thermoregulation in very-low-birth-weight infants during the golden hour: results and implications. *Adv Neonatal Care.* 2010;10(5):230–238.
3. Silverman WA, Sinclair JC. Temperature regulation in the newborn infant. *N Engl J Med.* 1966;274(2):92–94.
4. Sauer PJ, Dane HJ, Visser HK. New standards for neutral thermal environment of healthy very low birthweight infants in week one of life. *Arch Dis Child.* 1984;59(1):18–22.
5. Ellis J. Neonatal hypothermia. *J Neonatal Nurs.* 2005;11(2):76–82.
6. Lyon AJ, Pikaar ME, Badger P, et al. Temperature control in very low birthweight infants during first five days of life. *Arch Dis Child Fetal Neonatal Ed.* 1997;76(1):F47–F50.
7. Department of Reproductive Health and Research (RHR), World Health Organization. *Thermal Protection of the Newborn: A Practical Guide.* Geneva, Switzerland: World Health Organization; 1997.
8. Kumar V, Shearer JC, Kumar A, et al. Neonatal hypothermia in low resource settings: a review. *J Perinatol.* 2009;29(6):401–412.
9. McCall EM, Alderdice F, Halliday HL, et al. Interventions to prevent hypothermia at birth in preterm and/or low birth weight infants. *Cochrane Database Syst Rev.* 2018;2:CD004210. doi: 10.1002/14651858.CD004210.pub5
10. Zanelli S, Buck M, Fairchild K. Physiologic and pharmacologic considerations for hypothermia therapy in neonates. *J Perinatol.* 2011;31(6):377–386.
11. Thoresen M, Whitelaw A. Cardiovascular changes during mild therapeutic hypothermia and rewarming in infants with hypoxic–ischemic encephalopathy. *Pediatrics.* 2000;106(1):92–99.
12. Gebauer CM, Knuepfer M, Robel-Tillig E, et al. Hemodynamics among neonates with hypoxic-ischemic encephalopathy during whole-body hypothermia and passive rewarming. *Pediatrics.* 2006;117(3):843–850.
13. Kattwinkel J, Perlman JM, Aziz K, et al. Neonatal resuscitation: 2010 American heart association guidelines for cardiopulmonary resuscitation and emergency cardiovascular care. *Pediatrics.* 2010;126(5):e1400–e1413.
14. Doctor BA, O'Riordan MA, Kirchner HL, et al. Perinatal correlates and neonatal outcomes of small for gestational age infants born at term gestation. *Am J Obstet Gynecol.* 2001;185(3):652–659.
15. Hassan IA, Wickramasinghe YA, Spencer SA. Effect of limb cooling on peripheral and global oxygen consumption in neonates. *Arch Dis Child Fetal Neonatal Ed.* 2003;88(2):F139–F142.
16. Marks KH, Lee CA, Bolan CD Jr, et al. Oxygen consumption and temperature control of premature infants in a double-wall incubator. *Pediatrics.* 1981;68(1):93–98.
17. Hey EN. The relation between environmental temperature and oxygen consumption in the new-born baby. *J Physiol.* 1969;200(3):589–603.
18. Soll RF. Heat loss prevention in neonates. *J Perinatol.* 2008;28:S57–S59.
19. Glass L, Silverman WA, Sinclair JC. Effect of the thermal environment on cold resistance and growth of small infants after the first week of life. *Pediatrics.* 1968;41(6):1033–1046.
20. Jacobs SE, Berg M, Hunt R, et al. Cooling for newborns with hypoxic ischaemic encephalopathy. *Cochrane Database Syst Rev.* 2013;(1):CD003311.
21. Kasdorf E, Perlman JM. Hyperthermia, inflammation, and perinatal brain injury. *Pediatr Neurol.* 2013;49(1):8–14.
22. Shankaran S, Laptook AR, Pappas A, et al. Effect of depth and duration of cooling on death or disability at age 18 months among neonates with hypoxic-ischemic encephalopathy: a randomized clinical trial. *JAMA.* 2017;318(1):57–67.
23. Knobel R, Holditch-Davis D. Thermoregulation and heat loss prevention after birth and during neonatal intensive-care unit stabilization of extremely low-birthweight infants. *J Obstet Gynecol Neonatal Nurs.* 2007;36(3):280–287.
24. Bhatt DR, White R, Martin G, et al. Transitional hypothermia in preterm newborns. *J Perinatol.* 2007;27:S45–S47.
25. Vohra S, Roberts RS, Zhang B, et al. Heat Loss Prevention (HeLP) in the delivery room: a randomized controlled trial of polyethylene occlusive skin wrapping in very preterm infants. *J Pediatr.* 2004;145(6):750–753.
26. Lang N, Bromiker R, Arad I. The effect of wool vs. cotton head covering and length of stay with the mother following delivery on infant temperature. *Int J Nurs Stud.* 2004;41(8):843–846.
27. Symonds ME, Lomax MA. Maternal and environmental influences on thermoregulation in the neonate. *Proc Nutr Soc.* 1992;51(2):165–172.
28. Korones SB. An encapsulated history of thermoregulation in the neonate. *NeoReviews.* 2004;5(3):e78–e85.
29. Knobel RB. Fetal and neonatal thermal physiology. *Newborn Infant Nurs Rev.* 2014;14(2):45–49.
30. Erbani R, Degrugilliers L, Lahana A, et al. Failing to meet relative humidity targets for incubated neonates causes higher heat loss and metabolic costs in the first week of life. *Acta Paediatrica.* 2018;107:1177–1183.
31. Delanaud S, Decima P, Pelletier A, et al. Thermal management in closed incubators: new software for assessing the impact of humidity on the optimal incubator air temperature. *Med Eng Phys.* 2017;46:89–95.
32. Sinclair L, Crisp J, Sinn J. Variability in incubator humidity practices in the management of preterm infants. *J Paediatr Child Health.* 2009;45:535–540.

33. Sung MK, Lee EY, Chen J, et al. Improved care and growth outcomes by using hybrid humidified incubators in very preterm infants. *Pediatrics*. 2010;125(1):e137–145.

34. de Goffau MC, Bergman KA, de Vries HJ, et al. Cold spots in neonatal incubators are hot spots for microbial contamination. *Appl Environ Microbiol*. 2011;77(24):8568–8572.

35. Agren J, Sjors G, Sedin G. Ambient humidity influences the rate of skin barrier maturation in extremely preterm infants. *J Pediatr*. 2006;148(5):613–617.

36. Darmstadt GL, Kumar V, Yadav R, et al. Introduction of community-based skin-to-skin care in rural Uttar Pradesh, India. *J Perinatol*. 2006;26(10):597–604.

37. Sodemann M, Nielsen J, Veirum J, et al. Hypothermia of newborns is associated with excess mortality in the first 2 months of life in Guinea-Bissau, West Africa. *Trop Med Int Health*. 2008;13(8):980–986.

38. Belsches TC, Tilly AE, Miller TR, et al. Randomized trial of plastic bags to prevent term neonatal hypothermia in a resource-poor setting. *Pediatrics*. 2013;132(3):e656–e661.

39. Conde-Agudelo A, Díaz-Rossello JL. Kangaroo mother care to reduce morbidity and mortality in low birthweight infants. *Cochrane Database Syst Rev*. 2016;(8):CD002771.

40. Sheldon RE. The bowel bag: A sterile, transportable method for warming infants with skin defects. *Pediatrics*. 1974;53(2):267–269.

41. Thompson DN. Postnatal management and outcome for neural tube defects including spina bifida and encephalocoeles. *Prenat Diagn*. 2009;29(4):412–419.

5

Methods of Restraint

Margaret Mary Kuczkowski

Physical restraints are required for proper positioning for certain procedures. Infants may also need to be restrained to prevent accidental injury or interference with treatment (i.e., removal of feeding tubes, catheters). Always select the least restrictive but most appropriate restraint for the individual patient.

A. Definitions

1. Physical restraint: "Any manual method, physical or mechanical device, material or equipment that immobilizes a child or reduces his or her ability to move the arms, legs, body or head freely" (as defined by the Centers for Medicare and Medicaid Services [CMS] and The Joint Commission) (1,2)

B. Indications

1. Required for procedures that necessitate proper positioning to maintain asepsis and facilitate access to patient (IV placement, lumbar punctures, etc.) (1)
2. To reduce the risk of interference with treatment (removal of feeding tubes, IV access, mechanical ventilation, etc.) (2)
3. To prevent movement artifact for radiographic studies and MRI (3)
4. To prevent accidental injury

C. Contraindications

Restraints Should Not Be Utilized

1. When close observation of the patient could protect against potential injury or potential interference with treatment (1,2)
2. When a change in treatment or medication regimen could protect against potential injury or interference with treatment (1,2)

3. When modification of the patient's environment (decreased stimuli, appropriate developmental positioning, reduced noise) could protect against potential injury or interference with treatment (1,2)
4. When use of a restraint could compromise patient care, procedures, or emergency access (1)

D. Techniques

Restraints for Procedures/Positioning

Whole Body Restraints

1. **Mummy Restraint**
   a. **Purpose:** Safe temporary method for restraining infants for treatment or examination; allows unimpeded access to head and scalp; individual extremities can be released for access for examination or treatment (1,2)
   b. **Equipment**
      (1) Clean blanket or small sheet
      (2) Safety pins or other device for securing final blanket fold
   c. **Procedure** (1)
      (1) Open blanket or sheet.
      (2) Fold one corner toward the center.
      (3) Place infant on blanket, with shoulders at fold and feet toward opposite corner (**Fig. 5.1A**).
      (4) With infant's right arm flexed and midline, tuck right side of blanket across trunk and under left side of body (**Fig. 5.1B**).
      (5) Fold lower corner up toward head and tuck under left shoulder (**Fig. 5.1C**).
      (6) With infant's left arm flexed and midline, tuck left side of blanket across trunk and under right side of body. Be sure to secure arms under blanket (**Fig. 5.1D**).

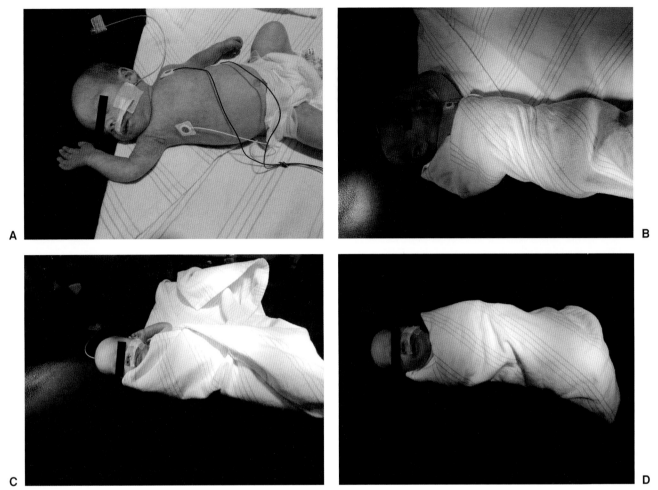

FIGURE 5.1 **A:** Mummy restraint: Steps (1)–(3). **B:** Mummy restraint: Step (4). **C:** Mummy restraint: Step (5). **D:** Mummy restraint: Step (6).

2. Commercial restraints for special procedures
   a. A "papoose board" is a flat padded board with canvas straps and Velcro closures and is often used for circumcisions in neonates.
   b. Specially designed sterile wraps to restrain newborn infants for umbilical venous catheterization or for lumbar punctures (**Fig. 5.2A–C**).
   c. Vacuum immobilization bags (MedVac Infant Immobilizer Bag, CFI Medical Solutions, Fenton, Michigan) are useful for performing MRI and CT scans in newborn infants and usually eliminate the need for sedation (3).

Extremity Restraints

1. **Extremity restraint (wrist or ankle) (Fig. 5.3)**
   a. **Purpose:** Immobilization of one or more extremities; protects infant from interfering with or removing treatment regimens (IV access, feeding tube, endotracheal tube, etc.)

   b. **Equipment**
      (1) Commercially available restraint (sheepskin and/or foam padding) for larger infants
          OR
      (2) Roll of gauze or gauze pads
      (3) Adhesive tape
      (4) Safety pins or other securing device
   c. **Procedure**
      (1) Open gauze and fold in half lengthwise to reinforce material.
      (2) Wrap wrist or ankle with gauze at least three times to create secure restraint. *Caution:* Do not wrap gauze too tight; this might interfere with distal circulation.
      (3) Use adhesive tape to ensure that gauze does not unravel.
      (4) Secure restraint to mattress, blanket, or light sandbag with safety pin. (1)
2. **Mitten Restraint**
   a. **Purpose:** Thumbless device to restrain or cover hand; eliminate infant's ability to grasp and possibly

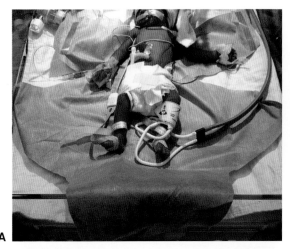

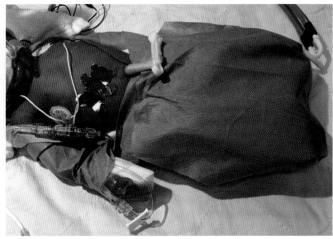

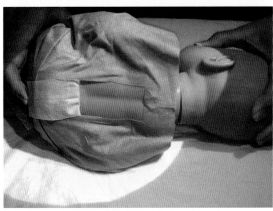

FIGURE 5.2 **A,B:** Neowrapi: Wrap to immobilize arms and legs before placement of umbilical catheters. (Patent pending; picture provided courtesy of M. Peesay, MD and C. Papageorgopoulos, BSN, RN.) **C:** Lumbar Wrapi: Wrap to immobilize baby prior to lumbar puncture. (Patent pending; picture provided courtesy of M. Peesay, MD and C. Papageorgopoulos, BSN, RN.)

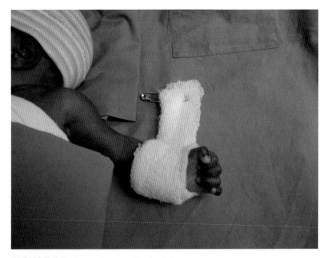

FIGURE 5.3 Extremity restraint (wrist).

dislodge necessary treatment regimens (IV access, feeding tube, endotracheal tube, etc.), prevent infant from scratching self or removing dressings, interfering with maintenance of skin integrity

b. **Equipment**
  (1) Commercial mittens OR stockinette material (cut to fit individual infant)
  (2) Adhesive tape
  (3) Safety pins or other securing device (optional)

c. **Procedure**
  (1) Place infant's hand inside mitten/stockinette.
  (2) Secure mitten/stockinette by applying tape to material and fastening around infant's wrist. *Caution:* Do not wrap tape too tight; this might interfere with distal circulation.
  (3) If using stockinette material, may need to tie end of stockinette in order to isolate fingers inside the stockinette material.
  (4) Secure restraint to mattress, blanket, or light sandbag with safety pin (optional) (2).

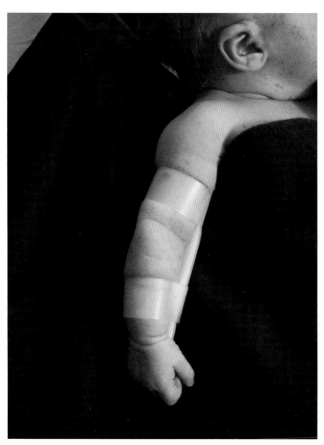

FIGURE 5.4 Elbow restraint.

3. **Elbow restraint (freedom splint) (Fig. 5.4)**
   a. **Purpose:** Reduces ability of infant to flex elbow
   b. **Equipment**
      (1) Commercially available restraints (sheepskin and/or foam padding) for larger infants
         OR
      (2) Foam-padded armboard
      (3) Adhesive tape
      (4) Additional padding material (i.e., cotton balls, gauze pads)
   c. **Procedure**
      (1) Cut pieces of tape (appropriate size; tape should not completely encircle extremity). Consider double backing the tape to eliminate the tape adhering to the skin.
      (2) Extend upper extremity.
      (3) Place armboard under elbow to eliminate the ability to flex joint.
      (4) Tape extremity securely to armboard. Tape should be applied above and below elbow joint.
      (5) Pad bony prominences with cotton as needed (2).

Restraints for Vascular Access

Restraints can be used to secure IV access and prevent accidental dislodgement.

1. **Equipment**
   a. Restraint device (i.e., armboard): Armboards vary in size; a larger infant may require an armboard that is 1 to 2 cm wider than the hand/foot and extends from the proximal joint to the distal joint. However, to maintain functional position and natural curvature of the hand at rest for long-term restraint, the armboard can be shorter in length to allow for curvature of fingers around the end of the board.
   b. Adhesive tape: Transparent tape is recommended for visualization of IV site especially during continuous infusion (may be double backed).
   c. Additional padding material (i.e., cotton balls, gauze pads).
2. **Procedure**
   a. Ensure that the infant's extremity is in a developmentally appropriate position.
   b. Assess skin integrity where restraint is to be applied.
   c. Apply restraint board using transparent tape. Do not allow tape to encircle extremity. Three pieces of tape should sufficiently restrain the extremity and allow for visualization of the tips of fingers (**Fig. 5.5**) or toes (**Fig. 5.6A,B**). The sequence of tape allows for functional positioning of thumb and ankle.
   d. Pad bony prominences and maintain natural curvature of extremities (especially the hand and fingers) (1).

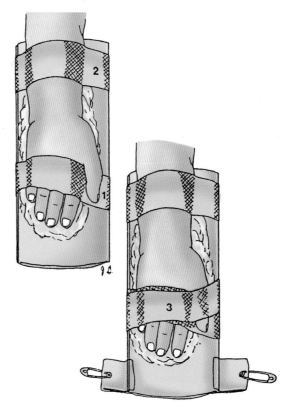

FIGURE 5.5 Restraint for vascular access—wrist and forearm. Tape is applied in order, *1* through *3*, as shown.

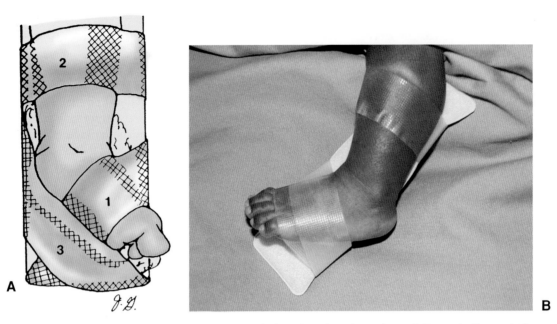

FIGURE 5.6 A: Restraint for vascular access—foot and ankle. Tape is applied in order, *1* through *3*, as shown. **B:** Foot and ankle restraint for vascular access on premature infant.

E. Precautions

1. Restraints should be a last resort after other reasonable alternatives have failed, including close observation, treatment and/or medication change, modification of environment, etc. Document use of alternative methods (1).

2. For restraints during procedures, proper techniques for analgesia, sedation, and distraction (pacifier, touch, sound, etc.) may be necessary in addition to the restraint (2).

3. Family education regarding the need, procedure, and time frame for the use of the restraint is required. Provide an opportunity for collaboration with the family. If possible, remove the restraints when the family is visiting (1).

4. Weigh equipment required for restraints (i.e., armboards) prior to use. If possible, maintain a list of the weights of common restraint materials in use when weighing infants for monitoring daily growth.

5. Evaluate the patient and proper use, placement, and position of restraint according to patient need, hospital policy, and regulatory agency requirement. Regulatory agencies such as The Joint Commission, CMS, and the U.S. Food and Drug Administration (FDA) Centers publish standards of medical care regarding the safe use and legal requirements for restraint implementation and maintenance (1,2).

6. Ensure that the infant is in a proper and functional position that promotes flexion and midline positioning of upper and lower extremities.

a. **Rationale:** Prevention of contractures and support of self-calming techniques of neonates (prone, side lying) (**Figs. 5.7** and **5.8**) (4,5).

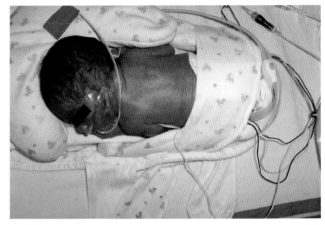

FIGURE 5.7 Prone positioning during procedures and at rest provides for improved breathing and sleep, lower expenditure of energy, and more stable physiologic functioning. Care must be taken to create positioning support of the trunk and hips.

7. Pad bony prominences and maintain natural curvature of extremities (especially the hand and fingers).

a. **Rationale:** Prevents contractures and neurovascular injury; preserves skin integrity; reduces friction and pressure to skin from restraint material (1).

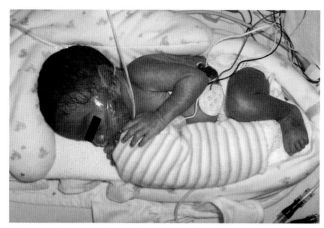

FIGURE 5.8 Side-lying positioning is the best alternative to prone for procedures and sleeping. This position allows for more midline positioning of the upper and lower extremities. Nesting support increases postural stability and decreases arching of the back.

8. When utilizing tape for securing an extremity to a board, use transparent tape when possible to allow for careful and complete assessment of the underlying skin. Do not apply tape too securely, as it may impede circulation. The use of double-backed tape may be helpful in areas that do not require adherence to the infant's skin. Tips of all digits should remain visible for assessment.
9. Restraints on the upper or lower extremities need to be assessed at least hourly (and/or according to hospital policy and regulatory agency requirement [The Joint Commission, CMS]) for
   a. Skin integrity, including excoriation, erythema, and edema
   b. Pulses
   c. Temperature
   d. Color
   e. Capillary refill
   f. Range of motion (ROM) (1,2).
10. Check for possible constriction by inserting a finger between infant's skin and the secured restraint (2).
   a. **Rationale:** Constriction from a tight restraint can cause neurovascular injury and impede circulation.
11. Specific assessments related to oxygenation, musculoskeletal system, and cardiorespiratory conditions need to be performed in relation to the restraint device and its usage (1).
12. Observe any treatment equipment for proper positioning and patency, especially in close proximity to the restraint device (kinked IV access, dislodgement of catheters, etc.) (1).
13. Attach restraint to a fixed location on bed (if necessary), maintaining the opportunity for quick release and regular vascular checks (safety pin, secure tucking, etc.). Do not attach restraint to equipment that can be moved (crib side rails, incubator doors), as injury may occur.

Quick release allows for mobility and access in an emergency (1,2).
14. Document restraint use and, if required, obtain physician order (see hospital policy and/or regulatory agency requirement [The Joint Commission, CMS]) (1,2).
15. Remove restraint at the earliest time possible.

F. Complications

1. Failure of restraint resulting in self-injury and/or interference with treatment
2. Neurovascular impairment (1)
3. Impairment of skin integrity (i.e., pressure ulcer formation, necrosis) (1)
4. Contractures or positional deformity/paralysis from prolonged immobility (1)
5. Limb injury (fracture or dislocation) from movement of infant without release of secured restraint or from securing restraint to movable object (e.g., crib side rails, incubator doors) (1)
6. Impairment or compromise of medical state, including oxygenation, musculoskeletal system, and cardiorespiratory conditions (1)
7. Increased agitation or irritability (1)
8. Extravasation injury leading to impairment of skin integrity, tissue necrosis, infection, and/or nerve and tendon damage (4)

G. Special Considerations

1. A temporary alternative to restraint usage during procedures is *therapeutic safe holding*. This is defined as the use of a secure, comfortable, temporary holding position that provides close physical contact with the parent or caregiver for 30 minutes or less and restricts the movement of the child for the clinical procedure (6). Staff must properly prepare the parent or caregiver and provide proper supervision throughout the procedure.
2. Proper Positioning
   Whenever possible during the use of the restraint or immediately following the use of the restraint the infant should be positioned with the following guidelines:
   • Upper extremities—flexed, midline, and contained
   • Head and neck—neutral and midline
   • Shoulders—rounded to allow upper extremities midline
   • Body—curved "C" position with rounded lower back
   • Lower extremities—flexed, midline, contained, and supported for foot bracing (5).
3. The American Academy of Pediatrics has outlined recommendations addressing infant sleep positioning to reduce the risk of sudden infant death syndrome. The recommendation states that, "hospitalized preterm infants should be kept predominantly in the supine position,

at least from postmenstrual age of 32 weeks onward, so that they become acclimated to supine sleeping before discharge" (5). Therefore, when returning the patient to a sleep and/or recovery position following a procedure, health care professionals should endorse and model this behavior for parents and caregivers whenever possible.

References

1. Perry AG, Potter PA, Ostendorf W. *Clinical Nursing Skills & Techniques*. 9th ed. St Louis, MO: Mosby/Elsevier; 2017.

2. Lippincott. *Lippincott Nursing Procedures*. 7th ed. Philadelphia, PA: Wolters Kluwer; 2016.

3. Mathur AM, Neil JJ, McKinstry RC, et al. Transport, monitoring, and successful brain MR imaging in unsedated neonates. *Pediatr Radiol*. 2008;38:260–264.

4. Ramasethu J. Prevention and management of extravasation injuries in neonates. *NeoReviews*. 2004;5(11):c491.

5. Drake E. Positioning the neonate for best outcomes. *National Association of Neonatal Nurses*. 2017. http://apps.nann.org/store/product-details?productId=45241425.

6. Kennedy R, Binns F. Therapeutic safe holding with children and young people in hospital. *Nurs Child Young People*. 2016;28(4):28–32.

CHAPTER

6

Aseptic Preparation

Ha-young Choi

A. Definitions

1. Aseptic technique: application of preventative measures used to minimize contamination by pathogens.
2. Antiseptic: relating to or denoting substances that prevent the growth of disease-causing microorganisms, usually refers to substances that may be applied to living tissues or cells.
3. Disinfectants: substances that are meant to destroy microorganisms on the surface of nonliving objects; are usually too strong or caustic to apply to living tissue.

B. Background

Adherence to proper aseptic technique and standard precautions are important in the health care setting, and especially so in the neonatal intensive care unit (NICU). These measures aim to protect patients and the health care workers and control the spread of infection. Patients in the NICU are particularly susceptible to nosocomial or hospital-acquired infection, with profound impacts on survival, outcomes, and costs of care.

Protocols and procedures for aseptic technique in NICUs are constantly being reevaluated and updated, and hand hygiene guidelines are routinely published by the U.S. Centers for Disease Control (CDC) (1,2). Hospital managers should continuously develop and update strict policies and regulations as well as quality improvement projects aimed to promote adherence to aseptic technique and hand hygiene (3).

C. Indications

1. Preparation of patient's skin and the hands of personnel prior to performing a procedure
   a. To remove transient flora, which is sometimes pathogenic flora that are transiently found on the skin, usually less than 24 hours, for example, *Escherichia coli*

   b. To decrease and temporarily suppress most resident skin flora, which is the usually low-virulence flora that survive and multiply on skin, for example, *Staphylococcus epidermidis*
2. Decontamination after a procedure
3. Maintenance of clean surgical sites

D. Standard Precautions

1. Universal precautions
   a. All human blood and certain human body fluids are treated as if known to be infectious for HIV, HBV, and other blood-borne pathogens.
   b. Universal precautions protect the caregiver and the patient, but remember it does not preclude the need for proper antisepsis, which is targeted at decreasing skin flora.
2. Core components (1)
   a. Use gloves when touching blood, body fluids, mucous membranes, or nonintact skin, and when handling items or surfaces soiled with blood or body fluids.
   b. Use a mask and eye protection during procedures that might generate splashing or droplets in the air.
   c. Use a gown or a plastic apron when splashing of blood or body fluid is likely.
   d. Wash hands carefully if they become contaminated with blood or body fluids.
   e. Take extraordinary care when handling needles and other sharp objects, and dispose of them in puncture-resistant containers.
   f. Exclude from patient care all personnel with exudative lesions or weeping dermatitis until these conditions have resolved.
3. Hand hygiene (1)
   a. Alcohol-based hand rubs are the most effective products for reducing the number of pathogenic microorganisms on the hands of health care providers (1).

(1) In order to be effective, products should contain at least 60% to 95% alcohol.

(2) Faster drying time leads to improved adherence (4,5).

(3) If hand disinfectants are not allowed to dry, alcohol-based disinfectant vapors can accumulate inside incubators (6).

b. Antiseptic soaps and detergents are the next most effective and nonantimicrobial soaps are the least effective. Soap and water are recommended in cases of:

(1) Visibly soiled hands

(2) Hospital outbreaks of contact with patients suspected to have *Clostridium difficile*, *Norovirus*, or *Bacillus anthracis*

(3) Before eating

(4) After using the restroom

c. Technique of hand hygiene:

(1) Remove all rings, watches, bracelets, etc.

(2) Roll up sleeves to the elbows.

(3) The CDC recommends *at least* 15 seconds of rubbing the solution on the hands, paying particular attention to the areas between the fingers, the thumb, and little finger.

d. In addition to hospital personnel, parents and visitors should also be taught to adhere to strict hand hygiene, as nosocomial infections can be spread by family members (7).

4. Gloves

a. Are not an alternative to hand hygiene.

b. The warm, wet skin surface under gloves offers an ideal environment for bacterial multiplication. Gloves are not completely impermeable to microorganisms.

c. Vinyl gloves may leak more readily than latex gloves (8).

d. Always clean hands before putting on and after removing gloves.

e. Change gloves during patient care if hands are moved from a contaminated body site (e.g., diaper area) to clean site (IV site or face).

f. Do not wear the same pair of gloves for the care of more than one patient.

5. Surgical hand antisepsis (1,2)

a. Before performing any procedure where sterile gloves will be worn.

b. Remove rings, watches, and bracelets before beginning the surgical hand scrub.

c. Remove debris from underneath fingernails using a nail cleaner under running water.

d. Performing surgical hand antisepsis using either an antimicrobial soap or an alcohol-based hand sanitizer with persistent activity is recommended before donning sterile gloves when performing surgical procedures.

e. When performing surgical hand antisepsis using an antimicrobial soap, scrub hands and forearms for the length of time recommended by the manufacturer, usually 2 to 6 minutes. Rapid multiplication of bacteria occurs under surgical gloves if hands are washed with a nonantimicrobial soap.

f. Long scrub times (e.g., 10 minutes) are not necessary. A scrub brush is not recommended.

g. When using an alcohol-based surgical hand-scrub product with persistent activity, follow the manufacturer's instructions.

h. Before applying the alcohol solution, prewash hands and forearms with a nonantimicrobial soap and dry hands and forearms completely.

i. When rinsing hands with water, keep hands and wrists elevated above forearms.

j. When drying hands after washing, use sterile towel and dry hands first before drying forearms.

k. After application of the alcohol-based product as recommended, allow hands and forearms to dry thoroughly before donning sterile gloves.

E. Proper Use of Antiseptics

No antiseptic is totally effective or without risk and there is no absolute consensus on the optimal antiseptic for use in neonates (9–11). The U.S. Food and Drug Administration (FDA) is awaiting further data on commonly used antiseptics (i.e., benzalkonium chloride, benzethonium chloride, chloroxylenol, ethyl alcohol, isopropyl alcohol, and povidone-iodine) so that the agency can make a safety and efficacy determination about these ingredients. While we await the data on these commonly used active ingredients, the FDA recommends that health care personnel continue to use currently available products, consistent with infection control guidelines (12).

1. Refer to **Table 6.1** and Section G for advantages and complications associated with each antiseptic option.

2. Always allow antiseptics and disinfectants to dry before starting procedure.

a. A drying time of at least 30 seconds is required for optimal effect.

b. Avoid removal of antiseptic from skin prior to the procedure—removal negates the residual slow-release effect.

c. After the procedure, remove iodine-containing antiseptics from all but the immediate area of the procedure to prevent absorption.

d. Contamination of instruments or sample with antiseptic may invalidate specimens taken for culture.

3. Ensure that skin is not visibly soiled prior to application of antiseptic. However, overly vigorous scrubbing of the skin prior to, or with antiseptics application may lead to skin breakdown without conferring extra benefit regarding antisepsis (13). Antiseptic should

TABLE 6.1 **A Comparison of Commonly Used Antiseptics**

CONSIDERATIONS	ALCOHOL (70–90%)	IODINE (1%)	IODOPHOR	CHLORHEXIDINE
1. Indications	Hand washing Skin preparation Minor procedures Preparation of external auditory canal	Surgical hand washing Skin preparation	Surgical hand washing Skin preparation	Hand washing (4%) Skin preparation (0.5% in 70% alcohol)
2. Side effects				
a. Nontoxic	Yes	Hypothyroidism	Hypothyroidism	Yes Local ototoxicity
b. Nonsensitizing	Yes	No	Yes	Yes
c. Nonirritating	Burns in preterm neonates	No	Yes	Yes
3. Mode of action	Protein denaturation	Oxidation	Oxidation	Cell wall disruption
4. Bactericidal	Yes	Yes	Yes	Yes
5. May be used with detergent	No	No	Yes	Yes
6. Persistent local action	No	Yes	Yes	Yes
7. Effective against				
a. Gram-positive bacteria	Yes	Yes	Yes	Yes
b. Gram-negative bacteria	Yes	Yes	Yes	Yes
c. Spores	No	No	No	No
d. Tubercle bacillus	Yes	Yes	No	No
e. Viruses	Lipophilic only	Yes	Yes	Yes
f. Fungi	Yes	Yes	Yes	Yes
8. Use associated with resistance	No	No	No	Contamination
9. Rapid action	Yes	Yes	No (4–5 min)	Yes
10. Easily inactivated by extraneous organic matter	Maybe (inactivated by nonbacterial protein)	Yes	No (good for crevice and fat penetration)	No

be applied gently but with some mild pressure, not enough to damage the fragile skin of the neonate.

F. Technique (▶ Video 6.1: Aseptic Preparation)

1. Preparation for a minor procedure
   a. Definition
      (1) Short duration (5 to 10 minutes); noncomplex.
      (2) Does not involve an area, such as the central nervous system (CNS), which is especially vulnerable to infection.
      (3) Does not require skin incision.
      (4) Includes blood drawing (not blood culture), placement of peripheral venous line.
   b. Preparation of personnel
      (1) Wear cap/beard cover if hair is likely to contaminate the field.
      (2) Perform hand hygiene as above using alcohol hand sanitizer or antimicrobial soap.
      (3) Wear clean gloves.
   c. Preparation of patient skin
      (1) If necessary, remove hair using small scissors or clippers, taking care not to nick skin. Do not shave the area, as this may irritate or nick the skin and increase the risk of infection (14).

(2) Apply antiseptic of choice (see **Table 6.1**).
  (a) Alcohol may be used, depending on patient age. Preparation with Iodophor may be optimal, but color tends to obscure underlying vessels.
  (b) Apply three times in circles progressing away from procedure site.
  (c) Apply with gentle friction.
  (d) Allow to dry. Do not wipe off antiseptic.
  (e) Never touch skin after application of antiseptic and before initiation of the procedure.
  (f) If using alcohol, reapply it prior to every attempt at procedure, as resident flora can quickly regenerate.
2. Preparation for a major procedure
  a. Definition of major procedure
    (1) Invasive or involving skin incision
    (2) Includes central line placement, cutdown, chest tube, lumbar puncture
    (3) Duration longer than 5 to 10 minutes
  b. Masks, drapes, and gowns. Clothing is an important barrier to microorganisms shed into the air from the skin and mucous membranes. In the United States, surgical masks and gowns must be registered by the FDA to demonstrate safety and efficacy
    (1) Put on cap and mask.
    (2) Follow procedure for surgical hand hygiene above.
    (3) Put on *sterile gown* with the aid *of an assistant* (**Fig. 6.1**).
    (4) Put on *sterile gloves,* without contaminating external *surface with* ungloved hand (**Fig. 6.2**).
      (a) An assistant in sterile attire may assist in putting on gloves.
      (b) Pull gloves well over sleeve ends; the permeable cotton cuffs should not be visible.

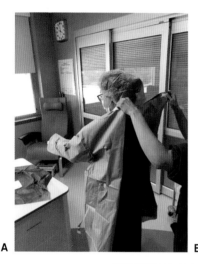
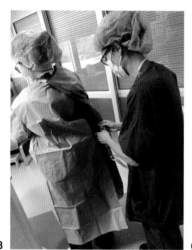
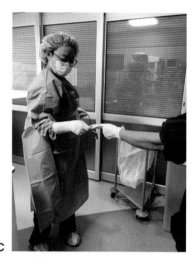
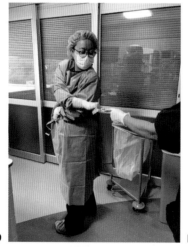
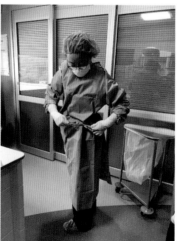

FIGURE 6.1 Technique for donning sterile surgical gown with the aid of an assistant. **A:** The assistant pulls gown over practitioner's shoulders, while touching only the inside of the gown, to secure gown behind the neck. **B:** Assistant ties the inside ties of the gown. **C:** Once sterile gloves have been donned, the practitioner hands tie to assistant, taking care to touch only the white half of the card, while assistant touches only colored half of the card. **D:** Practitioner and assistant turn in place in opposite directions, to encircle tie around practitioner. **E:** Once tie is completely around the practitioner, with gown now held closed, the practitioner can tug on the tie and separate tie from card, which remains in the hands of the assistant.

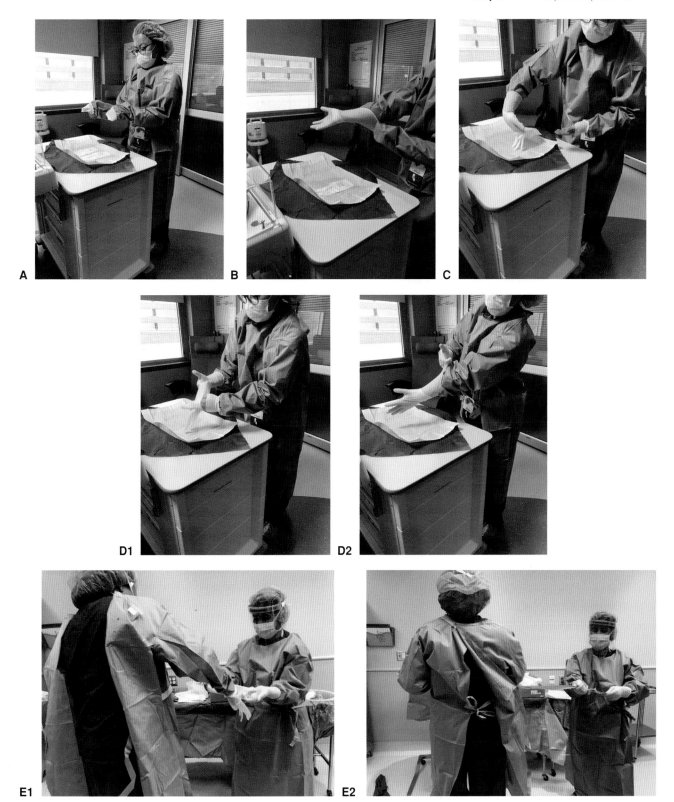

FIGURE 6.2 Proper technique for donning sterile gloves. **A:** Hands should remain inside the sleeves, brought to the ends of the sleeves. **B:** With nondominant hand still within the sleeve of the sterile gown, place opposite hand into glove, pulling ends completely over porous cloth cuffs. **C:** Lift the next glove by placing the gloved hand within the pocket formed by the fold. Take care not to touch the external, sterile surface of the gloved hand with the ungloved hand. **D1-2:** Pull glove completely over porous cotton cuffs. **E1-2:** Sterility is easier to maintain with the aid of an assistant who is wearing sterile attire.

3. Preparation of patient skin
   a. Prior to procedure, have assistant:
      (1) Wash area, if soiled, with soap and water.
      (2) If necessary, remove hair using small scissors or clippers, taking care not to nick skin. Do not shave the area, as this may irritate or nick the skin and increase the risk of infection (14).
   b. Apply antiseptic
      (1) Apply antiseptic with three separate sponges.
      (2) Start at center of expected procedural entry point, and apply in circular motion, creating gradually larger circles in a centrifugal manner, until at least 5 cm outside immediate area of procedure.
      (3) Alcohol (70%) should not be used as antiseptic for a major procedure.
   c. Allow antiseptic to dry. Do not wipe off antiseptic prior to procedure.
   d. Use a large-barrier drape to provide large sterile area around surgical site (2).

G. Complications/Precautions

1. Dry skin in health care providers caused by repeated use
   a. Moisturizing skin products or barrier creams after hand washing can decrease cracking of hands without compromising safety (15). Hand lotions approved for hospital use are recommended (1).
2. Hexachlorophene
   a. Not recommended for general use in neonates. May be used in term neonates during outbreaks of *Staphylococcus aureus* infections if other infection control measures are ineffective.
   b. Not recommended for bathing neonates—transcutaneous absorption with CNS vacuolation has been reported.
   c. Possible teratogenicity when used for hand washing by a pregnant staff member.
3. Iodine—see Iodophor
   a. Often dissolved in alcohol, therefore more likely to burn premature skin.
   b. Allergic contact dermatitis has been reported.
   c. Skin absorption/hypothyroidism.
4. Iodophor, for example, povidone-iodine
   a. Burns possible when allowed to pool under infant.
   b. Absorption through skin reported in neonates.
   c. Alteration of thyroid function may happen due to absorption of iodine through the skin (16,17). However, the high incidence of transient neonatal hypothyroidism observed in premature infants in Europe after routine skin cleansing with iodine has not been confirmed in North America. This difference in incidence may be due to the prior iodine status of the neonate (18).
   d. Some reports of increased false-positive rate of blood cultures compared to iodine or chlorhexidine (19,20).
5. Chlorhexidine
   a. Similarity in name and preparation has led to some confusion between chlorhexidine and hexachlorophene. These compounds are different in structure and properties.
   b. Sensorineural deafness when instilled into middle ear; ocular toxicity with direct exposure to eye.
   c. Burns possible when allowed to pool under infant (21).
   d. Absorption through skin and from umbilical stump (22,23). No associated pathology has been documented.
   e. Contamination with gram-negative organisms has been reported, in particular *Pseudomonas* and *Proteus* species (24).
   f. Aqueous chlorhexidine may be gentler on the skin than alcohol preparations (25). However, skin damage has been reported even with aqueous chlorhexidine (26).
   g. Acetate preparations may also be easier on the skin than alcohol preparations (27).
6. Alcohol
   a. Burns in premature infants (28).
   b. Transcutaneous absorption of alcohol (29).
   c. Exposure to high concentrations of alcohol vapors in incubators (6).
   d. Not sufficient antisepsis for major procedures.
7. Latex
   a. Sensitization and allergy can develop due to repeated exposures, both in health care workers and in patients with repeated exposures (30).
   b. In particular, latex should be avoided in infants with neural tube defects and genitourinary abnormalities, due to the high rates of sensitization in these populations (31).

References

1. Centers for Disease Control and Prevention (CDC). Core infection prevention and control practices for safe healthcare delivery in all settings—recommendations of the Healthcare Infection Control Practices Advisory Committee. https://www.cdc.gov/hicpac/recommendations/core-practices.html. Accessed March 15, 2017.
2. Centers for Disease Control and Prevention (CDC). Guidelines for the prevention of intravascular catheter-related infections. *Clin Infect Dis.* 2011;52(9):e162–e193.
3. McLean HS, Carriker C, Bordley WC. Good to great: quality-improvement initiative increases and sustains pediatric health care worker hand hygiene compliance. *Hosp Pediatr.* 2017;7(4):189–196.
4. Larson EL, Cimiotti J, Haas J, et al. Effect of antiseptic handwashing vs alcohol sanitizer on health care-associated

infections in neonatal intensive care units. *Arch Pediatr Adolesc Med.* 2005;159(4):377–383.

5. Sharma VS, Dutta S, Taneja N, et al. Comparing hand hygiene measures in a neonatal ICU: a randomized crossover trial. *Indian Pediatr.* 2013;50(10):917–921.

6. Hsieh S, Sapkota A, Wood R, et al. Neonatal ethanol exposure from ethanol-based hand sanitisers in isolettes. *Arch Dis Child Fetal Neonatal Ed.* 2018;103(1):F55–F58.

7. Morel AS, Wu F, Dell-Latta P, et al. Nosocomial transmission of methicillin-resistant Staphylococcus aureus from a mother to her preterm quadruplet infants. *Am J Infect Control.* 2002;30:170–173.

8. Phalen RN, Le T, Wong WK. Changes in chemical permeation of disposable latex, nitrile, and vinyl gloves exposed to simulated movement. *J Occup Environ Hyg.* 2014;11(11):716–721.

9. McDonnell G, Russell AD. Antiseptics and disinfectants: activity, action, and resistance. *Clin Microbiol Rev.* 1999;12(1):147–179.

10. Ponnusamy V, Venkatesh V, Clarke P. Skin antisepsis in the neonate: What should we use? *Curr Opin Infect Dis.* 2014;27(3):244–250.

11. Sathiyamurthy S, Banerjee J, Godambe SV. Antiseptic use in the neonatal intensive care unit—a dilemma in clinical practice: an evidence based review. *World J Clin Pediatr.* 2016;5(2):159–171.

12. U.S. Food & Drug Administration. FDA In Brief: FDA issues final rule on safety and effectiveness for certain active ingredients in over-the-counter health care antiseptic hand washes and rubs in the medical setting. Released December 19, 2017. https://www.fda.gov/newsevents/newsroom/fdainbrief/ucm589474.htm

13. Mimoz O, Lucet JC, Kerforne T, et al. Skin antisepsis with chlorhexidine-alcohol versus povidone iodine-alcohol, with and without skin scrubbing, for prevention of intravascular-catheter-related infection (CLEAN): an open-label, multicentre, randomised, controlled, two-by-two factorial trial. *Lancet.* 2015;386(10008):2069–2077.

14. Tanner J, Norrie P, Melen K. Preoperative hair removal to reduce surgical site infection. *Cochrane Database Syst Rev.* 2011;(11):CD004122.

15. Paula H, Hübner NO, Assadian O, et al. Effect of hand lotion on the effectiveness of hygienic hand antisepsis: implications for practicing hand hygiene. *Am J Infect Control.* 2017;45(8):835–838.

16. Aitken J, Williams FL. A systematic review of thyroid dysfunction in preterm neonates exposed to topical iodine. *Arch Dis Child Fetal Neonatal Ed.* 2014;99(1):F21–F28.

17. Kieran EA, O'Sullivan A, Miletin J, et al. 2% chlorhexidine-70% isopropyl alcohol versus 10% povidone-iodine for insertion site cleaning before central line insertion in preterm infants: a randomised trial. *Arch Dis Child Fetal Neonatal Ed.* 2018;103(2):F101–F106.

18. Parravicini E, Fontana C, Paterlini GL, et al. Iodine, thyroid function, and very low birth weight infants. *Pediatrics.* 1996;98(4 Pt 1):730–734.

19. Linder N, Prince S, Barzilai A, et al. Disinfection with 10% povidone-iodine versus 0.5% chlorhexidine gluconate in 70% isopropanol in the neonatal intensive care unit. *Acta Paediatr.* 2004;93(2):205–210.

20. Mimoz O, Karim A, Mercat A, et al. Chlorhexidine compared with povidone-iodine as skin preparation before blood culture. A randomized, controlled trial. *Ann Intern Med.* 1999;131(11):834–837.

21. Neri I, Ravaioli GM, Faldella G, et al. Chlorhexidine-induced chemical burns in very low birth weight infants. *J Pediatr.* 2017;191:262–265.e2.

22. Garland JS, Alex CP, Uhing MR, et al. Pilot trial to compare tolerance of chlorhexidine gluconate to povidone-iodine antisepsis for central venous catheter placement in neonates. *J Perinatol.* 2009;29(12):808–813.

23. Ng AL, Jackson C, Kazmierski M. Evaluation of antiseptic use in pediatric surgical units in the United Kingdom—Where is the evidence base?. *Eur J Pediatr Surg.* 2016;26(4):309–315.

24. Wishart MM, Riley TV. Infection with Pseudomonas maltophilia hospital outbreak due to contaminated disinfectant. *Med J Aust.* 1976;2(19):710–712.

25. Charles D, Heal CF, Delpachitra M, et al. Alcoholic versus aqueous chlorhexidine for skin antisepsis: The AVALANCHE trial. *CMAJ.* 2017;189(31):E1008–E1016.

26. Lashkari HP, Chow P, Godambe S. Aqueous 2% chlorhexidine induced chemical burns in an extremely premature infant. *Arch Dis Child Fetal Neonatal Ed.* 2012;97(1):F64.

27. Janssen LMA, Tostmann A, Hopman J, et al. 0.2% chlorhexidine acetate as skin disinfectant prevents skin lesions in extremely preterm infants: a preliminary report. *Arch Dis Child Fetal Neonatal Ed.* 2018;103(2):F97–F100.

28. Reynolds PR, Banerjee S, Meek JH. Alcohol burns in extremely low birthweight infants: still occurring. *Arch Dis Child Fetal Neonatal Ed.* 2005;90(1):F10.

29. Harpin V, Rutter N. Percutaneous alcohol absorption and skin necrosis in a preterm infant. *Arch Dis Child.* 1982;57(6):477–479.

30. Caballero ML, Quirce S. Identification and practical management of latex allergy in occupational settings. *Expert Rev Clin Immunol.* 2015;11(9):977–992.

31. Blumchen K, Bayer P, Buck D, et al. Effects of latex avoidance on latex sensitization, atopy and allergic diseases in patients with spina bifida. *Allergy.* 2010;65(12):1585–1593.

Analgesia and Sedation in the Newborn

Victoria Tutag-Lehr, Mirjana Lulic-Botica, Johanna M. Calo,
Gloria B. Valencia, and Jacob V. Aranda

A. Introduction

The human imperative to provide comfort and prevent pain in newborn babies is shared by many neonatal health caregivers. The American Academy of Pediatrics (AAP) Prevention and Management of Pain and Stress in the Neonate updated policy statement also emphasizes the need for effective prevention and treatment of pain in infants (1). Neurodevelopmental adverse effects of repetitive pain are greatest in premature infants, a complex population with high exposure to procedures and medications (2,3), with the most immature infants receiving the highest number of painful events (1). The assessment and management of pain in the newborn has greatly advanced during the past three decades (4,5). The need for procedural analgesia for neonates is well established (1–8). Consistency on the use of pain and sedation continues to vary among clinicians and practice site (9–11). Not all institutions have instituted preventative protocols with nonpharmacologic and pharmacologic therapies for painful procedures in newborns (10,11). A paucity of pharmacokinetic (PK) and pharmacodynamic (PD) data remains for many analgesics and sedatives secondary to the varying infant gestational ages and weights (12). Comorbid conditions, complex drug regimens, ethical issues, and genetic polymorphisms (13–17) complicate studies in critically ill neonates. For example, newborns and children who are CYP2D6 ultra metabolizers have experienced respiratory depression from therapeutic doses of codeine and tramadol (18,19). Due to the increased incidence of these cases, codeine and tramadol have an age restriction on many formularies (19). Neonatal pain management requires careful selection and dosing of medications, appropriate assessment and monitoring, and ability to promptly recognize and manage adverse effects (20–23). Improvements in neonatal pain management are driven by advances in developmental neurobiology, developmental PK and PD of analgesics, and the development of age-appropriate tools for pain assessment and by best evidence in clinical practice for this vulnerable population (14,22,23).

This chapter offers general guidelines for analgesia and sedation in newborn infants undergoing procedures that are frequently performed in the neonatal intensive care unit (1,7–9). Selection of the optimal sedative for the management of stress in ventilated infants remains less clear and is beyond the scope of this chapter (24–27).

B. Definitions

1. **Analgesia:** A condition in which nociceptive stimuli are perceived, but not interpreted as pain; usually accompanied by sedation without loss of consciousness (24).
2. **Conscious sedation:** A medically controlled state of depressed consciousness that allows protective reflexes to be maintained, retains the ability to maintain a patent airway independently and continuously, and permits appropriate responses by the patient (1).
3. **Deep sedation:** A medically controlled state of depressed consciousness or unconsciousness from which the patient is not easily aroused. It may be accompanied by a partial or complete loss of protective reflexes and includes the inability to maintain a patent airway independently and respond purposefully to stimulation (1).
4. **Tolerance:** The ability to resist the action of a drug or the requirement for increasing doses of a drug, with time, to achieve a desired effect (28,29).
5. **Withdrawal:** The development of a substance-specific syndrome that follows the cessation of, or reduction in, intake of a psychoactive substance previously used or administered regularly (24).

6. **Neonatal abstinence syndrome:** Onset of withdrawal symptoms in neonates upon cessation of an agent associated with physical dependence (29,30).

C. General Indications

1. Any condition or procedure known to be painful (see E) (1,12,17)
2. Physiologic indications consistent with perception of pain (9,21–23)
    a. Tachycardia
    b. Tachypnea
    c. Elevated blood pressure (with secondary increase in intracranial pressure)
    d. Decreased arterial oxygen saturation
    e. Hyperglycemia secondary to hormonal and metabolic stress responses
    f. Increased skin blood flow measured by laser Doppler in response to acute pain (6)
3. Behavioral indications consistent with perception of pain (9,21–23)
    a. Simple motor responses (i.e., withdrawal of an extremity from a noxious stimulus)
    b. Facial expressions (i.e., grimace)
    c. Altered cry (primary method of communicating painful stimuli in infancy)
    d. Agitation

D. Specific Indications

1. Analgesia
   In general, the potency of analgesic treatment selected should be related directly to the anticipated or assessed level of pain (1,8).
    a. Mild pain
        (1) Nonpharmacologic approaches (see H)
        (2) Local and/or topical anesthesia
        (3) Nonopioid analgesics (e.g., acetaminophen) (31,32)
    b. Moderate and severe pain
        (1) IV opioid analgesics (see E)
        (2) Local and/or topical anesthesia (7)
        (3) Benzodiazepines (see E)
        (4) γ-Aminobutyric acid analog—gabapentin (see E)
2. Sedation
   Sedatives when administered in conjunction with analgesics enhance the anticipated benefits. Because of the escalated risks associated with deep sedation, conscious sedation should be the usual clinical endpoint.
    a. Benzodiazepines (see E)
    b. Chloral hydrate (see E)
    c. Nonpharmacologic approaches (see H)

E. Precautions

1. The clinical assessment of pain in the newborn is imprecise. The Neonatal Pain Agitation and Sedation Scale (N-PASS) assesses ongoing pain, agitation, and sedation levels in term and premature neonates (22). Neonatal pain scales vary in content, utility, reliability, and ease of use and include physiologic, behavioral, and contextual parameters (see Appendix B.1) (21–23).
2. Physiologic and behavioral indicators of pain are nonspecific and are associated with many other factors. Ideally, a neonatal pain scale would be fast and easy to use; have reliability and validity for term, preterm, ventilated, and sedated neonates; be able to discriminate between other states (e.g., hunger); and account for confounding factors (e.g., medications, sepsis, cardiac disease) that may reduce the specificity of behavioral and physiologic responses. In reality, however, these scales show varying degrees of sensitivity and specificity (which markedly effects interpretation), a wide interrater variability of pain scores that can reduce the sensitivity, and behavioral responses of the preterm or neurologically impaired neonate (which can reduce the specificity of the pain assessment) (22,23).
3. Intubated neonates receiving muscle relaxants may have altered physiologic indicators and completely ablated behavioral indicators.
4. A high index of suspicion is required to identify newborn infants in pain (1,8,10,21).
5. When medicating patients, be aware that:
    a. There are numerous potential complications associated with analgesic and sedative agents (Appendix B.2) (25–33).
    b. Large inter- and intraindividual variations in response have been documented (34,35).
    c. Newborns have immature and deficient drug biotransformation and elimination capabilities, which impact on drug response and adverse effects (20,34–36). Data have been steadily accumulating on the PK/PD of sedatives and analgesics in the newborn (14–16,37–42). Neonates, especially premature neonates, have immature hepatic microsomal enzyme systems, which mature over 3 to 6 months (38–40). Many drugs, including morphine, are metabolized by these systems; therefore, these neonates will have significant increases in half-life (>50%) compared with adults and older children for these agents (38,39). The glomerular filtration rate (GFR) is decreased during the first week of life, affecting the elimination of active metabolites of opioids (e.g., morphine) (40,41). Preterm infants will primarily produce the M3G metabolite of morphine, which has antianalgesic properties and a longer half-life compared with morphine (40,41). Neonates have a large percentage

of body mass as water and a decreased plasma concentration of albumin and α-glycoprotein (14–16). These variables influence the PK/PD of sedatives, analgesics, and concomitant medications, which may interact with these agents (34,35).

    d. Medications must always be titrated slowly (1,8, 9,24).

    e. Coadministration of opioids, benzodiazepines, and other sedatives may result in greatly exaggerated respiratory depressant effects, including apnea (34). This combination may require a decrease in dosage of each medication.

    f. Drug-induced neurodevelopmental apoptosis in neonatal and pregnant animals is associated with exposure to sedatives, general anesthetics, ketamine, propofol, and opioid analgesics (27,42–44). Drug exposures longer than 3 hours were associated with widespread loss of neuronal cells and long-term negative effects on the animals' behavior or learning (43,44). An FDA warning of April 2017 advised delaying elective surgery in children younger than 3 years of age and pregnant women where medically appropriate (44). Labeling is now included with anesthetic and sedation products warning that exposure to these agents for lengthy periods of time or over multiple surgeries or procedures may negatively affect brain development in children younger than 3 years. Dexmedetomidine, an α-agonist sedative and analgesic, has neuroprotective properties, and is an alternative to neurotoxic agents (45).

6. Resuscitation equipment and medications should be immediately available. Be prepared to support ventilation and perform tracheal intubation if needed; respiratory depression is a common side effect of several analgesic and sedative agents (33,34).

7. Neonatal abstinence syndrome (NAS)

    a. Newborn infants who have developed tolerance to a sedative or analgesic agent, by either direct or in utero exposure, may exhibit symptoms of NAS upon abrupt cessation of the drug or administration of the appropriate reversal agent (e.g., naloxone or flumazenil) (28–30,46–49). For example, naloxone administered to opioid-dependent neonates may precipitate acute, severe withdrawal symptoms (29,30).

    b. The appropriate use of opioids allows the newborn to respond to clinical interventions with minimal adverse effects. Opioid-sparing agents include regional anesthesia, acetaminophen (31,32), and gabapentin (50). Currently, there are no data for use of NSAID analgesia in newborns (51). Combining opioids with either an NMDA-receptor antagonist or α₂-adrenergic agonist agent may decrease the incidence of opioid tolerance and withdrawal (47).

    c. Newborns with a history of in utero opioid exposure may have increased analgesic requirements (30). Due to the worldwide opioid epidemic, the number of infants with NAS has quadrupled over the past decade (48). More women continue to take opioids, benzodiazepines, amphetamines, SSRI antidepressants, inhalants, and other drugs throughout pregnancy. Polysubstance withdrawal symptoms in the newborn can be severe and difficult to manage (48,49). Severe neonatal agitation associated with polysubstance withdrawal may require management with adjunctive agents such as gabapentin (50). Gabapentin abuse is becoming prevalent throughout the United States among heroin users (48,49). In utero gabapentin exposure can cause neonatal irritability and agitation. Appendix B.3 contains NAS scoring tools and pharmacologic management.

    d. Chronic analgesic therapy with agents known to induce tolerance, such as opioids, requires gradual weaning, with close monitoring for evidence of withdrawal symptoms. Administration of semisynthetic opioids, such as fentanyl, produces tolerance more rapidly in infants and young children compared with the natural opioids (28). Tolerance may be produced within 3 to 5 days with fentanyl, compared with 1 to 2 weeks for morphine (28,33,34). In addition, it appears that tolerance will develop more rapidly if the opioid infusion is continuous rather than intermittent (46). Fentanyl is frequently used in neonates undergoing very painful procedures because of its rapid onset of analgesia, hemodynamic stability, and ability to prevent pain-induced increase in pulmonary vascular resistance (33,34,46).

    e. Changing opioids and cross-tolerance: The term cross-tolerance is used when repeated doses of a drug within a class cause tolerance not only to the administered drug, but also to drugs in the same structural class (28). Cross-tolerance between opioids in neonates is often incomplete; therefore, extreme caution must be used when changing from one opioid to another (28,33). When converting from one opioid to another, starting at half the conversion dose and titrating upward based on clinical effect is advised (28,33). Incomplete cross-tolerance may be related to conformational changes in opioid receptors (28).

8. When using analgesics for a painful procedure:

    a. Consider both the duration and the intensity of anticipated pain when selecting medications and methods. For example, short procedures with mild to moderate discomfort, such as lumbar puncture, may be best managed with topical and local anesthetics (1,7–9).

    b. Minimize the number of painful episodes. Coordinating and clustering the performance of multiple procedures at the same time may avoid the need for repeated administration of analgesics.

c. Ensure that oxygen, suction, airway, resuscitation equipment, and reversal agents are readily available.

d. Follow nothing-by-mouth guidelines for surgery.

e. Have a nurse or other professional not involved in the procedure constantly monitor respirations, pulse oximetry, heart rate, and level of consciousness.

9. Chloral hydrate is no longer regarded as a first-line, safe sedative for infants or young children (1,52). This agent must be used with caution in neonates (particularly premature neonates) secondary to the risk of hyperbilirubinemia, narrow therapeutic index, and accumulation of toxic metabolites (52). For these reasons, current recommendations are to use chloral hydrate in a single dose only if other agents are not appropriate or available. Chloral hydrate is no longer commercially available in the United States and in many other countries. Some hospital pharmacies compound chloral hydrate solutions from crystals (53).

F. Advantages and Disadvantages of Commonly Used Agents in the Pediatric Patient

Commonly used sedatives and analgesics for the pediatric patient are listed in Appendix B.4.

G. Complications

See Appendix B.4.

H. Nonpharmacologic Approaches

1. Swaddling and skin-to-skin contact during heel-stick procedures have been shown to reduce behavioral pain responses (1,9).

2. Breastfeeding is an effective analgesic for neonates undergoing acute painful procedures such as heel lance for routine metabolic screening (54). Breastfeeding infants have shown significantly reduced duration of crying during and after immunization.

3. Nonnutritive sucking has been demonstrated to significantly reduce crying in response to painful stimuli (1,9).

4. Sensorineural stimulation (SS), a method of gently stimulating the tactile, gustatory, auditory, and visual system simultaneously, has shown effectiveness at decreasing pain during minor procedures such as a heel lance. SS is achieved by looking at and gently talking to the infant, while stroking or massaging the face or back (1).

5. Sucrose (1,9,55)
   a. Infants who drank 2 mL of a 12% sucrose solution prior to blood collection via heel stick cried 50% less compared with control infants during the same

procedure. Infants who received sucrose on a pacifier prior to and during circumcision cried significantly less than the control group.

b. Two mL of 12% to 50% sucrose administered orally 2 minutes prior to the procedure is an effective neonatal analgesic with few adverse effects. However, there is one report of lower neurodevelopmental scores in preterm infants ($n = 103$; <31 weeks' gestational age) associated with repeated doses of sucrose for analgesia, although a later analysis showed that infants who received 10 or fewer doses of 24% sucrose over a 24-hour period were less at risk for poorer neurodevelopmental scores (56). Data are lacking on the neurodevelopmental outcomes of premature infants treated with repeated doses of sucrose.

c. The safe maximum dose of sucrose is unknown (55). Studies have given three doses: prior, during, and after the procedure (55,56). Document sucrose doses on the newborn's medication administration record as with any other analgesic.

d. The analgesic effect of 24% sucrose may be less effective after 46 weeks' postconceptual age (55). Higher sucrose concentrations such as 50%, 75% may be required for older infants. The analgesic efficacy of oral sucrose in infants exposed to opioids in utero is controversial (57). Oral sucrose exhibited an analgesic effect during heel lance in infants exposed in utero to methadone that was comparable to control infants (57).

I. Contraindications

1. There are no absolute contraindications to using analgesia and/or sedation when deemed clinically appropriate.

2. Be aware of the potential side effects associated with the specific agents selected and take proper precautions.

References

1. AAP Committee on Fetus and Newborn and Section on Anesthesiology and Pain Medicine. Prevention and management of procedural pain in the neonate: An update. *Pediatrics.* 2016;137(2):e20154271.
2. Ranger M, Chau CMY, Garg A, et al. Neonatal pain-related stress predicts cortical thickness at age 7 years in children born very preterm. *PLoS ONE.* 2013;8(10):e76702.
3. Johnston C, Barrington KJ, Taddio A, et al. Pain in Canadian NICUs: Have we improved over the past 12 years? *Clin J Pain.* 2011;27(3):225–232.
4. Anand KJS, Hickey PR. Pain and its effects in the human neonate and fetus. *N Engl J Med.* 1987;317:1321–1329.
5. Simons SH, van Dijk M, Anand KS, et al. Do we still hurt newborn babies? A prospective study of procedural pain and analgesia in neonates. *Arch Pediatr Adolesc Med.* 2003;157:1058–1064.

6. Tutag Lehr V, Cortez J, Grever W, et al. Randomized placebo controlled trial of sucrose analgesia on neonatal skin blood flow and pain response during heel lance. *Clin J Pain.* 2015;31(5):451–458.

7. Tutag Lehr V, Taddio A. Practical approach to topical anesthetics in the neonate. *Semin Perinatol.* 2007;31:323.

8. Anand KJ, Johnston CC, Oberlander TF, et al. Analgesia and local anesthesia during invasive procedures in the neonate. *Clin Ther.* 2005;27:844–876.

9. Spence K, Henderson-Smart D, New K, et al. Evidenced-based clinical practice guideline for management of newborn pain. *J Paediatr Child Health.* 2010;46(4):184–192.

10. Wallace H, Jones T. Managing procedural pain on the neonatal unit: Do inconsistencies still exist in practice? *J Neonatal Nursing.* 2017;23(3):119–126.

11. Harrison D, Sampson M, Reszel J, et al. Too many crying babies: A systematic review of pain management practices during immunizations on YouTube. *BMC Pediatr.* 2014;14:134.

12. Zimmerman KO, Smith PB, Benjamin DK, et al. Sedation, analgesia, and paralysis during mechanical ventilation of premature infants. *J Pediatr.* 2017;180:99–104.

13. Warrier I, Du W, Natarajan G, et al. Patterns of drug utilization in a neonatal intensive care unit. *J Clin Pharmacol.* 2006;46:449–455.

14. van den Anker JN, Schwab M, Kearns GL. Developmental pharmacokinetics. *Handbook Exp Pharmacol.* 2011;205:51–75.

15. Matic M, Norman E, Rane A, et al. Effect of UGT2B7 −900G>A (−842G>A; rs7438135) on morphine glucuronidation in preterm newborns: Results from a pilot cohort. *Pharmacogenomics.* 2014;15(12):1589–1597.

16. Ku LC, Smith PB. Dosing in neonates: Special considerations in physiology and trial design. *Pediatr Res.* 2015;77:2–9.

17. Janvier A, Lantos J; POST Investigators. Ethics and etiquette in neonatal intensive care. *JAMA Pediatr.* 2014;168(9):857–858.

18. Madadi P, Ross CJ, Hayden MR, et al. Pharmacogenetics of neonatal opioid toxicity following maternal use of codeine during breastfeeding: A case-control study. *Clin Pharmacol Ther.* 2009;85(1):31–35.

19. Throckmorton D. FDA media briefing on new warnings about the use of codeine and tramadol in certain children and nursing mothers. *Center for Drug Evaluation and Research.* April 20, 2017. https://www.fda.gov/NewsEvents/Newsroom/PressAnnouncements/ucm553285.htm. Accessed March 3, 2019.

20. Du W, Lehr VT, Lieh-Lai M, et al. An algorithm to detect adverse drug reactions in the neonatal intensive care unit. *J Clin Pharmacol.* 2013;53(1):87–95.

21. Walker SM. Neonatal pain. *Paediatr Anaesth.* 2014;24(1):39–48.

22. Hummel P, Puchalski M, Creech SD, et al. Clinical reliability and validity of the N-PASS: Neonatal pain, agitation and sedation scale with prolonged pain. *J Perinatol.* 2008;28:55–60.

23. Stevens B, Johnston C, Taddio A, et al. The premature infant pain profile: Evaluation 13 years after development. *Clin J Pain.* 2010;26:813–830.

24. Aranda JV, Carlo W, Hummel P, et al. Analgesia and sedation during mechanical ventilation in neonates. *Clin Ther.* 2005;27:877–899.

25. Anand KJ, Barton BA, McIntosh N, et al. Analgesia and sedation in preterm neonates who require ventilatory support: Results of the NOPAIN trial. Neonatal Outcome and prolonged analgesia in neonates. *Arch Pediatr Adolesc Med.* 1999;153:331–338.

26. McPherson C, Grunau RE. Neonatal pain control and neurologic effects of sedatives in preterm infants. *Clin Perinatol.* 2014;41(1):209–227.

27. Lei X, Guo Q, Zhang J. Mechanistic insights into neurotoxicity induced by anesthetics in the developing brain. *Int J Mol Sci.* 2012;13:6772–6799.

28. Suresh S, Anand KJS. Opioid tolerance in neonates: A state of the art review. *Paediatr Anaesth.* 2001;11:511–521.

29. Franck L, Vilardi J. Assessment and management of opioid withdrawal in ill neonates. *Neonatal Netw.* 1995;14:39–48.

30. Anand KJ, Campbell-Yeo M. Consequences of prenatal opioid use for newborns. *Acta Paediatr.* 2015;104(11):1066–1069.

31. Ohlsson A, Shah PS. Paracetamol (acetaminophen) for prevention or treatment of pain in newborns. *Cochrane Database Syst Rev.* 2016;10:CD011219.

32. Ceelie I, de Wildt SN, van Dijk M, et al. Effect of intravenous paracetamol on postoperative morphine requirements in neonates and infants undergoing major non-cardiac surgery: A randomized controlled trial. *JAMA.* 2013;309(2):149–154.

33. Witt N, Coynor S, Edwards C, et al. A guide to pain assessment and management in the neonate. *Curr Emerg Hosp Med Rep.* 2016;4:1–10.

34. Cote CJ, Karl HW, Notterman DA, et al. Adverse sedation events in pediatrics: Analysis of medications used for sedation. *Pediatrics.* 2000;106:633–644.

35. Morris FH Jr, Abramowitz PW, Nelson PS, et al. Risk of adverse drug events in neonates treated with opioids and the effect of a bar-code-assisted medication administration system. *Am J Health Syst Pharm.* 2011;68:57–62.

36. Aguado-Lorenzo V, Weeks K, Tunstall P, et al. Accuracy of the concentration of morphine infusions prepared for patients in a neonatal intensive care unit. *Arch Dis Child.* 2013;98:975–979.

37. Krekels EH, Tibboel D, de Wildt SN, et al. Evidence-based morphine dosing for postoperative neonates and infants. *Clin Pharmacokinet.* 2014;53:553–563.

38. Hines RN. Developmental expression of drug metabolizing enzymes: Impact on disposition in neonates and young children. *Int J Pharm.* 2013;452:3–7.

39. Barrett DA, Barker DP, Rutter N, et al. Morphine, morphine-6-glucuronide, morphine-3-glucuronide pharmacokinetics in new born infants receiving diamorphine infusions. *Br J Clin Pharmacol.* 1996;41:531–537.

40. Bhat R, Abu-Harb M, Chari G, et al. Morphine metabolism in acutely ill preterm newborn infants. *J Pediatr.* 1992;120:795–799.

41. Vieux R, Hascoet JM, Merdariu D, et al. Glomerular filtration rate reference values in very preterm infants. *Pediatrics.* 2010;125:e1186–e1192.

42. Filan PM, Hunt RW, Anderson PJ, et al. Neurologic outcomes in very preterm infants undergoing surgery. *J Pediatr.* 2012;160:409–414.

43. Xiong M, Zhang L, Li J, et al. Propofol-induced neurotoxicity in the fetal animal brain and developments in modifying these effects–an updated review of propofol fetal exposure in laboratory animal studies. *Brain Sciences.* 2016;6(2):11. doi:0.3390/brainsci6020011

44. U.S. Food & Drug Administration (FDA). FDA drug safety communication: FDA review results in new warnings about using general anesthetics and sedation drugs in young children

and pregnant women. April 27, 2017. https://www.fda.gov/Drugs/DrugSafety/ucm554634.htm. Accessed March 3, 2019.

45. Li J, Xiong M, Nadavaluru PR, et al. Dexmedetomidine attenuates neurotoxicity induced by prenatal propofol exposure. *J Neurosurg Anesthesiol.* 2016;28:51–64.

46. Frank LS, Vilardi J, Durand D, et al. Opioid withdrawal in neonates after continuous infusions of morphine or fentanyl during extracorporeal membrane oxygenation. *Am J Crit Care.* 1998;7:364–369.

47. Yaster M. Multi modal analgesia in children. *Eur J Anaesthesiol.* 2010;27:851–857.

48. Hall ES, Wexelblatt SL, Crowley M, et al. A multicenter cohort study of treatments and hospital outcomes in neonatal abstinence syndrome. *Pediatrics.* 2014;134(2):e527–e534.

49. Johnson MR, Nash DR, Laird MF, et al. Development and implementation of a pharmacist-managed, neonatal and pediatric, opioid-weaning protocol. *J Pediatr Pharmacol Ther.* 2014;19(3):165–173.

50. Sacha GL, Foreman MG, Kyllonen K, et al. The use of gabapentin for pain and agitation in neonates and infants in a neonatal ICU. *J Pediatr Pharmacol Ther.* 2017;22(3):207–211.

51. Aranda JV, Salomone F, Valencia GB, et al. Non-steroidal anti-inflammatory drugs in newborns and infants. *Pediatr Clin North Am.* 2017;64:1327–1340.

52. American Society of Health-System Pharmacists. Chloral hydrate oral solution and capsules. *Drugs No Longer Available Bulletin.* November 5, 2012.

53. Hill GD, Walbergh DB, Frommelt PC. Efficacy of reconstituted oral chloral hydrate from crystals for echocardiography sedation. *J Am Soc Echocardiogr.* 2016;29(4):337–340.

54. Shah PS, Herbozo C, Aliwalas LL, et al. Breastfeeding or breast milk for procedural pain in neonates. *Cochrane Database Syst Rev.* 2012;12:CD004950.

55. Stevens B, Yamada J, Ohlsson A, et al. Sucrose for analgesia in newborn infants undergoing painful procedures. *Cochrane Database Syst Rev.* 2016;(7):CD001069.

56. Johnston CC, Filion F, Snider L, et al. How much sucrose is too much sucrose? *Pediatrics.* 2007;119:226.

57. Marceau JR, Murray H, Nanan RK. Efficacy of oral sucrose in infants of methadone maintained mothers. *Neonatology.* 2010;97(1):67–70.

Physiologic Monitoring

CHAPTER

8

Temperature Monitoring

Neha Kumbhat and Melissa Scala

Infants, especially premature infants, are born with an insufficient ability to generate heat and have immature compensatory systems to prevent heat loss to the environment. A thermoneutral environment is a narrow range of environmental temperature in which the infant maintains a normal body temperature without increasing the metabolic rate and hence oxygen consumption. Maintaining a thermoneutral environment allows infants' caloric consumption to be utilized for growth rather than maintaining temperature (1). Immediately after birth an infant's temperature falls by 2° to 3°C; maintaining normothermia after delivery may reduce rates of mortality and morbidity, especially in premature infants (2).

Accurate temperature measurements are important to:

1. Guide best care to maintain a thermoneutral environment for the infant.
2. Alert caregivers to changes in infant clinical status. Temperature dysregulation may be a sign of sepsis.

Temperature monitoring may be done intermittently or continuously; both are commonly used in the neonatal intensive care unit (NICU). The site of measurement may be core (rectum, esophagus, or tympanic) or surface (skin, axilla). The axillary route is most common and preferred, especially for preterm neonates. The various methods are discussed further in this chapter.

INTERMITTENT TEMPERATURE MONITORING

A. Equipment

1. **Mercury in glass thermometer**
   a. The mercury glass thermometer remains the historical standard for noninvasive clinical temperature measurements.
   b. It has been the benchmark against which the newer methods of detecting temperature have been tested.

c. However, mercury in all of its forms is toxic and in an effort to decrease the amount of mercury in the waste stream, the AAP in 2001 recommended phasing out mercury-containing thermometers (3).
   d. Mercury thermometers should be avoided.
2. **Electronic digital thermometer (Fig. 8.1)**

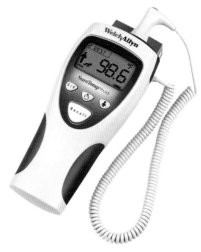

FIGURE 8.1 Electronic thermometers: Probe thermometer. (Courtesy of Welch Allyn, New York, USA.)

   a. Electronic digital thermometers are widely used.
   b. The electronic digital thermometer is designed to determine infant temperature by measuring the heat radiating from an adjacent blood vessel.
   c. The probe is made of a thermistor or thermocouple.
   d. Temperature is sensed by the probe, processed electronically, and displayed digitally. An audible signal marks the end of the determination time period. The determination time period is usually less than 45 seconds with a resolution of 0.1°C.
   e. Many of these thermometers are used with a probe cover.

B. Locations

1. Electronic thermometers are used in two locations—axillary and rectal.
2. The mean difference between axillary and rectal temperature varies widely and may differ by up to 1.2°C. Axillary temperatures are found to be less accurate estimates of core temperature and are generally lower than rectal temperatures.
3. Preterm infants have a smaller mean difference in temperature between axillary and rectal measurements (4,5).

C. Techniques

Electronic thermometers are used with a disposable sensor head cover, if included with the thermometer, and particularly if thermometers will be used for multiple patients or in multiple locations.

1. **Rectal temperatures:** Depth of insertion is important to obtain core temperature without trauma to the rectum.
   a. In order to measure the core temperature, insert the probe into the rectum gently up to 2 to 2.5 cm.
   b. Many thermometers in common usage report accurate temperature measurement with insertion of 1 cm in infants (www.welchallyn.com).
   c. If using a disposable thermometer with a metal tip, insert thermometer until metal tip is just inside the rectum.
2. **Axillary temperatures:** For noninvasive approximation of the core temperature, place the probe in the axilla. **Figure 8.2** shows correct method to take an axillary temperature.

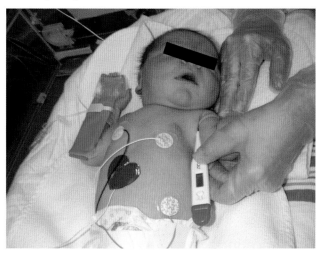

FIGURE 8.2 Axillary temperature being taken with an electronic probe thermometer. The probe is held perpendicular to the patient, and the arm is held securely against the side of the chest.

   a. Hold the infant's arm adjacent to his or her side so that the entire probe tip is in the cup of the axilla.

   b. Temperatures obtained via this method will correlate within a mean of 0.27°C (range: −0.13° to +0.67°C) (4).
   c. Although the correlation of axillary temperature with rectal temperature is imperfect, axillary is the most frequent location for temperature monitoring in the NICU for ease of use and reduced infant discomfort and complication (4).

D. Limitations and Complications

1. Inaccurate reading: Incorrect probe placement may reduce measurement reliability.
2. Infant discomfort may occur with measurement in both rectal and axillary locations (6–8).
3. Rare cases of rectal perforation resulting in pneumoperitoneum and peritonitis have been reported in the literature (9,10).

ADDITIONAL INTERMITTENT TEMPERATURE MONITORING

A. Equipment

1. **Infrared electronic thermometer**
   a. Infrared sensors detect energy radiating from the site of measurement (i.e., tympanic membrane for aural thermometers or skin site over the temporal artery).
   b. This mode of temperature measurement is less painful to infants than digital methods in rectal or axillary locations (6).

B. Locations

1. **Aural:** Tympanic membrane thermometers measure temperature by measuring the heat radiating from the tympanic membrane, using infrared radiation (IR).
   a. For an accurate measurement, the device needs to have a direct and consistent view of the tympanic membrane.
   b. Two anatomic factors in neonates that may affect tympanic thermometer accuracy include (1) the shape of the external auditory canal and (2) the angle between the tympanic membrane and the external auditory canal. This issue can be addressed by the concurrent use of an otoscope with the tympanic clinical thermometer (11).
   c. Due to mechanical difficulties, tympanic membrane thermometers are less frequently used in the NICU.

2. **Temporal artery:** Temporal artery thermometers measure the temperature of the skin over the temporal artery.
   a. Similar correlation with axillary temperatures is found when compared to rectal temperatures for infants cared for in open cribs.
   b. Readings may be affected by care in an incubator.
   c. Accuracy may increase with postmenstrual age (12).
   d. Readings are affected by care in an incubator leading to inaccurate results. They are less commonly used.

C. Technique

1. **Aural**
   a. After applying the disposable cover to the sensor head, gently insert the tapered end into the ear canal.
   b. Concurrent use of an otoscope might afford better visualization of the tympanic membrane. While holding the unit steady, depress the trigger.
   c. Remove from the ear canal and read the temperature. Temperature is detected in less than 2 seconds.
2. **Temporal artery**
   a. Check to see that the probe is clean.
   b. Attach a probe cover.
   c. Place the probe in the center of the forehead and depress the button.
   d. While holding the button depressed and the probe against the skin, swipe laterally across the forehead.
   e. Quickly place the probe against the skin behind the ear on the upper neck.
   f. Release the button with the probe still in contact with the skin on the neck.
   g. Lift device and read the digitally displayed temperature.

D. Limitations and Complications

1. Inaccurate readings.
2. **Aural:** Technically difficult in newborns. Inconsistent correlation with rectal or axillary measurements (12,13).
3. **Temporal artery:** Mixed results when accuracy compared to digital axillary thermometers (14,15).
4. Reduced accuracy with care in incubator, lower gestational age, and sweating patient (12).

CONTINUOUS TEMPERATURE MONITORING

A. Background

1. An intermittent measurement of temperature tells us how well the baby is maintaining that temperature,

without any information about the energy being used to achieve that thermal balance. The baby could be overcoming the effects of thermal stress by using more energy (**Fig. 8.3**).

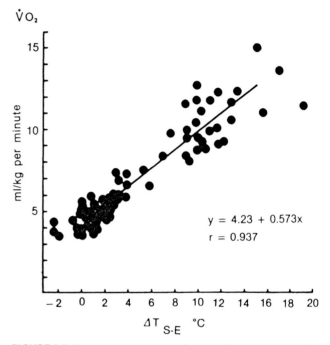

FIGURE 8.3 Oxygen consumption as a function of temperature gradient between skin and environment. (From Adamsons K Jr, Gandy GM, James LS. The influence of thermal factors upon oxygen consumption of the newborn human infant. *J Pediatr.* 1965;66(3):495–508. Copyright © 1965 Elsevier. With permission.)

2. A preterm infant normally has a central–peripheral temperature difference of 0.5° to 1°C. An increase in this difference above 2°C is indicative of cold stress and occurs prior to a fall in central temperature (16). A high central temperature with a wide central–peripheral gap can be seen in septic babies (17).
3. Several clinical trials have demonstrated a protective effect of hypothermia in term neonates with hypoxic ischemic encephalopathy (HIE) and continuous temperature monitoring plays an important role in controlled hypothermia as a treatment for HIE (see Chapter 50) (18).

B. Indications

1. Continuous temperature monitoring and servocontrol for whole body cooling (**Fig. 8.4**).
2. Automatic control of heater output of radiant warmer or incubator.

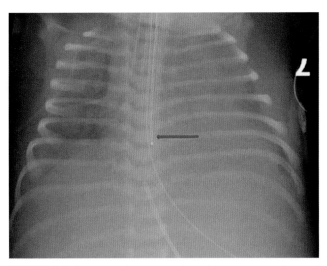

FIGURE 8.4 Chest x-ray showing esophageal temperature probe, used for servocontrolling of cooling blanket in whole body cooling protocol. The *blue arrow* points to the esophagel probe.

C. Contraindications

1. Caution should be used when using rectal continuous temperature probe in preterm infants as risk of tissue damage/perforation of GI tract is higher in this population (19,20).

D. Equipment Specifications

Two types of probes available: thermocouple and thermistor.

1. **Thermocouple probes**
   a. Thermocouple probes are less expensive and more widely used.
   b. A thermocouple probe is a very small bead made up of the junction of two dissimilar metals.
   c. The beads generate a very small voltage proportional to the temperature.
2. **Thermistors probes**
   a. Thermistors detect temperature as a change in resistance. (The thermocouple and thermistor are not interchangeable.)
   b. Battery-powered interface devices are available that allow the use of thermocouple probes with the thermistor-compatible monitor.
   c. The resolution is up to 0.1°C and the temperature is displayed in both Fahrenheit and Centigrade.

E. Monitors for Thermistor and Thermocouple Probes

1. **Monitors using thermistors** are identified as Yellow Springs Instrument Co. (YSI) 400- or YSI 700-compatible.
   a. YSI 400-compatible probes are single-element devices.
   b. YSI 700-compatible probes are dual-element devices.

c. YSI 400 and YSI 700 probes are physically identical and are available in the same configurations but are electrically different and will not work interchangeably.
2. **Monitors using thermocouple probes** are identified as such, and the probe connection is different from the thermistor type.
3. Probes for both thermistors and thermocouples are available in different configurations for different sites. For example:
   a. Surface skin probe
   b. Tympanic membrane thermocouple probe

F. Precautions

1. Do not apply skin probes to broken or bruised skin.
2. Do not apply skin probes over clear plastic dressings.
3. Do not use fingernails to remove skin surface probes.
4. Do not force core probes during insertion.
5. Do not reuse disposable probes.
6. Shield skin probe with reflective pad if used with radiant warmer or heat lamp.
7. When using servocontrol mechanisms for environmental control, take intermittent temperatures at other sites to monitor effectiveness.

G. Technique

1. Skin surface probe (**Table 8.1**)

TABLE 8.1 Sites for Temperature Monitoring

SITES	RANGE (°C)	APPLICATION
Surface		
1. Abdomen	36.0–36.5	Servocontrol
2. Axillary	36.5–37.0	Noninvasive approximation of core temperature
Core		
1. Esophageal	36.5–37.5 33.5	Reliable reflection of changes Target temperature in whole body cooling protocols
2. Rectal	36.5–37.5 34–35	Slow reflection of changes Target temperature in head cooling protocols associated with mild systemic hypothermia

a. Skin site should be dried prior to application. Site may be cleaned with sterile water or saline wipes prior to drying if debris is present. Wiping the skin with alcohol may improve adhesion but concern exists for irritation and absorption of alcohol through immature skin.

b. Cover probe with a reflective cover pad (foil-covered foam adhesive pad, incorporated in the disposable probe) (**Fig. 8.5**). Probe must be covered with an aluminum foil disk to reflect back the added heat from devices such as radiant warmers, phototherapy lights, infrared warming lights, and any other external radiant heat-generating sources (21).

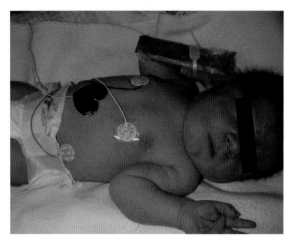

FIGURE 8.5 Skin probe properly placed on infant (note that probe has protective foil cover and lies flat on the skin surface).

c. The ideal site for application of the skin probe is not known, although the abdominal skin and flank are generally acceptable (21).

d. Ensure that skin probe is free of contact with bed (**Fig. 8.6**).

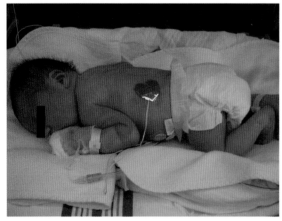

FIGURE 8.6 Newborn infant with skin probe free of contact from bed surface.

2. Application of core probe (see **Table 8.1**)
   a. Choose probe size according to site (i.e., rectum or esophagus).

b. Esophageal probe
   (1) Does not need lubrication prior to placement, but may need to be warmed to be more pliable prior to insertion.
   (2) Estimate the length of insertion needed to place the tip of the probe in the lower third of the esophagus. Measure the distance from the nose to the tragus of the ear and then from the ear to the xiphoid and subtract 2 cm from the total (see **Fig. 8.4**).
   (3) Insert probe through nostril until the desired length is reached.

c. Rectal probe
   (1) Lubricate probe before placing in rectum.
   (2) Probe should be placed approximately 3 cm beyond anal sphincter; further advancement will increase risk of perforation.

d. Do not force either probe.

3. Connect the probe to the monitor.

4. Monitor energy output changes.

5. Reposition or replace the probe if temperature recorded does not correlate with that recorded using an electronic thermometer. Skin surface temperature will be cooler than core temperature.

H. Complications

1. Skin irritation by probe or adhesive heat shield
2. Tissue trauma caused by core temperature probe includes:
   a. Rectal or colonic perforation
   b. Esophageal or gastric perforation
   c. Pneumoperitoneum
   d. Peritonitis
3. Unshielded skin probes or loosely adherent probes may cause unsafe environmental temperatures when the probes are used to servoregulate temperatures of incubators or radiant warmers. (**Table 8.2**)

NEWER ADVANCES IN DEVELOPMENT

Many temperature monitoring systems are being developed for use in low resource countries. Several temperature monitoring systems described in the section that follows are currently in development and/or in early use, and not routinely used in most NICUs.

A. Thermospot Temperature Indicator

1. A low-cost, reusable continuous temperature indicator especially designed for use in resource-limited countries where caregivers may have limited education.
2. The indicator is a small, flexible sticker that is applied to the infant's skin (**Fig. 8.7**).

TABLE 8.2 **Potential Pitfalls of Servocontrolled Heating Devices**

	SKIN < CORE	SKIN > CORE
Increased heater output	Cold stress Shock (vasoconstricted) Hypoxia Acidosis	Dislodged probe Servo fails to shut off Vasodilators (e.g., tolazoline) Shock (vasodilated)
Decreased heater output	Probe uninsulated (radiant heat)	
Servocontrol malfunction	Fever, overheating	
Internal cold stress	Unheated endotracheal oxygen, exchange transfusion	

Note: Changes in heater output may not be indicated; therefore, it is necessary to intermittently monitor the infant's core temperature (axillary optimal).

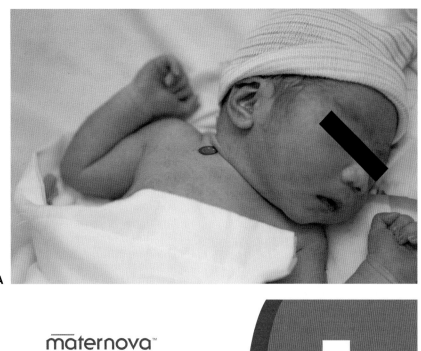

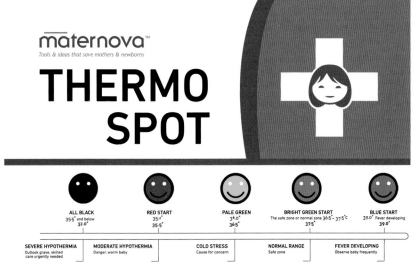

FIGURE 8.7 Thermospot temperature indicator (**A**) with picture of the scale (**B**). (Courtesy of Maternova, Inc.)

3. An LCD screen changes color according to the infant's temperature. The color varies from light green (normothermia) to black (hypothermia) to blue (hyperthermia) (22).

B. Wireless Thermistor Device

1. Hypothermia and hyperthermia is often missed in low- and middle-income countries where understaffed hospitals are unable to continuously monitor the infant's temperature.
2. A wireless thermistor device was created and tested in hospitals in Malawi.
3. It is a silicone armband that is attached to the infants' upper arm with the thermistor situated in the axilla.
4. The temperature data is transmitted via Bluetooth to an android device.
5. This device is low cost, reusable, user-friendly, and easily sanitized, attributes required in low- and middle-income countries (23).

C. Wearable Temperature Sensors

1. Dols and Chen (24) incorporated a negative temperature coefficient (NTC) Mon-A-Therm 90045 temperature sensor into a comfortable belt and isolated using soft cotton foam to limit influences of environmental temperatures. This belt is wrapped around the infant and the temperature is displayed on a screen.
2. Bempu, a light-up temperature-monitoring bracelet fits on a baby's wrist; it sounds an alarm and flashes orange if babies are too cold, so mothers can warm them against their skin or swaddle them. So far, the device has helped an estimated 10,000 newborns, mostly in India but also in 25 other countries (25).

References

1. Sherman TI, Greenspan JS, St. Clair N, et al. Optimizing the neonatal thermal environment. *Neonatal Netw.* 2006;25(4):251–260.
2. Wilson E, Maier R, Norman M, et al. Admission hypothermia in very preterm infants and neonatal morbidity. *J Pediatr.* 2016;175:61–67.
3. Goldman LR, Shannon MW; AAP Committee on Environmental Health. Technical report: Mercury in the environment: Implications for pediatricians. *Pediatrics.* 2001;108:197–205.
4. Hissink Muller PC, Van Berkel LH, De Baeufort AJ. Axillary and rectal temperature measurements poorly agree in newborn infants. *Neonatology.* 2008;94(1):31–34.
5. Lantz B, Ottosson C. Using axillary temperature to approximate rectal temperature in newborns. *Acta Paediatrica.* 2015;104:766–770.
6. Duran R, Vatansever U, Acunas B, et al. Comparison of temporal artery, mid-forehead skin and axillary temperature

recordings in preterm infants <1500 g of birthweight. *J Paediatr Child Health.* 2009;45:444–447.
7. Sim MA, Leow SY, Hao Y, et al. A practical comparison of temporal artery thermometry and axillary thermometry in neonates under different environments. *J Paediatr Child Health.* 2016;52(4):391–396.
8. Carr EA, Wilmoth ML, Eliades AB, et al. Comparison of temporal artery to rectal temperature measurements in children up to 24 months. *J Pediatr Nurs.* 2011;26(3):179–185.
9. Greenbaum EI, Carson M, Kincannon WN, et al. Hazards of temperature taking. *Br Med J.* 1970;3:4–5.
10. Greenbaum EI, Carson M, Kincannon WN, et al. Rectal thermometer-induced pneumoperitoneum in the newborn. *Pediatrics.* 1969;44:539–542.
11. Latman NS. Clinical thermometry: Possible causes and potential solutions to electronic, digital thermometer in accuracies. *Biomed Instrum Technol.* 2003;37(3):190–196.
12. Syrkin-Nikolau ME, Johnson KJ, Colaizy TT, et al. Temporal artery temperature measurement in the neonate. *Am J Perinatol.* 2017;34:1026–1031.
13. Craig JV, Lancaster GA, Taylor S, et al. Infrared ear thermometry compared with rectal thermometry in children: A systematic review. *Lancet.* 2002;360:603–609.
14. Siberry GK, Diener-West M, Schappell E, et al. Comparison of temple temperatures with rectal temperatures in children under two years of age. *Clin Pediatr (Phila).* 2002;41:405–415.
15. Robertson-Smith J, McCaffrey FT, Sayers R, et al. A comparison of mid-forehead and axillary temperatures in newborn intensive care. *J Perinatol.* 2015;35(2):120–122.
16. Lyon AJ, Pikaar ME, Badger P, et al. Temperature control in very low birthweight infants during first five days of life. *Arch Dis Child Fetal Neonatal Ed.* 1997;76:F47–F50.
17. Leante-Castellanos JL, Martínez-Gimeno A, Cidrás-Pidré M, et al. Central-peripheral temperature monitoring as a marker for diagnosing late-onset neonatal sepsis. *Pediatr Infect Dis J.* 2017;36(12):e293–e297.
18. Jacobs SE, Berg M, Hunt R, et al. Cooling for newborns with hypoxic ischaemic encephalopathy. *Cochrane Database Syst Rev.* 2013;(1):CD003311.
19. Tarnowaska A, Potocka K, Marcinski A, et al. Iatrogenic complications due to the nasogastric and rectal cannula in neonates. *Med Sci Monit.* 2004;10(3):46–50.
20. Su BH, Lin HY, Chiu HY, et al. Esophageal perforation: A complication of nasogastric tube placement in premature infants. *J Pediatr.* 2009;154:460.
21. Joseph RA, Derstine S, Killian M. Ideal site for skin temperature probe placement on Infants in the NICU: A review of literature. *Adv Neonatal Care.* 2017;17(2):114–122.
22. Pejaver RK, Nisarga R, Gowda B. Temperature monitoring in newborns using thermospot. *Indian J Pediatr.* 2004;71(9): 795–796.
23. David M, Muelenar AA, Muelenar P, et al. Distributed thermistor for continuous temperature monitoring of malnourished infants at risk for hypothermia. *Ann Glob Health.* 2017;83(1):9.
24. Chen W, Dols S, Oetomo SB, et al. Monitoring body temperature of newborn infants at neonatal intensive care units using wearable sensors. In *Proceedings of the Fifth International Conference on Body Area Networks.* Corfu Island, Greece; 2010:188–194.
25. Tanlgasalam V, Bhat BV, Adhisivam B, et al. Hypothermia detection in low birth weight neonates using a novel bracelet device. *J Matern Fetal Neonatal Med.* 2018;4:1–4.

Cardiorespiratory Monitoring

M. Kabir Abubakar

CARDIAC MONITORING

Monitoring of heart rate, oxygenation, and respiration is necessary to ensure physiologic stability for most infants in the neonatal intensive care unit (NICU). To be effective, monitoring needs to be continuous, noninvasive, accurate, and resistant to movement with few false alarms in both spontaneously breathing infants and those needing respiratory support. Progress in microchip and computer technology has facilitated the development of bedside monitors that can integrate multiple monitoring parameters into a single system. This chapter covers the fundamentals of cardiac and respiratory monitoring.

A. Purpose

1. Provide reliable, continuous, noninvasive, and accurate monitoring of neonatal cardiac activity
   a. Provide trends of heart rate over time
   b. Monitor beat-to-beat heart rate variability (1,2)
2. To allow continuous evaluation and surveillance of critically ill neonates
3. To provide early warning of potentially significant changes in heart rate by identification of heart rates above or below certain preset alarm limits

B. Background

1. Electrical activity of the heart is detected using impedance technology via skin surface electrodes (3).
2. The low-level electrical signal is amplified and filtered to eliminate interference and artifacts.
3. The electrical signal, defined in millivolts, is displayed as an electrocardiogram (ECG) tracing.
4. R-wave detection from the QRS complex is used to calculate heart rate.
5. The typical three-lead configuration (i.e., leads I, II, III) provides alternative vectors for ECG analysis.

C. Contraindications

None

D. Limitations

1. The three-lead ECG is most useful for long-term continuous cardiac monitoring; more detailed cardiac evaluation (i.e., assessment of hypertrophy or axis) or the identification of abnormal cardiac rhythms will require complete 12-lead ECG with rhythm strip.
2. Close proximity of electrodes in extremely small infants may interfere with signal detection.

E. Equipment

Hardware—Specifications

1. The monitoring system should have the appropriate frequency response and sensitivity to track the fast and narrow QRS complex of the neonate accurately
2. Heart rate is processed on a beat-to-beat basis with a short updating interval
3. Default heart rate alarm limits should be tailored to the neonatal population
   a. Low heart rate (bradycardia) limit of 100 beats/min (Note: Some term infants may have resting heart rates of 80 to 100 beats/min, requiring lower bradycardia alarm settings)
   b. High heart rate (tachycardia) limit of 180 to 200 beats/min
4. Monitor displays
   a. Cathode-ray tube (CRT)
      (1) Has high resolution and definition
      (2) Display can be either color or monochrome and more easily seen from different angles. CRT displays are no longer in common use

because of the improved quality and resolution of liquid crystal displays (LCD)

  b. LCD
    (1) Flat, thin display monitor
    (2) Now have improved resolution for fast and narrow QRS complex of the neonate
    (3) Back-lighting is necessary for viewing in low-light environments
    (4) Unlike CRT, viewing angle is critical
5. Heart rate displayed as alphanumeric part of waveform display or in a separate numerical display window
6. Recorder (optional)
  a. Electronic memory
    (1) Real-time ECG
    (2) Delayed ECG—stored retrospective display used primarily for review of a short time interval prior to and during the occurrence of an alarm. Many systems now have the ability to store information (both numerical data and waveforms) for extended periods of time (up to 7 days) for later review
  b. Printed record of ECG trend information
    (1) Typically used to document selected segments of ECG tracings such as periods associated with alarms or abnormal rhythms
    (2) Monitors may have dedicated printers (often integrated into monitor cases)
    (3) Central monitoring stations can provide remote access to information from all networked monitor units with printing capabilities
7. Units available for both bedside and transport monitoring (**Figs. 9.1** and **9.2**)

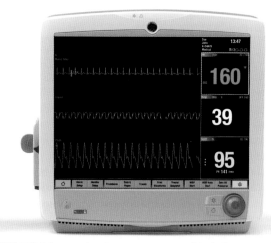

FIGURE 9.1 Typical multiparameter neonatal bedside monitor. (© 2019 GE Healthcare. All Rights Reserved.)

  a. Transport monitors typically smaller and battery powered
  b. Similar capabilities regarding parameter availability, but monitor specific

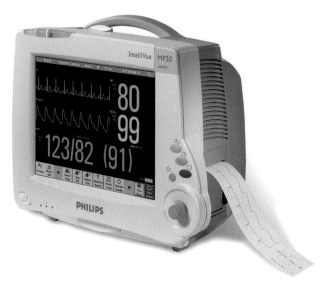

FIGURE 9.2 Typical multiparameter neonatal transport monitor with integrated printer. (Courtesy of Royal Philips.)

  c. Some monitors now have the ability to have modules that can be removed from the main monitor and used for transport then plugged back into the main monitor to allow for continuous recording without loss of memory data during transport.

Consumables—Specifications

1. Disposable neonatal ECG electrodes
  a. Patient contact surfaces of electrodes are coated in adhesive electrolyte gel, which acts as conductive medium between the patient and the metal lead while preventing direct patient contact with the metal.
  b. Typical commercially available neonatal leads incorporate silver–silver-chloride electrodes directly onto paper, foam, or fabric bodies with integrated lead wires; these are available in different sizes and forms designed for use in neonates of different gestations.
  c. Less commonly, adhesive electrode pads are separate from lead wires, which connect to the electrodes via clips.
  d. ECG limb plate electrodes may be used in extremely low–birth-weight infants with a small chest surface area and sensitive skin and when the application of chest leads would interfere with resuscitation or the performance of other procedures. Use of electrode gel as a conductor at the skin interface (rather than alcohol pads) is imperative in such cases. All neonatal leads should be latex, phthalate, and mercury free.
2. Characteristics to consider in electrode selection
  a. Adherence to skin of an active infant
  b. Quality of signal attained
  c. Minimal skin irritation
  d. Ease of removal using water or adhesive remover without damage to or removal of skin

e. Performance in the warm, moist environment of an infant incubator

f. Adhesive–skin interaction under overhead infant warmers

3. Lead wires and patient cable

   a. All cables should be clean and the insulation should be free of nicks or cuts.

   b. Lead wires should lock or snap into the patient cable, preventing easy disconnections.

   c. If using electrodes that attach via clips, use infant/pediatric lead wires with small electrode clips—standard adult-size clips will place too much torsion on the infant electrode, tugging on the skin, and possibly peeling off the electrode.

F. Precautions

1. Do not leave alcohol wipes under electrodes as conductors.

2. Do not apply electrodes to broken or bruised skin.

3. Avoid placing electrodes directly on the nipples.

4. Select the smallest appropriate/effective electrode for patient monitoring to minimize skin exposure and limit potential complications from irritation/adhesives.

5. Do not apply electrodes to clear film plastic dressings—dressing will act as an insulator between the skin and the electrode.

6. To avoid skin damage, do not use fingernails to remove electrodes.

7. Secure the patient cable to the patient's environment to prevent excessive traction.

8. Use only monitors that have been checked for safety and performance regularly—usually indicated by a dated sticker on the monitor from biomedical engineering.

9. Do not use monitors with defects such as exposed wires, broken or dented casing, broken knobs or controls, or cracked display.

10. Monitor alarms should prompt immediate patient assessment.

    a. Note alarm indication (i.e., tachycardia or bradycardia).

    b. Treat patient condition as necessary or correct the source of any false alarm.

    c. If alarm is silenced or deactivated during the course of patient evaluation, it should be reactivated prior to leaving the patient's bedside.

G. Techniques

1. Familiarize yourself with the monitor prior to patient use

2. Electrode and lead wire placement: Although you should refer to the monitor manufacturer's placement instructions, general electrode placement guidelines follow

a. Skin preparation: Skin should be clean and dry to provide the best electrode-to-skin interface.

   (1) Wipe skin with an alcohol pad (use a normal saline swab in extremely low–birth-weight infants with sensitive skin) and allow to dry thoroughly

   (2) Avoid the use of tape to secure electrodes—for optimal performance and proper electrical interface, electrodes must adhere directly to skin

b. Basic three-lead configuration for electrode placement (for electrodes with integrated lead wires) **(Fig. 9.3)**

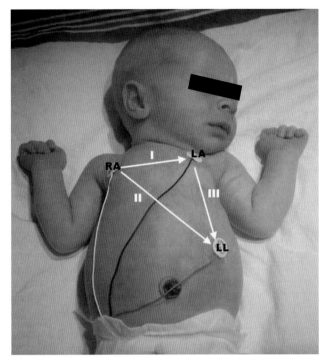

FIGURE 9.3 Basic electrode placement and lead vectors for optimal ECG signal detection. Right arm/left arm positions also provide maximal signal for impedance pneumography. Electrodes RA, LA and LL record the electrical activity of the heart in relation to themselves and also correspond with each other to form leads I (RA to LA), II (RA to LL) and III (LL to LA) as indicated by the arrows.

   (1) Right arm (white): Right lateral chest at level of the nipple line

   (2) Left arm (black): Left lateral chest at level of the nipple line

   (3) Left leg (red or green): Left lower rib cage

   (4) Although this configuration allows the use of the same electrodes to monitor both ECG and respiration, optimal ECG signal may be obtained when the right arm lead is at the right midclavicle and the left leg lead is at the xiphoid (4)

c. If not using electrodes with integrated wires, place electrode pads in basic three-lead configuration as above, then connect lead wires via electrode clips

   (1) White lead (right arm) to right chest electrode

   (2) Black lead (left arm) to left chest electrode

   (3) Red or green lead (left leg) to left lower rib cage electrode

3. Turn monitor on—most monitors will conduct an automatic self-test
4. Connect the patient cable to the monitor
5. Select the lead that provides the best signal and QRS size (lead II is the usual default) (**Fig. 9.4**)

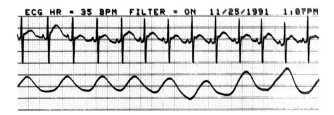

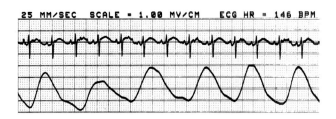

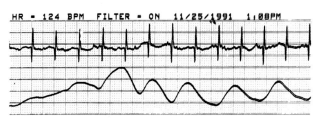

FIGURE 9.4 Typical ECG tracings: Lead I (**top**), lead II (**middle**), and lead III (**bottom**).

a. Ensure that heart rate correlates to QRS complexes seen on display—make sure that the QRS detector is not counting high or peaked T or P waves
6. Verify that low and high heart rate alarms are set appropriately

H. Complications

1. Skin lesions (rare)
   a. Irritation from alcohol—may occur with even short-term application to immature skin. (This can be alleviated by using normal saline swab to clean the skin in extremely low–birth-weight infants.)
   b. Trauma caused by rubbing with excessive vigor during skin preparation
   c. Irritation from incorrectly formulated electrode gel
   d. Secondary effects of skin breakdown
      (1) Cellulitis or abscess formation
      (2) Increased transepidermal water losses

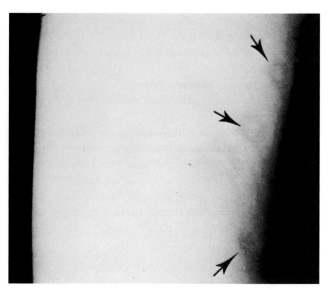

FIGURE 9.5 Arrows show residual hyperpigmented marks on the extremities present more than 1 year after application of ECG leads for cardiorespiratory monitoring.

   (3) Hypo- or hyperpigmented marks at sites of prior irritation or inflammation (**Fig. 9.5**)
2. Erroneous readings caused by artifacts (**Table 9.1**) (5)

TABLE 9.1 Steps to Minimize Artifact Interference

PROBLEM	TREATMENT
Poor electrode contact/ connection	1. Gently clean skin with alcohol wipe (or saline) and allow to dry prior to electrode reapplication. 2. Check electrode/cable connections.
Dried Electrode	Replace
Equipment interference	1. Systematically turn off one piece of adjacent equipment at a time while observing monitor for improvement in signal quality. 2. After source of interference is identified, increase distance between that equipment and patient while rerouting power cords and cables as necessary. 3. If above maneuver is unsuccessful, replace equipment.
60-Hz interference	1. Follow procedure for poor electrode contact. 2. Replace patient cable. 3. If 1 and 2 are unsuccessful, try an alternate monitor.

   a. Electrical interference
      (1) Sixty-cycle electrical interference (frequency of typical power lines)

(2) Interference from other equipment used in the patient's immediate environment

(3) Electrical spike may be generated when certain types of polyvinyl chloride tubing are mechanically deformed by infusion pump devices—spikes appear as ectopic beats on the monitor (rare) (6)

b. Decreased signal amplitude with motion artifact
c. Poor electrode contact or dried electrode gel
d. Incorrect vectors because of inaccurate lead placement (**Fig. 9.6**)
e. Inappropriate sensitivity settings

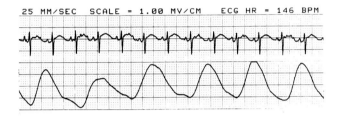

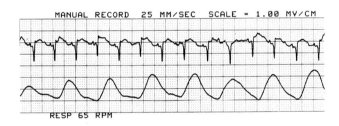

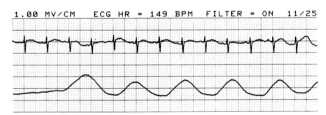

FIGURE 9.6 Normal P-, QRS-, and T-wave detection. **Top:** Lead II tracing with electrodes properly placed. Note normal P-, QRS-, and T-wave detection. **Middle:** Lead II tracing with electrodes close together on anterior chest wall. Note altered QRS- and decreased T-wave amplitude. **Bottom:** Lead II tracing with electrodes placed lateral on the abdomen. Note decreased wave amplitude and flattened P wave.

3. Monitor or cable failure
   a. Hardware or software failure
   b. Cable disconnection
4. Alarm failure
   a. False alarms (either tachycardia or bradycardia) resulting from inaccurate interpretation of heart rate
   b. Inappropriate alarm parameters for patient

RESPIRATORY MONITORING

A. Purpose

1. Reliable and accurate monitoring of neonatal respiratory activity
   a. Trending of respiratory activity over time
   b. Detection of apnea and tachypnea
2. Assessment and surveillance of critically ill neonates
3. To provide early warning of potentially significant changes in respiratory rate by identifying respiratory rates above or below preset alarm limits

B. Background

1. Measurement of transthoracic impedance is the most commonly used method for determining respiratory rate (7)
   a. A low-level, high-frequency signal is passed through the patient's chest via surface electrodes
      (1) Typically utilizes the same electrodes as are used for cardiac monitoring
      (2) Signal path usually from right arm (white) to left arm (black) electrodes, although some monitors may use right arm (white) to left leg (red or green) (**Fig. 9.7**)

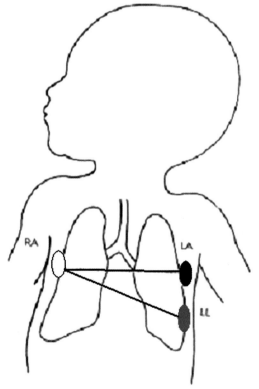

FIGURE 9.7 Transthoracic impedance pneumography: Diagrammatic representation of the path of the high-frequency signal between chest wall electrodes. Most monitors transmit signal right arm (*white*) → left arm (*black*), less commonly right arm (*white*) → left leg (*red*).

b. Impedance to the high-frequency signal is measured
   (1) Impedance is the electrical resistance to the signal
   (2) Changes in lung inflation cause an alteration in the density of the chest cavity, which is detected as a change in impedance
   (3) Changes in impedance modulate a proportional change in the amplitude of the high-frequency signal
c. The change in impedance, as seen by the modulation of the high-frequency signal, is detected and quantified by the monitor and recorded as breaths per minute
d. The monitor has an impedance threshold limit below which changes in impedance are not counted as valid respiratory activity—cardiac pumping with associated changes in pulmonary blood flow will also cause changes in thoracic impedance (usually much smaller changes than those associated with respiration)

C. Contraindications

None

D. Equipment

Hardware—Specifications

1. Equipment is the same as that for cardiac monitoring; multiparameter monitors incorporate both cardiac and respiratory monitoring into single units.
2. Respiratory monitoring parameters.
   a. Low-level threshold (for impedance) for breath validation should not be below 0.2 to minimize cardiogenic artifact.
   b. Coincidence alarm with rejection applies when respiratory rate being detected is equal to the heart rate activity being detected by the cardiac portion of the system.
   c. Default limits should be tailored to the neonatal population.
      (1) Adjustable apnea time-delay setting (length of apnea in seconds before alarming).
      (2) Typical apnea time delay is 15 to 20 seconds.

Consumables—Specifications

Same as for cardiac monitor

E. Precautions

1. Include previously discussed precautions for cardiac monitoring.

2. Muscular activity may be interpreted as respiration, resulting in failure to alarm during an apneic episode (see section G3a below).

F. Technique

1. Same as for cardiac monitor.
2. Ensure that the respiratory waveform correlates to the true initiation of inspiration.
3. Move right and left arm electrodes up toward the axillary area if detection of respiration is poor due to shallow breathing.
4. Set desired low and high respiratory rate and apnea delay alarm limits.

G. Complications

1. Skin lesions (see H1 under Cardiac Monitoring)
2. Monitor or cable failure
   a. Hardware or software failure
   b. Cable disconnection
3. Alarm failure
   a. False-positive "respiratory" signal in the absence of effective ventilation
      (1) Chest wall movement with airway obstruction (obstructive apnea)
      (2) Nonrespiratory muscular action (i.e., stretching, seizure, or hiccups) producing motion artifact (**Fig. 9.8**)

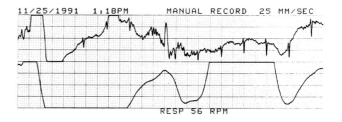

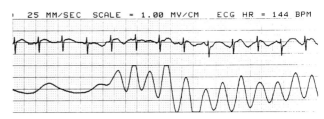

FIGURE 9.8 Tracings of artifacts affecting ECG/respiratory tracings. **Top:** Loose electrode affected by motion. **Bottom:** Motion artifact caused by patient's moving arm coming in contact with chest electrodes (note change in respiratory frequency signal).

b. False apnea alarm despite normal respiratory activity
  (1) Improper sensitivity not detecting present respiratory activity
  (2) Incorrect electrode placement
  (3) Loose electrodes
c. Inappropriate alarm parameters for patient
4. Accurate assessment of respiratory rate not practical when using high-frequency ventilatory modes
5. Respiratory rate measurement may not be accurate when using upper arm limb leads in extremely low–birth-weight infants

CARDIORESPIROGRAPH MONITORING

A. Definition

1. Graphical representation of heart rate and respiratory rate over time

B. Purpose

1. Monitoring of infants for identification and quantification of heart rate and respiratory activity, with detection of apnea, periodic breathing, and bradycardia
2. Identification of chronologic relationships between bradycardia and apnea events
3. Many systems also provide continuous S_pO_2 information to allow correlation with desaturation events

C. Background

1. Heart rate is plotted graphically as beats per minute (y-axis) versus time (x-axis).
2. Respiratory waveform is compressed to allow display of time range.
3. Short-term trending allows constant updating as the oldest information is displaced (typically based on a 2-minute window of time).
4. Time relationship between heart rate and respiratory activity is maintained.
   a. Allows for visualization of entire apnea episodes and identification of precipitating factors (e.g., a drop in respiratory rate may precede bradycardia).
5. Inclusion of S_pO_2 allows identification of temporal relationship for desaturation events (S_pO_2 is plotted in the same fashion as the heart rate on a second y-axis).

D. Contraindications

None

E. Equipment

Standard features of most neonatal monitors

EMERGING TECHNOLOGIES

A. Background

Given the known limitations and potential complications of current methods for cardiac/respiratory monitoring in neonates (i.e., ECG and impedance technologies), research continues to find alternate techniques for monitoring with similar or improved reliability.

B. Techniques Under Review

1. Wireless monitoring using photoplethysmography (8).
   a. Utilizes optical probe to detect/record heart and/or respiratory rates.
   b. Can eliminate the need for skin electrodes and wires utilizing abdominal belt/band and electronic data receiver.
   c. Preliminary data suggest similar data reliability to traditional electrode-based cardiac/respiratory monitoring systems.
2. Piezoelectric transducer sensors (9).
   a. Sensors placed in proximity to infant (i.e., under infant) detect an acoustic cardiorespiratory signal from which heart rate and breathing rate are calculated.
   b. Minute movements made by the body are monitored via a transducer that converts the body movements into electrical signals to report the presence or absence of respiration and normal heart rate.
   c. Preliminary data suggest the noninvasive device avoids skin irritation while providing accurate monitoring.
   d. May be affected by "noise" from nearby equipment.
3. Chest electrical impedance tomography (EIT): Functional EIT may be helpful in monitoring regional lung ventilation in mechanically ventilated patients. This uses electrodes placed around the chest either individually with equal spacing around the chest circumference or are integrated into electrode belts or stripes. Very small alternating electrical currents are applied through pairs of electrodes while the resulting voltages are measured on the remaining electrodes. The data generated are then used to calculate impedance changes associated with spontaneous breathing or mechanical ventilation and provide information on respiratory effort and regional lung ventilation and perfusion (10).

C. Implications

Although preliminary reports regarding such alternative monitoring devices are encouraging, additional research regarding reliability and safety will be required before such applications gain widespread acceptance.

References

1. Javorka K, Lehotska Z, Kozar M, et al. Heart rate variability in newborns. *Physiol Res.* 2017;66(Supplementum 2):S203–S214.
2. Di Fiore JM, Poets CF, Gauda E, et al. Cardiorespiratory events in preterm infants: interventions and consequences. *J Perinatol.* 2016;36(4):251–258.
3. Di Fiore JM. Neonatal cardiorespiratory monitoring techniques. *Semin Neonatol.* 2004;9:195–203.
4. Baird TM, Goydos JM, Neuman MR. Optimal electrode location for monitoring the ECG and breathing in neonates. *Pediatr Pulmonol.* 1992;12:247–250.
5. Jacobs MK. Sources of measurement error in noninvasive electronic instrumentation. *Nurs Clin North Am.* 1978;13:573–587.
6. Sahn DJ, Vaucher YE. Electrical current leakage transmitted to an infant via an IV controller: an unusual ECG artifact. *J Pediatr.* 1976;89:301–302.
7. Hintz SR, Wong RJ, Stevenson DK. Biomedical engineering aspects of neonatal monitoring. In: Martin RJ, Fanaroff AA, Walsh MC, eds. *Fanaroff and Martin's Neonatal-Perinatal Medicine: Diseases of the Fetus and Infant.* 8th ed. Philadelphia, PA: Mosby; 2006:609.
8. De D, Mukherjee A, Sau A, et al. Design of smart neonatal health monitoring system using SMCC. *Healthc Technol Lett.* 2016;4(1):13–19.
9. Sato S, Ishida-Nakajima W, Ishida A, et al. Assessment of a new piezoelectric transducer sensor for noninvasive cardiorespiratory monitoring of newborn infants in the NICU. *Neonatology.* 2010;98(2):179–190.
10. Frerichs I, Amato MB, van Kaam AH, et al. Chest electrical impedance tomography examination, data analysis, terminology, clinical use and recommendations: consensus statement of the TRanslational EIT developmeNt stuDy group. *Thorax.* 2017;72(1):83–93.

Blood Pressure Monitoring

M. Kabir Abubakar

Blood pressure (BP) monitoring is an integral part of neonatal care for both critically ill and stable newborn infants. Recognizing and treating abnormal blood pressure states can have significant prognostic implications in neonatal intensive care. The ideal blood pressure–monitoring system should be easy to set up, reliable, and give continuous information or enable measurements to be made at frequent intervals with minimal disruption to the infant. Neonatal BP monitoring may be performed by either noninvasive or invasive methods (1–4).

NONINVASIVE (INDIRECT) METHODS

Noninvasive BP measurement can be done using

1. Auscultatory measurement (manual noninvasive) or
2. Oscillatory arterial BP measurement (automatic non-invasive)

AUSCULTATORY MEASUREMENT (MANUAL NONINVASIVE)

Utilized for intermittent BP measurements; is simple and inexpensive, but now often not used in neonates because of the availability of automated methods of blood pressure measurement.

A. Background

1. This technique uses a BP cuff, insufflator, manometer, and stethoscope.
2. The sphygmomanometer uses a pneumatic cuff to encircle the upper arm or leg and a pressure gauge (manometer) to register the pressure in the cuff.
3. There are two types of manometers:
   a. Mercury (mercury column)
   b. Aneroid (mechanical air gauge)
4. The encircling pneumatic cuff is inflated to a pressure higher than the estimated systolic pressure in the

underlying artery. The cuff pressure compresses the artery and stops blood flow.
5. A stethoscope placed distal to the cuff, over the occluded artery, will pick up the Korotkoff sounds as the cuff is deflated and the pressure of the cuff decreases to the point at which blood flow resumes through the artery.
6. Korotkoff sounds are the noise generated by blood flow returning to the compressed artery and originate from a combination of turbulent blood flow and oscillations of the arterial wall. The sounds have been classified into five phases:
   a. Phase I: Appearance of clear tapping sounds corresponding to the appearance of a palpable pulse
   b. Phase II: Sounds become softer and longer
   c. Phase III: Sounds become crisper and louder
   d. Phase IV: Sounds become muffled and softer
   e. Phase V: Sounds disappear completely. The fifth phase is thus recorded as the last audible sound.
7. An 8- to 9-MHz Doppler device can be used in place of a stethoscope. This device will detect only systolic BP levels.

B. Indications

1. Measurement of BP in larger stable infants or when invasive BP measurement is not required or is unavailable.
2. When only intermittent BP measurements are required.

C. Contraindications

1. Severe edema in the limb to be measured will muffle the Korotkoff sounds.
2. Decreased perfusion, ischemia, infiltrate, or injury in the limb used for measurement.
3. Peripheral venous/arterial catheter in the limb used for measurement.

TABLE 10.1 Sources of Error in Indirect Blood Pressure Measurements

PROBLEM	EFFECT ON BLOOD PRESSURE	PRECAUTION
Defective manometer 1. Air leaks 2. Improper valve function 3. Dry, degraded, or cracked tubing 4. Loss of mercury	Falsely low values	1. Check level of mercury at zero cuff pressure 2. Check for cleared definition of meniscus 3. Verify that pressure holds when tightened. Check tubing for cracks
Inappropriate cuff size		Verify appropriately sized cuff
1. Too narrow 2. Too wide	1. Falsely high values 2. Falsely low values	
Cuff applied loosely	Falsely high values owing to ballooning of bag and narrowing of effective surface	Apply cuff snugly
Cuff applied too tightly	Inaccurate reading owing to impedance of flow through artery	Apply cuff snugly without undue pressure
Rapid deflation of cuff	1. Falsely low values owing to inaccurate detection of beginning of sounds or 2. Falsely high values owing to inadequate equilibration between cuff pressure and manometer pressure	Deflate cuff at rate of 2–3 mm Hg/sec
Active or agitated patient	Variable	Recheck when patient is quiet

D. Limitations

1. Provides only intermittent BP measurements.
2. Manual measurement cumbersome or impossible in small infants.
3. Accuracy depends on ability to recognize Korotkoff sounds and may be user dependent.
4. Pressure may not be detectable in low-perfusion states or shock. Do not assume that it is simply an equipment problem; use clinical correlation.
5. Pressure is not detectable or is inaccurate when the baby is actively moving or agitated.
6. Measures only systolic and diastolic BP; mean BP measurement not available.
7. Can be used only to measure pressure in the upper arm or thigh.
8. The Korotkoff sound method tends to give values for systolic pressure that are lower than the true intra-arterial pressure, and diastolic values that are higher.
9. Inaccurate measurements (Table 10.1).

E. Equipment

1. Neonatal cuff (Table 10.2). Select a cuff that will fit comfortably around the upper arm or thigh; the inflatable bladder should completely encircle the extremity without overlapping. The width should be 90% of the limb circumference at the midpoint (5)
2. Mercury manometer or aneroid-type gauge
3. Appropriate-sized stethoscope with diaphragm or Doppler system

TABLE 10.2 Neonatal Cuff

CUFF NO. (SIZE)	LIMB CIRCUMFERENCE (CM)
1	3–6
2	4–8
3	6–11
4	7–13
5	8–15

From American Academy of Pediatrics Task Force Pressure Control: Report. *Pediatrics*. 1977;59:797.

F. Precautions (Table 10.1)

1. Carefully select the appropriate cuff size, because incorrect size can significantly alter the BP recorded (6).
   a. Cuff too small: BP will be higher than actual BP.
   b. Cuff too large: BP will be lower than actual BP.
2. Check functional integrity of manometer.
3. Check integrity of cuff for leaks.
4. Check speed of cuff deflation: If deflation is too rapid, accuracy may be compromised.
5. Patient must be quiet and still during measurements.
6. For optimal infection control, use disposable cuff for each patient.

G. Technique

1. Place the infant supine, with the limb fully extended and level with the heart.
2. Measure the limb circumference and select the appropriate size cuff for the limb.
   a. Neonatal cuffs are marked with the size range (**Table 10.2**).
   b. When the cuff is wrapped around the limb, the end of the cuff should line up with the range mark (**Fig. 10.1**).

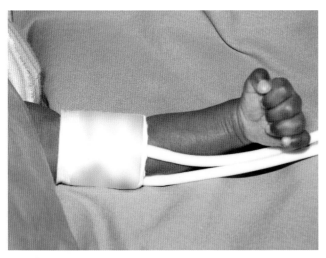

FIGURE 10.1 Cuff of correct size applied to upper arm.

   c. If the end of the cuff falls short of the range mark, the cuff size is too small.
   d. If the end of the cuff falls beyond the range mark, the cuff size is too large.
3. Apply the cuff snugly to the bare limb, above the elbow or knee joint.
4. Place the stethoscope or Doppler over the brachial artery for the upper arm or over the popliteal artery for the thigh.
5. Inflate the cuff rapidly to a pressure 15 mm Hg above the point at which the brachial pulse disappears.
6. Deflate the cuff slowly.

7. The pressure at which a sound is first heard is the systolic pressure (Korotkoff I). The pressure at which silence begins corresponds to the diastolic pressure (Korotkoff V). The pressure should be measured to the nearest 2 mm Hg.

In patients in whom the sounds do not disappear, the point at which the sounds change abruptly to a muffled tone can be accepted as an approximation of the diastolic pressure but will be slightly higher than true diastolic pressure.

H. Complications

1. Perfusion in the limb may be compromised if the cuff is not completely deflated.
2. Prolonged or repeated cuff inflation has been associated with ischemia, purpura, and/or neuropathy.
3. Cuff inflation will interfere with pulse oximetry measurement in the same limb.
4. Nosocomial infection may result from using the same cuff for more than one patient.

OSCILLOMETRIC MEASUREMENT OF ARTERIAL BLOOD PRESSURE (AUTOMATIC NONINVASIVE)

A. Background

The oscillometric or noninvasive blood pressure (NIBP)–monitoring technique offers a method for measuring all arterial blood pressure parameters (systolic, diastolic, mean, heart rate) (7–15). The underlying principle of this method is that the arterial wall oscillates when blood flows in pulsatile fashion through a vessel. These oscillations are transmitted to a cuff placed around the limb. As the pressure within the cuff is reduced, the pattern of oscillations changes (**Fig. 10.2**). When arterial pressure is just above the cuff pressure, there is a rapid increase in the amplitude of the oscillations and this is taken as systolic pressure. The point at which the amplitude of the oscillations is maximal coincides with the mean arterial pressure. Diastolic pressure is recorded when there is a sudden decrease in oscillations. Although many types of monitors use the same basic technique, the integration of the oscillometric method within an NIBP algorithm may differ substantially between manufacturers.

1. This technique employs a BP cuff interfaced to a computerized BP monitor.
2. A pneumatic cuff is used in the same fashion as with the auscultatory technique.
3. The monitor employs a miniature computer-controlled air pump and a bleed valve to control inflation and deflation of the cuff.

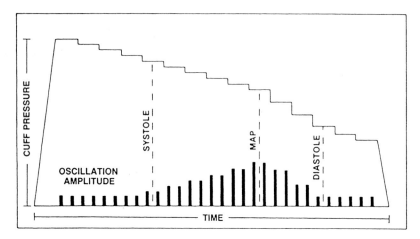

FIGURE 10.2 Determination sequence for oscillometric measurement.

4. A pressure transducer interfaced to the cuff tubing senses the inflation pressure of the cuff and oscillations transmitted to the cuff by the underlying artery.
5. The system will inflate the cuff to a level above the point at which no pulsations are detected.
6. As the cuff is being deflated to the level of the systolic pressure, oscillations from the arterial wall are transmitted to the cuff. A transducer measures static pressure and pressure oscillations received and transmitted by the cuff.
7. The systolic pressure is assigned the value of the cuff pressure at the time oscillations were initially detected.
8. Mean arterial pressure is generally the lowest cuff pressure with the greatest average oscillation amplitude. The diastolic value is determined by the lowest cuff pressure when there is a sudden decrease in oscillations.
9. Heart rate values are calculated by computing the mean value of the time interval between pulsations.
10. Higher detection sensitivity allows this technique to be used on parts of the extremities where auscultatory methods are not possible (i.e., forearm and lower leg).

B. Indications

1. Measurement of BP in stable infants or when invasive BP measurement is not required or is unavailable.
2. When only intermittent BP measurements are required.

C. Contraindications

1. Severe edema in the limb to be measured; will affect result
2. Decreased perfusion, ischemia, infiltrate, or injury in limb
3. Peripheral venous/arterial catheter in place in limb

D. Limitations

1. Provides only intermittent BP measurements.
2. Pressure may not be detectable in low-perfusion states or shock. Do not assume that it is simply an equipment problem; use clinical correlation.
3. Pressure is not detectable or may be inaccurate in neonates who are restless or having seizures.
4. Inaccurate measurements (**Table 10.1**).

E. Equipment

1. Neonatal NIBP monitor—display should include systolic, diastolic, mean, and heart rate values (**Fig. 10.3**).

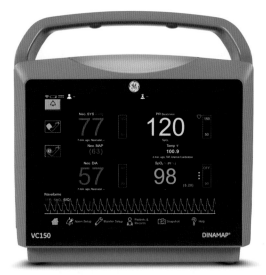

FIGURE 10.3 Oscillometric BP monitor. (© 2019 GE Healthcare. All Rights Reserved.)

2. Neonatal cuff (designed for use with the specific monitor)—cuff may be single-tube or double-tube type, provided the appropriate adapter is used. Neonatal cuff sizes range from 1 to 5 (**Table 10.2**).

F. Precautions

1. Incorrect cuff size can significantly alter the BP value obtained; therefore, careful selection of cuff size is very important.
   a. An oversized cuff will yield lower BP values; an undersized cuff will produce higher BP values.
2. Patient must be still during measurements.
3. For optimal infection control, cuffs should be for single-patient use only.
4. Oscillometric BP measurement may lose accuracy in very hypotensive states; this needs to be taken into consideration in such patients (16,17).

G. Technique

1. Become familiar with the monitor and the equipment to be used. Be aware of the normal BP changes with gestational and postnatal age (18).
2. Measure the circumference of the extremity where the cuff is to be applied. Select the appropriately sized cuff for the limb (**Fig. 10.1**).
3. Apply the cuff snugly to the limb. The cuff can be applied over a thin layer of clothing if necessary; however, a bare limb is recommended.
4. Attach the monitor air hoses to the cuff. The limb from which pressure is to be measured should be level with the heart.
5. Turn the monitor on and ensure that it passes the power-on self-test before proceeding.
6. Press the appropriate button to start a blood pressure determination cycle.
7. If the values obtained from the initial cycle are questionable, repeat the measurement. Multiple readings with similar values yield the optimal assurance of accuracy.
8. If readings are still questionable after repeating the cycle, reposition the cuff and repeat the measurement.
9. Periodic inspection of the cuff and extremity is critical to avoid problems such as cuff detachment or shift in extremity position.
10. Most NIBP systems can be programmed by the user to measure BP automatically at user-determined intervals. The interval between measurements should be long enough to ensure adequate circulation and minimize trauma to the limb and skin distal to the cuff.
11. In infants with suspected congenital heart disease, BP should be measured in all four extremities or at least the right arm and a leg for pre- and postductal comparison.

H. Complications

1. Perfusion in the limb may be compromised if the cuff is not completely deflated.
2. Repeated continuous cycling may cause ischemia, purpura, and/or neuropathy in the extremity.
3. Cuff inflation will interfere with pulse oximetry measurement and IV infusion in the same limb.
4. Nosocomial infection may arise from using the same cuff for more than one patient.

CONTINUOUS BLOOD PRESSURE MONITORING (INVASIVE)

A. Purpose

Intra-arterial direct BP monitoring is considered to be the "gold standard" for measuring BP. It provides continuous real-time beat-to-beat blood pressure readings allowing clinicians to observe and react to rapid changes in BP in critically ill neonates. The pressure waveforms produced can be analyzed, allowing further information about the patient's cardiovascular status. It has the added advantage of permitting access for repeated arterial blood sampling in critically ill neonates.

B. Background

1. BP measurement is obtained from the vascular system via a catheter that has been introduced into an artery, either the umbilical artery in the neonate or a peripheral artery (Chapters 31 and 33).
2. The pressure waveform of the arterial pulse is transmitted by a column of noncompressible bubble-free fluid to a pressure transducer where it is converted to an electrical signal. This electrical signal is then processed, amplified, and converted into a visual display by a microprocessor. An understanding of the physical principles involved in these processes is important in order to reduce errors and accurately interpret the waveform displayed.
3. A BP transducer is a device that converts mechanical forces (pressure) to electrical signals. There are two major types of transducers.
   a. **Strain gauge pressure transducer:** Composed of metal strands or foil that is either stretched or released by the applied pressure on the diaphragm.
      (1) Applied pressure causes a proportional and linear change in electrical resistance.
      (2) Problems associated with strain gauges include drift due to temperature changes (departure from the real signal value), fragility, and cost.
   b. **Solid-state pressure transducer (semiconductor):** Composed of a silicon chip that undergoes electrical resistance changes because of the applied pressure.
      (1) Lower cost, accurate, and disposable.
      (2) Because of the miniature integration on the silicone chip, the circuitry necessary to minimize temperature drift is incorporated in the device.

4. Miniature transducer-tipped catheters are available that do not depend on fluid-filled lines for the transmission of pressure. Microtransducer catheters in general have better fidelity characteristics, but at a much higher cost than conventional fluid-filled systems and are currently not generally available for neonatal use.

5. The standard medical BP transducer output rating is 5 μV/V/mm Hg. The pressure monitor processes the electrical signal generated by the transducer and converts it to BP units in either millimeters of mercury or kilopascals, including generation of systolic, diastolic, and mean values. The monitor provides a user-friendly numerical and graphical display allowing beat-to-beat measurement of pressure and also allows analysis of the waveform. Analysis can be clinical (e.g., morphology, determining the position of the dicrotic notch or "swing" that can give information regarding filling status and cardiac output) or computerized.

C. Indications

To continuously monitor intravascular pressure

1. In very small or unstable infants, particularly those with severe hypotension, on inotropic support.
2. During major procedures that could cause or exacerbate cardiovascular instability.
3. To monitor infants on ventilator support or extracorporeal membrane oxygenation.
4. Allow frequent arterial blood sampling.

D. Contraindications

None absolute, except for those specific to catheter placement

E. Limitations

1. The pulse pressure waveform measured in the peripheral artery is narrower and taller than that in the proximal aorta. Thus, systolic BP in the peripheral arteries can read higher than that in proximal aorta. This amplification is greater in patients with increased vascular tone or on inotropic therapy.
2. Very small-diameter catheters may result in underreading of systolic BP.

F. Equipment

There are five components of the intra-arterial BP-monitoring system (**Figs. 10.4** and **10.5**). Commercial pressure-monitoring kits have most components integrated.

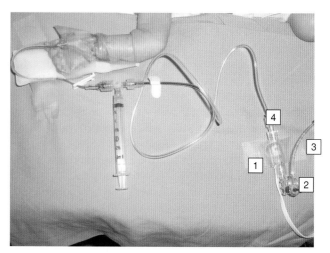

FIGURE 10.4 Representative disposable BP transducer setup. (*1*) Pressure transducer; (*2*) integral continuous flush device; (*3*) infusion port (connects to infusion pump); (*4*) high-pressure tubing.

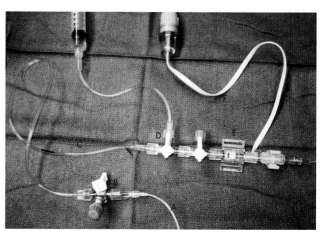

FIGURE 10.5 Disposable blood pressure transducer setup with closed-loop system for sampling. **A:** Umbilical arterial catheter. **B:** Stopcock with special valve to draw blood samples. **C:** High-pressure tubing. **D:** Stopcock attached to heparinized saline flush syringe. **E:** Stopcock for zeroing transducer. **F:** Pressure transducer. **G:** Transducer cable. **H:** Tubing with continuous heparinized saline infusion from infusion pump.

1. Intra-arterial catheter: May be an umbilical arterial catheter (Chapter 31) or peripheral arterial catheter (Chapter 33).
2. Pressure-monitoring tube: Fluid-filled tubing to couple arterial cannula to the pressure transducer. This tubing should be short (not to exceed 100 to 120 cm from the transducer to the patient connection) and stiff (low compliance to reduce damping of pressure wave). A three-way tap is incorporated in the tubing to allow the system to be zeroed and blood samples taken.
3. Pressure transducer with cable to signal processor.
4. Neonatal physiologic monitor (multiparameter-monitoring system).
   a. Minimum configuration should have the capability of displaying systolic, diastolic, and mean pressures and heart rate.

b. It should have provision for high and low alarm settings.

5. Mechanical infusion device (infusion pump) with syringe and tubing to deliver heparinized saline (usually 1 U heparin/mL of fluid at 1 mL/hr; in infants weighting less than 750 g, a rate of 0.8 mL/hr may be used through the umbilical arterial catheter). Pressurized IV bag should not be used.

6. Some disposable pressure-monitoring kits offer closed-loop systems for sampling (**Fig. 10.5**).
   a. The system employs a mechanism for aspirating and holding a fixed amount of blood in the pressure tubing rather than in a syringe.
   b. The distal end is equipped with a small chamber with a rubber septum that allows a self-guiding short blunt syringe adapter to penetrate and aspirate blood for the sample.
   c. The initial volume pulled back is sufficient to ensure that the blood drawn into the sample chamber is greater than the catheter/distal tubing volume and is not diluted by the fluid being infused. The absence of stopcocks at the distal end eliminates a possible site for contamination. In addition, the blood pulled back is conserved, and the amount of fluid used to flush the sample line is reduced.

G. Technique

For catheter placement, see Part 5 of the book, "Vascular Access."

1. Familiarize yourself with the bedside monitor and the pressure zero/calibration procedure. To maintain accuracy, the pressure transducer is exposed to atmospheric pressure to calibrate the reading to zero. This is done in several ways depending on the particular transducer.

2. If using discrete components, assemble the pressure-monitoring circuit, maintaining the sterile integrity.
   a. A basic circuit configuration will consist of a transducer dome, flush device, stopcock, pressure tubing, and an optional arterial extension set (short length of pressure tubing, <12 inches in length, inserted between the catheter and the pressure tubing).
   b. Ensure that all the Luer-Lock connections are tight and free of any defects.
   c. If possible, avoid the use of IV tubing components in the pressure-monitoring circuit.

3. Set up the infusion pump that will be used for the continuous infusion through the flush device. Continuous flush devices limit flow rates to 3 or 30 mL/hr, depending on the model (19–22). For neonatal arterial lines, the infusion pump supplying the flush device should be set to 0.5 to 3 mL/hr and should never exceed the flow rating of the flush device. When pump flow exceeds the flush device rating, it will cause an occlusion alarm in most IV pumps. A pump flow rate of 1 mL/hr is recommended for most arterial lines.

4. For circuit priming, use the solution that will be used for the continuous infusion. Prime the circuit slowly to avoid trapping air bubbles in the flush device inlet. Ensure that the entire circuit and all the ports are fluid filled and bubble free.

5. If using disposable transducers, connect the reusable interface cable to the transducer and to the monitor. Turn the monitor on.

6. Secure the transducer at the patient's reference level, defined as the midaxillary line (heart level). If using transducer holders, level the reference mark on the holder at the patient's reference level.

7. Connect the distal end of the circuit to the patient's catheter, ensuring that the catheter hub is filled with fluid and is bubble free.

8. Start the infusion pump. The pump rate cannot exceed the flow rate of the flush device.

9. Open the stopcock connected to the transducer to air (shut off to the patient, open to atmosphere).

10. Zero/calibrate the monitor according to the manufacturer's instructions.

11. Close the stopcock connected to the transducer (open to the patient).

12. Set the monitor pressure waveform scale to one that accommodates the entire pressure wave.

13. Observe the waveform obtained. If the wave appears to be damped (flattened, poorly defined, with slow rise time), check the circuit for air bubbles starting at the distal end (**Fig. 10.6**). If no air bubbles are detected, then gently flush the catheter.

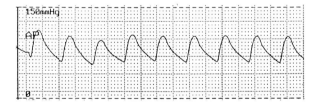

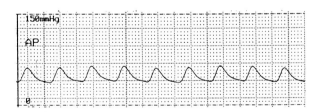

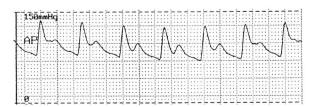

FIGURE 10.6 Arterial pressure waveforms: normal arterial waveform (**top**); dampened arterial waveform (**middle**); arterial waveform with spike caused by catheter whip or inappropriate tubing (**bottom**). (Note that figure demonstrates waveform appearance only and not actual pressure values.)

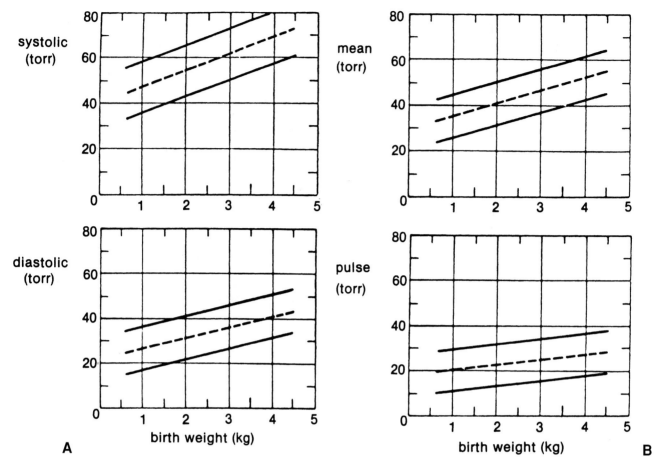

FIGURE 10.7 Pressures obtained by direct measurement through umbilical artery catheter in healthy newborn infants during first 12 hours of life. Broken lines represent linear regressions; solid lines represent 95% confidence limits. **A:** Systolic pressure (**top**) and diastolic pressure (**bottom**). **B:** Mean aortic pressure (**top**) and pulse pressure (systolic–diastolic pressure amplitude) (**bottom**). (Reprinted with permission from Versmold HT, Kitterman JA, Phibbs RH, et al. Aortic blood pressure during the first 12 hours of life in infants with birth weight 610 to 4,220 grams. *Pediatrics*. 1981;67(5):607–613. Copyright © 1981 by the AAP.)

14. Once a stable pressure reading is obtained, set the alarm limits. Mean arterial pressure value is optimally used to set alarm limits (**Fig. 10.7**).
15. Zero the transducer every 8 hours.
16. When blood samples are drawn from the line, flushing should be done gently with a syringe using a minimal amount of heparinized saline solution.

H. Complications (Table 10.3)

1. Defective transducer
2. Cracked Luer-Lock connections, causing leaks, low pressure readings, or blood to back up in the line
3. Air bubbles in the line
4. Malfunctioning infusion pump not providing continuous flush, causing the line to clot off
5. Defective reusable transducer interface cable (disposable transducer system)

6. Erroneous readings caused by the transducer not being properly set at the patient's reference level. Lower readings occur when the transducer is high; higher readings occur when the transducer is lower than the patient's reference level.
7. Problems associated with catheters
8. Tip of the catheter lodging against the wall of the vessel (will cause the pressure wave to flatten and the pressure to rise slowly as a result of the continuous infusion)
9. Transducer not zeroed to atmosphere (static pressure trapped by stopcock valve and a syringe stuck in the port that should be opened to air). This will cause lower or negative pressure readings.
10. Loss of blood if stopcock is left open and third port is not capped
11. Fluid overload if a pressurized IV bag is used instead of an infusion pump and the fast flush mode is used to clear the line (20)

TABLE 10.3 Trouble-Shooting for Intravascular Pressure Monitoring

PROBLEM	CAUSE	PREVENTION	TREATMENT
Damped pressure tracing	Catheter tip against vessel wall	Usually unavoidable	Reposition catheter while observing waveform
	Partial occlusion of catheter tip by clot	Use continuous infusion of normal saline or ½ normal saline with 1 Unit heparin/mL of fluid	Remove line if possible. If line removal is not an option, then aspirate clot with syringe and flush with heparinized saline
	Clotting in stopcock or transducer, or blood in system	Flush catheter carefully after blood withdrawal and re-establish continuous infusion; back-flush stopcocks to remove blood	Change components
Abnormally high or low readings	Change in transducer level. A 10 cm change in height will alter the pressure reading by 7.5 mm Hg. Note: If the cannula is inserted into the radial artery, raising the hand will not affect the measurement as long as the transducer is maintained level with the heart[a]	Maintain the transducer at the same level as the patient's heart	Recheck patient and transducer positions
	Leaks in transducer system	Assemble transducer carefully, ensuring that dome is attached snugly; use Luer-Lock fittings and disposable stopcocks	Check all fittings, transducer dome, and stopcock connections
	External vascular compression	Secure catheter firmly without putting tape circumferentially on extremity	Loosen tape, securing catheter in place
	Strained transducer	Attention to stopcocks when aspirating to module	Replace transducer
	High intrathoracic pressure secondary to mechanical ventilation; reduces venous return and cardiac output	Be aware of problem	Use minimal amount of mean airway pressure required to achieve optimal ventilation
Damped pressure without improvement after flushing	Air bubbles in transducer connector tubing	Flush transducer and tubing carefully when setting up system and attaching to catheter; handle system carefully	Check system, rapid flush, attach syringe to transducer, and aspirate bubble
No pressure reading available	Transducer not open to catheter or settings on monitor amplifiers incorrect–still on zero, cal, or off	Follow routine, systematic steps for setting up system and pressure measurements	Check system–stopcocks, monitor, and amplifier setup

[a]Data from Ward M, Langton JA. Blood pressure measurement. *Cont Edu Anaesth Crit Care Pain*. 2007;7(4):122–126.

References

1. Nuntnarumit P, Yang W, Bada-Ellzey HS. Blood pressure measurements in the newborn. *Clin Perinatol*. 1999;26(4):981–986.
2. Seri I, Evans J. Controversies in the diagnosis and management of hypotension in the newborn infant. *Curr Opin Pediatr*. 2001;13:116–123.
3. Short BL, Van Meurs K, Evans JR; Cardiology Group. Summary proceedings from the cardiology group on cardiovascular instability in preterm infants. *Pediatrics*. 2006;117(3 Pt 2):S34–S39.
4. de Boode WP. Clinical monitoring of systemic hemodynamics in critically ill newborns. *Early Hum Dev*. 2010;86(3):137–141.
5. Ogedegbe G, Pickering T. Principles and techniques of blood pressure measurement. *Cardiol Clin*. 2010;28(4):571–586.

6. Stebor AD. Basic principles of noninvasive blood pressure measurement in infants. *Adv Neonatal Care.* 2005;5(5):252–261.

7. Pickering TG, Hall JE, Appel LJ, et al. Recommendations for blood pressure measurement in humans and experimental animals: Part 1: blood pressure measurement in humans: a statement for professionals from the Subcommittee of Professional and Public Education of the American Heart Association Council on High Blood Pressure Research. *Hypertension.* 2005;45(1):142–161.

8. O'Shea J, Dempsey EM. A comparison of blood pressure measurements in newborns. *Am J Perinatol.* 2009;26(2): 113–116.

9. Dasnadi S, Aliaga S, Laughon M, et al. Factors influencing the accuracy of noninvasive blood pressure measurements in NICU infants. *Am J Perinatol.* 2015;32(7):639–644.

10. Lalan S, Blowey D. Comparison between oscillometric and intra-arterial blood pressure measurements in ill preterm and full-term neonates. *J Am Soc Hypertens.* 2014;8(1):36–44.

11. Alpert BS, Quinn D, Gallick D. Oscillometric blood pressure: a review for clinicians. *J Am Soc Hypertens.* 2014;8(12): 930–938.

12. Troy R, Doron M, Laughon M, et al. Comparison of noninvasive and central arterial blood pressure measurements in ELBW infants. *J Perinatol.* 2009;29(11):744–749.

13. Takci S, Yigit S, Korkmaz A, et al. Comparison between oscillometric and invasive blood pressure measurements in critically ill premature infants. *Acta Paediatr.* 2012;101(2):132–135.

14. Dannevig I, Dale HC, Liestol K, et al. Blood pressure in the neonate: three non-invasive oscillometric pressure monitors compared with invasively measured blood pressure. *Acta Paediatrica.* 2005;94(2):191–196.

15. Meyer S, Sander J, Gräber S, et al. Agreement of invasive versus non-invasive blood pressure in preterm neonates is not dependent on birth weight or gestational age. *J Paediatr Child Health.* 2010;46(5):249–254.

16. Engle WD. Blood pressure in the very low birth weight neonate. *Early Hum Dev.* 2001;62(2):97–130.

17. Weindling AM, Bentham J. Blood pressure in the neonate. *Acta Paediatr.* 2005;94(2):138–140.

18. Vesoulis ZA, El Ters NM, Wallendorf M, et al. Empirical estimation of the normative blood pressure in infants <28 weeks gestation using a massive data approach. *J Perinatol.* 2016;36(4): 291–295.

19. Morray J, Todd S. A hazard of continuous flush systems for vascular pressure monitoring in infants. *Anesthesiology.* 1983;58:187–189.

20. Barbeito A, Mark JB. Arterial and central venous pressure monitoring. *Anesthesiol Clin.* 2006;24(4):717–735.

21. Pinsky MR. Functional hemodynamic monitoring. *Crit Care Clin.* 2015;31(1):89–111.

22. Romagnoli S, Romano SM, Bevilacqua S, et al. Dynamic response of liquid-filled catheter systems for measurement of blood pressure: precision of measurements and reliability of the Pressure Recording Analytical Method with different disposable systems. *J Crit Care.* 2011;26(4):415–422.

11

Continuous Blood Gas Monitoring

M. Kabir Abubakar

Adequate monitoring of oxygenation and acid base status is an important and necessary component in the management of critically ill neonates in the intensive care unit. This provides information that is fundamental to the diagnosis of respiratory and metabolic disorders and to assess the effect of therapeutic interventions. Traditionally, arterial blood gas analysis has been used as the gold standard because it provides data on hydrogen ion content of the blood (pH), arterial oxygen tension (PaO_2), partial pressure of carbon dioxide ($PaCO_2$), a calculation of the bicarbonate ion (HCO_3), and base deficit. However, arterial blood gas sampling requires invasive procedures and provides only intermittent data. There are now noninvasive methods including pulse oximetry, transcutaneous PO_2 and CO_2 monitoring, and interesting developments in continuous intra-arterial blood gas analysis (in those patients who already have an indwelling arterial catheter) that supplement traditional intermittent blood gas analysis. These provide real-time continuous dynamic data on the patient's respiratory status, thus can be used to provide early warning and immediately evaluate the efficacy of clinical interventions in the NICU.

PULSE OXIMETRY

Pulse oximetry has remained the most common method of continuous oxygen monitoring in clinical care. It is noninvasive, easy to use, readily available, and able to provide continuous monitoring of arterial oxygen saturations and pulse rate.

A. Definitions

1. Arterial oxyhemoglobin saturation measured by arterial blood gas analysis is referred to as SaO_2.
2. Arterial oxyhemoglobin saturation measured noninvasively by transcutaneous pulse oximetry is referred to as SpO_2.

B. Background

1. Principles of oxygen transport
   a. Approximately 98% of the oxygen in the blood is bound to hemoglobin.

   The amount of oxygen content in the blood is related directly to the amount of hemoglobin in the blood, amount of oxygen bound to the hemoglobin, and to the partial pressure of unbound, dissolved oxygen in the blood (PaO_2) (1). The relationship of arterial PO_2, in near-term infants, to percent saturation measured by pulse oximetry is shown in **Figure 11.1**.

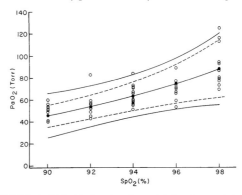

FIGURE 11.1 Individual PaO_2 values for each infant (*empty circles*) at each studied SpO_2 plus mean (*solid circles*) and 95% prediction limits (*solid lines*) at each SpO_2: *Broken lines* represent estimated 2 SD limits for PaO_2 at studied SpO_2 values based on shape of oxyhemoglobin dissociation curve and PaO_2 versus SpO_2 data from normal preterm infants. (Reprinted from Brockway J, Hay WW Jr. Prediction of arterial partial pressure of oxygen with pulse oxygen saturation measurements. *J Pediatr.* 1998;133(1):63-66. © 1998 Elsevier. With permission.)

   b. The relationship between blood PaO_2 and the amount of oxygen bound to hemoglobin is presented graphically as an oxygen–hemoglobin affinity curve (**Fig. 11.2**). Percent oxygen saturation is calculated using the formula

$$\frac{Oxyhemoglobin}{Oxhyhemoglobin + Deoxyhemoglobin} \times 100$$

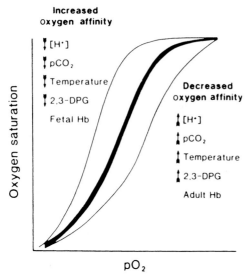

FIGURE 11.2 Factors affecting hemoglobin–oxygen affinity. 2,3-DPG, 2,3-diphosphoglycerate. (Reprinted by permission from Nature: Hay WW Jr. Physiology of oxygenation and its relation to pulse oximetry in neonates. *J Perinatol*. 1987;7(4):309–319. Copyright © 1987 Springer Nature.)

2. Principles of pulse oximetry
   a. Based on the principles of spectrophotometric oximetry and plethysmography (2).
   b. Arterial saturation and pulse rate are determined by measuring the absorption of selected wavelengths of light.

   Oxygenated hemoglobin (oxyhemoglobin) and reduced hemoglobin (deoxyhemoglobin) absorb light as known functions of wavelengths. By measuring the absorption levels at different wavelengths of light, the relative percentages of these two constituents and SpO_2 are calculated.
   c. A sensor composed of two light-emitting diodes (LEDs) as light sources and one photodetector as a light receiver is employed. The photodetector is an electronic device that produces a current proportional to the incident light intensity (2,3).

   There are two methods of sending light through the measuring site: transmission and reflectance. In the transmission method, the emitter and photodetector are opposite of each other with the measuring site in between. In the reflectance method, the emitter and photodetector are next to each other on the measuring site. The light bounces from the emitter to the detector across the measuring site. The transmission method is the most common type used and is discussed here.
   (1) One LED emits red light with an approximate wavelength of 660 nm.
      Red light is absorbed selectively by deoxyhemoglobin.

   (2) The other LED emits infrared light with an approximate wavelength of 925 nm.
      Infrared light is absorbed selectively by oxyhemoglobin.
   d. The different absorption of the wavelengths when transmitted through tissue, pulsatile blood, and nonpulsatile blood are utilized (**Fig. 11.3**).

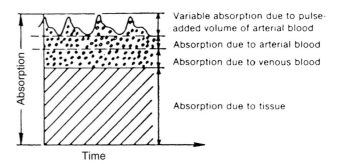

FIGURE 11.3 Tissue composite showing dynamic as well as static components affecting light absorption. (Reprinted by permission from Springer: Wukitch MW, Petterson MT, Tobler DR, et al. Pulse oximetry: Analysis of theory, technology and practice. *J Clin Monit*. 1988;4(4):290–301. Copyright © 1988 Little, Brown and Company.)

   (1) The photodetector measures the level of light that passes through without being absorbed.
   (2) During the absence of pulse (diastole), the detector establishes baseline levels for the wavelength absorption of tissue and nonpulsatile blood.
   (3) With each heartbeat, a pulse of oxygenated blood flows to the sensor site.
   (4) Absorption during systole of both the red and the infrared light is measured to determine the percentage of oxyhemoglobin.
   (5) Because the measurements of the change in absorption are made during a pulse (systole), these pulses are counted and displayed as pulse rate. In addition, the pulse oximeter also displays a plethysmographic waveform which can help clinicians distinguish an artifactual signal from the true signal.

C. Indications

1. Noninvasive continuous or intermittent arterial oxygen saturation and heart rate monitoring
2. To monitor oxygenation in infants suffering from conditions associated with
   a. Hypoxia
   b. Apnea/hypoventilation
   c. Cardiorespiratory disease
   d. Bronchopulmonary dysplasia

3. To monitor response to therapy
   a. Resuscitation
      Pulse oximetry is a necessary adjunct to monitoring in the delivery room. With the use of pulse oximetry, SpO$_2$ values can be obtained within 1 minute after birth (**Fig. 11.4**) (4–8)

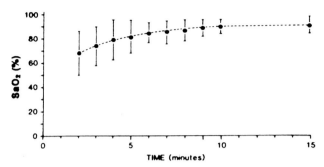

FIGURE 11.4 Mean arterial oxygen saturation (S$_a$O$_2$) values measured by pulse oximetry from the time of cord clamping. Values are means ± SD. (Reprinted by permission from Springer: House JT, Schultetus RR, Gravenstein N. Continuous neonatal evaluation in the delivery room by pulse oximetry. *J Clin Monit*. 1987;3(2):96–100. Copyright © 1987 Little, Brown and Company, Inc.)

   b. Monitoring effectiveness of positive pressure ventilation or during placement of an endotracheal tube
4. To monitor side effects of other therapy
   a. Endotracheal tube suctioning
   b. Positioning for laryngoscopy, spinal tap, and other procedures
5. For extremely low–birth-weight infants <1,000 g (9–11)
   It is optimal to use pulse oximetry for oxygen monitoring in the very low–birth-weight infant because of its noninvasiveness. Pulse oximetry can be used reliably in very low–birth-weight infants with acute as well as chronic lung disease (9–11).
6. Pulse oximetry also offers an advantage for precise fraction of inspired oxygen (F$_I$O$_2$) control during neonatal anesthesia because of the short response time to changes in SpO$_2$ (10).
7. Screening tool for critical congenital heart disease and infant car seat testing in the newborn

D. Limitations

1. Decreased accuracy when arterial saturation is <65%.
   Pulse oximetry will overestimate SpO$_2$ at this level; therefore, blood gas confirmation is imperative (9–11).
2. Not a sensitive indicator for hyperoxemia (10).

Pulse oximeter accuracy does not allow for precise estimation of PaO$_2$ at saturations >90%. Small changes in O$_2$ saturation (1% to 2%) may be associated with large changes in PaO$_2$ (6 to 12 mm Hg) (10).

3. Because pulse oximeters rely on pulsatile fluctuations in transmitted light intensity to estimate SpO$_2$, they are all adversely affected by movement (9–11).
   In some cases, the pulse oximeter may calculate an SpO$_2$ value for signals caused by movement, or it may reject the signal and not update the display. Usually, pulse rate output from the oximeter will reflect the detection of nonarterial pulsations, indicating either "0" saturation or "low-quality signal" (3). Advances in microprocessor technology have led to improved signal processing, which makes it possible to minimize motion artifact and monitor saturation more accurately during motion or low-perfusion states (10).
4. Significant levels of carboxyhemoglobin or methemoglobin can yield erroneous readings (carboxyhemoglobin absorbs light at the 660-nm wavelength). However, carboxyhemoglobin levels of <3% will not affect the accuracy of the instrument.
5. SpO$_2$ may be overestimated in darkly pigmented infants although this is not always consistent (10–13).
6. Erroneous readings can occur in the presence of high fetal hemoglobin (14).
   A smaller effect on accuracy is noted when fetal hemoglobin levels are <50% (14). With a predominance of fetal hemoglobin, an SpO$_2$ of >92% may be associated with hyperoxemia (14). However, whereas saturations may appear adequate, PaO$_2$ may be low enough to produce increased pulmonary vascular resistance (SpO$_2$/PaO$_2$ curve shift to the left).
   Infants with chronic lung disease and prolonged oxygen dependence are older and have less fetal hemoglobin; therefore, SpO$_2$ readings obtained from these patients may be more accurate than those obtained from neonates with acute respiratory disorders at an earlier age (14). The same situation exists in infants who have undergone exchange transfusion because of decreased levels of fetal hemoglobin.
7. Light sources that can affect performance include surgical lights, xenon lights, bilirubin lamps, fluorescent lights, infrared heating lamps, and direct sunlight.
   Although jaundice does not account for variability in pulse oximeter accuracy (15), phototherapy can interfere with accurate monitoring. Therefore, appropriate precautions should be taken, such as covering the probe with a relatively opaque material (1).
8. Do not correlate SpO$_2$ values with laboratory hemoximeters (15).
   Most laboratory oximeters measure fractional oxygen saturation (all hemoglobin including dysfunctional

hemoglobin) as opposed to functional oxygen saturation (oxyhemoglobin and deoxyhemoglobin excluding all dysfunctional hemoglobin).

Use of normal adult values for hemoglobin, 2,3-diphosphoglycerate, and, in some cases, $PaCO_2$ can lead to errors in the algorithm used to calculate SaO_2 with some blood gas analysis instruments (15).

9. Although pulse oximeters can detect hyperoxemia, it is important that type-specific alarm limits are set to avoid hypo or hyperoxemia (2,16).

10. Pulse oximeters rely on detecting pulsatile flow in body tissues; therefore, a reduction in peripheral pulsatile blood flow produced by peripheral vasoconstriction results in an inadequate signal for analysis (2). Some oximeters can provide a pulsatility index to indicate the degree of tissue perfusion in the extremity.

11. Pulse oximeters average their readings over several seconds depending on oximeter type and internal algorithm settings. Oximeters with a long averaging time may not be able to detect acute and transient changes in SpO_2 (3).

12. Venous congestion may produce venous pulsations, which can produce low readings.

13. The pulse oximeter only provides information about oxygenation. It does not give any indication of the patient's carbon dioxide elimination.

In summary, it is optimal to make some correlation between SpO_2 and PaO_2 throughout a reasonable range of SpO_2 (lower, 85% to 88%; higher, 95% to 97%) before relying completely on SpO_2 for oxygen and/or respirator management (14,16).

E. Equipment

1. Manufacturer-specific sensor and monitor with
   a. Display of SpO_2 and pulse rate and a pulse indicator
   b. Adjustable alarm limits for SpO_2 and pulse rate
   c. Battery-powered operation
2. Neonatal sensor, either disposable or reusable
   a. Disposable sensors have become the standard for infection and quality control
   b. Disposable neonatal sensors are available in different sizes, depending on the site to be used

F. Precautions

1. Use only with detectable pulse.
   Cardiopulmonary bypass with nonpulsating flow, inflated blood pressure cuff proximal to the sensor, tense peripheral edema, hypothermia, low-perfusion state secondary to shock or severe hypovolemia, and

significant peripheral vasoconstriction may interfere with obtaining accurate readings (9).

2. Assess the sensor site every 3 to 4 hours to be certain that the adherent bandage is not constricting the site and that the skin is intact.
3. Whenever possible, the SpO_2 sensor should not be on the same extremity as the blood pressure cuff.
   When the cuff is inflated, the SpO_2 sensor will not detect a pulse, will not update SpO_2 values, and will alarm.
4. Malpositioned sensor: When a probe is not placed symmetrically, it can allow some light from the LED emitters to reach the photodetector in the sensor without going through the tissue at the monitoring site and will therefore produce falsely low readings. This is called the penumbra effect.
5. To avoid possible transfer of infection most pulse oximetry probes are single patient use only although there are probes designed to be cleaned and reused, follow manufacturer's instructions for the particular probe being used.

G. Technique

1. Familiarize yourself with the system before proceeding.
2. Select an appropriate sensor and apply it to the patient.
   a. Finger, toe, lateral side of the foot, across the palm of the hand or wrist. (Placing the sensor in a position matching that of the arterial line, if present, may avoid discrepancies caused by intracardiac or ductal shunts when trying to correlate SpO_2 with arterial PaO_2, i.e., match a postductal arterial line with a postductal pulse oximetry position.)
   b. For neonates 500 g to 3 kg, anterolateral aspect of a foot (**Fig. 11.5**) (1).

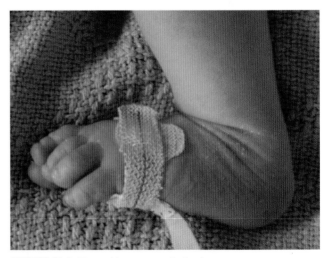

FIGURE 11.5 Disposable sensor applied to foot.

c. For infants weighing >3 kg, use the palm, wrist, thumb, great toe, or index finger (1).

d. Align the LEDs (light source) and the detector so they are directly opposite each other.

e. Reusable sensors should be applied with nonadhesive elastic wrap.

f. Tighten sensor snugly to the skin but not so as to impede circulation. The probe should then be left in place for several seconds until extremity movement stops and the signal is stable.

g. Secure the sensor to the site to prevent tugging or movement of the sensor independent of the body part.

h. Cover the sensor to reduce the effect of intense light levels, direct sunlight, or phototherapy.

3. Attach the sensor to the system interconnecting cable and turn on the monitor (Attaching the sensor to the baby before connecting the cable to the monitor that is already turned on will shorten the time taken for data acquisition and display of SpO_2 information.) (6).

4. Modern pulse oximeters have internal system autocalibration during start-up; so no other calibration is needed.

5. After a short interval, if all connections are correct, the monitor will display the pulse detected by the sensor. If the pulse level is adequate, it will display SpO_2 and pulse rate. If the pulse indicator is not synchronous with the patient's pulse rate, reposition the probe. After repositioning the sensor, if the pulse detector is still not indicating properly, change the sensor site and ensure that there is adequate perfusion to the site.

6. Once reliable operation is achieved, set the high and low alarm limits for SpO_2.

a. Although pulse oximeters can detect hyperoxemia, it is important that type-specific alarm limits are set and a low specificity is accepted (16,17). Alarm limits are determined by gestational age, presence of acute or chronic lung disease, cardiac disease, and risk of retinopathy of prematurity (18).

b. The optimal alarm limit, defined as having a sensitivity of 95% or more, associated with maximal specificity, will differ depending on which particular monitor is used.

Note that SpO_2 is a more sensitive indicator of hypoxemia and decreased tissue oxygenation than is PaO_2. Lower alarm limits should be individualized to alert the user when the oxygenation requirements of the given patient are not met.

H. Complications

1. Management based on erroneous readings caused by a misapplied sensor or conditions affecting instrument performance.

2. Limb ischemia if sensor applied too tightly, particularly in an extremely preterm infant or an edematous limb.

TRANSCUTANEOUS BLOOD GAS MONITORING

Transcutaneous measurements of oxygen and carbon dioxide are useful in the neonatal intensive care unit because they provide continuous and relatively noninvasive estimation of these parameters to supplement arterial blood gas measurements.

A. Definitions

1. Transcutaneous measurement of oxygen is referred to as $P_{tc}O_2$.

2. Transcutaneous measurement of carbon dioxide is referred to as $P_{tc}CO_2$.

B. Purpose

1. Noninvasive blood gas monitoring of PO_2 and PCO_2
2. Trending of PO_2 and PCO_2 over time

C. Background

1. Transcutaneous monitoring measures skin-surface PO_2 and PCO_2 to provide estimates of arterial partial pressure of oxygen and carbon dioxide. The devices increase tissue perfusion by heating the skin and then electrochemically measuring the partial pressure of oxygen and carbon dioxide.

2. Accomplished by two electrodes contained in a heated block that maintains the electrodes and the skin directly beneath it at a constant temperature (**Fig. 11.6**) (19).

a. Arterialized capillary oxygen levels are more accurately measured by heating the skin to establish hyperemia directly beneath the sensor.

b. The electrodes are covered with an electrolyte solution and sealed with a semipermeable plastic membrane.

3. A modified Clark electrode is used to measure oxygen.

a. It produces an electrical current that is proportional to PO_2.

b. Measured current is converted to PO_2 and then corrected for temperature.

4. A Severinghaus-type electrode is used to measure CO_2.

a. pH-sensitive glass electrode.

b. CO_2 diffuses from the skin surface through the membrane. The CO_2 changes the pH of the electrolyte solution bathing the electrode.

c. The measured pH is converted to PCO_2 and then corrected for temperature.

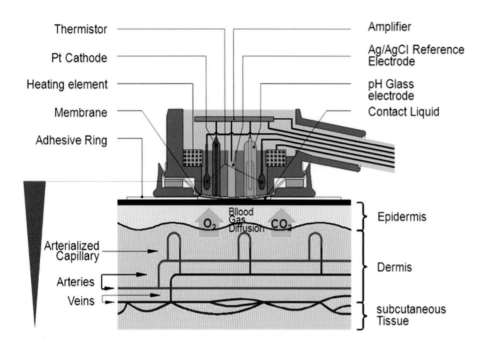

FIGURE 11.6 Principle of cutaneous PO_2 measurement by heated oxygen sensor. Cross section of cutaneous oxygen sensor (©2015 Radiometer Medical ApS and HemoCue AB. All rights reserved).

Conversion of electric current and pH to PO_2 and PCO_2, respectively, is based on conversion equations adjusted by a two-point calibration. This is part of the setup and calibration process.

D. Indications

1. To approximate arterial PaO_2 and $PaCO_2$ for respiratory management (19)
   a. To monitor the effect of therapeutic ventilatory maneuvers particularly in infants who have combined oxygenation and ventilation problems
   b. For stabilization and monitoring during transport
2. To reduce the frequency of arterial blood gas analysis (19,20)
3. To determine by a noninvasive and continuous method the regional arterial oxygen tension (19,20)
4. To infer regional arterial blood flow (e.g., in the lower limbs of infants with duct-dependent coarctation of the aorta) (19,20)

E. Contraindications

1. Skin disorders (e.g., epidermolysis bullosa, staphylococcal scalded skin syndrome)
2. Relative contraindications
   a. The extremely low–birth-weight infant (19,20)
   b. Severe acidosis
   c. Significant anemia
   d. Decreased peripheral perfusion
   e. $P_{tc}O_2$ may underestimate PaO_2 (19,20)

F. Equipment—Specifications

1. Transcutaneous monitor components
   a. Dual electrode
   b. Electrode cleaning kit
   c. Electrolyte and membrane kit
   d. Contact solution
   e. Double-sided adhesive rings
   f. Calibration gas cylinders with delivery apparatus
2. Digital display shows values for $P_{tc}O_2$, $P_{tc}CO_2$, and site of sensor (**Fig. 11.7**)

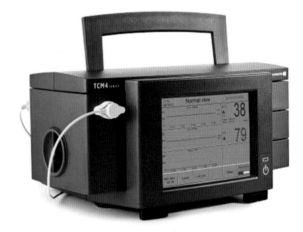

FIGURE 11.7 Combined transcutaneous PO_2/PCO_2 and SpO_2 monitor. (Courtesy of Radiometer.)

Monitor with controls for both high and low alarm limits, and for electrode temperature. The monitor may also have a site placement timer that will alarm as an indication to change the site of the electrode.

G. Precautions

1. Be aware that
   a. Equilibration requires approximately 20 minutes after the electrode is placed, with the response time for $P_{tc}O_2$ being much faster than that for $P_{tc}CO_2$. Therefore, management changes based on transcutaneous values should be guided by values that have been consistent for at least 5 minutes.
   b. Periodic correlation with PO_2 from appropriate arterial sites is recommended (19,20).
   c. $P_{tc}O_2$ may underestimate PaO_2 in the infant with hyperoxemia (PaO_2 >100 mm Hg), with reliability of $P_{tc}O_2$ measurement decreasing as PaO_2 increases (19,20).
   d. $P_{tc}O_2$ may underestimate PaO_2 in older infants with bronchopulmonary dysplasia (21,22).
   e. Pressure on the sensor (e.g., infant lying on sensor) may restrict blood supply, resulting in falsely low $P_{tc}O_2$ values.
   f. Manufacturers' parts are not interchangeable. Only supplies of the same brand and designated for the monitor should be used.
2. To avoid skin burns, change electrode location *at least* every 4 hours.
3. $P_{tc}O_2$ may underestimate PaO_2 in the presence of
   a. Severe acidosis.
   b. Severe anemia.
   c. Decreased peripheral perfusion.

H. Technique

1. Familiarize yourself with the system before proceeding.
2. Perform routine electrode maintenance, if there is any question as to the status of the electrode.
   a. Remove the membrane, rinse the electrode with deionized water, and dry with a soft lint-free tissue or gauze.
   b. Clean the electrode using the solution provided in the cleaning kit; abrasive compounds or materials should never be used (they will permanently damage the electrode).
   c. Rinse the electrode with deionized water, and dry with lint-free tissue.
   d. Apply the electrolyte solution.
   e. Place a new membrane on the electrode. Avoid finger contact, and always handle the membrane inside its protective package or with plastic tweezers.
3. Perform two-point gas calibration using the device-specific apparatus, as per manufacturer's instruction.
4. Use an alcohol pad to clean and degrease the skin site where the sensor is to be placed.
5. Apply double-sided adhesive ring to the sensor.

6. Apply one drop of contact solution to the skin site.
7. Peel the protective backing from the adhesive ring, place the sensor on the skin over the contact solution, and press the sensor to the skin.
   a. For best results, place the sensor on a location with good blood flow.
      (1) Appropriate sites include the lateral abdomen, anterior or lateral chest, volar aspect of the forearm, inner upper arm, inner thigh, or posterior chest (**Fig. 11.8**) (21).

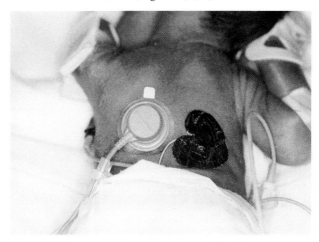

FIGURE 11.8 Cutaneous PO$_2$/PCO$_2$ sensor applied to the back.

   (2) Although large differences between pre- and postductal PaO_2 values are uncommon in premature infants with hyaline membrane disease, preductal location of the electrode is optimal for prevention of hyperoxemia (22).
   b. Choose a site devoid of hair.
   c. Avoid bony prominences.
   d. Avoid areas with large surface blood vessels (**Fig. 11.8**).
8. Secure the sensor cable to prevent tugging of the electrode when the cable is manipulated.
9. Allow 15 to 20 minutes for site equilibration before taking readings.
10. Note the time at which the sensor was placed on the skin, so that the site can be changed after a 4-hour period (maximum site time). When changing the sensor site:
    a. Use an alcohol pad to help loosen the adhesive and peel gently from the skin.
    b. Inspect the skin site for signs of sensitivity to heat or to the adhesive. In the event of skin irritation, either lower the sensor temperature or change the site more frequently; mild erythema after sensor removal is typical.
    c. Peel adhesive ring off the sensor.
    d. Flush the membrane surface with deionized water.
    e. Gently blot excess water and dry the sensor.
    f. Recalibrate if instructed to do so by the manufacturer's guidelines.
       Most manufacturers recommend recalibration every 4 to 8 hours.

TABLE 11.1 Poor Correlation of $P_{tc}O_2$ and PaO_2

PROBLEM	TECHNICAL SOLUTION	CLINICAL
$P_{tc}O_2 < PaO_2$ 1. Improper calibration 2. Insufficient warm-up period after electrode application 3. Insufficient heating temperature	1. Recalibrate 2. Allow longer warm-up period 3. Increase heating temperature	1. Presence of shock 2. Use with high-dose dopamine 3. Obstructive heart disease with hypoperfusion 4. Edema 5. Severe hypothermia
$P_{tc}O_2 > PaO_2$ 1. Improper calibration 2. Reading taken immediately after electrode application 3. Air bubble beneath membrane or leak to atmosphere 4. Excessive heating temperature	1. Recalibrate 2. Allow longer warm-up period 3. Reapply electrode 4. Attempt calibration at lower temperature	1. Right-to-left ductal shunt with preductal electrode and postductal arterial sample

11. Remember that response time for gas measurements is slow and values will not always immediately reflect physiologic changes.
    a. Average 90% response time for O_2 is 15 to 20 seconds.
    b. Average 90% response time for CO_2 is 60 to 90 seconds.
12. Complications.
13. Skin blisters or burns (23).
14. Management based on erroneous readings if the unit was not calibrated properly or site precautions were not adhered to (Table 11.1).

CONTINUOUS UMBILICAL ARTERY PO$_2$ MONITORING (24,25)

The following method for monitoring PO$_2$ and the subsequent method for monitoring blood gases are included for completeness. The editors are not aware of any current commercial source of the equipment in the United States.

A. Purpose

1. Continuous arterial PO$_2$ monitoring from the umbilical artery.
   Continuous PaO$_2$ monitoring through the umbilical artery offers a means for determining precise data on a continuous basis.
2. Trending of PaO$_2$ over time.

B. Background

1. Dual-purpose biluminal catheter.
   a. A miniature polarographic bipolar oxygen electrode is incorporated into the tip of a bilumen umbilical catheter.

   b. The small lumen contains the wires for the electrode.
   c. The larger lumen can be used for blood sampling, infusion, blood pressure monitoring, and sampling for instrument calibration.
   d. The electrode is covered by a gas-permeable membrane, under which is a layer of dried electrolyte. The probe is packed dry and is then activated before use. Water vapor from the activating (hydrating) solution diffuses through the membrane to form a thin layer of liquid electrolyte on the surface of the electrode.
   e. While it is in the artery, the electrode will produce an electrical current proportional to the PO$_2$ in the blood.
   f. The device is calibrated to the PO$_2$ value obtained from a blood sample drawn from the catheter.

C. Contraindications

1. Previous history of or evidence of compromise to the vascular supply of the lower extremities or the buttock area
2. History of previous complications related to an umbilical arterial line
3. Peritonitis
4. Necrotizing enterocolitis
5. Omphalitis
6. Omphalocele

D. Equipment

Previously commercially available monitoring systems have been withdrawn from the market recently because of high production costs.

E. Precautions

See also Chapter 31.

1. This specialized catheter is stiffer and has a wider outer diameter than other umbilical artery catheters. There is the theoretical possibility of a higher rate of failure to insert the catheter and potential increase in rates of vascular injury and thrombosis.
2. Failure to insert this catheter does not imply that insertion of other arterial catheters will be unsuccessful.
3. The electrode may fail to activate or may lose activation.
4. The catheter should be removed slowly to ensure that physiologic vasospasm occurs with removal.

F. Technique

1. Use sterile procedure.
2. Prepare the catheter according to the manufacturer's instructions.
3. 4-Fr catheters are recommended for infants weighing <1,500 g.
4. The technique for placement/insertion is the same as that used for the placement of conventional umbilical artery catheters (see Chapter 31).
5. Verify catheter position by radiography.
6. Draw blood sample for calibration.
7. Calibrate the monitor according to the manufacturer's instructions.

G. Complications

Same as for umbilical artery catheterization. See Chapter 31.

CONTINUOUS UMBILICAL ARTERY PO_2, PCO_2, pH, AND TEMPERATURE BLOOD GAS MONITORING (26–32)

A. Purpose

1. Continuous arterial blood gas monitoring from the umbilical artery.

    Continuous blood gas monitoring through the umbilical artery offers a means for determining precise data on a continuous basis.
2. Trending of blood gas data over time.

B. Background

1. A very thin, multiparameter, single-use disposable fiberoptic sensor

    a. Measures pH, PCO_2, PO_2, and temperature directly
    b. Introduced into the bloodstream via the umbilical artery catheter
    c. Port allows blood sampling, blood pressure monitoring, and drug infusion
2. Calculated parameters include bicarbonate, base excess, and oxygen saturation
3. Delivers continuous ventilation, oxygenation, and acid balance information, while also conserving blood volume by reducing blood sampling

C. Contraindications

1. Previous history or evidence of compromise to the vascular supply of the lower extremity or the buttock area
2. History of previous complications related to an umbilical arterial line
3. Peritonitis
4. Necrotizing enterocolitis
5. Omphalitis
6. Omphalocele

D. Equipment

Previously commercially available monitoring systems have been withdrawn from the market recently because of high production costs.

E. Precautions

1. The fiberoptic sensor may fail as a result of excessive kinking during sensor insertion into the umbilical artery catheter.
2. The sensor should be removed slowly to ensure that there is no microthrombus release if heparinization of the catheter was suboptimal.
3. See also Chapter 31.

F. Technique

1. Use sterile procedure.
2. Insert umbilical artery catheter (see Chapter 31).
3. Verify catheter position by radiography.
4. Calibrate sensor following the manufacturer's instructions.
5. Introduce the sensor into the umbilical artery catheter following the manufacturer's instructions.

G. Complications

Same as for umbilical artery catheterization; see Chapter 31.

References

1. Hay WW. Physiology of oxygenation and its relation to pulse oximetry in neonates. *J Perinatol.* 1987;7:309–319.

2. Tin W, Lal M. Principles of pulse oximetry and its clinical application in neonatal medicine. *Semin Fetal Neonatal Med.* 2015;20(3):192–197.

3. Jubran A. Pulse oximetry. *Crit Care.* 2015;19:272.

4. Sahni R. Continuous noninvasive monitoring in the neonatal ICU. *Curr Opin Pediatr.* 2017;29(2):141–148.

5. Davis PG, Dawson JA. New concepts in neonatal resuscitation. *Curr Opin Pediatr.* 2012;24:147–153.

6. Dawson JA, Morley CJ. Monitoring oxygen saturation and heart rate in the early neonatal period. *Semin Fetal Neonatal Med.* 2010;15(4):203–207.

7. Kapadia V, Wyckoff MH. Oxygen therapy in the delivery room: what is the right dose? *Clin Perinatol.* 2018;45(2):293–306.

8. Rabi Y, Dawson JA. Oxygen therapy and oximetry in the delivery room. *Semin Fetal Neonatal Med.* 2013;18(6): 330–335.

9. Solevåg AL, Solberg MT, Šaltytė-Benth J. Pulse oximetry performance in mechanically ventilated newborn infants. *Early Hum Dev.* 2015;91(8):471–473.

10. Hay WW Jr, Rodden DJ, Collins SM, et al. Reliability of conventional and new pulse oximetry in neonatal patients. *J Perinatol.* 2002;22(5):360–366.

11. McVea S, McGowan M, Rao B. How to use saturation monitoring in newborns. *Arch Dis Child Educ Pract Ed.* 2019;104(1):35–42.

12. Bohnhorst B, Peter CS, Poets CF. Pulse oximeters' reliability in detecting hypoxemia and bradycardia: comparison between a conventional and two new generation oximeters. *Crit Care Med.* 2000;28(5):1565–1568.

13. Foglia EE, Whyte RK, Chaudhary A, et al. The effect of skin pigmentation on the accuracy of pulse oximetry in infants with hypoxemia. *J Pediatr.* 2017;182:375–377.

14. Anderson JV. The accuracy of pulse oximetry in neonates: effects of fetal hemoglobin and bilirubin. *J Perinatol.* 1987;7:323.

15. Hay WW Jr, Brockway J, Eyzaguirre M. Neonatal pulse oximetry: accuracy and reliability. *Pediatrics.* 1989;83:717–722.

16. Bachman TE, Newth CJL, Iyer NP, et al. Hypoxemic and hyperoxemic likelihood in pulse oximetry ranges: NICU observational study. *Arch Dis Child Fetal Neonatal Ed.* 2018. pii: fetalneonatal-2017-314448.

17. Shiao SY, Ou CN. Validation of oxygen saturation monitoring in neonates. *Am J Crit Care.* 2007;16(2):168–178.

18. Saugstad OD, Aune D. In search of the optimal oxygen saturation for extremely low birth weight infants: a systematic review and meta-analysis. *Neonatology.* 2011;100:1–8.

19. Sandberg KL, Brynjarsson H, Hjalmarson O. Transcutaneous blood gas monitoring during neonatal intensive care. *Acta Paediatr.* 2011;100(5):676–679.

20. Tobias JD. Transcutaneous carbon dioxide monitoring in infants and children. *Paediatr Anaesth.* 2009;19(5):434–444.

21. Palmisano BW, Severinghaus JW. Transcutaneous PCO and PO: a multicenter study of accuracy. *J Clin Monit.* 1990;6:189–195.

22. Pearlman SA, Maisels MJ. Preductal and postductal transcutaneous oxygen tension measurements in premature newborns with hyaline membrane disease. *Pediatrics.* 1989;83:98–100.

23. Golden SM. Skin craters—a complication of transcutaneous oxygen monitoring. *Pediatrics.* 1981;67:514–516.

24. Fink SE. Continuous P_aO_2 monitoring through the umbilical artery. *Neonat Intensive Care.* 1990;3:16–19.

25. Menzel M, Henze D, Soukup J, et al. Experiences with continuous intra-arterial blood gas monitoring. *Minerva Anestesiol.* 2001;67(4):325–331.

26. Weiss IK, Fink S, Harrison R, et al. Clinical use of continuous arterial blood-gas monitoring in the pediatric intensive care unit. *Pediatrics.* 1999;103:440–445.

27. Coule LW, Truemper EJ, Steinhart CM, et al. Accuracy and utility of a continuous intra-arterial blood-gas monitoring system in pediatric patients. *Crit Care Med.* 2001;29: 420–426.

28. Meyers PA, Worwa C, Trusty R, et al. Clinical validation of a continuous intravascular neonatal blood gas sensor introduced through an umbilical artery catheter. *Respir Care.* 2002;47(6):682–687.

29. Rais-Bahrami K, Rivera O, Mikesell GT, et al. Continuous blood gas monitoring using an in-dwelling optode method: comparison to intermittent arterial blood gas sampling in ECMO patients. *J Perinatol.* 2002;22(6):472–474.

30. Rais-Bahrami K, Rivera O, Mikesell GT, et al. Continuous blood gas monitoring using an in-dwelling optode method: clinical evaluation of the Neotrend® sensor using a Luer stub adaptor to access the umbilical artery catheter. *J Perinatol.* 2002;22(5):367–369.

31. Ganter M, Zollinger A. Continuous intravascular blood gas monitoring: development, current techniques, and clinical use of a commercial device. *Br J Anaesth.* 2003;91(3):397–407.

32. Tobias JD, Connors D, Strauser L, et al. Continuous pH and Pco_2 monitoring during respiratory failure in children with the Paratrend 7 inserted into the peripheral venous system. *J Pediatr.* 2000;136(5):623–627.

End-Tidal Carbon Dioxide Monitoring

M. Kabir Abubakar

CAPNOGRAPHY

Capnography or end-tidal carbon dioxide ($P_{et}CO_2$) monitoring is the continuous and noninvasive measurement of CO_2 in exhaled respiratory gas. Capnography has become an increasingly valuable tool in airway and ventilation monitoring during intensive care and anesthesia. It is a useful adjunct tool in the management of ventilated infants, providing information about CO_2 production, pulmonary perfusion, alveolar ventilation, respiratory patterns, and the elimination of CO_2 from the lungs. If ventilation and perfusion are well matched, with no alveolar disease, $P_{et}CO_2$ will approximate $PaCO_2$.

A. Definitions

1. Capnography is the continuous analysis and graphical representation over time of CO_2 concentrations in exhaled respiratory gases. A capnograph is the measuring instrument that displays the waveform or the capnogram.
2. Capnometry refers to numerical measurement or analysis of CO_2 concentrations. A capnometer is a device that measures and displays the breath-to-breath numeric values of CO_2.

B. Purpose

1. Noninvasive continuous analysis and recording of CO_2 during tidal breathing (1)
2. $P_{et}CO_2$ monitoring (2)
3. Additional confirmation of endotracheal tube placement (3)
4. To monitor the quality of cardiopulmonary resuscitation and indicate return of spontaneous circulation (4)

C. Background

1. CO_2 may be measured in a gas sample by several techniques. Infrared and colorimetric technology are the most commonly used methods in clinical practice:
   a. Infrared technology: The most commonly used technique in capnography. CO_2 absorbs specific wavelengths of infrared light. The amount of CO_2 in a gas sample can be determined by comparing the measured absorbance of infrared light by that gas with the absorbance of a known standard.
   b. Colorimetry: Used primarily for small disposable $P_{et}CO_2$ detectors for verification of endotracheal tube placement. A pH-sensitive nontoxic chemical indicator strip is housed in a clear dome; the strip changes color from purple to yellow in the presence of exhaled CO_2; the color change is reversible and changes from purple to yellow with each exhaled breath in correctly intubated patients.
   c. Molecular correlation spectrography.
   d. Raman spectrography.
   e. Mass spectrography.
   f. Photoacoustic spectrography.
2. Capnographic devices incorporate one of the two types of analyzers: mainstream and sidestream (5–8).
   a. With a mainstream analyzer, the sensor is attached directly to an optical adapter that is in line with the endotracheal tube.
   b. With a sidestream analyzer, a low–deadspace adapter is placed in line with the endotracheal tube and gas is aspirated continuously to the analyzer for measurement.

D. Indications

1. Evaluation of the exhaled CO_2, specifically $P_{et}CO_2$, which is the maximum partial pressure of CO_2 exhaled

during a tidal breath just prior to the beginning of inspiration (designated $P_{et}CO_2$) (5–11).

2. Monitoring the severity of pulmonary disease and evaluating response to therapy, particularly therapy intended to change the ratio of deadspace to tidal volume (12) or to improve the matching of ventilation to perfusion (*V/Q*) (13).

3. Accurate and continuous graphic reflection of CO_2 elimination when weaning ventilator support (12,14).

4. Continued monitoring of the integrity of the ventilatory circuit (15).

5. Use of capnography in combination with pulse oximetry can allow for additional monitoring to detect airway obstruction or subclinical degrees of respiratory depression in the sedated patient (16).

6. Verifying that tracheal rather than esophageal intubation has taken place (3,17,18).

E. Contraindications

There are no absolute contraindications to capnography in the mechanically ventilated infant, but consideration should be given to the amount of deadspace and weight that will be added to the breathing circuit by these devices.

F. Limitations (5,18,19)

1. The composition of the respiratory gas mixture may affect the capnogram; the infrared spectrum of CO_2 has some similarities to the spectra for both oxygen and nitrous oxide (most available capnographs have a correction factor already incorporated into the calibration).

2. Rapid changes in respiratory rate and tidal volume may lead to measurement error, depending on the frequency response of the capnograph; different capnographs may have different frequency response times.

3. Contamination of either the monitor or the sampling system by secretions, blood, or condensation may lead to inaccurate results.

4. Large deadspace affects $P_{et}CO_2$ measurements. The difference between $P_{et}CO_2$ and $PaCO_2$ increases as deadspace volume increases and may vary within the same patient over time.

5. The $P_{et}CO_2$ adapter can add to the deadspace and resistance of the respiratory circuit, particularly in small infants.

6. $P_{et}CO_2$ measurements may not provide an accurate correlation with $PaCO_2$ in infants with nonhomogeneous lung disease and, therefore, cannot be substituted for $PaCO_2$ analyses in preterm infants during this critical period (20–22).

7. The presence of large endotracheal tube leaks in ventilated neonates can lead to underestimation of the $P_{et}CO_2$ value (23).

8. Acute pulmonary hypoperfusion during cardiac surgery may be associated with a sudden decrease in $P_{et}CO_2$ and mimic accidental endotracheal extubation (24).

G. Equipment

1. Use adaptors specifically designed for neonatal application.

2. For mainstream capnography, an airway adapter is needed, along with a reusable sensor attachment.

3. For sidestream capnography, an airway adapter with sampling tube is used (**Fig. 12.1**).

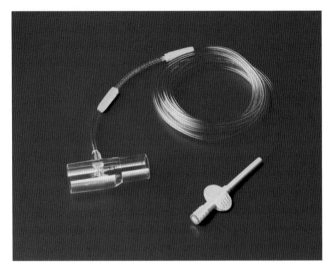

FIGURE 12.1 Infant sidestream low–deadspace adapter with sample tubing. (© Drägerwerk AG & Co. KGaA, Lubeck. All rights reserved.)

4. Sidestream technology can be used with nasal prongs in spontaneously breathing patients.

5. Capnograph or capnometer.

H. Precautions

1. In the mainstream adapter, prevent condensation in the airway adapter.

2. In the sidestream adapter, prevent fluid (water) buildup in the sampling tube. A microstream device is preferred for neonatal patients with low flow ventilation circuits because of the deadspace of the sampling tubing and sampling rate.

3. For both mainstream and sidestream, when adding bulk to the endotracheal tube, extra attention should be given to properly securing the position of the endotracheal tube.

4. Tidal volume measurements may be affected if the $P_{et}CO_2$ adapter is placed between the endotracheal tube and the ventilator flow sensor.

I. Technique

1. Familiarize yourself with the system before proceeding.
2. Follow manufacturer's instructions for equipment calibration.
3. Attach the adapter in line with the endotracheal tube and the ventilator T piece (both sidestream and mainstream) **(Fig. 12.2)**.

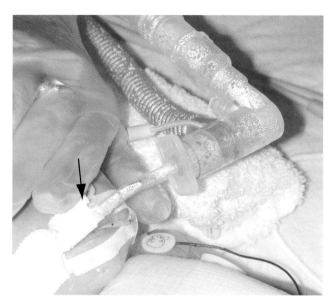

FIGURE 12.2 Infant sidestream low–deadspace adapter (*arrow*) in line with endotracheal tube.

4. For mainstream capnography, connect the sensor to the airway adapter.
5. For sidestream capnography, connect the sampling tube to the analyzer.

J. Complications

1. With mainstream analyzers, the use of too large an airway tube adapter together with the weight of the probe may introduce an excessive amount of not only airway deadspace, but bulk and weight to the endotracheal tube increasing the risk of tube kinking or dislodgement.
2. With sidestream capnography, a low–deadspace adapter allows for less bulk and weight; however, care must be taken not to pull excessively on the sample line that is connected to the measurement instrument (7,8,23).

COLORIMETRIC CARBON DIOXIDE MEASUREMENT

Colorimetry provides a quick qualitative measure of CO_2 in a gas sample. This method uses a pH-sensitive chemical indicator (similar to a litmus paper) in a plastic housing that is attached between the endotracheal tube and the ventilator circuit or positive-pressure delivery device. The pH-sensitive indicator changes color when exposed to CO_2 (usually from purple to yellow, depending on the device). The response time is sufficiently fast to detect exhaled CO_2 within 1 or 2 breaths. Colorimetric end-tidal CO_2 detection is simple and requires no power but does not provide waveform or quantification of CO_2.

A. Indications

1. For confirmation of endotracheal tube placement.
2. International consensus statements on neonatal resuscitation recommend that endotracheal tube placements be additionally verified by using clinical signs and detection of exhaled CO_2 (25).

B. Procedure

1. Immediately following endotracheal intubation, attach calorimetric CO_2 detector to endotracheal tube adaptor and continue positive-pressure ventilation with T-piece resuscitator or self-inflating bag.
2. Within one to two breaths, the indicator color should change from purple to yellow with every exhalation if the tube is within the trachea and not in the esophagus. Some CO_2 detectors have a small plastic strip that needs to be removed for the gas to flow through.
3. Remove the CO_2 detector before attaching the ventilator circuit.
4. Only use devices meant for neonatal patients. Larger devices with a bigger deadspace may dilute the CO_2 coming from the patient resulting in poor detection of exhaled CO_2.

C. Limitations

1. This device is not very sensitive when CO_2 output is low, as may be the case in patients with cardiac arrest and minimal CO_2 excretion and in very preterm infants during initial resuscitation (3,24–27).
2. Devices are for single patient use only.

References

1. Walsh BK, Crotwell DN, Restrepo RD. Capnography/capnometry during mechanical ventilation: 2011. *Respir Care.* 2011;56(4):503–509.
2. Galia F, Brimioulle S, Bonnier F, et al. Use of maximum end-tidal CO_2 values to improve end-tidal CO_2 monitoring accuracy. *Respir Care.* 2011;56:278–283.

3. Wyllie J, Carlo WA. The role of carbon dioxide detectors for confirmation of endotracheal tube position. *Clin Perinatol.* 2006;33:111–119.

4. Sandroni C, De Santis P, D'Arrigo S. Capnography during cardiac arrest. *Resuscitation.* 2018;132:73–77.

5. Paiva EF, Paxton JH, O'Neil BJ. The use of end-tidal carbon dioxide (ETCO$_2$) measurement to guide management of cardiac arrest: a systematic review. *Resuscitation.* 2018;123:1–7.

6. Kugelman A, Golan A, Riskin A, et al. Impact of continuous capnography in ventilated neonates: a randomized, multi-center study. *J Pediatr.* 2016;168:56–61.

7. Lightdale JR, Goldmann DA, Feldman HA, et al. Microstream capnography improves patient monitoring during moderate sedation: a randomized, controlled trial. *Pediatrics.* 2006;117:e1170–e1178.

8. Hawkes GA, Kelleher J, Ryan CA, et al. A review of carbon dioxide monitoring in preterm newborns in the delivery room. *Resuscitation.* 2014;85(10):1315–1319.

9. Lopez E, Mathlouthi J, Lescure S, et al. Capnography in spontaneously breathing preterm infants with bronchopulmonary dysplasia. *Pediatr Pulmonol.* 2011;46(9):896–902.

10. Bhat YR, Abhishek N. Mainstream end-tidal carbon dioxide monitoring in ventilated neonates. *Singapore Med J.* 2008; 49(3):199–203.

11. Wu CH, Chou HC, Hsieh WS, et al. Good estimation of arterial carbon dioxide by end-tidal carbon dioxide monitoring in the neonatal intensive care unit. *Pediatr Pulmonol.* 2003;35:292–295.

12. Trevisanuto D, Giuliotto S, Cavallin F, et al. End-tidal carbon dioxide monitoring in very low birth weight infants: correlation and agreement with arterial carbon dioxide. *Pediatr Pulmonol.* 2012;47:367–372.

13. McSwain SD, Hamel DS, Smith PB, et al. End-tidal and arterial carbon dioxide measurements correlate across all levels of physiologic dead space. *Respir Care.* 2010;55(3):288–293.

14. Frankenfield DC, Alam S, Bekteshi E, et al. Predicting dead space ventilation in critically ill patients using clinically available data. *Crit Care Med.* 2010;38(1):288–291.

15. Ortega R, Connor C, Kim S, et al. Monitoring ventilation with capnography. *N Engl J Med.* 2012;367:e27.

16. Hamel DS, Cheifetz IM. Do all mechanically ventilated pediatric patients require continuous capnography? *Respir Care Clin N Am.* 2006;12:501–513.

17. Gowda H. Question 2. Should carbon dioxide detectors be used to check correct placement of endotracheal tubes in preterm and term neonates? *Arch Dis Child.* 2011;96:1201–1203.

18. Schmölzer GM, O'Reilly M, Davis PG, et al. Confirmation of correct tracheal tube placement in newborn infants. *Resuscitation.* 2013;84:731–737.

19. Siobal MS. Monitoring exhaled carbon dioxide. *Respir Care.* 2016;61:1397–1416.

20. Molloy EJ, Deakins K. Are carbon dioxide detectors useful in neonates? *Arch Dis Child Fetal Neonatal Ed.* 2006;91:F295–F298.

21. Aliwalas LL, Noble L, Nesbitt K, et al. Agreement of carbon dioxide levels measured by arterial, transcutaneous and end tidal methods in preterm infants < or = 28 weeks gestation. *J Perinatol.* 2005;25(1):26–29.

22. Lopez E, Grabar S, Barbier A, et al. Detection of carbon dioxide thresholds using low-flow sidestream capnography in ventilated preterm infants. *Intensive Care Med.* 2009;35(11):1942–1949.

23. Schmalisch G. Current methodological and technical limitations of time and volumetric capnography in newborns. *Biomed Eng Online.* 2016;15(1):104.

24. Misra S, Koshy T, Mahaldar DA. Sudden decrease in end tidal carbon dioxide in a neonate undergoing surgery for type B interrupted aortic arch. *Ann Card Anaesth.* 2011;14: 206–210.

25. Wyckoff MH, Aziz K, Escobedo MB, et al. Part 13: Neonatal resuscitation: 2015 American Heart Association Guidelines Update for Cardiopulmonary Resuscitation and Emergency Cardiovascular Care (Reprint). *Pediatrics.* 2015;136(Suppl 2): S196–S218.

26. Schmolzer GM, Poulton DA, Dawson JA, et al. Assessment of flow waves and colorimetric CO$_2$ detector for endotracheal tube placement during neonatal resuscitation. *Resuscitation.* 2011;82:307–312.

27. Karlsson V, Sporre B, Hellström-Westas L, et al. Poor performance of main-stream capnography in newborn infants during general anesthesia. *Paediatr Anaesth.* 2017;27:1235–1240.

CHAPTER

13

Transcutaneous Bilirubin Monitoring

Caitlin Drumm

A. Background

1. Jaundice occurs in most newborn infants. The majority of neonatal jaundice is benign; however, 10% of term and 25% of near-term infants develop hyperbilirubinemia requiring phototherapy (1). A high level of unconjugated bilirubin is potentially toxic to the nervous system, causing bilirubin encephalopathy and kernicterus (2).

2. The American Academy of Pediatrics (AAP) recommends that universal screening for hyperbilirubinemia, with either a total serum bilirubin (TSB) or a transcutaneous bilirubin (TCB), be performed prior to hospital discharge for all newborns. Universal screening should be combined with a determination of clinical risk factors and a targeted follow-up plan (3,4).

3. Visual assessment of jaundice, although clinically important, may not be accurate (5,6).

4. Transcutaneous bilirubinometers measure the yellowness of reflected light from the skin and subcutaneous tissues to provide an objective *noninvasive* measurement of the degree of neonatal jaundice and thereby predict the approximate TSB.

5. Transcutaneous bilirubinometers are predominantly used for *screening* for significant hyperbilirubinemia in term and near-term newborn infants and should be used as a tool to determine whether a TSB should be measured (2).

6. Two transcutaneous bilirubinometers are currently used in the United States. Although these instruments use different technologies and algorithms, their underlying principles of operation are similar. Both bilirubinometers provide TCB measurements that correlate well with TSB values at levels <15 mg/dL, in term and late preterm newborn infants; but wider variations have been noted at higher bilirubin levels (7,8).

   a. Konica Minolta/Air-Shields JM-103 jaundice meter (Dräger Medical, Telford, Pennsylvania) (6,9) **(Fig. 13.1)**.

   b. BiliChek noninvasive bilirubin analyzer (Children's Medical Ventures/Respironics, Norwell, Massachusetts) (6,8).

   c. The JM-105 jaundice meter (Dräger Medical, Telford, Pennsylvania) was cleared by the U.S. Food and Drug Administration in November 2014, but has not yet undergone comprehensive study in the United States (10).

   d. Two other transcutaneous bilirubinometers, the Bilitest BB77 (Bertocchi SRL Elettromedicali, Cremona, Italy) and BiliMed (Medick SA, Paris, France), are used in Europe but are not approved for use in the United States (11,12).

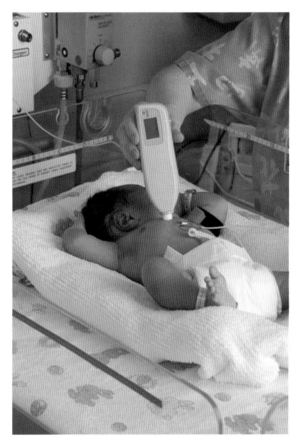

FIGURE 13.1 Use of the Konica Minolta/Air-Shields JM-103 jaundice meter on the sternum.

B. Indications

1. TCB may be obtained:
   a. As part of universal predischarge assessment between 1 and 4 days of life in term and near-term newborn infants, to assess the risk of development of severe hyperbilirubinemia, by using the hour-specific bilirubin nomogram (**Figs. 13.2** and **13.3**) (3,4,13). The AAP recommends routine predischarge bilirubin screening of all newborns.
   b. As a screening tool to help determine whether a TSB should be measured.
   c. For repeated noninvasive measurement of progression of jaundice in term or near-term newborn infants.

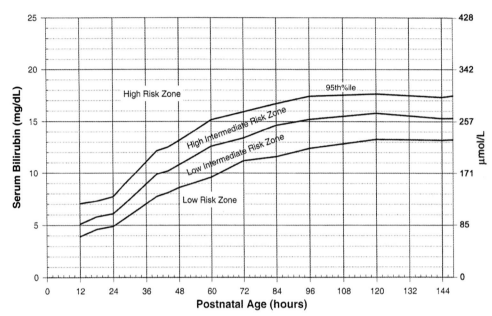

FIGURE 13.2 Nomogram for designation of risk in 2,840 well newborns at 36 or more weeks' gestational age with birth weight of 2,000 g or more or 35 or more weeks' gestational age and birth weight of 2,500 g or more based on hour-specific serum bilirubin values (3,9). (Reprinted with permission from American Academy of Pediatrics Subcommittee on Hyperbilirubinemia. Management of hyperbilirubinemia in the newborn infant 35 or more weeks of gestation. *Pediatrics*. 2004;114(1):297–316. Erratum: *Pediatrics*. 2004;114(4):1138. Copyright © 2004 by the AAP.)

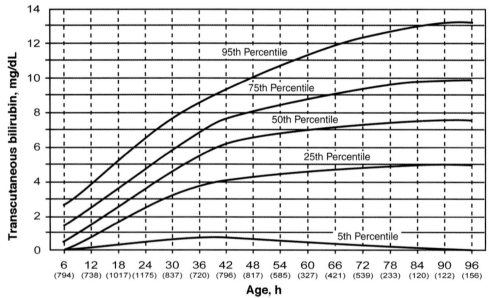

FIGURE 13.3 Nomogram showing smoothed curves for the 5th, 25th, 50th, 75th, and 95th percentiles for TCB measurements among healthy newborns (gestational age ≥35 weeks). A total of 9,397 TCB measurements were obtained for 3,894 newborns. The number of infants studied at each interval is shown in parentheses. (Reprinted with permission from Maisels MJ, Kring E. Transcutaneous bilirubin levels in the first 96 hours in a normal newborn population of ≥35 weeks' gestation. *Pediatrics*, 2006;117(4):1169–1173. Copyright © 2006 by the AAP.)

d. When clinical jaundice is noted in the first 24 hours of life.

e. When jaundice appears excessive for the infant's age.

2. Many studies indicate that the TCB level generally underestimates TSB in term and late-preterm infants, particularly at high TSB levels (>10 mg/dL). To avoid false negatives (i.e., missing a TSB approaching or exceeding treatment threshold), it is recommended to check a TSB in the following situations (4):

   a. The TCB value is at 70% of the TSB level recommended for the use of phototherapy.

   b. The TCB value is above the 75th percentile on the Bhutani nomogram.

   c. The TCB value is >13 mg/dL at follow-up after hospital discharge.

3. TSB (in addition to other studies to determine underlying pathology) should be obtained when (3,4):

   a. Infant is receiving phototherapy or the TSB is rising rapidly.

   b. TSB value approaching exchange transfusion levels or not responding to phototherapy.

   c. Infant has an elevated direct bilirubin level.

   d. Jaundice is present at or beyond age 3 weeks.

   e. In sick or premature (<35 weeks' gestation) infants.

C. Limitations

1. TCB measurement is a *screening tool* and should not be used for treatment decisions, but rather to select those infants who should undergo TSB measurement (2).

2. A TSB should always be obtained when therapeutic intervention is being considered (2).

3. Many studies have shown that the TCB measurement tends to underestimate the TSB value, particularly when the TSB exceeds 10 mg/dL (3).

4. The two large studies evaluating the BiliChek device and the JM-103 device included few patients with TSB values >15 mg/dL. The accuracy of TCB measurement in this range has not been evaluated adequately (7,8).

5. All TCB devices are not the same. Significant variations can occur among instruments (11). New instruments should be validated against hospital laboratory measurements.

6. TCB measurements systematically underestimate the TSB value if the infant is being treated with phototherapy or has received an exchange transfusion and should not be used within 24 hours of either of these therapies (3,6,14–17):

   a. Phototherapy alters the chemical structure of bilirubin in the subcutaneous tissues, making it more water soluble. Measurement of TCB in infants undergoing phototherapy is not reliable because the large decrease in subcutaneous bilirubin may not yet be reflected in the serum (15,16). Correlation coefficients have been found to decrease to as low as 0.33 in infants undergoing phototherapy for longer than 48 hours (15).

   b. Correlation between TCB and TSB has been shown to return to pre-phototherapy levels once off treatment for 24 hours. After 24 hours, the correlation coefficients have been shown to improve to 0.8, with further improvement to 0.84 by 48 hours posttreatment (18).

   c. The use of a photo-opaque patch on the forehead to shield the skin may allow for continued measurement of TCB levels in term infants undergoing phototherapy. Good agreement has been shown between serum bilirubin levels and TCB measured from the patched area, and is most effective in following trends in bilirubin values in infants undergoing phototherapy (14).

7. Measurements should not be made on skin that is bruised, covered with hair, or has a birthmark. Localized edema and poor tissue perfusion may also alter TCB readings (19).

8. TCB measurements may decrease the need for multiple TSB measurements in late preterm infants; little information is available in very preterm infants, in whom measurements may be less reliable (14,16,19).

D. Equipment

TCB monitors currently in use in the United States include:

1. Konica Minolta/Air-Shields JM-103 jaundice meter (Dräger Medical, Telford, Pennsylvania) (**Figs. 13.1 and 13.4**)

   a. Determines the yellowness of subcutaneous tissue by measuring the difference between optical densities for light in the blue and green wavelengths.

   b. Measurement probe has two optical paths.

   c. By calculating the difference between the optical densities, the parts common to the epidermis and dermis are deducted. As a result, the difference can be obtained for subcutaneous tissue only.

   d. Theoretically allows for measurement of degree of yellowness of skin and subcutaneous tissue with minimal influence of melanin pigment and skin maturity.

   e. Linear correlation of this measurement with TSB allows for conversion to TSB by the meter, which is indicated digitally.

2. BiliChek noninvasive bilirubin analyzer (Children's Medical Ventures/Respironics, Norwell, Massachusetts)

   a. Noninvasive device consisting of light source, microspectrophotometer, fiberoptic probe, and microprocessor control circuit. The BiliChek also requires the use of a disposable calibration tip with each measurement.

   b. Uses entire spectrum of visible light reflected by the skin.

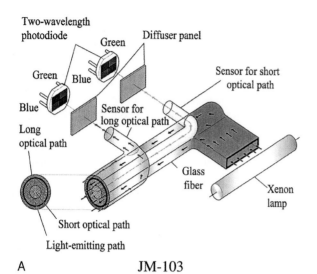

A   JM-103

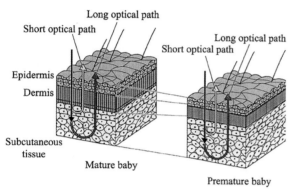

B   JM-103

FIGURE 13.4 The JM-103 jaundice meter determines the yellowness of the subcutaneous tissue by measuring the difference in optical densities for reflected light in the blue (450 nm) and green (550 nm) wavelengths. When the jaundice meter probe is pressed against the forehead or sternum a xenon lamp flashes and the emitted light scatters, is absorbed by the skin and subcutaneous tissue, and then returns to the measuring probe where it is collected by photodiodes. There is a linear correlation between the difference in optical density of the reflected light and TSB. This allows for conversion to TSB, which is then displayed on the jaundice meter screen. (Reprinted with permission of Walter de Gruyter and Company from Yasuda S, Itoh S, Isobe K, et al. New transcutaneous jaundice device with two optical paths. 2005;35(1):81–88. Permission conveyed through Copyright Clearance Center, Inc.)

   c. White light is transmitted into the skin and the reflected light is collected for analysis.
   d. Algorithms take into account the effect of hemoglobin, melanin, and dermal thickness.
   e. Absorption of light due to bilirubin in the capillary bed and subcutaneous tissue is isolated by spectral subtraction.

E. Special Circumstances/Considerations

1. Hospital protocols should include the conditions under which TCB and TSB levels are to be obtained (2). Protocols for training and recertification of TCB users should be in place.

2. Only TSB measurements should be performed in infants with jaundice severe enough to warrant exchange transfusion (see C) (8).
3. TCB is less accurate in infants undergoing phototherapy; therefore, serum levels are preferred for monitoring bilirubin values in such infants (see C) (3,6,13,15).
4. Race/skin color: TCB readings obtained by the Bili-Chek have been found to correlate with TSB values in White, Black, Asian, Hispanic, Indigenous African, and Indian infants (8,15,20). In Black infants, TCB readings obtained by the JM-103 correlate less closely with TSB values, with the TCB generally being greater than the TSB (7,21).

F. Techniques

1. Calibrate the TCB device according to manufacturer specifications. New devices should be correlated with serum samples before use.
2. Measure TCB by pressing the trigger button and gently pressing the tip to the infant's forehead or sternum until the device indicates that reading is complete.
   a. Some studies have shown that TCB measurements from the sternum correlated slightly better with TSB levels than TCB measurements from the forehead, possibly as a result of the exposure of the forehead to ambient light. Other studies indicate both sites to be equivalent (7,22).
   b. The difference between TCB and TSB has been found to be significantly greater in nurseries where more than one location (e.g., both chest and forehead) were used for TCB assessment, when compared to nurseries where either chest or forehead was used alone. Therefore, nursery protocols should establish one exclusive site for TCB measurement, whether that be the forehead or the chest (21).
   c. Measurements must be taken in a consistent manner with regard to placement of the probe and amount of pressure applied to the device. Inter- and intraoperative variability may be minimized with proper training (7).
   d. Measurement of the TCB using the BiliChek system takes approximately 20 to 80 seconds. This time is required for the monitor to make five measurements that are averaged to provide one TCB value. The JM-103 takes approximately 10 seconds to obtain its dual measurements and calculate the TCB value.
3. BiliChek individual calibration tips are made of disposable plastic. The manufacturer recommends against repeated use of the disposable probes.

G. Complications

No complications have been reported from the use of TCB monitors, except for the risk of inappropriate use, the possibility of underestimation of the level of jaundice (see C and E), or overestimation of the level of jaundice leading to unnecessary blood draws to determine the TSB level.

H. Effectiveness

TCB measurement has been shown to decrease the number of heel pricks in some studies but has not changed the length of hospital stay or number of newborns requiring phototherapy. TCB monitoring has been shown to reduce the number of infants readmitted for phototherapy (23).

References

1. Sarici SU, Serdar MA, Korkmaz A, et al. Incidence, course, and prediction of hyperbilirubinemia in near-term and term newborns. *Pediatrics*. 2004;113(4):775–780.
2. American Academy of Pediatrics Subcommittee on Hyperbilirubinemia. Neonatal jaundice and kernicterus. *Pediatrics*. 2001;108(3):31.
3. American Academy of Pediatrics Subcommittee on Hyperbilirubinemia. Management of hyperbilirubinemia in the newborn infant 35 or more weeks of gestation. *Pediatrics*. 2004;114:297.
4. Maisels MJ, Bhutani VK, Bogen D, et al. Hyperbilirubinemia in the Newborn Infant >/ = 35 weeks' gestation: an update with clarifications. *Pediatrics*. 2009;124:1193–1198.
5. Szabo P, Wolf M, Bucher HU, et al. Detection of hyperbilirubinaemia in jaundiced full-term neonates by eye or bilirubinometer? *Eur J Pediatr*. 2004;163(12):722–727.
6. Maisels MJ. Transcutaneous bilirubinometry. *NeoReviews*. 2006;7(5):e217–e225.
7. Maisels MJ, Ostrea EM, Touch S, et al. Evaluation of a new transcutaneous bilirubinometer. *Pediatrics*. 2004;113: 1628–1635.
8. Bhutani VK, Gourley GR, Adler S, et al. Noninvasive measurement of total serum bilirubin in a multiracial predischarge newborn population to assess the risk of severe hyperbilirubinemia. *Pediatrics*. 2000;106:e17.
9. Yasuda S, Itoh S, Isobe K, et al. New transcutaneous jaundice device with two optical paths. *J Perinat Med*. 2003;31:81–88.
10. Jones DF, McRea AR, Kowles JD, et al. A prospective comparison of transcutaneous and serum bilirubin within brief time intervals. *Clin Pediatr (Phila)*. 2017;56(11):1013–1017.
11. De Luca D, Zecca E, Corsello M. Attempt to improve transcutaneous bilirubinometry: a double-blind study of Medick BiliMed versus Respironics Bilicheck. *Arch Dis Child Fetal Neonatal Ed*. 2008;93:F135–F139.
12. Bertini G, Pratesi S, Consenza E, et al. Transcutaneous bilirubin measurement: evaluation of Bilitest. *Neonatology*. 2008;93:101–105.
13. Bhutani VK, Johnson L, Sivieri EM. Predictive ability of a predischarge hour-specific serum bilirubin for subsequent significant hyperbilirubinemia in healthy term and near-term newborns. *Pediatrics*. 1999;103(1):6–14.
14. Zecca E, Barone G, DeLuca D, et al. Skin bilirubin measurement during phototherapy in preterm and term newborn infants. *Early Human Dev*. 2009;85:537–540.
15. Mahajan G, Kaushal RK, Sankhyan N, et al. Trancutaneous bilirubinometer in assessment of neonatal jaundice in Northern India. *Indian Pediatr*. 2005;42:41–45.
16. Nanjundaswamy S, Petrova A, Mehta R, et al. Transcutaneous bilirubinometry in preterm infants receiving phototherapy. *Am J Perinatol*. 2005;22(3):127–131.
17. Grabehenrich J, Grabenhenrich L, Buhrer C, et al. Transcutaneous bilirubin after phototherapy in term and preterm infants. *Pediatrics*. 2014;134(5):1324–1329.
18. Tan KL, Dong F. Transcutaneous bilirubinometry during and after phototherapy. *Acta Paediatrica*. 2003;92:327–331.
19. Willems WA, van den Berg LM, de Wit H, et al. Transcutaneous bilirubinometry with the Bilicheck® in very premature newborns. *J Mat Fetal Neonatal Med*. 2004;16:209–214.
20. Slusher TM, Angyo IA, Bode-Thomas F, et al. Transcutaneous bilirubin measurements and serum total bilirubin levels in Indigenous African infants. *Pediatrics*. 2004;113:1636–1641.
21. Taylor JA, Burgos AE, Flaherman V, et al. Discrepancies between transcutaneous and serum bilirubin measurements. *Pediatrics*. 2015;135(2):224–231.
22. Ebbesen F, Rasmussen LM, Wimberley PD. A new transcutaneous bilirubinometer, BiliChek®, used in the neonatal intensive care unit and the maternity ward. *Acta Paediatr*. 2002;91:203–211.
23. Peterson JR, Okorodudu AO, Mohammad AA, et al. Association of transcutaneous bilirubin testing in hospital with decreased readmission rate for hyperbilirubinemia. *Clinical Chem*. 2005;51:540–544.

Amplitude-Integrated EEG (aEEG)

Nathalie El Ters, Stephanie S. Lee, and Amit M. Mathur

Conventional EEG (cEEG) in neonates remains the gold standard for EEG monitoring but requires skilled personnel to apply leads and interpret the EEG. Longitudinal studies can be challenging because of the high maintenance requirements of cEEG leads and the concern for skin breakdown in newborns. Amplitude-integrated EEG (aEEG) is a limited-channel modality that has the benefit of easy lead application and interpretation by clinicians. The EEG signal is recorded using one or two channels consisting of two or four electrodes, respectively, placed in the C3-P3, C4-P4 areas of the newborn's head. The raw EEG signal is amplified, filtered by attenuating frequencies below 2 Hz and above 15 Hz to minimize muscle artifact, noise and electrical interference, compressed and displayed in a semi-logarithmic scale alongside the raw EEG **(Fig. 14.1)** (1).

INDICATIONS FOR aEEG MONITORING

A. Seizures

1. The true incidence of seizures in newborns is difficult to estimate due to the atypical presentation and subclinical nature of these events, especially in the preterm infants.
2. The reported incidence in term infants ranges between 1 and 5 per 1,000 newborns (2).

B. Population At-Risk

1. Hypoxic ischemic encephalopathy (HIE) (3)
2. Brain injury in acutely ill neonates (severe persistent pulmonary hypertension [PPHN], congenital heart defects requiring cardiopulmonary bypass, ECMO)
3. CNS infection
4. Intracranial bleeds, perinatal strokes, and venous sinus thrombosis

5. Inborn errors of metabolism, genetic syndromes involving the central nervous system
6. Preterm infants with high-grade intraventricular hemorrhage (IVH) or encephalopathy

C. Equipment

1. **aEEG monitors:** These are freestanding machines that are easy to set up and use.
   a. Currently available aEEG comes with a seizure detection algorithm and an optional software for automated background classification.
   b. The RecogniZe (Natus Medical Inc., San Carlos, CA) algorithm detects areas of regularity in an

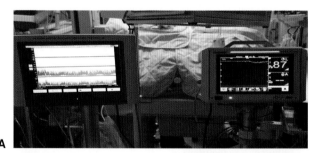

A

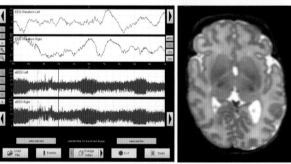

B

FIGURE 14.1 A: aEEG machine recording at the bedside of a preterm infant. **B:** Three hours of aEEG with 10 seconds of EEG from a preterm infant at term equivalent age, whose brain MRI at term was normal and his aEEG tracing shows normal continuous background with mature sleep–wake cycling.

EEG waveform, using at least five similar consecutive waves with wavelengths that are equivalent to a frequency of 14 Hz or less, peak-to-peak amplitude greater than 5 μV and at least 21 seconds of continuous detection, or 26 seconds of discontinuous detection, in 1 minute of EEG signal.

2. **Types of electrodes**
   a. Subdermal needle electrodes
   b. Gold cup electrodes
   c. Hydrogel electrodes

D. Procedure

1. **Preparation of the skin and application of the electrodes**
   a. Using a cotton swab, the skin is gently cleaned with Nuprep gel (Weaver and Company, Aurora, CO, USA)
      (1) Nuprep is a mildly abrasive cleansing gel that effectively cleans the surface of the skin in order to achieve lower impedance.
      (2) This step is used with subdermal needles, hydrogel, and gold cup electrodes.
   b. *Applying gold cup electrodes*
      (1) This method uses a conductive paste and a paper tape to fix the electrodes in place.
      (2) Collodion is not used in this population due to its toxic properties, and it is usually used to glue down gold cup electrodes.
      (3) This may affect the quality of the recordings and the stability of the electrodes, especially in a humidified and warm environment such as in an incubator.
   c. *Applying subdermal needles*
      (1) Clean the scalp around the insertion sites with an antiseptic solution appropriate for gestational age.
      (2) Insert the needle electrodes at the insertion sites subdermally. The needles should be angled downward.
      (3) Secure the electrodes with a tape over the needles.
   d. *Applying hydrogel electrodes*
      (1) Hydrogel electrodes are an alternative to gold cup and subdermal needles in aEEG recordings when used with adequate skin preparation (4), and they have replaced gold cup and subdermal needle electrodes in continuous aEEG monitoring in the neonatal intensive care unit.
      (2) Hydrogel electrodes have the advantage of increased stickiness on the preterm skin especially in a humidified environment, and they have a flat surface that can decrease the pressure point on the skin when the infant's head

lies on them. In addition, hydrogel electrodes are sterile and disposable.

2. **Placement of electrodes**
   a. Electrodes are placed in the P3-P4 positions for single-channel positions and C3-P3 and C4-P4 for two-channel.
      (1) Electrode positions are based on the International 10–20 system for newborns, as shown in **Figure 14.2** (5).

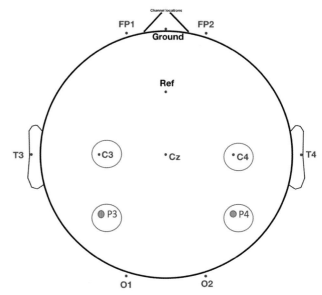

FIGURE 14.2 The electrode positions are adopted according to the International 10–20 system for the newborn. For two-channel recordings, electrode positions are placed in F3-P3 and F4-P4 positions or C3-P3 and C4-P4 positions.

   (2) The electrode locations are determined by specific measurements between the landmarks of the skull.
   (3) The numbers 10 and 20 refer to the measurements between the electrodes as 10% or 20% of the total front–back distance or total right–left distance of the head.
   (4) The reference electrode is positioned in the midline on the forehead.
   b. Most aEEG machines are accompanied by an electrode placement tape or measuring device that helps with electrode placement at C3-P3 and C4-P4 locations. The measuring device is placed between the tragus and the sagittal suture. Two arrows indicate the position of C3 and P3 on the left, C4 and P4 on the right.

3. **Impedance**
   a. Continuous monitoring of electrode impedance is critical to all EEG recordings.
      (1) The most important advancement in aEEG digital monitoring is the introduction of simultaneous display of raw EEG signal and continuous impedance monitoring.

(2) These two components allow clinicians and staff to detect artifact and alert them about improper electrode contact.

b. An impedance detector, incorporated within the device, alerts the staff about the quality of the tracings and about the location of the loose electrode.

(1) High impedance makes the EEG signal unreliable and will prevent triggering of the seizure detection algorithm. Ideally impedance should be <10 Ω although values of 10 to 20 Ω are acceptable. If poor impedance is detected, remove the electrode and perform a gentle cleaning of the underlying area before applying it again.

4. **One-channel versus two-channel**

a. Two-channel aEEG recordings allow clinicians to compare between the right and left hemispheres, detecting asymmetries or underlying focal abnormalities (6). This function cannot be achieved with single channel which detects the electrical activity across the cerebral hemispheres.

b. Using single-channel aEEG, without raw single-channel EEG for confirmation, individual seizure detection is less than 50% (7).

(1) In a study comparing single-channel aEEG alone, two-channel aEEG alone, and two-channel aEEG with continuous raw EEG, the authors found a higher sensitivity and specificity for detecting seizures when aEEG is read simultaneously with raw EEG (8).

(2) Most new digital monitors display both the aEEG and the simultaneous raw EEG trace allowing a more specific interpretation of possible seizure events.

5. **Duration of recordings**

a. There is no definite guideline for the duration of aEEG.

b. Earlier analysis of aEEG in neonates relied on 3- to 4-hour recordings of aEEG as described in literature (1,9,10).

c. The American Clinical Neurophysiology Society guidelines indicate that the duration of conventional EEG recording is determined by the indication of EEG (3).

(1) The committee recommends monitoring infants at risk for seizures for at least 24 hours.

(2) If seizures are detected, monitoring should continue until patient is seizure free for at least 24 hours.

E. Complications

1. No major complications were reported with the application of aEEG in newborns. Skin irritation is always a concern with electrode application.

2. This potential complication should always be monitored for by clinicians and nurses to prevent pressure ulcers and skin infection.

F. Special Circumstances

1. It is very important to be aware of some situations where the electrode positions may have to be adjusted in the setting of skin lacerations due to a scalp electrode, forceps, or vacuum-assisted delivery.

2. The interelectrode distance is very important in determining the amplitude of the background; therefore a reduction in distance between the electrodes will result in a reduction of the background amplitude.

3. Scalp swelling such as with a cephalohematoma, hydrops, or subgaleal hemorrhage will decrease EEG amplitude.

4. Asymmetric scalp edema may lead to an asymmetry in the EEG backgrounds.

INTERPRETATION OF aEEG TRACINGS

A. Background Classification

1. The classification of the aEEG background is based on patterns described in term infants with HIE and in premature infants.

2. Hellstrom-Westas (1) proposed a classification that applies to all newborns regardless of their gestational ages or state of illness. It consists of five patterns (**Fig. 14.3**).

a. **Continuous:** Minimum amplitude between 5 and 10 µV and maximum amplitude between 10 and 50 µV.

b. **Discontinuous:** Minimum amplitude variable and <5 µV and maximum amplitude >10 µV.

c. **Burst suppression:** Minimum amplitude with minimum variability at 0 to 2 µV and intermittent bursts with amplitude >25 µV. There are two patterns in this state. BS+ represents high-frequency bursts (≥100/hr), and BS− represents low-frequency bursts (<100/hr).

d. **Low voltage:** Minimum and maximum amplitudes are of a low voltage (at or below 5 µV).

e. **Inactive, flat:** Inactive pattern with voltage below 5 µV.

B. Sleep–Wake Cycling

1. Sleep–wake cycling (SWC) is characterized by the presence of cyclical variations of broad bandwidths (representing deep quiet sleep) alternating with narrower ones (representing awake alert state and active sleep).

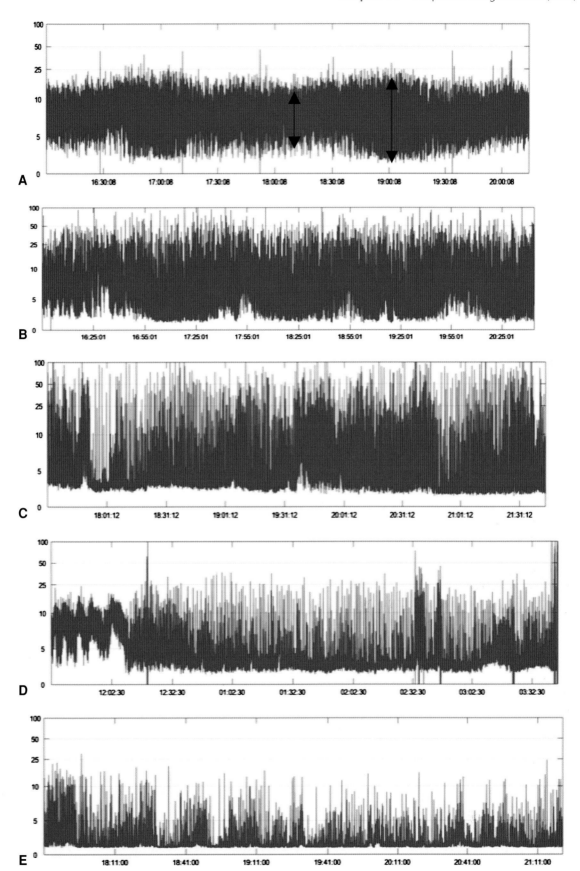

FIGURE 14.3 Classification of aEEG backgrounds. **A,B:** Discontinuous background. **C:** Burst suppression with high burst density (BS+). **D:** Burst suppression with low burst density (BS–). **E:** Inactive and flat tracing.

2. There are three different patterns of SWC in a newborn (1).
   a. **No SWC:** No variations of the bandwidth are noted on aEEG tracings.
   b. **Imminent or immature SWC:** The lower border amplitude of the aEEG displays initial variations but not fully discrete between the stages as seen with the more mature aEEG tracings.
   c. **Developed SWC:** Discrete sinusoidal variations on aEEG tracings with alternating continuous and discontinuous activity, with cycle duration greater or equal to 20 minutes.

C. Seizure Recognition

1. aEEG can be useful in detecting electrographic seizures. Seizures are most often subclinical in the newborn with no clinical signs; continuous monitoring using aEEG in a high-risk population (i.e., infants with HIE, meningitis, or IVH) helps in earlier identification of seizure events.
2. Seizures can be easily identified on aEEG by pattern recognition.
   a. Seizures are displayed on the monitor as an abrupt change in the baseline (transient rise of the minimum, maximum, or both).
      (1) This is due to a change in EEG frequency and amplitude.
      (2) Single seizures appear as isolated changes in the backgrounds of aEEG recordings (**Fig. 14.4**).

b. Seizures on raw EEG are characterized by the sudden appearance of an abnormal electrical event, lasting 10 seconds or more, with evolving, repetitive waveforms that gradually build up and then decline in frequency, morphology, or amplitude.
   (1) Status epilepticus is commonly recognized as a sawtooth pattern on a continuous background (**Fig. 14.5**).
   (2) Status epilepticus can also present as a continuous rise of the baseline.

3. Currently, there are software programs installed on commercially available systems that provide automatic detection of seizures.
   a. These programs are not accurate and they are affected by movement and noise (11).
   b. They are always used in conjunction with the clinical judgment of the physician who still needs to review the aEEG trend and the accompanying raw EEG trace.
   c. In addition, aEEG has a lower sensitivity and specificity for seizure detection compared to conventional EEG, especially if the seizures originate from a remote area and if they are of short duration and amplitude (8,12).

D. Effect of Medications on aEEG

1. Sedatives and antiepileptic drugs depress the background and the SWC on aEEG.

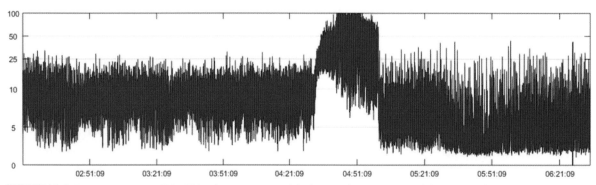

FIGURE 14.4 Seizure patterns on aEEG. aEEG with a transient rise of the lower and upper margins of the tracing indicating a seizure.

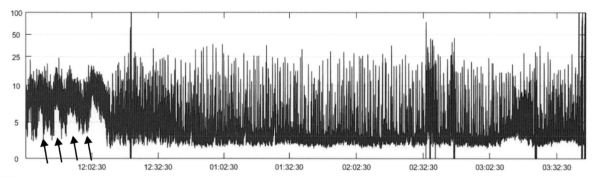

FIGURE 14.5 Seizure patterns on aEEG. aEEG with repetitive seizures recorded in the beginning of the tracing (*arrows*) followed by a burst suppression pattern.

a. There is an additive effect of multiple sedatives on the aEEG depression (13). In infants with HIE, midazolam infusion was found to have a depressive effect on aEEG background (14).

b. This suppression was brief and resolved within 2 hours in infants with mild HIE while it persisted for infants who suffered from a more profound and severe injury.

2. Some studies have also shown that surfactant administration can cause marked depression on aEEG for up to 10 minutes in preterm infants, but the mechanism for this is unclear (15,16).

E. Effect of Gestational Age

1. Burdjalov et al. found that the presence of SWC had the strongest correlation with postconceptional age (9), and its presence indicates cerebral maturation and a higher level of integrity between the different central nervous system functions.

2. This has been expanded upon across multiple studies showing that the presence of SWC in preterm babies matures with age (17,18). Several investigators (1,9,10, 19) have shown that the bandwidth span gets narrower with age in preterm infants, indicating a greater degree of maturation.

F. Recognition of Artifacts

1. **High impedance**
   a. The most important advancement in aEEG digital monitoring is the (1) introduction of simultaneous display of raw EEG signal and (2) continuous impedance monitoring.
   b. These two important components allow clinicians and staff to detect artifact and alert them about improper electrode contact.

2. **Environmental artifact**
   a. State arousal during nursing cares (patting artifact) leads to a transient rise of the minimum amplitude of a discontinuous background, which can be misinterpreted as an epileptic event.
      (1) The raw EEG in these cases is very helpful in delineating the true nature of these events.
      (2) Timing of nursing cares and administration of medications should be annotated.
   b. The interelectrode distance is very important because any changes in this measure affects the amplitude of the EEG signal. The guideline for electrode placement should be closely followed to avoid problems.
   c. High-frequency ventilation may shift the amplitude upward, and the EEG signal may show monorhythmic activity with a high frequency identical to that of the high-frequency ventilation. ECG

artifacts and muscle activity may falsely elevate the baseline, and affect the interpretation of the background.
   (1) Simultaneous interpretation of the original EEG signal is necessary to reveal the exact cause of the unexpected findings.
   (2) A cEEG recording is sometimes needed to accurately evaluate the background and identify artifacts (20,21).

G. Limitations

1. aEEG is a bedside neuromonitoring tool commonly used in neonatal intensive care units, due to its easy application and interpretation by clinical neonatologists.
   a. The application takes few minutes and does not require highly skilled personnel.
   b. The most important step is the placement of the electrodes in their corresponding positions.
   c. Despite these advantages, aEEG has many limitations.
      (1) The main limitation is that aEEG only covers the centro-parietal area of the brain, excluding the frontal, temporal, and occipital regions.
      (2) The time-compressed nature of the aEEG tracings and the centro-parietal location of the electrodes may lead to missing seizures with low amplitude, brief duration (12), and focal ones from remote areas of the brain like the occipital region (22).

2. Nevertheless, aEEG remains easily accessible in neonatal intensive care units and can be used in different clinical contexts, in conjunction with conventional EEG, and other imaging modalities.
   a. While this tool demonstrated great usefulness in monitoring of babies with HIE, it is also being increasingly used in preterm babies for research purposes, for predicting short- and long-term outcomes.
   b. aEEG background patterns, the number of bursts/hr, and the presence or absence of cyclicity were studied in the first few days of life, and abnormalities detected on the background are found to be correlated with poor neurodevelopmental outcomes (23,24).

References

1. Hellstrom-Westas L, Rosén I, de Vries LS, et al. Amplitude-integrated EEG classification and interpretation in preterm and term infants. *NeoReviews.* 2006;7(2):e76–e87.

2. Vasudevan C, Levene M. Epidemiology and aetiology of neonatal seizures. *Semin Fetal Neonatal Med.* 2013;18(4):185–191.

3. Shellhaas RA, Chang T, Tsuchida T. The American clinical neurophysiology society's guideline on continuous electroencephalography monitoring in neonates. *J Clin Neurophysiol.* 2011;28(6):611–617.

4. Foreman SW, Thorngate L, Burr RL, et al. Electrode challenges in amplitude-integrated electroencephalography (aEEG): research application of a novel noninvasive measure of brain function in preterm infants. *Biol Res Nurs.* 2011;13(3):251–259.

5. Tao JD, Mathur AM. Using amplitude-integrated EEG in neonatal intensive care. *J Perinatol.* 2010;30 Suppl:S73–S81.

6. Shah DK, Lavery S, Doyle LW, et al. Use of 2-channel bedside electroencephalogram monitoring in term-born encephalopathic infants related to cerebral injury defined by magnetic resonance imaging. *Pediatrics.* 2006;118(1):47–55.

7. Shellhaas RA, Soaita AI, Clancy RR. Sensitivity of amplitude-integrated electroencephalography for neonatal seizure detection. *Pediatrics.* 2007;120(4):770–777.

8. Shah DK, Mackay MT, Lavery S, et al. Accuracy of bedside electroencephalographic monitoring in comparison with simultaneous continuous conventional electroencephalography for seizure detection in term infants. *Pediatrics.* 2008;121(6):1146–1154.

9. Burdjalov VF, Baumgart S, Spitzer AR. Cerebral function monitoring: a new scoring system for the evaluation of brain maturation in neonates. *Pediatrics.* 2003;112(4):855–861.

10. Thornberg E, Thiringer K. Normal pattern of the cerebral function monitor trace in term and preterm neonates. *Acta Paediatr Scand.* 1990;79(1):20–25.

11. Lawrence R, Mathur A, Nguyen The Tich S, et al. A pilot study of continuous limited-channel aEEG in term infants with encephalopathy. *J Pediatr.* 2009;154(6):835.e1–841.e1.

12. Hellstrom-Westas L. Comparison between tape-recorded and amplitude-integrated EEG monitoring in sick newborn infants. *Acta Paediatr.* 1992;81(10):812–819.

13. Bell AH, Greisen G, Pryds O. Comparison of the effects of phenobarbitone and morphine administration on EEG activity in preterm babies. *Acta Paediatr.* 1993;82(1):35–39.

14. van Leuven K, Groenendaal F, Toet MC, et al. Midazolam and amplitude-integrated EEG in asphyxiated full-term neonates. *Acta Paediatr.* 2004;93(9):1221–1227.

15. Skov L, Hellström-Westas L, Jacobsen T, et al. Acute changes in cerebral oxygenation and cerebral blood volume in preterm infants during surfactant treatment. *Neuropediatrics.* 1992;23(3):126–130.

16. Bell AH, Skov L, Lundstrøm KE, et al. Cerebral blood flow and plasma hypoxanthine in relation to surfactant treatment. *Acta Paediatr.* 1994;83(9):910–914.

17. Sisman J, Campbell DE, Brion LP. Amplitude-integrated EEG in preterm infants: maturation of background pattern and amplitude voltage with postmenstrual age and gestational age. *J Perinatol.* 2005;25(6):391–396.

18. Olischar M, Klebermass K, Kuhle S, et al. Reference values for amplitude-integrated electroencephalographic activity in preterm infants younger than 30 weeks' gestational age. *Pediatrics.* 2004;113(1 Pt 1):e61–e66.

19. Zhang D, Liu Y, Hou X, et al. Reference values for amplitude-integrated EEGs in infants from preterm to 3.5 months of age. *Pediatrics.* 2011;127(5):e1280–e1287.

20. Toet MC, van der Meij W, de Vries LS, et al. Comparison between simultaneously recorded amplitude integrated electroencephalogram (cerebral function monitor) and standard electroencephalogram in neonates. *Pediatrics.* 2002;109(5):772–779.

21. Rennie JM, Chorley G, Boylan GB, et al. Non-expert use of the cerebral function monitor for neonatal seizure detection. *Arch Dis Child Fetal Neonatal Ed.* 2004;89(1):F37–F40.

22. Rakshasbhuvankar A, Paul S, Nagarajan L, et al. Amplitude-integrated EEG for detection of neonatal seizures: a systematic review. *Seizure.* 2015;33:90–98.

23. Kidokoro H, Kubota T, Hayashi N, et al. Absent cyclicity on aEEG within the first 24 h is associated with brain damage in preterm infants. *Neuropediatrics.* 2010;41(6):241–245.

24. Hellstrom-Westas L, Klette H, Thorngren-Jerneck K, et al. Early prediction of outcome with aEEG in preterm infants with large intraventricular hemorrhages. *Neuropediatrics.* 2001;32(6):319–324.

Blood Sampling

CHAPTER
15

Vessel Localization

Suna Seo

TRANSILLUMINATION

A. Indication

Failure to locate an accessible artery or vein under normal lighting conditions for

1. Puncture for sampling (1–3)
2. Vessel cannulation (4,5)

B. Contraindications

None

C. Precautions

Verify that the light source equipment has an intact heat-absorbing glass and infrared and UV filters (6).

D. Equipment

1. Transillumination source
   a. High-intensity cold source with a fiberoptic cable (Fig. 15.1)
   b. Light-emitting diode (LED) (Fig. 15.2) (4,5)
   c. Otoscope light may be used in some instances (Fig. 15.3) (1)
2. Alcohol swab
3. Sterile glove or disposable plastic covers

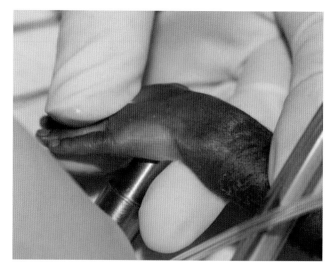

FIGURE 15.1 Fiberoptic transilluminator placed on the palmar surface to visualize veins on the dorsum of hand.

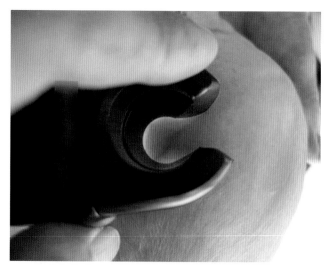

FIGURE 15.2 LED transilluminator positioned to visualize a scalp vein. (Courtesy of Veinlite by Translite, Sugar Land, Texas.)

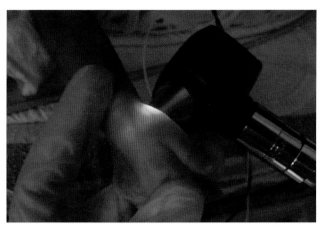

FIGURE 15.3 Otoscope placed on the palmar surface to visualize cephalic vein.

E. Technique

1. Clean end of light source with an alcohol swab. Cover with sterile glove or disposable plastic cover.
2. Dim light in room. Some residual light is necessary to visualize operating field.
3. Set light source at low intensity and increase as needed for visualization.
4. Position probe to transilluminate vessel.
5. Identify vessel as a dark, linear structure (**Figs. 15.4** and **15.5**).

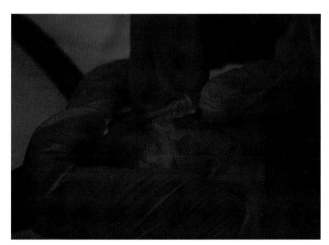

FIGURE 15.4 Transilluminator placed on the palmar surface to visualize the veins on the dorsum during IV insertion.

6. Compensate for distortion if light is not directly opposite the puncture site.
7. Do not maintain contact between light source and extremity for long periods of time.

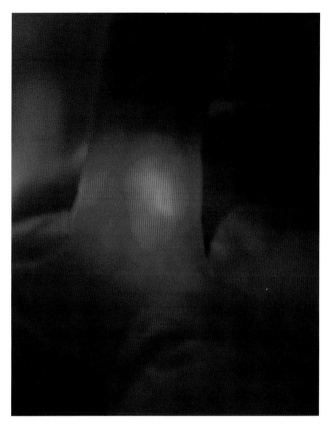

FIGURE 15.5 Transilluminator placed posteriorly to visualize the posterior tibial artery.

F. Complications

1. Thermal burns from light probe (**Figs. 15.6** and **15.7**) (6–10)
2. Contamination from breach of sterile technique

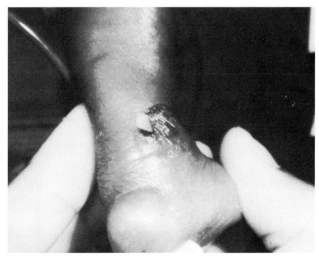

FIGURE 15.6 Burn from transilluminator.

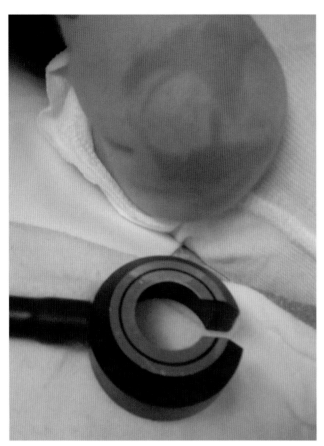

FIGURE 15.7 Superficial burn after prolonged transillumination.

ULTRASONOGRAPHY

A. Background

The use of portable ultrasound (US) as an adjunct tool for neonatal percutaneously inserted central catheter (PICC) (11) placement and percutaneous central venous catheter (CVC) placement (12–15) has increased with the advent of smaller neonatal probes, and growing knowledge and experience of US.

B. Indication

To locate artery or vein for vessel cannulation with real-time visualization of the needle entry in the vein and relationship to surrounding structures (11–18).

C. Contraindications

None

D. Precautions

The difference between veins and arteries can be subtle in neonates. Veins are usually collapsible and arteries are pulsatile (16).

E. Equipment

1. High-frequency (>10 MHz), small (<30-mm width), linear US probe
2. Doppler function (screening for thrombosis and occlusion)
3. Zoom function
4. Sterile gel
5. Sterile probe cover

F. Technique

1. Place a sterile cover over the probe, and use sterile lubricant on the probe.
2. Use your nondominant hand to hold and position the US probe (**Fig. 15.8**).

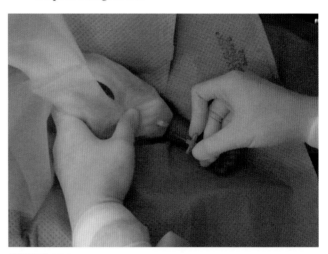

FIGURE 15.8 US probe positioned perpendicular to vein to access for PICC placement.

3. Optimize probe orientation, placing the target vessel in the center of the screen.
   a. Short-axis or transverse view: Probe is placed transverse to the direction of the vessel, which is seen in cross-section (**Fig. 15.9A**).
   b. Long-axis or sagittal view: Probe follows the direction of the vessel, which is seen in its length. Following the vein's path, identify valves, stenosis, or thrombosis (**Fig. 15.9B**).
   c. Out-of-plane where the needle crosses the US beam perpendicularly.
   d. In-plane where the needle stays in the US beam (**Fig. 15.9C**).

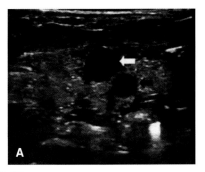 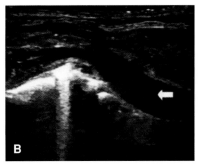 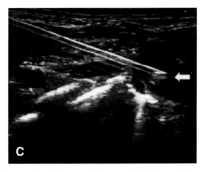

FIGURE 15.9 **A:** Transverse, out-of-plane view shows the cross-section of the internal jugular vein (*white arrow*) and the carotid artery (*black arrow*). The relative compression of the vessel and pulsed Doppler control of vascular flux can help identify the vein and the artery, respectively. **B:** The sagittal view shows the subclavian vein (SCV) (*white arrow*) in plane and the overlying pleura (*black arrow*) and lung. **C:** Sagittal view, in plane, with the needle (*black arrow*) tip (*white arrow*) placed in the SCV. Aspiration of blood can confirm correct placement. (Reprinted with permission from Lausten-Thomsen U, Merchaoui Z, Dubois C, et al. Ultrasound-guided subclavian vein cannulation in low birth weight neonates. *Pediatr Crit Care Med.* 2017;18(2):172–175.)

4. Position the handheld transducer probe perpendicular to a vein.
5. The needle tip should always be in the field of view during the procedure.

G. Complications

None

NEAR-INFRARED VISUALIZATION

A. Background

The infrared light source emits a harmless, near-infrared light, which is absorbed by the blood. Tissues surrounding the blood reflect the light and this image is captured by a digital video camera and processed. A green LED adds contrast to the image, which is then directly projected onto the surface of the skin in real time. This device requires no patient contact and has no heat, radiation, or laser eye safety issues (19–21).

Near-infrared visualization may be helpful for vein preservation, but the benefit has not been correlated to vein cannulation. Cost effectiveness and necessary training requirements are yet to be determined. Although systematic reviews and meta-analyses have not shown overall benefit of using near-infrared light devices, the device may be useful for patients with difficulties in successful cannulation (22,23).

B. Indication

1. To locate an accessible artery or vein for
   a. Phlebotomy
   b. Vessel cannulation

C. Contraindications

None

D. Equipment

Direct projection vascular imaging device

E. Technique

1. Position the head unit at 90 degrees and approximately 13 in (33 cm) above the target location.
2. Focus the device.
3. Switch to and utilize alternate modes.
   a. Universal
   b. Inverse
   c. Resize
   d. Fine Detail

References

1. Goren A, Laufer J, Yativ N, et al. Transillumination of the palm for venipuncture in infants. *Pediatr Emerg Care.* 2001;17(2):130–131.
2. Mattson D, O'Connor M. Transilluminator assistance in neonatal venipuncture. *Neonatal Netw.* 1986;5:42–45.
3. Dinner M. Transillumination to facilitate venipuncture in children. *Anesth Analg.* 1992;74:467.
4. Hosokawa K, Kato H, Kishi C, et al. Transillumination by light-emitting diode facilitates peripheral venous cannulations in infants and small children. *Acta Anaesthesiol Scand.* 2010;54:957–961.
5. John J. Transillumination for vascular access: old concept, new technology. *Pediatr Anesth.* 2007;17:189–190.
6. Sumpelmann R, Osthaus WA, Irmler H, et al. Prevention of burns caused by transillumination for peripheral venous access in neonates. *Pediatr Anaesth.* 2006;16:1094–1098.

7. Perman MJ, Kauls LS. Transilluminator burns in the neonatal intensive care unit: a mimicker of more serious disease. *Pediatr Dermatol.* 2007;24:168–171.

8. Keroack MA, Kotilainen HR, Griffin BE. A cluster of atypical skin lesions in well-baby nurseries and a neonatal intensive care unit. *J Perinatol.* 1996;16:370–373.

9. Sajben FP, Gibbs NF, Friedlander SF. Transillumination blisters in a neonate. *J Am Acad Dermatol.* 1999;41:264–265.

10. Withey SJ, Moss AL, Williams GJ. Cold light, heat burn. *Burns.* 2000;26:414–415.

11. Johnson KN, Thomas T, Grove J, et al. Insertion of peripherally inserted central catheters in neonates less than 1.5 kg using ultrasound guidance. *Pediatr Surg Int.* 2016;32(11):1053–1057.

12. Lausten-Thomsen U, Merchaoui Z, Dubois C, et al. Ultrasound-guided subclavian vein cannulation in low birth weight neonates. *Pediatr Crit Care Med.* 2017;18(2):172–175.

13. Breschan C, Graf G, Jost R, et al. A retrospective analysis of the clinical effectiveness of supraclavicular, ultrasound-guided brachiocephalic vein cannulations in preterm infants. *Anesthesiology.* 2018;128(1):38–43.

14. Oulego-Erroz I, Alonso-Quintela P, Terroba-Seara S, et al. Ultrasound-guided cannulation of the brachiocephalic vein in neonates and preterm infants: a prospective observational study. *Amer J Perinatol.* 2018;35(05):503–508.

15. Brasher C, Malbezin S. Central venous catheters in small infants. *Anesthesiology.* 2018;128(1):4–5.

16. Detaille T, Pirotte T, Veyckemans F. Vascular access in the neonate. *Best Pract Res Clin Anaesthesiol.* 2010;24:403–418.

17. Fidler HL. The use of bedside ultrasonography for PICC placement and insertion. *Adv Neonatal Care.* 2011;11:52–53.

18. Merchaoui Z, Lausten-Thomsen U, Pierre F, et al. Supraclavicular approach to ultrasound-guided brachiocephalic vein cannulation in children and neonates. *Front Pediatr.* 2017;5:211.

19. Hess HA. A biomedical device to improve pediatric vascular access success. *Pediatr Nurs.* 2010;36:259–263.

20. Perry AM, Caviness AC, Hsu D. Efficacy of a near-infrared light device in pediatric intravenous cannulation: a randomized controlled trial. *Pediatr Emerg Care.* 2011;27(1):5–10.

21. Phipps K, Modic A, O'Riordan MA, et al. A randomized trial of the vein viewer versus standard technique for placement of peripherally inserted central catheters (PICCs) in neonates. *J Perinatol.* 2012;32:498–501.

22. Conversano E, Cozzi G, Pavan M, et al. Impact of near infrared light in pediatric blood drawing centre on rate of first attempt success and time of procedure. *Ital J Pediatr.* 2018;44(1):60.

23. Park JM, Kim MJ, Yim HW, et al. Utility of near-infrared light devices for pediatric peripheral intravenous cannulation: a systematic review and meta-analysis. *Eur J Pediatr.* 2016;175(12):1975–1988.

16

Venipuncture

Amber M. Dave

A. Indications

1. Blood sampling
   a. Routine laboratory tests, particularly if the volume of blood required is larger than can be obtained by capillary sampling (≥1.5 ml)
   b. Blood culture
   c. Central hematocrit
   d. Preferred (over capillary sample) for certain studies (1,2)
      (1) Ammonia, lactate, or pyruvate level (arterial optimal)
      (2) Drug levels
      (3) Cross-matching blood
      (4) Hemoglobin/hematocrit
      (5) Karyotype
      (6) Coagulation studies
2. Administration of medications

B. Contraindications

1. Use of deep vein in the presence of coagulation defect
2. Local infection and/or inflammation at puncture site
3. Femoral or internal jugular vein (see G)
4. External jugular vein in infants with respiratory distress, intracranial hemorrhage, or raised intracranial pressure

C. Precautions

1. Observe universal precautions.
2. When sampling from neck veins, place infant in head-down position to avoid cranial air embolus. Do not use neck veins in infants with intracranial bleeding or increased intracranial pressure.
3. Remove tourniquet before removing needle (to minimize hematoma formation).
4. Apply local pressure with dry gauze to produce hemostasis (usually 2 to 3 minutes).
5. Avoid using alcohol swab to apply local pressure (painful, impairs hemostasis).

D. Special Considerations for Neonates

1. Conserve sites to preserve limited venous access by using distal sites first whenever possible
2. Use small needle or scalp vein butterfly. A 23-gauge needle is the best. Hemolysis or clotting may occur with a 25-gauge or smaller needle
3. Avoid use of chlorhexidine in infants <2 months old
4. Choice of veins in order of preference (Fig. 16.1)
   a. Dorsum of hands
   b. Dorsum of feet
   c. Basilic, cephalic, or cubital veins in the antecubital fossa
   d. Greater saphenous vein at the ankle
   e. Vein in center of the volar aspect of the wrist
   f. Proximal greater saphenous vein
   g. Scalp
   h. Neck
5. Pain control
   a. Lidocaine–prilocaine topical anesthetic cream applied 30 minutes prior to procedure, if time allows (3,4)
   b. Oral sucrose solution (12% to 25%) provides quick and effective pain control for venipuncture (4,5)
   c. Heel lancing can be more painful and may require more punctures than venipuncture in infants (3,6)

E. Equipment

1. Gloves
2. A 23-gauge venipuncture needle (Fig. 16.2)
3. Syringe with volume just larger than sample to be drawn

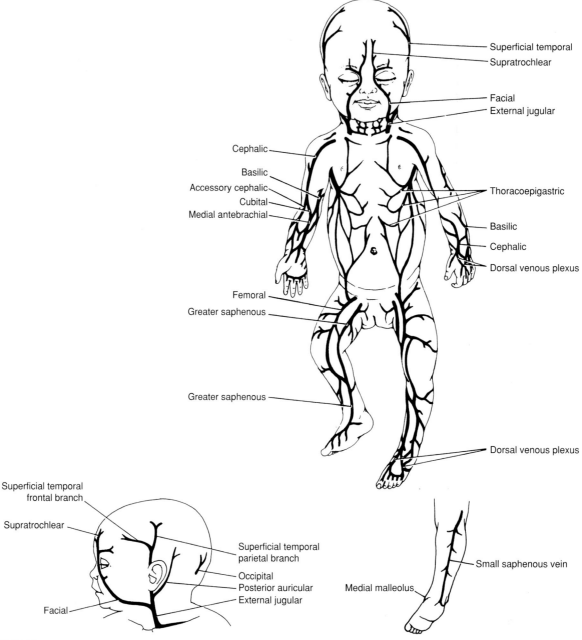

FIGURE 16.1 The superficial venous system in the neonate.

4. Antiseptic swabs—70% alcohol or povidone–iodine solution or 0.5% chlorhexidine in 70% alcohol for infants >2 months old
5. Gauze pads
6. Appropriate containers for specimens
7. For blood culture
   a. Antiseptic: Povidone–iodine solution preparation (three swabs); or 0.5% chlorhexidine in 70% alcohol (for infants >2 months old)
   b. Sterile gloves
   c. Blood culture bottle(s)
   d. Transfer needle
8. Tourniquet or sphygmomanometer cuff

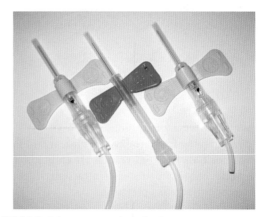

FIGURE 16.2 Safety-engineered needles for venipuncture.

F. Technique

General Venipuncture

1. Perform hand hygiene and prepare materials.
2. Locate the appropriate vessel. Use transillumination if necessary (see Chapter 15). Warm extremity with heel warmer or warm washcloth if circulation is poor.
3. Apply anesthetic cream if time permits, and/or administer sucrose solution if possible.
4. Restrain infant appropriately, such as by swaddling, leaving only the extremity of the site of venipuncture exposed.
5. Prepare area with antiseptic (see Chapter 6). Allow to dry for at least 30 seconds.
6. Occlude vein proximally using either
   a. Tourniquet made with two rubber bands looped together (Fig. 16.3).
   b. Or using forefinger and thumb to encircle the extremity or use forefinger and middle finger as a tourniquet (Fig. 16.4A)

7. Remove occlusion device and replace to promote optimal vein distension.
8. Syringe collection: Check syringe function and attach to needle. Penetrate skin first and position for entry of vein (Fig. 16.4A,B).
   a. Puncture the skin 3 to 5 mm distal to the vein to allow good access without pushing the vein away.
   b. If possible, insert needle at area where vessel bifurcates to avoid "rolling" of veins.
   c. Angle of entry 15 to 30 degrees.
   d. Bevel up preferred for optimal blood flow (less chance of needle occlusion by vein wall).
   e. Direct needle in the direction of blood flow (towards the heart). If the needle enters alongside the vein rather than into it, withdraw the needle slightly without removing it completely, and adjust angle into the vessel.
9. Release tourniquet.
10. Collect sample by gentle suction, to prevent occlusion by vein wall and to avoid hemolysis.

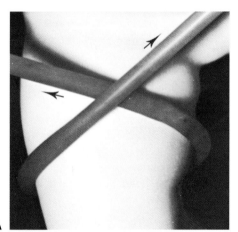
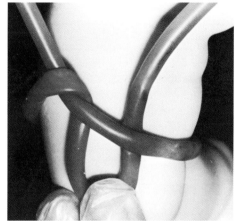
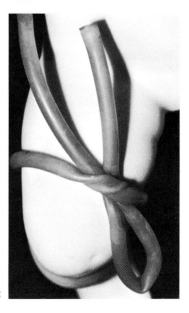

FIGURE 16.3 Correct application of a tourniquet for quick release.

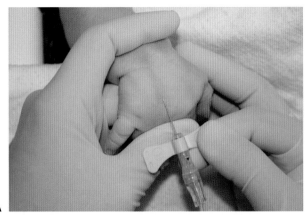 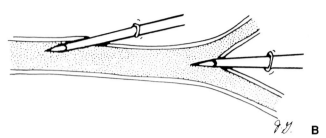

FIGURE 16.4 A: Venipuncture technique. Note position of fingers with forefinger occluding vein proximally. **B:** Needle penetrating skin a short distance from site of venipuncture.

11. Remove needle and apply local pressure with dry gauze for 1 to 3 minutes or until complete hemostasis.
12. Remove remaining povidone–iodine solution or chlorhexidine solution with sterile saline or water wipe.

Drip Technique

1. Cut the extension tubing of the 23-gauge butterfly needle catheter at 1 to 2 cm length (**Fig. 16.2**).
2. Follow steps 1 to 8, as above.
3. Insert the needle in the vein as in step 8, but without a syringe attached to the needle.
4. Collect the drops of blood directly into specimen container (**Fig. 16.5**).

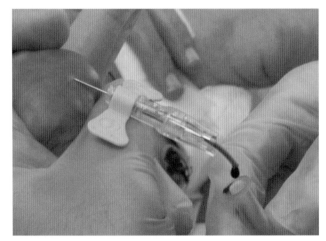

FIGURE 16.5 Drip technique of blood collection.

5. Short sterile hypodermic needles (23 or 24 gauge) may also be used to collect blood samples by the drip method but are sometimes less successful because the blood may pool at the hub of the needle and clot.

6. Drip method cannot be used for blood culture or coagulation studies (6).

Scalp Vein

1. Locate the frontal, superficial temporal, or posterior auricular scalp veins (**Fig. 16.1**).
2. Shaving the site may be necessary to allow for proper visualization.
3. Use scalp vein needle set or 23-gauge butterfly.
4. Occlude vein proximally with finger by placing digital pressure at the base of the vein.
5. Feel for a pulse to avoid entering an artery.
6. Use a shallow angle (15 to 20 degrees). Apply traction to the scalp with the nondominant hand to prevent rolling of the vessel.
7. Catheter should be directed in the same direction as the blood flow (toward the heart).
8. See F, "General Venipuncture."

Proximal Greater Saphenous Vein (7)

1. This technique should be used rarely—only if blood samples are essential and cannot be obtained by venipuncture from other sites.
2. Use only in older infants or in term neonates without evidence of coagulopathy.
3. Have assistant hold infant's thighs abducted with knees and hips slightly flexed.
4. Locate femoral triangle (**Fig. 16.6A**).
   a. **Proximal boundary:** Inguinal ligament.
   b. **Lateral boundary:** Medial border of sartorius muscle.
   c. **Medial boundary:** Lateral border of adductor longus muscle.
5. Enter skin and then vein at point medial to the arterial pulsation, approximately two-thirds along the line from inguinal ligament to apex of triangle (**Fig. 16.6B**).

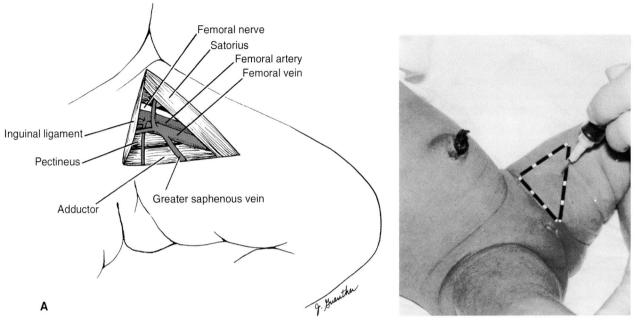

FIGURE 16.6 A: Anatomy of the femoral triangle as defined in the text. (Adapted from Plaxico DT, Bucciarella RL. Greater saphenous vein venipuncture in the neonate. *J Pediatr*. 1978;93(6):1025–1026. Copyright © 1978 Elsevier. With permission.) **B:** Position of the femoral triangle on the abducted thigh.

a. Use relatively steep angle (45 to 60 degrees).
b. After entering skin, advance 1 to 4 mm while applying gentle suction until blood return is achieved.
6. See F, "General Venipuncture."

External Jugular Vein

1. Position infant in head-down position with head extended and rotated away from selected vessel (**Fig. 16.7**).

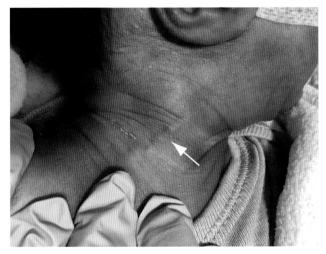

FIGURE 16.7 Infant positioned for puncture of external jugular vein (white arrow).

2. Prepare skin over sternocleidomastoid muscle with antiseptic.
3. Flick infant's heel to induce crying and optimize vein distension.

4. Visualize external jugular vein running from angle of jaw to posterior border of sternocleidomastoid in its lower third.
5. Puncture vessel where it runs across the anterior border of the sternocleidomastoid muscle.
6. See F, "General Venipuncture."

G. Complications (8–11)

1. Hemorrhage with coagulation defect or puncture of deep vein
2. Venous thrombosis or embolus, limb ischemia, and arteriovenous fistula with puncture of large, deep vein (9)
3. Laceration of adjacent artery
4. During femoral vein puncture
    a. Reflex arteriospasm of femoral artery with gangrene of extremity (10)
    b. Penetration of peritoneal cavity
    c. Septic arthritis of hip (11)
    d. Arteriovenous fistula (9)
5. During internal jugular puncture
    a. Laceration of carotid artery
    b. Pneumothorax/subcutaneous emphysema
    c. Interference with ventilation due to positioning
    d. Raised intracranial pressure to head-down position aggravating intraventricular hemorrhage
6. During scalp vein puncture:
    a. Laceration of artery
    b. Corneal abrasion or other eye damage if rubber band used improperly

References

1. Baral J. Use of a simple technique for the collection of blood from premature and full-term babies. *Med J Aust.* 1968;1:97.
2. Kayiran SM, Ozbek N, Turan M, et al. Significant differences between capillary and venous complete blood counts in the neonatal period. *Clin Lab Haematol.* 2003;25:9–16.
3. Shah VS, Ohlsson A. Venepuncture versus heel lance for blood sampling in term neonate. *Cochrane Database Syst Rev.* 2011;(10):CD001452.
4. Biran V, Gourrier E, Cimerman P, et al. Analgesic effects of EMLA cream and oral sucrose during venepuncture in preterm infants. *Pediatrics.* 2011;128(1):e63–e70.
5. Stevens, B, Yamada J, Ohlsson A, et al. Sucrose for analgesia in newborn infants undergoing painful procedures. *Cochrane Database Syst Rev.* 2016;(7):CD001069.
6. Ogawa S, Ogihara T, Fujiwara E, et al. Venepuncture is preferable to heel lance for blood sampling in term neonate. *Arch Dis Child Fetal Neonatal Ed.* 2005;90(5):F432–F436.
7. Plaxico DT, Bucciarelli RL. Greater saphenous vein venipuncture in the neonate. *J Pediatr.* 1978;93:1025–1026.
8. Ramasethu J. Complications of vascular catheters in the neonatal intensive care unit. *Clin Perinatol.* 2008;35:199–222.
9. Gamba P, Tchaprassian Z, Verlato F, et al. Iatrogenic vascular lesions in extremely low birth weight and low birth weight neonates. *J Vasc Surg.* 1997;26(4):643–646.
10. Kantr RK, Gorton JM, Palmieri K, et al. Anatomy of femoral vessels in infants and guidelines for venous catheterizations. *Pediatrics.* 1989;83:1020–1022.
11. Asnes RS, Arendar GM. Septic arthritis of the hip: a complication of venipuncture. *Pediatrics.* 1966;38:837–841.

Arterial Puncture

Amber M. Dave

A. Indications (1,2)

1. Sampling for arterial blood gas determination
2. Sampling for routine laboratory test when venous and capillary sampling are not suitable or unobtainable
3. Sampling for ammonia, lactate, or pyruvate level
4. To obtain a large quantity (≥1.5 mL) of blood from an infant

B. Contraindications

1. Coagulation defects, thrombocytopenia
2. Circulatory compromise in the extremity
3. Inappropriate artery
   a. Femoral artery
   b. Use of radial artery if collaterals are inadequate (see Allen test described under Radial Artery Puncture)
   c. Ulnar artery (poor collaterals)
4. Infection and/or inflammation in sampling area
5. When cannulation of that vessel is anticipated
6. Use of peripheral arteries on the ipsilateral arm in an infant with congenital heart disease requiring a shunt via the subclavian artery

C. Precautions

1. Perform arterial sampling only when venous or capillary sampling is inappropriate or unobtainable.
2. Use smallest possible (23- to 27-gauge) needle to minimize trauma to vessel and to prevent hematoma formation.

3. Avoid laceration of the artery caused by puncturing both sides of arterial wall in exactly opposite locations.
4. Remove excess heparin and air bubble from the blood gas syringe. If a small bubble gets into the sample, point the tip of the syringe up, expel the air bubble immediately, and cap syringe.
5. Guarantee hemostasis at the end of the procedure. Pressure must be applied even if an attempt is unsuccessful or results in an inadequate sample.
6. Check distal circulation after puncture.
   a. Arterial pulse
   b. Capillary refill time
   c. Color and temperature
7. Take action to reverse arteriospasm, if necessary. (See Chapter 36.)

D. Selection of Arterial Site

1. Peripheral site preferred.
2. Radial artery preferred if ulnar collateral intact (see Allen test below).
3. Posterior tibial artery satisfactory.
4. Dorsalis pedis artery is often small or absent, but may be accessible in some infants.
5. Brachial artery *only if indication is urgent and peripheral arterial or umbilical artery access is not available* because of risk of injury to the adjacent median nerve, and the risk of ischemia due to the absence of collaterals at this site (3).
6. Temporal artery should be avoided because of risk of neurologic damage (4,5).
7. Ulnar artery should be avoided because of the risk of impaired circulation to the hand due to poor collateral circulation or damage to the ulnar or the median nerve.

E. Equipment

1. Sterile gloves
2. Sterile needle
   a. A 23- to 25-gauge venipuncture needle, preferably a safety-engineered needle
   b. A butterfly needle with extension tubing is often easier to use
3. Appropriate syringes, including a preheparinized blood gas syringe
4. Antiseptic for skin preparation: Povidone-iodine solution or 0.5% chlorhexidine in 70% alcohol (for infants >2 months old); sterile water or sterile saline wipe to remove antiseptic at end of procedure
5. Gauze pads
6. High-intensity fiberoptic light for transillumination (optional) and a sterile glove to cover (see Chapter 15)
7. Bedside ultrasound, if available
8. Oral sucrose solution (24% to 25%) or eutectic mixture of local anesthetics (EMLA) for pain control, if possible (6,7)

F. Technique (▶ Video 17.1: Radial Artery Blood Sampling)

General Principles (1,2)

1. Transillumination may assist location of vessel (see Fig. 15.5) (8). Use of ultrasound guidance may decrease the number of attempts, increase success when performed by an experienced practitioner, and decrease the risk of hematoma formation or ischemia (9,10).
2. Give sucrose or apply EMLA cream if time allows.
3. Perform hand hygiene and prepare materials.
4. Wear sterile gloves.
5. Attach syringe to needle.
6. Designate nondominant hand as nonsterile and use this hand to support extremity and site of puncture.
7. With sterile hand, clean the site with povidone-iodine or 0.5% chlorhexidine, allow it to dry for at least 30 seconds.
8. Position needle for arterial puncture against direction of blood flow.
   a. Keep angle of entry shallow for superficial vessels at 15 to 30 degrees; use 45-degree angle for deeper arteries. Keep bevel of needle up.
   b. Penetrate the skin first slightly proximal to the best point of pulsation, and then puncture artery to minimize trauma to vessel.
   c. Apply gentle suction on syringe as soon as blood flow is observed; maintain needle in same position until all blood samples have been collected.
   d. If no blood flow is obtained or blood flow ceases, adjust depth of penetration or the angle of the needle. If resistance is encountered, withdraw needle cautiously until blood returns. Be patient and gentle—artery may spasm when needle is introduced, or with multiple attempts.
   e. Use fresh needle and repeat skin preparation if withdrawal from skin is necessary.
9. Apply firm, local pressure for 1 to 3 minutes to achieve complete hemostasis and avoid hematoma formation.
10. Inspect fingers for circulatory compromise (11,12).
11. Remove povidone-iodine from skin using sterile water or sterile saline wipe at end of procedure.

Radial Artery Puncture

1. Locate radial and ulnar arteries at proximal wrist crease (**Fig. 17.1**).
   a. Radial artery is lateral to flexor carpi radialis tendon.
   b. Ulnar artery is medial to flexor carpi ulnaris tendon.
2. The effectiveness of the modified Allen test (described below) for assessing the adequacy of collateral supply to the hand has not been adequately studied in neonates and suffers from poor interobserver reliability. Transillumination is a valuable adjunct and use of ultrasound has also been reported (13).
   a. Elevate infant's hand.
   b. Occlude both radial and ulnar arteries at wrist.
   c. Massage palm toward wrist.
   d. Release occlusion of ulnar artery only.
   e. Look for color to return to hand in <10 seconds, indicating adequate collateral supply.
   f. Do not puncture radial artery if color return takes more than 15 seconds.
3. Slightly extend supine wrist, avoiding hyperextension, which may occlude the vessel (**Fig. 17.2**) (2).
4. See F, "General Principles."
5. Puncture the skin at the level of proximal crease and penetrate artery at 15 to 30 degrees with bevel up (**Fig. 17.3** and **Fig. 17.4**).

Posterior Tibial Puncture

1. Locate artery by palpation or transillumination between Achilles tendon and medial malleolus (**Fig. 17.5**; see also Fig. 15.5). Puncture the artery just posterior to medial malleolus.
2. See F, "General Principles."

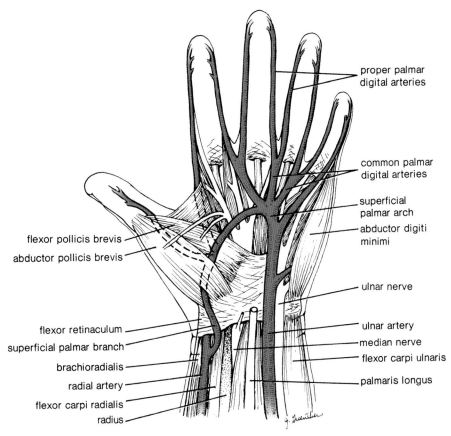

proper palmar digital arteries

common palmar digital arteries

superficial palmar arch

abductor digiti minimi

ulnar nerve

ulnar artery

median nerve

flexor carpi ulnaris

palmaris longus

flexor pollicis brevis

abductor pollicis brevis

flexor retinaculum

superficial palmar branch

brachioradialis

radial artery

flexor carpi radialis

radius

FIGURE 17.1 Anatomy of the major arteries of the wrist and hand.

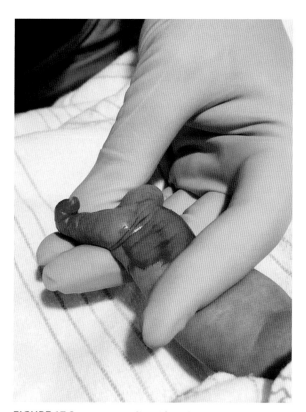

FIGURE 17.2 Positioning of hand for radial artery puncture.

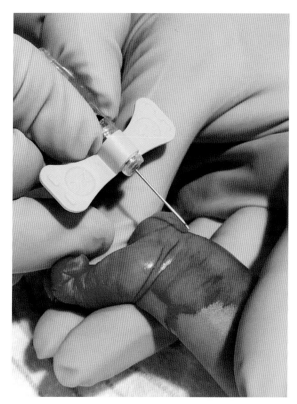

FIGURE 17.3 Angle of needle entry.

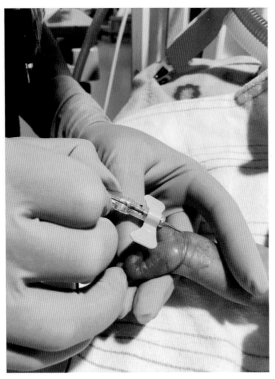

FIGURE 17.4 Lateral view of radial artery puncture site.

Dorsalis Pedis Puncture

1. Locate artery by palpation or transillumination on dorsum of foot between extensor hallucis longus and extensor digitorum longus tendons (**Fig. 17.6**). It

can be located between the first and second meta-tarsals in the dorsal midfoot between the first and second toes.
2. See F, "General Principles."

Brachial Artery Puncture

1. Locate the artery by palpation or transillumination along the medial margin of the biceps muscle at the bend of elbow and enter the artery at or above the level of anterior cubital fossa.
2. See F, "General Principles."

G. Complications (12)

See Chapter 33 for complications of arterial cannulation.

1. Distal ischemia from arteriospasm, thrombosis, or embolism
2. Hemorrhage or hematoma
3. Nerve damage (14)
    a. Median nerve (brachial artery puncture)
    b. Posterior tibial nerve
    c. Femoral nerve
4. Extensor tendon sheath injury, resulting in "false corti-cal thumb" (15)
5. Pseudoaneurysm following brachial artery puncture (16)

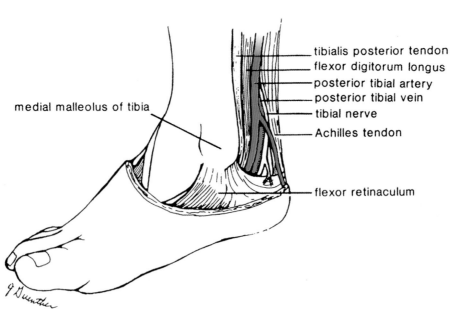

FIGURE 17.5 Anatomic relations of the posterior tibial artery.

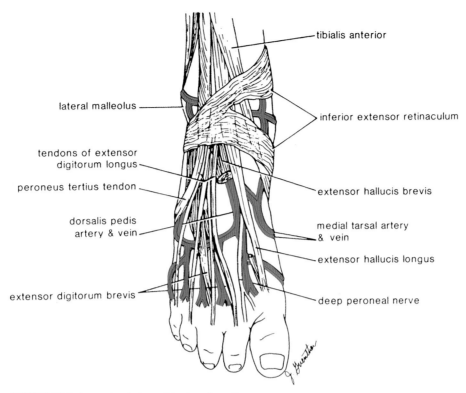

FIGURE 17.6 Anatomic relations of the dorsalis pedis artery.

References

1. Smith AD. Arterial blood sampling in neonates. *Lancet.* 1975;1:254–255.
2. Shaw JC. Arterial sampling from the radial artery in premature and full-term infants. *Lancet.* 1968;2:389–390.
3. Okeson GC, Wulbrecht PH. The safety of brachial artery puncture for arterial blood sampling. *Chest.* 1998;114:748–751.
4. Bull MJ, Schreiner RL, Garg BP, et al. Neurologic complications following temporal artery catheterization. *J Pediatr.* 1980;96:1071–1073.
5. Simmons MA, Levine RL, Lubchenco LO, et al. Warning: serious sequelae of temporal artery catheterization. *J Pediatr.* 1978;92:284.
6. Acharya AB, Annamali S, Taub NA, et al. Oral sucrose analgesia for preterm infant venipuncture. *Arch Dis Childhood Fetal Neonatal Ed.* 2004;89:F17–F18.
7. Stevens B, Yamada J, Ohlsson A, et al. Sucrose for analgesia in newborn infants undergoing painful procedures. *Cochrane Database Syst Rev.* 2016;(7):CD001069.
8. Wall PM, Kuhns LR. Percutaneous arterial sampling using transillumination. *Pediatrics.* 1977;59:1032–1035.
9. Gao YB, Yan JH, Gao FQ, et al. Effects of ultrasound-guided radial artery catheterization: an updated meta-analysis. *Am J Emerg Med.* 2016;33(1):50–55.
10. Aouad-Maroun M, Raphael CK, Sayyid SK, et al. Ultrasound-guided arterial cannulation for paediatrics. *Cochrane Database Syst Rev.* 2016;(9):CD011364.
11. Noreng MF. Blood flow in the radial artery before and after arterial puncture. *Acta Anaesthesiol Scand.* 1986;30:281–282.
12. Gillies ID, Morgan M, Sykes MK, et al. The nature and incidence of complications of peripheral artery puncture. *Anaesthesia.* 1979;34:506–509.
13. Barone JE, Madlinger RV. Should an Allen test be performed before radial artery cannulation? *J Trauma.* 2006;61:468–470.
14. Pape KE, Armstrong DL, Fitzhardinge PM. Peripheral median nerve damage secondary to brachial arterial blood gas sampling. *J Pediatr.* 1978;93:852–856.
15. Skogland RR, Giles EJ. The false cortical thumb. *Am J Dis Child.* 1986;140:375–376.
16. Landau D, Schreiber R, Szendro G, et al. Brachial artery pseudoaneurysm in a premature infant. *Arch Dis Child Fetal Neo Ed.* 2003;88:F152–F153.

Capillary Blood Sampling

Catherine M. Brown

A. Purpose

To obtain capillary blood samples that provide accurate laboratory results with minimal discomfort and potential for injury/infection.

B. Background

Capillary blood sampling is the most frequently performed skin-breaking procedure in neonatal intensive care units (1). It is an easily mastered, minimally invasive procedure that, when performed with proper technique and equipment, provides laboratory results that are comparable to arterial samples (2,3). The only exception to this is a complete blood count (CBC), where capillary samples have a higher hemoglobin (Hgb), hematocrit (Hct), red blood cell (RBC) count, and white blood cell (WBC) count when compared to venous samples (4). The advantage of capillary sampling is that repeated testing may be carried out, and peripheral veins may be saved for IV access.

C. Indications

1. Capillary blood gas sampling
2. Routine laboratory analysis (standard hematology, chemistries, toxicology/drug levels) requiring a limited amount of blood in which minimal cell lysis does not alter results
3. Newborn metabolic screen

D. Contraindications

1. Edema, because interstitial fluid dilutes the sample and gives inaccurate results
2. Injury or anomalies that preclude putting pressure on the foot

3. Areas that are bruised or injured by multiple previous heelsticks
4. Poor perfusion
5. Local infection
6. Peripherally inserted central catheter (PICC) or peripheral IV catheter in the foot

E. Limitations

1. Venous or arterial blood rather than capillary samples should be used for
   a. Blood cultures, which require sterile technique
   b. Tests in which even a minimal amount of hemolysis will compromise results
   c. Special tests such as coagulation studies (newer coagulation tests that require only a few drops of blood are still not widely available)
   d. Laboratory tests that require more than 1.5 mL of blood

F. Equipment

1. Gloves
2. Heel-warming device (see G)
3. Antiseptic (povidone-iodine/saline or chlorhexidine gluconate [CHG] swab)
   a. Cleanse site with povidone-iodine for those <32 weeks' gestation or CHG swab in infants who are ≥32 weeks' gestational age (5).
4. Pad or other means of protecting bed linens
5. Heel-lancing device (see G). Use appropriate size for infant (Table 18.1)
6. Specimen collector as appropriate
   a. Serum separators
   b. Hematology tubes
   c. Capillary blood gas tube
   d. Newborn metabolic screen filter paper
   e. DNA card

TABLE 18.1 Examples of Automated Heel-Lancing Products Based on Infant Size

INFANT SIZE	AVAILABLE PRODUCTS	INCISION DEPTH/LENGTH
<1,000 g	Tenderfoot Micropreemie	0.65 mm/1.40 mm
Low birthweight and preemie >1,000 g	Tenderfoot Preemie/BD Quikheel Preemie	0.85 mm/1.75 mm
Term to 3–6 mo	Tenderfoot Newborn/ BD Quikheel Infant	1.0 mm/2.50 mm
6 mo–2 yr	Tenderfoot Toddler	2.0 mm/3.00 mm

7. Capillary tubes for blood transfer to lab tubes if appropriate
8. Small adhesive bandage or gauze wrap

G. Heel-Lancing Devices and Heel Warmers

1. **Automated heel-lancing device:** Encased, spring-loaded, retractable blade that provides a controlled and consistent width and depth of incision for blood testing.
   a. Incision depths range from 0.65 to 2 mm for micro-preemies through toddlers (Tenderfoot, International Technidyne Corporation, Edison, New Jersey) and from 0.85 to 1 mm for preemies and newborns (BD Quikheel Lancet, BD Vacutainer Systems, Franklin Lakes, New Jersey) (see **Table 18.1**).
   b. The controlled depths avoid damage to the calcaneus (6–8) while providing greater yield with less pain, hemolysis, and laboratory-value error (6,9). The shallower devices can be used to obtain small samples from larger infants who require frequent point-of-care glucose testing (10).
   c. Nonautomated (manual) stylet-type lancets and spring-loaded needle puncture devices designed for adult glucose testing are not appropriate for infants (9).
2. **Heel warmer:** Chemically activated packet to heat heel prior to capillary testing. If heel warming is used, a commercial prepackaged unit provides controlled temperature. The warmer should be applied for 5 minutes and then removed prior to heelstick. Warming of the heel is not always required (11). Please follow the procedure at your facility with regard to warming the heel prior to capillary puncture.

H. Precautions

1. Site
   a. Appropriate sites for capillary heelsticks are on the outer aspects of the heel making sure to avoid the calcaneus.
   b. Do not use the end of the heel. The calcaneus is superficial at this site, and there is an increased risk of osteomyelitis (6).
   c. Do not use fingertips, toes, or earlobes of babies.
2. Hand position
   a. Do *not* squeeze the heel. Squeezing the heel results in greater pain, lower blood yield, and increased cell lysis.
3. Collection
   a. If using capillary tubes for blood transfer, it is essential to determine whether the tube contains substances such as anticoagulants, which may have the potential to interfere with lab results. Do not use tubes containing anticoagulants for newborn metabolic screens, or DNA cards.
   b. Scoop-shaped collectors provided with mini–lab tubes are used to guide blood drops to the specimen tube. Avoid repeated "scooping" along the surface of the foot. Microclots that form in blood on the skin can alter lab results.

I. Technique

1. Identify site; the preferred areas for capillary heel testing are the outer aspects of the heel (**Fig. 18.1**).

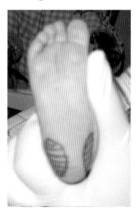

FIGURE 18.1 Appropriate sites for capillary heelstick sampling are along the sides of the heels.

   a. Vary sites to prevent bruising and skin damage.
   b. The plantar surface can be used in term and late preterm infants if the preferred areas are compromised by previous frequent testing (**Fig. 18.2**). The acceptable skin-to-calcaneal perichondrium distance is 2.2 mm or more to avoid complications (6).

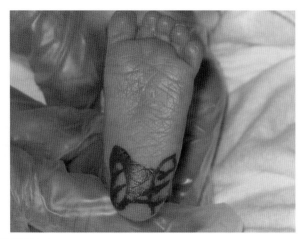

FIGURE 18.2 Alternative site for capillary heelstick sampling. If frequent sampling has rendered the sides of the heels unsuitable, the plantar surface between them can be used. Do not incise the end of the heel.

2. Apply heel warmer for 5 minutes. Remove just before procedure.
3. Provide comfort measures: Facilitated tucking/swaddling and the use of pacifiers combined with administration of a concentrated sucrose solution result in less measurable pain and faster resolution of discomfort in the infant following the procedure (12) (Fig. 5.1). Kangaroo care 30 minutes prior to and during procedure has shown a reduction in pain scores for stable premature infants (13).
4. Wash hands and put gloves on.
5. Cleanse site with povidone-iodine wipe for those <32 weeks' gestation or CHG swab in infants who are ≥32 weeks' gestational age (14).
6. Position hand with fingers along the calf and thumb at ball of foot to stabilize. Apply pressure along calf toward heel (Fig. 18.3).

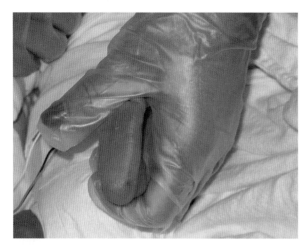

FIGURE 18.3 Position for hand and automated lancing device. Position heel in the apex of the angle of the thumb and forefinger with fingers along the calf and thumb along the ball of the foot. Place automated lancing device in appropriate position. Apply pressure along the calf with counterpressure by the thumb. Do not squeeze the heel.

7. Prepare automated device by removing release clip.
8. Place automated device on site, line up arrow to desired puncture location and activate.
9. Apply pressure to leg with counterpressure to ball of foot with an upward motion of the fingers along the calf and a forward motion of the thumb on the plantar surface of the foot, and allow blood drop to form.
10. Wipe away first drop of blood with gauze or clean wipe.
11. Using capillary action (the ability of a liquid to flow into a smaller tube without assistance), fill blood gas tube, holding tube horizontally (Fig. 18.4).

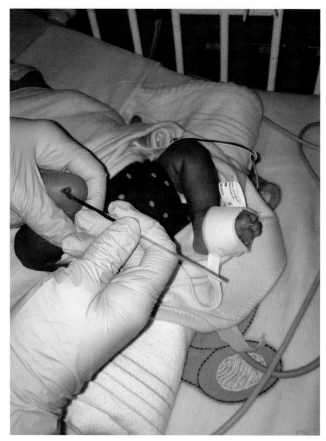

FIGURE 18.4 Capillary blood gas sampling.

12. Release pressure, allowing capillaries to refill.
13. Guide blood drops into tube or collect with capillary tube for transfer to laboratory tube.
14. If blood stops flowing, wipe site to remove clot with CHG or saline swab, gauze, or clean wipe; ensure time for capillary refill; and then reapply pressure to leg. If blood does not flow, choose another site and repeat procedure or consider venipuncture.
15. When samples have been collected, apply pressure to puncture site and wrap with gauze or apply adhesive bandage. Remove povidone-iodine from skin with saline wipe.
16. Continue comfort measures.

J. Specimen Handling

1. Collect blood gas sample first, then hematology samples, and then chemistry/toxicology samples.
2. Ensure that blood gas samples are free of air bubbles.
   a. Place the tube horizontally so that the blood is drawn by capillary action and does not collect air bubbles that can alter results. Apply caps to ends of tube.
   b. Capillary blood gas samples should be analyzed within 10 minutes or should be kept horizontally on ice for up to 1 hour, and the tube must be rolled prior to analysis. Consult institution laboratory for guidance on blood gas sample storage and transport.
3. Flick side of hematology microtube during collection process to activate anticoagulant and prevent clotting.
4. Newborn metabolic screen: Follow specific collection guidelines (14)
   a. Minimum 24 to 48 hours after birth.
   b. Integrity of collection medium: Avoid touching filter paper, as oils from finger can compromise results.
   c. Single (no overlapping) drops on filter paper. Position infant so that incision is in the dependent position, allowing a large drop of blood to form. Blood should drop freely onto designated circle on filter paper. Repeat for each circle (**Fig. 18.5**).
   d. Do not apply blood to filter paper using capillary tubes that contain anticoagulants or other materials that can interfere with lab results.

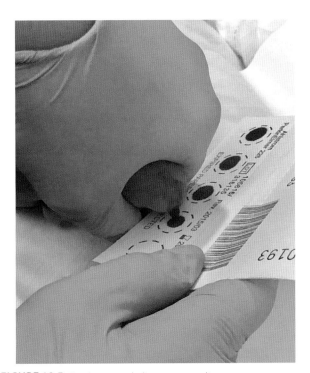

FIGURE 18.5 Newborn metabolic screen sampling.

K. Complications

1. Pain
2. Infection (cellulitis, abscess, perichondritis, osteomyelitis) (**Fig. 18.6**) (15,16)
3. Tissue loss and scarring
4. Calcified nodules (17)

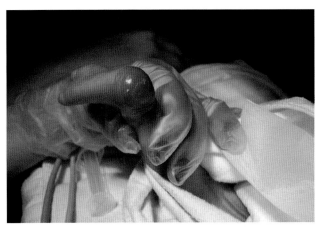

FIGURE 18.6 Cellulitis of heel—complication of capillary heelstick sampling.

L. Inaccurate Laboratory Results

1. Hyperkalemia secondary to excessive hemolysis.
   a. Use proper technique and procedures to minimize cell lysis.
2. Erroneous blood gas results.
   a. Ensure that sample is free of air bubbles.
   b. Avoid delay in analysis.
   c. Use proper technique and procedures to minimize cell lysis.

References

1. Courtois E, Droutman S, Magny JF, et al. Epidemiology and neonatal pain management of heelsticks in intensive care units: EPIPPAIN 2, a prospective observational study. *Int J Nurs Stud.* 2016;59:79–88.
2. Richter S, Kerry C, Hassan N, et al. Capillary blood gas as a substitute for arterial blood gas: a meta-analysis. *Br J Hosp Med (Lond).* 2014;75:136–142.
3. Goenka A, Bhoola R, McKerrow N. Neonatal blood gas sampling methods. *South Afr J Child Health.* 2012;6:3–9.
4. Kayiran SM, Ozebek N, Turan M, et al. Significant differences between capillary and venous complete blood counts in the neonatal period. *Clin Lab Haematol.* 2003;25:9–16.
5. Chapman AK, Aucott SW, Milstone AM. Safety of chlorhexidine gluconate used for skin antisepsis in the preterm infant. *J Perinatol.* 2012;32:4–9.
6. Arena J, Emparanza JI, Nogues A, et al. Skin to calcaneus distance in the neonate. *Arch Dis Child Fetal Neonatal Ed.* 2005;90:F328–F331.

7. Kazmierczak SC, Robertson AF, Briley KP. Comparison of hemolysis in blood samples collected using an automatic incision device and a manual lancet. *Arch Pediatr Adolesc Med.* 2002;156:1072–1074.

8. Vertanen H, Fellman V, Brommels M, et al. An automatic incision device for obtaining blood samples from the heels of preterm infants causes less damage than a conventional manual lancet. *Arch Dis Child Fetal Neonatal Ed.* 2001;84:328–331.

9. Shah V, Taddio A, Kulasekaran K, et al. Evaluation of a new lancet device (BD QuickHeel) on pain response and success of procedure in term neonates. *Arch Pediatr Adolesc Med.* 2003;157(11):1075–1078.

10. Folk LA. Guide to capillary heelstick blood sampling in infants. *Adv Neonatal Care.* 2007;7:171–178.

11. Janes M, Pinelli J, Landry S, et al. Comparison of capillary blood sampling using an automated incision device with and without warming the heel. *J Perinatol.* 2002;22:154–158.

12. Yin T, Yang L, Lee TY, et al. Development of atraumatic heel-stick procedures by combined treatment with non-nutritive sucking, oral sucrose, and facilitated tucking: a randomized control trial. *Int J Nurs Stud.* 2015;52:1288–1299.

13. Johnston C, Campbell-Yeo M, Disher T, et al. Skin to skin care for procedural pain in neonates. *Cochrane Database Syst Rev.* 2017;2:CD008.

14. Bryant K, Horns K, Longo N, et al. A primer on newborn screening. *Adv Neonatal Care.* 2004;4(5):306.

15. Abril Martin JC, Aguilar Rodriguez L, Albinana Cilvetti J. Flatfoot and calcaneal deformity secondary to osteomyelitis after heel puncture. *J Pediatr Orthop B.* 1999;8:122–124.

16. Lauer BA, Altenburgher KM. Outbreak of staphylococcal infections following heel puncture for blood sampling. *Am J Dis Child.* 1981;135:277–278.

17. Rho NK, Youn SJ, Park HS, et al. Calcified nodule on the heel of a child following a single heel stick in the neonatal period. *Clin Exp Dermatol.* 2003;28:502–503.

Miscellaneous Sampling

19

Lumbar Puncture

Marko Culjat

A. Indications

1. Initial diagnosis of central nervous system (CNS) infections.
   a. Bacterial and fungal infections.

   The inclusion of lumbar puncture (LP) as part of sepsis workup depends on the timing of presumed sepsis (early- vs. late-onset sepsis), prematurity, maternal status (intrapartum antibiotic prophylaxis [IAP], diagnosis of chorioamnionitis), and clinical symptoms (1). While there are differing approaches among health care providers, most sources recommend the following:
   - In a setting of presumed early-onset sepsis, all newborns with overt signs of sepsis should undergo full evaluation, including LP.
   - If newborn is well appearing, but mother was diagnosed with chorioamnionitis or received inadequate IAP in a setting of prolonged rupture of membranes, LP does not need to be performed (2,3).
   - In a setting of late-onset sepsis, LP is always recommended, since approximately one-third of culture-confirmed meningitis will have a negative blood culture (1). The approach of obtaining a CSF culture only if blood culture is positive is not appropriate.
   - In practice, these recommendations are often modified based on clinical stability of the infant (4).
   b. Diagnosis of congenital infections. Diagnostic evaluations in a setting of possible congenital herpes simplex and syphilis infections are needed (5,6). Other infections include toxoplasmosis, cytomegalovirus, and lately, Zika virus (7).
2. Monitor efficacy of meningitis treatment.

   While there is some controversy on whether to repeat an LP in older infants being treated for meningitis, this approach might be beneficial in VLBW infants since approximately 10% of cases have a positive repeat CSF culture despite apparently adequate antimicrobial treatment (4,8,9).
3. Drainage of CSF in communicating hydrocephalus associated with intraventricular hemorrhage, presenting with signs of increased intracranial pressure (ICP) or worsening ventriculomegaly (see Section B.1) (10).
   a. Serial drainage of 10 to 15 mL/kg of CSF via LP for a limited number of days (usually <3) has been implemented in patients with worsening ventriculomegaly and developing signs of ICP, with cutoff values for ventricular index and diagonal ventricular size varying among practitioners (10–14).
   b. A meta-analysis of four studies found no evidence to support repeated CSF removal in infants at risk of or developing posthemorrhagic hydrocephalus if there are no signs of increased ICP (15).
4. Diagnostic workup of metabolic disease (16,17).
5. Diagnosis of CSF spread in patients with leukemia (18).
6. CSF instillation of chemotherapeutic agents (19).

B. Contraindications

1. Increased ICP: In the neonate with open cranial sutures, increased ICP in a setting of space-occupying intracranial lesions or meningitis rarely results in transtentorial or cerebellar herniation. However, herniation can occur after LP in the presence of elevated ICP, even when the sutures are open (20,21). If signs of significantly increased ICP exist (rapidly declining or severely depressed level of consciousness, abnormal posturing, cranial nerve palsies, tense anterior fontanel, abnormalities in heart rate, respirations, or blood pressure without other cause), neuroimaging should be performed before LP. Open fontanels may mitigate development of papilledema until late in the clinical course (22).

2. Uncorrected thrombocytopenia or bleeding diathesis (23).
3. Infection of the skin or underlying tissue at or near the puncture site.
4. Lumbosacral anomalies, suspected or confirmed by imaging.
5. Clinical instability where risk of the procedure outweighs the benefit.

C. Equipment

All equipment must be sterile, apart from mask and cap.
    Prepackaged LP kits are available. Recommended equipment includes:

1. Mask, and optional cap and sterile gown
2. Sterile gloves
3. Povidone-iodine swabs (×3)
4. Aperture drape and sterile towels
5. Beveled spinal needle with stylet—usually two sizes available:
    a. Small: 25 gauge, 1 inch in length
    b. Large: 22 gauge, 1.5 inch in length
6. Three or more collection vials with caps
7. Adhesive bandage, gauze

D. Precautions

1. Monitor vital signs and oxygen saturation. Increasing supplemental oxygen during the procedure could prevent hypoxemia (24). However, the prudent approach would be to adjust the FiO_2 to keep monitored oxygen saturation within institutional reference ranges. Avoid flexion of the neck, in either the sitting or recumbent positions, since it does not increase interspinous spaces but significantly increases the risk of airway obstruction (25–29). Lateral recumbent position with flexed knees has been associated with significant, but temporary desaturation episodes (28,29).
2. Use strict aseptic technique (see Chapter 6).
3. Always use a needle with stylet while penetrating the skin, to avoid development of intraspinal epidermoid tumor (30,31).
4. Once the needle tip is past the skin, prevent traumatic tap caused by overpenetration by advancing the needle slowly, either in a "stylet-out" or "stylet-in" technique (see Section E.9) (32–34). Topical anesthetics and eutectic mixtures applied prior to the procedure might reduce the incidence of traumatic tap (33,34) by reducing pain (35) and struggling of the infant (36,37). However, due to inadequate evidence regarding safety and effectiveness, no unequivocal clinical recommendations can be made (see Section E.4) (38).

5. Never aspirate CSF with a syringe. Even a small amount of negative pressure can increase the risk of intracranial subdural hemorrhage or cerebellar herniation.
6. Palpate landmarks accurately to adequately determine L3–L4 and L4–L5 interspaces (lower interspace should be used for preterm infants; see Section E.3). Mean level of termination of the spinal cord falls at the L3–L4 level at 23 to 27 gestational weeks; L3 level at 28 to 34 gestational weeks; L2–L3 level at 35 to 40 gestational weeks. The spinal cord termination level reaches mean adult levels of L1–L2 by 2 months post-term (39).
7. Communicate clearly with your assistant.

E. Technique (▶ Video 19.1: Lumbar Puncture)

1. Obtain informed consent (see Chapter 3).
2. Proper positioning of the infant is key to a successful LP. The sitting position with hip flexion provides the widest interspinous spaces, with the second best position being lateral decubitus with hip flexion (25–27). Instruct the assistant to restrain the infant in the appropriate position (**Figs. 19.1** and **19.2**).

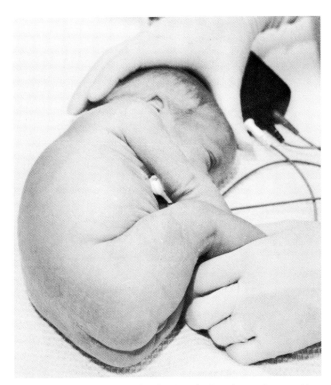

FIGURE 19.1 Restraining infant for LP in the lateral recumbent position. Neck should not be flexed. (*continued*)

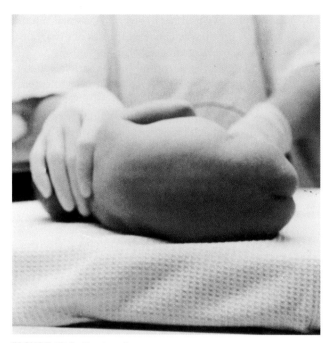

FIGURE 19.1 (*Continued*)

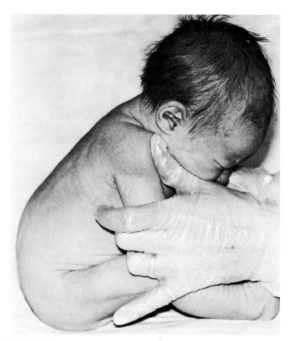

FIGURE 19.2 Restraining infant for LP in the sitting position.

3. Palpate the superior aspect of the iliac crests. An imaginary, intercristal or Tuffier line, drawn between the iliac crests is traditionally said to cross the spinal column at the level of L4 vertebra or L4–L5 interspace. However, the line can cross as low as L5 vertebra in neonates (40).

Careful palpation of the crests and the spinal column is important for proper identification of interspinous spaces. The preferred sites for LP are L3–L4 and L4–L5 (**Fig. 19.3**). Use the lower space for extremely premature infants (<28 gestational weeks).

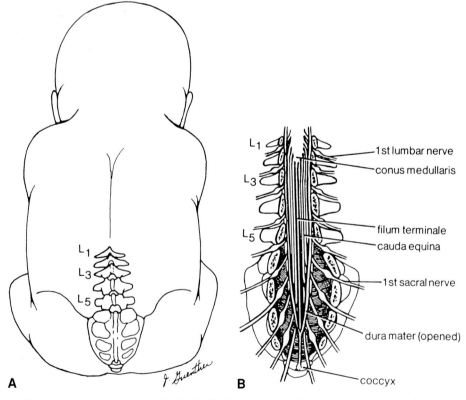

FIGURE 19.3 **A:** Externally palpable anatomic landmarks. **B:** Vertebral bodies removed to show anatomy of spinal cord in lumbosacral area in relation to external landmarks.

4. Pain control. Several guidelines and recommendations exist to guide procedural pain management in newborns (41–43).

   a. Use of eutectic mixture of local anesthetics (EMLA) is the only pain control measure studied specifically for LP (35). The study showed blunting of physiologic markers of pain (heart rate, and behavioral pain score) during insertion and withdrawal of the needle, when 1 g of EMLA was applied over 1 sq in (~2.5 × 2.5 cm) for 60 to 90 minutes. Most studies that assessed pain control with EMLA applied the mixture to the puncture site 30 to 90 minutes prior to the procedure (41,44). A Cochrane review (45) was not able to support any clinical recommendations regarding effectiveness or safety of topical anesthetics in needle-related pain control in neonates; there were significantly higher rates of local redness, swelling, and blanching after application of EMLA. Other studies indicate that EMLA is safe for premature infants as young as 30 weeks' (46) and 26 weeks' gestation (47). If there are multiple daily applications of EMLA, checking methemoglobin levels is recommended (44,46). A significant increase in methemoglobin (>5%) or clinical symptoms (cyanosis) can rarely be seen in premature infants (in ~1%), and after a prolonged application (3 hours or longer) or high doses (3.5 g) in older infants (47).

   b. Fentanyl could be considered for pain control during LP. An intravenous dose of 0.5 to 2 mcg/kg is effective in controlling procedural pain. The major side effect is chest wall rigidity, seen after rapid administrations of >1 mcg/kg/dose, which can be managed by a paralytic drug, such as vecuronium, or naloxone (41). Slow administration of fentanyl over 3 to 5 minutes is recommended.

   c. Oral sucrose given immediately prior to the procedure has been shown to be effective in reducing procedural pain from heal lance, venipuncture, and intramuscular injections in preterm and term infants (48). No study showed effective pain control with sucrose during an LP. Effects of sucrose on long-term neurodevelopmental outcomes remain unclear (41), but there is a suggested association between poorer short-term motor outcomes and multiple sucrose doses given in the first week of life to infants born at less than 31 weeks' gestation (49).

   d. Subcutaneous application of lidocaine has not been consistently demonstrated to reduce a pain response during an LP (41). It is known to cause burning pain during the subcutaneous application, so its value is questionable in control of needle-related pain in this setting.

5. Prepare for aseptic procedure (see Chapter 6).

6. Clean/disinfect the lumbar area three times with povidone-iodine swabs. Begin at the desired interspace and swab in enlarging circles to include the iliac crests. Allow antiseptic to dry.

7. Drape, placing the aperture over the LP site, leaving the infant's face exposed. Consider using a transparent aperture drape, as it does not obstruct the view of the patient.

8. Insert the needle in the midline of the chosen interspace. Verbalize to your assistant when you are about to insert the needle.

   a. Hold a finger (in sterile glove) on the spinous process above the chosen interspace to aid in locating the puncture site if the infant moves.

   b. Angle the needle slightly cephalad toward the umbilicus to avoid the spinous processes (**Fig. 19.4**). One study determined that a 65- to 70-degree angle of entry would be appropriate, regardless of gestational age (25).

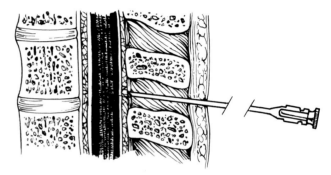

FIGURE 19.4 Inserting spinal needle in slightly cephalad direction to avoid vertebral bodies.

   c. If resistance is met, withdraw the needle slightly and redirect more cephalad, as you are most likely hitting the superior aspect of the spinous process.

9. Advance the needle slowly to a depth of approximately 1 to 1.5 cm in a term infant, less in a preterm infant. Approximate depth of insertion, in millimeters, can be calculated using the formula: $2.5 \times$ (weight in kg) + 6 (25).

   a. Once you pass the skin, you can either remove the stylet and advance the needle slowly until you get CSF flow ("stylet-out" technique); or advance the needle with the stylet in place while frequently removing the stylet to check for CSF flow ("stylet-in" technique). The "stylet-out" technique has an increased success rate of LP on first attempt, but it is unclear whether it carries increased risk of developing iatrogenic intraspinal epidermoid tumor (33).

   b. A change in resistance as the needle passes through dura (**Fig. 19.5**) is difficult to appreciate in newborns.

   c. Wait for fluid after removing the stylet or advancing the needle, as the flow may be slow.

   d. If no fluid is obtained, rotate the needle to reorient the bevel and clear a potential obstruction of the bevel by the spinal nerve roots. If no fluid is obtained, place the stylet back into the needle and

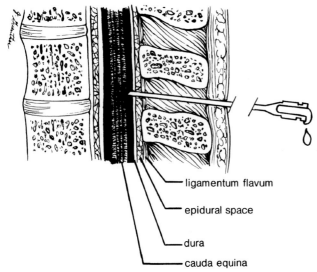

ligamentum flavum

epidural space

dura

cauda equina

FIGURE 19.5 Needle has penetrated the dura, and stylet has been removed to allow free flow of spinal fluid.

remove the needle. Attempt the procedure using an adjacent interspace, using a new needle with stylet for each attempt. Be cautious if moving to a higher interspace, since the spinal conus might be low, depending on the gestation age of the infant.

10. Allow CSF to flow passively into the collection tubes. Do not aspirate with a syringe. If indicated, opening pressure measurement is possible in a quiet infant.
    a. Collect 1 mL of CSF in each of three to four tubes.
    b. Send a sample for bacterial culture. Even 0.5 mL would be adequate for the culture.
    c. Send the clearest sample for cell count, which is usually the last tube.
    d. Send the remainder for desired chemical studies.
    e. If LP was traumatic, you should see clearing of CSF in subsequent collection tubes.

11. For treatment of hydrocephalus, remove 10 to 15 mL/kg of CSF, or collect until CSF flow ceases, up to 10 minutes (10–14).

12. Always replace the stylet before removing the needle to prevent entrapment of spinal nerve roots in the extra-dural space. Remove the needle, and place an adhesive bandage over the puncture site.

13. Remove all povidone-iodine from the skin using a saline wipe.

F. Complications

In neonates, most common complications include:

1. Transient hypoxemia from positioning for the procedure. This can be seen in up to 60% of cases and depends on the method of positioning used—most

commonly seen with the lateral recumbent position with flexed knees (27–29).

2. Traumatic, or bloody, tap is seen in up to one-third of neonatal LPs, secondary to a puncture of the epidural venous plexus on the posterior surface of the vertebral body (33,34). This might make the interpretation of cell counts, glucose, and protein level more difficult.

3. Other complications that have been described in neonates are rare, but potentially clinically detrimental. They include:
   a. Intraspinal epidermoid tumor from epithelial tissue introduced into the spinal canal (30,31).
   b. Symptomatic epidural CSF collection (50). While epidural CSF collection might be frequent (one report notes that 63% of newborns developed an epidural CSF collection after an LP (51)), it is rarely clinically significant. The same report notes complete reabsorption of the fluid collection within 10 days after an LP.
   c. Percutaneous CSF leak (52).
   d. Cerebellar herniation secondary to sudden intracranial decompression. This is an extremely rare complication in neonates, usually occurring when an underlying intracranial process is present (20,21).
   e. Iatrogenic meningitis. One study reports three cases of iatrogenic meningitis in approximately 22,000 neonatal and early infant LPs. The symptoms developed within 72 hours of the procedure (53). While rare, this complication can be difficult to treat, and can lead to significant neurodevelopmental delay.
   f. Epidural abscess (54).
   g. Vertebral osteomyelitis (54).
   h. Meningitis secondary to traumatic LP performed during bacteremia (55,56). A theoretical risk of bacterial transfer via a traumatic LP during bacteremia exists. However, apart from individual reports showing an association between the two, no clear pathophysiologic connection has been shown.
   i. Intramedullary hemorrhage secondary to spinal cord puncture (see discussion in Section E.3 regarding cord termination in preterm infants) (57).
   j. In older children and adults, headache is the most common complication following LP, occurring in up to 40% of patients (58). There is no clear evidence that headache occurs in infants.
   k. Other potential complications described in older children and adults are rare, with a combined estimated incidence of <0.3% (58). Even though not described in literature, these complications might develop in the newborn:
      • Subdural and epidural hematoma (59,60) are more common in children than adults, possibly secondary to higher elasticity and poorer adherence of the arachnoid to the dura in children (61). They can

lead to compression of the subarachnoid space, decreasing the success rate of subsequent LPs (61).
- Subarachnoid hematoma (60,62).
- Aspiration.
- Cardiopulmonary arrest.
- Discitis (63).
- Spinal cord abscess (64).
- Acute spondylitis (65).
- Sixth nerve palsy caused by removal of excessive CSF with resulting traction on the nerve (66).

References

1. Ku LC, Boggess KA, Cohen-Wolkowiez M. Bacterial meningitis in the infants. *Clin Perinatol.* 2015;42(1):29–45.
2. Verani JR, McGee L, Schrag SJ. Prevention of perinatal group B Streptococcal disease: Revised guidelines from CDC, 2010. *MMRW Recomm Rep.* 2010;59(RR10):1–36.
3. Baker CJ, Byington CL, Polin RA; Committee on Infectious Diseases, Committee on Fetus and Newborn. Recommendations for the prevention of perinatal group B Streptococcal (GBS) disease. *Pediatrics.* 2011;128(3):611–616.
4. Stoll BJ, Hansen N, Fanaroff AA, et al. To tap or not to tap: high likelihood of meningitis without sepsis among very low birth weight infants. *Pediatrics.* 2004;113:1181–1186.
5. Workowski KA, Bolan GA. Sexually transmitted diseases treatment guidelines. *MMRW Recomm Rep.* 2015;64 (RR-03):1–137.
6. Kimberlin DW, Baley J; Committee on Infectious Diseases, Committee on Fetus and Newborn. Guidance on management of asymptomatic neonates born to women with active genital herpes lesions. *Pediatrics.* 2013;131:e635–e646.
7. Staples JE, Dziuban EJ, Fischer M, et al. Interim guidelines for the evaluation and testing of infants with possible congenital Zika virus infection. *MMRW Morb Mortal Wkly Rep.* 2016;65(3):63–67.
8. Greenberg RG, Benjamin DK Jr, Cohen-Wolkowiez M, et al. Repeat lumbar puncture in infants with meningitis in the neonatal intensive care unit. *J Perinatol.* 2011;31:425–429.
9. Kimberlin DW. Meningitis in the neonate. *Curr Treat Options Neurol.* 2002;4:239–248.
10. Whitelaw A. Intraventricular hemorrhage and posthemorrhagic hydrocephalus: pathogenesis, prevention and future interventions. *Semin Neonatol.* 2001;6:135–146.
11. McCrea HJ, Ment LR. The diagnosis, management, and postnatal prevention of intraventricular hemorrhage in the preterm neonate. *Clin Perinatol.* 2008;35:777–792.
12. Whitelaw A, Evans D, Carter M, et al. Randomized clinical trial of prevention of hydrocephalus after intraventricular hemorrhage in preterm infants: brain-washing versus tapping fluid. *Pediatrics.* 2007;119:e1071–e1078.
13. Soul JS, Eichenwald E, Walter G, et al. CSF removal in infantile posthemorrhagic hydrocephalus results in significant improvement in cerebral hemodynamics. *Pediatr Res.* 2004;55:872–876.
14. Ventriculomegaly Trial Group. Randomized trial of early tapping in neonatal posthaemorrhagic ventricular dilatation: Results at 30 months. *Arch Dis Child.* 1994;70:F129–F136.
15. Whitelaw A, Lee-Kelland R. Repeated lumbar or ventricular punctures in newborns with intraventricular hemorrhage. *Cochrane Database Syst Rev.* 2017;4:CD000216.
16. Hyland K, Arnold LA. Value of lumbar puncture in the diagnosis of genetic metabolic encephalopathies. *J Child Neurol.* 1999;14(Suppl 1):S9–S15.
17. Hoffman GF, Surtees RA, Wevers RA. Cerebrospinal fluid investigations for neurometabolic disorders. *Neuropediatrics.* 1998;29:59–71.
18. Arber DA, Borowitz MJ, Cessna M, et al. Initial diagnostic workup of acute leukemia: Guideline from the College of American Pathologists and the American Society of Hematology. *Arch Pathol Lab Med.* 2017;141(10): 1342–1393.
19. Kerr JZ, Berg S, Blaney SM. Intrathecal chemotherapy. *Crit Rev Oncol Hematol.* 2001;37(3):227–236.
20. Thibert RL, Burns JD, Bhadelia R, et al. Reversible uncal herniation in a neonate with a large MCA infarct. *Brain Dev.* 2009;31(10):763–765.
21. Kalay S, Öztekin O, Tezel G, et al. Cerebellar herniation after lumbar puncture in galactosemic newborn. *AJP Rep.* 2011;1(1):43–46.
22. Rigi M, Almarzouqi SJ, Morgan ML, et al. Papilledema: epidemiology, etiology, and clinical management. *Eye Brain.* 2015;7:47–57.
23. New H, Berryman J, Bolton-Maggs PHB, et al. Guidelines on transfusion for fetuses, neonates and older children. *Br J Haematol.* 2016;175:784–828.
24. Fiser DH, Gober GA, Smith CE, et al. Prevention of hypoxemia during lumbar puncture in infancy with preoxygenation. *Pediatr Emerg Care.* 1993;9:81–83.
25. Ouelgo-Erroz I, Mora-Matilla M, Alonso-Quintela P, et al. Ultrasound evaluation of lumbar spine anatomy in newborn infants: implications for optimal performance of lumbar puncture. *J Pediatr.* 2014;165:862–865.
26. Oncel S, Gunlemez A, Anik Y, et al. Positioning of infants in the neonatal intensive care unit for lumbar puncture as determined by bedside ultrasonography. *Arch Dis Child Fetal Neonatal Ed.* 2013;98:F133–F135.
27. Abo A, Chen L, Johnston P, et al. Positioning for lumbar puncture in children evaluated by bedside ultrasound. *Pediatrics.* 2010;125:e1149–e1153.
28. Weisman LE, Merenstein GB, Steenbarger JR. The effect of lumbar puncture position in sick neonates. *Am J Dis Child.* 1983;137:1077–1079.
29. Gleason CA, Martin RJ, Anderson JV, et al. Optimal position for a spinal tap in preterm infants. *Pediatrics.* 1983;71:31–35.
30. Ziv ET, Gordon McComb J, Krieger MD, et al. Iatrogenic intraspinal epidermoid tumor: two cases and a review of the literature. *Spine (Phila Pa 1976).* 2004;29:E15–E18.
31. Gardner DJ, O'Gorman AM, Blundell JE. Intraspinal epidermoid tumour: late complication of lumbar puncture. *CMAJ.* 1989;141(3):223–225.
32. Murray MJ, Arthurs OJ, Hills MH, et al. A randomized study to validate a midspinal canal depth nomogram in neonates. *Am J Perinatol.* 2009;26:733–738.
33. Nigrovic LE, Kuppermann N, Neuman MI. Risk factors for traumatic or unsuccessful lumbar puncture in children. *Ann Emerg Med.* 2007;49:762–771.

34. Baxter AL, Fisher RG, Burke BL, et al. Local anesthetic and stylet styles: factors associated with resident lumber puncture success. *Pediatrics*. 2006;117:876–881.

35. Kaur G, Gupta P, Kumar A. A randomized trial of eutectic mixture of local anesthetics during lumbar puncture in newborns. *Arch Pediatr Adolesc Med*. 2003;157:1065–1070.

36. Pinheiro JMB, Furdon S, Ochoa LF. Role of local anesthesia during lumbar puncture in neonates. *Pediatrics*. 1993;91:379–382.

37. Porter FL, Miller JP, Cole FS, et al. A controlled clinical trial of local anesthesia for lumbar punctures in newborns. *Pediatrics*. 1991;88:663–669.

38. Foster JP, Taylor C, Spence K. Topical anaesthesia for needle-related pain in newborn infants. *Cochrane Database Syst Rev*. 2017;2:CD010331.

39. Barson AJ. The vertebral level of termination of the spinal cord during normal and abnormal development. *J Anat*. 1970;106:489–497.

40. van Schoor A, Bosman MC, Bosenberg AT. The value of Tuffier's line for neonatal neuraxial procedures. *Clin Anat*. 2014;27(3):350–375.

41. Anand KJ, Johnston CC, Oberlander TF, et al. Analgesia and local anesthesia during invasive procedures in the neonate. *Clin Ther*. 2005;27(6):844–876.

42. American Academy of Pediatrics, Committee on Fetus and Newborn, Committee on Drugs, Section on Anesthesiology, Section on Surgery, Canadian Paediatric Society, Fetus and Newborn Committee. Prevention and management of pain and stress in neonate. *Pediatrics*. 2000;105:454–461.

43. Lim Y, Godambe S. Prevention and management of procedural pain in the neonate: an update, American Academy of Pediatrics, 2016. *Arch Dis Child Educ Pract Ed*. 2017;102:254–256.

44. Weise KL, Nahata MC. EMLA for painful procedures in infants. *J Pediatr Health Care*. 2005;19(1):42–47.

45. Foster JP, Taylor C, Spence K. Topical anaesthesia for needle-related pain in newborn infants. *Cochrane Database of Syst Rev*. 2017;(2):CD010311.

46. Essink-Tebbes CM, Wuis EW, Liem KD, et al. Safety of lidocaine-prilocaine cream application four times a day in premature neonates: a pilot study. *Eur J Pediatr*. 1999;158(5):421–423.

47. Taddio A, Ohlsson A, Einarson TR, et al. A systematic review of lidocaine-prilocaine cream (EMLA) in the treatment of acute pain in neonates. *Pediatrics*. 1998;101(2):E1.

48. Stevens B, Yamada J, Ohlsson A, et al. Sucrose for analgesia in newborn infants undergoing painful procedures. *Cochrane Database Syst Rev*. 2016;7:CD001069.

49. Johnston CC, Filion F, Snider L, et al. Routine sucrose analgesia during the first week of life in neonates younger than 31 weeks' postconceptional age. *Pediatrics*. 2002;110(3):523–528.

50. Amini A, Liu JK, Kan P, et al. Cerebrospinal fluid dissecting into epidural space after lumbar puncture causing cauda equine syndrome: review of literature and illustrative case. *Childs Nerv Syst*. 2006;22:1639–1641.

51. Kiechl-Kohlendorfer U, Unsinn KM, Schlenck B, et al. Cerebrospinal fluid leakage after lumbar puncture in neonates: incidence and sonographic appearance. *AJR Am J Roentgenol*. 2003;181(1):231–234.

52. Lagae D, Yamagouse Tchameni Y, Gudinchet F, et al. Percutaneous cerebrospinal fluid leak in a preterm infant following lumbar puncture. *Swiss Society of Neonatology*. August 2017:1–16. https://www.neonet.ch/files/6614/9967/6384/COTM_08_2017.pdf.

53. Samoui H, Hariga D, Hajj N, et al. [Iatrogenic meningitis after diagnostic lumbar puncture: 3 case reports in the paediatric children's hospital of tunis] [Article in French]. *Bull Soc Pathol Exot*. 2011;104(1):10–13.

54. Bergman I, Wald ER, Meyer JD, et al. Epidural abscess and vertebral osteomyelitis following serial lumbar punctures. *Pediatrics*. 1983;72:476–480.

55. Teele DW, Dashefsky B, Rakusan T, et al. Meningitis after lumbar puncture in children with bacteremia. *N Engl J Med*. 1981;305(18):1079–1081.

56. Wintergerst U, Daumling S, Belohradsky BH. [Meningitis following lumbar puncture in bacteremia?] [Article in German]. *Monatsschr Kinderheilkd*. 1986;134(11):826–828.

57. Tubbs RS, Smyth MD, Wellons JC 3rd, et al. Intramedullary hemorrhage in a neonate after lumbar puncture resulting in paraplegia: a case report. *Pediatrics*. 2004;113:1403–1405.

58. Evans RW. Complications of lumbar puncture. *Neurol Clin*. 1998;16:83–105.

59. Adler MD, Comi AE, Walker AR. Acute hemorrhagic complication of diagnostic lumbar puncture. *Pediatr Emerg Care*. 2001;17:184–188.

60. Hart IK, Bone I, Hadley DM. Development of neurological problems after lumbar puncture. *Br Med J*. 1988;296:51–52.

61. Muthusami P, Robinson AJ, Shroff MM. Ultrasound guidance for difficult lumbar puncture in children: pearls and pitfalls. *Pediatr Radiol*. 2017;47(7):822–830.

62. Blade J, Gaston F, Montserrat E, et al. Spinal subarachnoid hematoma after lumbar puncture causing reversible paraplegia in acute leukemia. *J Neurosurg*. 1983;58:438–439.

63. Bhatoe HS, Gill HS, Kumar N, et al. Post lumbar puncture discitis and vertebral collapse. *Postgrad Med J*. 1994;70:882–884.

64. Bertol V, Ara JR, Oliveros A, et al. Neurologic complications of lumbar spinal anesthesia: spinal and paraspinal abscess. *Neurology*. 1997;48:1732–1733.

65. Lintermans JP, Seyhnaeue V. Spondolytic deformity of the lumbar spine and previous lumbar punctures. *Pediatr Radiol*. 1977;5:181–182.

66. Hofer JE, Scavone BM. Cranial nerve VI palsy after dural-arachnoid puncture. *Anesth Analg*. 2015;120(3):644–646.

CHAPTER

20

Subdural Tap

Aaron Mohanty

A. Indications (1–7)

1. The most common indication for subdural tap is drainage of subdural collection to relieve increased intracranial pressure.
2. Subdural taps also are indicated to sample subdural fluid for cytologic, biochemical, and microbiologic studies.

B. Contraindications

1. Overlying infected scalp.
2. Uncorrected bleeding diathesis or thrombocytopenia.
3. Closed fontanelle with nonseparated sutures.
4. Performing subdural taps in the absence of radiologic imaging like CT, ultrasound, and MRI scans (**Fig. 20.1**) can no longer be justified unless the investigations cannot be performed due to nonavailability or in a life-threatening situation.

C. Principles

1. The subdural tap is performed through an open fontanelle (usually anterior fontanelle) or through the open or splayed sutures (**Fig. 20.2**).
   a. In patients with previous bone defects like burr holes, the subdural tap can be performed through the bone defect.
   b. Thus, the tap is uncommon after 6 to 9 months of age when the sutures and fontanelles close.
2. It is essential to enter the subdural space without injuring the underlying pia or cortex and to avoid any traversing veins in the subdural space.
   a. The tap site should correspond to the thickest location of the subdural collection as demonstrated in the imaging studies.
   b. If the collection is noncontiguous and the collection needs to be drained from different sites, the tap sites should be carefully identified depending on the

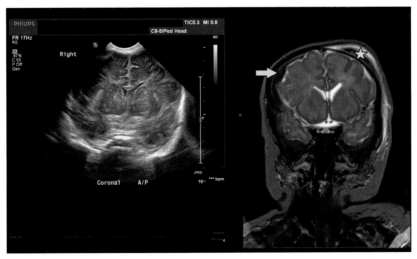

FIGURE 20.1 Subdural collections can be difficult to detect on ultrasound and are more readily apparent on MRI. LEFT: Conventional transcranial ultrasound on a neonate with seizure, coronal view. RIGHT: MRI brain, T2-weighted sequence coronal view, performed on the same neonate 1 day before the ultrasound. A subdural hemorrhage spans the right frontal convexity, shown as hypointense T2-weighted signal abnormality (*arrow*). Large scalp hematoma is also present (*asterisk*), which extends across the coronal suture consistent with subgaleal hematoma. (Images courtesy Dr. Arash Zandieh, MedStar Georgetown University Hospital)

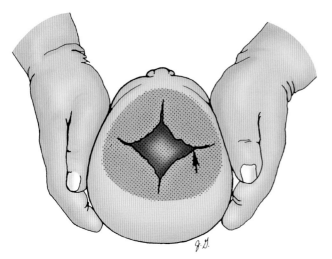

FIGURE 20.2 Position and restraint for subdural tap. Stippling demonstrates area to be prepared for procedure. An *arrow* indicates site for needle puncture.

location of the subdural collection and the suture or bone defect.

3. The most ideal location for the subdural tap is the lateral edge of the anterior fontanelle away the midline.
   a. The side of the tap depends on the thickness of the subdural collection; the side with thicker collection is preferred.
   b. If the thickness is equal on both sides, tapping from the right side is preferred as the right brain is nondominant in the majority of the population.
4. Unlike the ventricles, the subdural space is located very superficial under the bone.
   a. Considering this, the needle should not extend more than 0.5 cm into the intracranial space.
   b. The bevel of the needle should be inserted at 45- to 60-degree angle and directed laterally.
      (1) This allows a longer length of the needle to be in the subdural space that reduces needle pullout during the procedure.
      (2) Inadvertent advancement is a concern in a crying or irritable child who is not properly restrained.
   c. Some prefer to use a hemostat clipped to the shaft of the needle to identify the exact depth to prevent advancement into the cerebral cortex.
5. The cerebral cortical veins conglomerate medially as they approach the sagittal sinus and pass through the subdural space. Thus, the most lateral part of the anterior fontanelle is often the ideal location for the tap.
6. Drainage of a large amount of fluid rapidly can cause acute subdural bleeding or cortical hemorrhages due to sudden decompression.
   a. The subdural fluid is usually drained slowly as it drips from the tube.
   b. A gentle and controlled aspiration with a 2- or 3-mL syringe is sometimes preferred to reduce the duration of the tap.

c. The risks of needle pullout in an irritable infant with spontaneous drainage versus a reduced tap time by slow aspiration with a 2-mL syringe should be taken into account during the tap.

7. The amount of subdural fluid removed during a tap should be limited to 15 to 20 mL in one setting. Repeated taps can be performed at intervals if more fluid is required to be drained. A lax anterior fontanelle in an infant often indicates that the required amount has been reached.

8. If multiple taps are required, the site of the tap can be changed by taking into account the location of the fluid and the fontanelle. This is done to prevent development of a cutaneous track and CSF leak.

D. Equipment

1. Povidone-iodine solution (povidone-iodine–soaked sticks can be used)
2. Sterile drapes
3. 21- and 23-gauge butterfly needles
4. Sterile gauze swabs
5. Sterile gloves
6. Face mask
7. At least three sterile specimen tubes with occluding caps
8. Adhesive dressings
9. Safety razor
10. Sterile saline or water

E. Technique[1]

1. Obtain informed consent.
2. Place the infant in a supine position, with the head stabilized in a neutral position either by soft rolls or with the help of an assistant (see **Fig. 20.2**).
   a. Restrain the infant with a blanket (see Mummy Restraint in Chapter 5).
   b. The surgeon/operator stands behind the head overlooking the frontal region.
3. Mark the subdural tap site and the midline.
   a. It is essential that the tap site is well marked as it is possible that the landmarks can be missed after the scalp preparation.
   b. The region of the tap is often shaved using a safety razor, though, shaving is not considered essential. It is sometimes advantageous to shave a localized area at the needle entry site because this serves as a marker when introducing the needle.
   c. Alternatively, the tap site can be marked with a skin marker. The midline is also marked well, acting as a reference for the location of the sagittal sinus.

---

[1]For the purpose of the description, we will describe the steps of performing a subdural tap through the right side of the anterior fontanelle.

4. Usually sedation is not required for the procedure.
   a. However, if necessary, local anesthetic can be injected at the site.
   b. Caution should be taken not to enter the intracranial compartment during the injection as there is no underlying skull bone at the tap site.
5. Wear the face mask, wash hands using antiseptic soap, and wear sterile gloves.
6. Prepare the scalp with povidone-iodine solution paint, and allow it to dry.
   a. Usually a wide area of preparation is ideal; covering up to the midline and laterally up the temporal region.
   b. Place sterile drapes around the tap site.
   c. It is sometimes useful only to drape the posterior aspect and leave the anterior aspect uncovered, as it allows identification of the landmarks (nose, mid-pupillary line, lateral canthus) during the procedure.
7. Confirm the location of the entry site again, by palpating the lateral edge of the anterior fontanelle. This step is essential for avoiding the midline and the sagittal sinus.
8. Take the 21-gauge (or 23-gauge) scalp vein needle and introduce the tip through the scalp into the subdural space at a 45- to 60-degree angle by holding it firmly at the wings and directing it away from the midline laterally or toward the thickest part of the collection.
   a. It can be helpful to clip a small hemostat to the shaft of the needle, at about 0.5 cm from the tip to limit the depth of the needle tip. Others pinch the needle between the thumb and the index finger at 0.5 cm from the tip to limit the depth (**Fig. 20.3**).

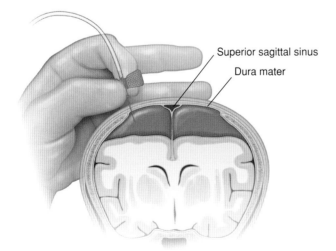

FIGURE 20.3 Coronal section of anatomic drawing showing subdural needle penetrating the dura in a patient with bilateral convexity subdural fluid collections. Operator's fingers are placed for maximal stabilization of the needle.

b. The needle may be advanced in the subcutaneous tissue for few millimeters before puncturing the dura to prevent a CSF leak post tap.
9. The entry into subdural space is usually accompanied by emergence of subdural fluid through the tube.
   a. Often a slight "giving way" sensation is felt as the needle enters the subdural space.
   b. It is essential that the needle is held in place without any movement during rest of the procedure.
   c. It is advantageous to support the hand with the rest of the fingers rested on the scalp.
10. Allow the subdural fluid to slowly drip out from the other end of the tube; collect the fluid in at least three different tubes for evaluation (one for cytologic, one for biochemical, and the third for culture). Additional tubes may be used if more studies are required.
11. In a restless infant, it can be prudent to use a 2- or 3-mL syringe to gently aspirate the fluid to reduce the overall length of the procedure.
    a. The risks of needle pullout in an irritable infant during a spontaneous drainage versus a reduced tap time by slow aspiration with a 2-mL syringe should be considered during the tap.
    b. The tube attached to the scalp vein facilitates attaching and removing the syringe several times during the procedure without disturbing the needle tip.
12. The procedure should be discontinued once 15 to 20 mL is reached or when the anterior fontanelle is lax and soft.
13. Pull out the needle and apply gentle pressure for about a minute or two to prevent any spontaneous leaks through the track.
    a. A sterile occlusive dressing is adequate after the procedure.
    b. Remove excess povidone-iodine from the scalp by using a sterile saline or water wipe.
14. If no subdural fluid is obtained during the tap, remove the needle, check the entry point and landmarks, and correlate them again with the imaging studies.
15. If the entry site was correct and no fluid could be drained, the tap can be attempted at another site.

F. Complications

1. **Subdural bleeding**
   a. This is the most worrisome complication, usually from the needle tip injuring the cortex or a traversing vein.
   b. If frank blood exits, the procedure is stopped, and an urgent CT scan is performed.
2. **Infection:** This is usually uncommon unless the child is undergoing repeated taps.
3. **Subdural fluid leak**
   a. A gentle but sustained external pressure often prevents the fluid leak following the tap.

b. Advancing the needle through the subcutaneous tissue for few millimeters before puncturing the dura often prevents the CSF leak.

4. **Seizures:** These result from subdural bleeding or trauma to the cortex.

5. **Brain injury and intraparenchymal injury:** Inadvertent advancement of the needle tip into cortex and repeated attempts at aspiration during a tap can result in cortical injury.

References

1. Hobbs C, Childs AM, Wynne J, et al. Subdural hematoma and effusion in infancy: an epidemiological study. *Arch Dis Child.* 2005;90:952–955.

2. Mahapatra AK, Bhatia R, Banerji AK, et al. Subdural empyema in children. *Indian Pediatr.* 1984;21:561–567.

3. Kanu OO, Nnoli C, Olowoyeye O, et al. Infantile subdural empyema: the role of brain sonography and percutaneous subdural tapping in a resource-challenged region. *J Neurosciences in Clin Pract.* 2014;5:355–359.

4. Wang X, Zhang X, Cao H, et al. Surgical treatments for infantile purulent meningitis complicated by subdural effusion. *Med Sci Monit.* 2015;21:3166–3171.

5. Vinchon M, Joriot S, Jissendi-Tchofo P, et al. Postmeningitis subdural fluid collection in infants: changing pattern and indications for surgery. *J Neurosurg Pediatrics.* 2006;104:383–387.

6. Brill CB, Jarath V, Black P. Occipital interhemispheric acute subdural hematoma treated by lambdoid suture tap. *Neurosurgery.* 1985;16:247–251.

7. Melo JRT, Dirocco FR, Bourgeois M, et al. Surgical options for treatment of traumatic subdural hematomas in children younger than 2 years of age. *J Neurosurg Pediatrics.* 2014;13:456–461.

Suprapubic Bladder Aspiration

Jane Germano

A. Indications (1–8)

1. To obtain urine for culture

   Suprapubic bladder aspiration is considered the most reliable method of obtaining urine for culture in infants and children <2 years old. In this age group, the distended bladder is located intra-abdominally. Any number of bacteria in urine obtained by this method is considered significant and likely to be indicative of urinary tract infection. Contamination with skin flora can occur but should be avoidable with careful skin preparation. Although bladder catheterization has a higher success rate, it also has a much higher false-positive rate than suprapubic aspiration (2–4). Reported success rates for suprapubic aspiration vary widely, from 23% to 97% (2,4,8,9). With careful attention to performing the procedure when the infant has a full bladder, success is generally 89% to 95%, even in very–low-birth-weight infants (9,10). The use of portable ultrasound (9,11–13) or transillumination (14) to determine bladder size can increase the chance of success.

B. Contraindications (4,7,8,10)

1. Empty bladder as a result of recent void or dehydration.

   A full bladder is essential for success of the procedure and avoidance of complications.
2. Skin infection over the puncture site.
3. Distention or enlargement of abdominal viscera (e.g., dilated loops of bowel, massive hepatomegaly).
4. Genitourinary anomaly or enlargement of pelvic structures (e.g., ovarian cyst, distention of vagina or uterus).
5. Uncorrected thrombocytopenia or bleeding diathesis.

C. Equipment

All equipment must be sterile, except transillumination light or ultrasound equipment.

1. Gloves
2. Gauze sponges and cup with iodophor or chlorhexidine antiseptic solution or prepared antiseptic-impregnated swabs
3. 3-mL syringe
4. 22–24-gauge × 1.5-in (40-mm) needle
5. Pain control (15–20)
   a. Oral 24% sucrose solution: 0.5 to 1 mL preterm infants, 2 mL term infants
   b. Eutectic Mixture of Local Anesthetics (EMLA) cream composed of 2.5% lidocaine and 2.5% prilocaine; with occlusive dressing
6. Transillumination light or portable ultrasound (optional)

D. Precautions

1. Use strict aseptic technique (see Chapter 6).
2. Delay the procedure if the infant has urinated in the last hour.
3. If the infant is systemically ill, do not delay antibiotic therapy to wait for further urine production.
4. Correct bleeding diathesis before the procedure. Consider catheterization as an alternative.
5. Be certain of landmarks. Do not insert the needle over the pubic bone or off the midline.
6. Aspirate urine using only gentle suction. The use of too much suction can draw the bladder mucosa to the needle, obstructing the collection of urine and increasing the risk of injury to the bladder.

E. Technique

1. If time permits, apply local anesthetic (EMLA) cream 0.5 to 1 g to a 1- to 2-cm area just above pubic bone in the midline and cover with occlusive dressing 1 hour prior to procedure (17,18).
2. Determine the presence of urine in the bladder.
   a. Verify that the diaper has been dry for at least 1 hour.
   b. Palpate or percuss the bladder.
   c. Optionally, use transillumination light (14) or portable ultrasound guidance (5,11–13).
3. Have an assistant restrain the infant in the supine, frog-leg position.
4. Remove occlusive dressing if EMLA was used.
5. To avoid reflex urination, ask assistant to
   a. Place the tip of a finger in the anus and apply pressure anteriorly in a female infant, or
   b. Pinch the base of the penis gently in a male infant.
6. Locate landmarks. Palpate the top of the pubic bone. The site for needle insertion is 1 to 2 cm above the symphysis pubis in the midline (**Fig. 21.1**).
7. Wash hands thoroughly and put on gloves.
8. Clean the suprapubic area (including the area over pubic bone) three times with antiseptic solution.
9. Have assistant provide oral sucrose to infant to decrease pain/ discomfort (see Chapter 7) (21,22).
10. Palpate the symphysis pubis, and insert the needle (with syringe attached) 1 to 2 cm above the pubic symphysis in the midline (**Fig. 21.2**).
    a. Maintain the needle perpendicular to table or directed slightly caudad.
    b. Advance the needle 1 to 3 cm. A slight decrease in resistance may be felt when the bladder is penetrated.

11. Aspirate gently, as the needle is slowly advanced, until urine enters the syringe. Do not advance the needle more than 3 cm.
    a. Withdraw the needle if no urine is obtained.
    b. Do not probe with the needle or attempt to redirect it to obtain urine.
    c. Wait at least 1 hour before attempting to repeat the procedure.
12. Withdraw the needle after urine is obtained. Apply gentle pressure over the puncture site with sterile gauze to stop any bleeding.
13. Transfer urine to a sterile container to send for culture.

F. Complications

Minor transient hematuria is the most commonly reported complication, occurring in <1% to 10% of cases (6). Serious complications are very rare, occurring in ≤0.2% of cases (10).

1. Bleeding
   a. Transient macroscopic hematuria (blood-tinged urine) (6)
   b. Gross hematuria (6,19,20)
   c. Abdominal wall hematoma (20)
   d. Bladder wall hematoma (6,23)
   e. Pelvic hematoma (24)
   f. Hemoperitoneum (25)
2. Infection
   a. Abdominal wall abscess (26,27)
   b. Sepsis (28,29)
   c. Osteomyelitis of pubic bone (30)
3. Perforation
   a. Bowel (27,31)
   b. Pelvic organ (31)

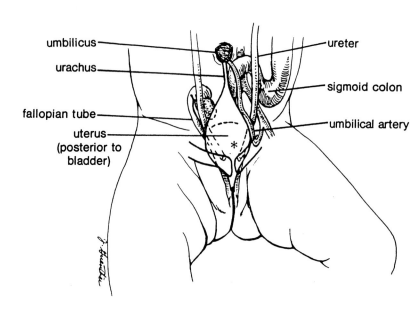

FIGURE 21.1 The bladder in the neonate, with immediate anatomical relations. An *asterisk* indicates approximate site for needle insertion.

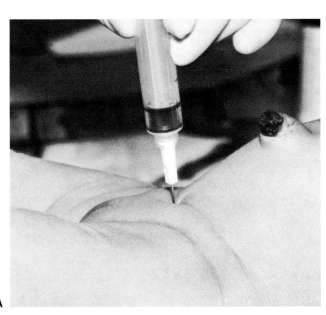

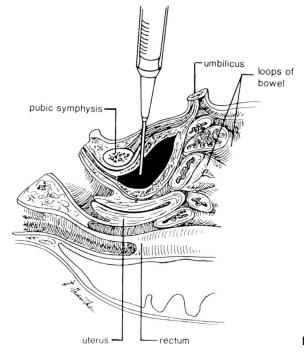

A

B

FIGURE 21.2 A: Insertion of needle 1 to 2 cm above symphysis pubis. **B:** Midline sagittal section to emphasize the intra-abdominal position of the full bladder in the neonate and its posterior anatomic relations.

References

1. Arshad M, Seed PC. Urinary tract infection in the infant. *Clin Perinatol.* 2015;42:17–28.
2. Eliacik K, Kanik A, Yavascan O, et al. A comparison of bladder catheterization and suprapubic aspiration methods for urine sample collection from infants with suspected urinary tract infection. *Clin Peditr (Phila).* 2016;55(9):819–824.
3. Phillips B. Towards evidence based medicine for paediatricians. Urethral catheter or suprapubic aspiration to reduce contamination of urine samples in young children? *Arch Dis Child.* 2009;94:736–739.
4. Schmidt B, Copp HL. Work-up of pediatric urinary tract infection. *Urol Clin North Am.* 2015;42(4):519–526.
5. Ozkan B, Kava O, Akdağ R, et al. Suprapubic bladder aspiration with or without ultrasound guidance. *Clin Pediatr.* 2000;39:625–626.
6. Pollack CV, Pollack ES, Andrew ME. Suprapubic bladder aspiration versus urethral catheterization in ill infants: success, efficiency and complication rates. *Ann Emerg Med.* 1994;23:225–230.
7. Roberts KB; Subcommittee on Urinary Tract Infection, Steering Committee on Quality Improvement and Management. Urinary Tract Infection: Clinical practice guideline for the diagnosis and management of the initial UTI in febrile infants and children 2 to 24 months. *Pediatrics.* 2011;128(3):595–610.
8. Tobiansky R, Evans N. A randomized controlled trial of two methods for collection of sterile urine in neonates. *J Paediatr Child Health.* 1998;34:460–462.
9. Gochman RF, Karasic RB, Heller MB. Use of the portable ultrasound to assist urine collection by suprapubic aspiration. *Ann Emerg Med.* 1991;20(6):631–635.
10. Barkemeyer BM. Suprapubic aspiration of urine in very low birth weight infants. *Pediatrics.* 1993;92:457–459.
11. Chu RW, Wong YC, Luk SH, et al. Comparing suprapubic urine aspiration under real time ultrasound guidance with conventional blind aspiration. *Acta Paediatr.* 2002;91:512–516.
12. Munir V, Barnett P, South M. Does the use of volumetric bladder ultrasound improve the success rate of suprapubic aspiration of urine? *Pediatr Emerg Care.* 2002;18:346–349.
13. Garcia-Neito V, Navarro JF, Sanchez-Almeida ES, et al. Standards for ultrasound guidance of suprapubic bladder aspiration. *Pediatr Nephrol.* 1997;11:607–609.
14. Buck JR, Weintraub WH, Coran AG, et al. Fiberoptic transillumination: a new tool for the pediatric surgeon. *J Pediatr Surg.* 1977;12:451–463.
15. Lefrak L, Burch K, Caravantes R, et al. Sucrose analgesia: identifying potentially better practices. *Pediatrics.* 2006;118:S197–S202.
16. El-Naggar W, Yiu A, Mohamed A, et al. Comparison of pain during two methods of urine collection in preterm infants. *Pediatrics.* 2010;125:1224–1229.
17. Nahum Y, Tenenbaum A, Isaiah W, et al. Effect of eutectic mixture of local anesthetics (EMLA) for pain relief during suprapubic aspiration in young infants: a randomized, controlled trial. *Clin J Pain.* 2007;23:756–759.
18. Kozer E, Rosenbloom E, Goldman D, et al. Pain in infants who are younger than 2 months during suprapubic aspiration and transurethral bladder catheterization: a randomized, controlled trial. *Pediatrics.* 2006;118:e51–e56.
19. Carlson KP, Pullon DH. Bladder hemorrhage following transcutaneous bladder aspiration. *Pediatrics.* 1977;60:765.

20. Lanier B, Daeschner CW. Serious complication of suprapubic aspiration of the urinary bladder. *J Pediatr.* 1971;79:711.

21. Krishnan L. Pain relief in neonates. *J Neonatal Surg.* 2013;2(2):19.

22. Stevens B, Yamada J, Ohlsson A, et al. Sucrose for analgesia in newborn infants undergoing painful procedures. *Cochrane Database Syst Rev.* 2016;7:CD001069.

23. Morell RE, Duritz G, Oltorf C. Suprapubic aspiration associated with hematoma. *Pediatrics.* 1982;69:455–457.

24. Mandell J, Stevens PS. Supravesical hematoma following suprapubic urine aspiration. *J Urol.* 1978;119:286.

25. Kimmelstiel FM, Holgersen LO, Dudell GG. Massive hemoperitoneum following suprapubic bladder aspiration. *J Pediatr Surg.* 1986;21(10):911–912.

26. Moustaki M, Stefos E, Malliou C, et al. Complications of suprapubic aspiration in transiently neutropenic children. *Pediatr Emerg Care.* 2007;23(11):823–825.

27. Polnay L, Fraser AM, Lewis JM. Complication of suprapubic bladder aspiration. *Arch Dis Child.* 1975;50:80–81.

28. Mustonen A, Uhari M. Is there bacteremia after suprapubic aspiration in children with urinary tract infection? *J Urol.* 1978;119:822–823.

29. Pass RF, Waldo FB. Anaerobic bacteremia following suprapubic bladder aspiration. *J Pediatr.* 1979;94:748–750.

30. Wald ER. Risk factors for osteomyelitis. *Am J Med.* 1985;78:206–212.

31. Weathers WT, Wenzl JE. Suprapubic aspiration: perforation of a viscus other than the bladder. *Am J Dis Child.* 1969;117:590–592.

Bladder Catheterization

Jane Germano

A. Indications (1–4)

1. To obtain urine for culture, particularly when suprapubic collection is contraindicated and when clean-catch specimen is unsatisfactory.

   Although suprapubic bladder aspiration is considered the most reliable method of obtaining urine for culture in infants and young children (see Chapter 21), bladder catheterization is an acceptable alternative method. Bladder catheterization has been shown to be less painful than suprapubic bladder aspiration in girls and uncircumcised boys and has a higher success rate, especially if the practitioner is inexperienced in bladder aspiration (5). However, urine samples collected by catheterization have a higher false-positive rate than suprapubic aspiration (6–8), and catheterization can introduce bacteria colonizing the distal urethra into the bladder, causing a urinary tract infection (see F). The diagnosis of urinary tract infection cannot be made reliably by culturing urine collected in a bag (9–11).
2. To monitor precisely the urinary output of a critically ill patient
3. To quantify bladder residual
4. To relieve urinary retention (e.g., in neurogenic bladder) (12)
5. To instill contrast agent to perform cystourethrography (13)

B. Contraindications (1,3)

Contraindications include pelvic fracture, urethral trauma, and blood at the meatus. In the presence of uncorrected bleeding diathesis, potential risks and benefits must be considered.

C. Equipment

All equipment must be sterile. Commercial prepackaged urinary drainage kits, with or without collection burettes for closed drainage, are available.

1. Gloves
2. Gauze sponges and cup with iodophor antiseptic solution (not containing alcohol), or
3. Prepared antiseptic-impregnated swabs
4. Towels for draping
5. Surgical lubricant
6. Cotton-tipped applicators
7. Urinary catheter

   Silicone urinary drainage catheters are available in 3.5, 5, 6.5, and 8 French (Fr) sizes. A 3.5- or 5-Fr umbilical catheter may be substituted for a urinary catheter
8. Sterile container for specimen collection or collection burette for continuous closed drainage

D. Precautions

1. Use strict aseptic technique.
2. Use adequate lighting.
3. Try to time the procedure for when the infant has not recently voided (1 to 2 hours after the last wet diaper). Portable ultrasound can be helpful in determining when there is sufficient urine present in the bladder, reducing the chance of an unsuccessful attempt (14,15).
4. Avoid vigorous irrigation of the perineum in preparation for catheterization. This may increase the risk of introducing bacteria into the urinary tract.
5. Avoid separating the labia minora too widely, to prevent tearing of the fourchette.
6. Use the smallest-diameter catheter to avoid traumatic complications. A 3.5-Fr catheter is recommended for

infants weighing <1,000 g and a 5-Fr catheter is recommended for larger infants.

7. If the catheter does not pass easily, do not use force. Suspect obstruction and abandon the procedure.

8. To avoid coiling and knotting, insert the catheter only as far as necessary to obtain urine.

9. If urine is not obtained in a female infant, recheck the location of the catheter by visual inspection or by radiographic examination. It may have passed through the introitus into the vagina.

10. Remove the catheter as soon as possible, to avoid infectious complications.

11. If the catheter cannot be removed easily, do not use force. Consult urology, as catheter knots can occur.

E. Technique

Male Infant (1,11,16,17)

1. Set up equipment and squeeze a small amount of lubricant onto a sterile field.

2. Restrain the infant supine in the frog-leg position.

3. Wash hands thoroughly and put on sterile gloves.

4. Stabilize the shaft of the penis with the nondominant hand. This hand is now considered contaminated.

5. If the infant is uncircumcised, gently retract the foreskin just enough to expose the meatus. Do not attempt to lyse adhesions. The young male infant has physiologic phimosis, and the foreskin cannot be fully retracted (16). If the foreskin is tightly adherent, attempt to line up the preputial ring and the meatus.

6. Apply gentle pressure at the base of the penis to avoid reflex urination.

7. Using the free hand for the rest of the procedure, clean the glans three times with antiseptic solution. Begin at the meatus and work outward and down the shaft of the penis.

8. Drape sterile towels across the lower abdomen and across the infant's legs.

9. Place the wide end of the catheter into the specimen container.

10. Lubricate the tip of the catheter well.

11. Move the specimen container and catheter onto the sterile drape between the infant's legs.

12. Gently insert the catheter through the meatus just until urine is seen in the tube (**Fig. 22.1**).

    a. During insertion, apply gentle upward traction on the penile shaft to prevent kinking of the urethra (see **Fig. 22.1**).

    b. If the meatus cannot be visualized, insert the catheter through the preputial ring in a slightly inferior direction. If there is any question about catheter position, abandon the procedure.

    c. If resistance is met at the external sphincter, hold the catheter in place, applying minimal pressure. Generally, spasm will relax after a brief period, allowing easy passage of catheter. If not, suspect obstruction and abandon the procedure.

    d. Do not move the catheter in and out. This will increase the risk of urethral trauma.

    e. Do not insert extra tubing length in an attempt to stabilize a catheter to be left indwelling. This will increase the risk of trauma and knotting.

13. Collect specimen for culture.

14. If the catheter is to remain indwelling, connect the catheter immediately to a closed sterile system for urine collection. Tape the tube securely to the inner thigh.

15. If the catheter is to be removed, gently withdraw it when urine flow ceases.

16. Remove iodophor solution completely using a wet gauze or towel after procedure.

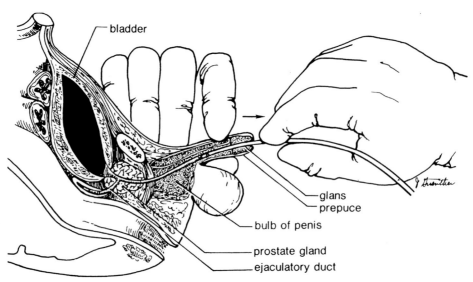

FIGURE 22.1 Anatomic drawing demonstrating bladder catheterization in the male.

Female Infant (1,16–18)

1. Follow steps 1 through 3 of technique for male infant.
2. Retract the labia minora.
   a. Use sterile gauze sponges with nondominant hand, or
   b. Have an assistant retract the labia with two cotton-tipped applicators (**Fig. 22.2**).

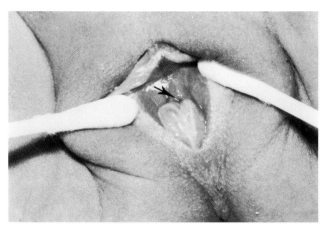

FIGURE 22.2 External genitalia in the female. Retraction of labia majora and minora with cotton-tipped applicators. An *arrow* indicates urethral meatus.

3. Using the free hand for the rest of the procedure, cleanse the area between the labia minora three times with antiseptic solution.
   a. Swab in an anterior-to-posterior direction to avoid drawing fecal material into the field.

4. Follow steps 8 through 11 of the technique for the male infant.
5. Visualize the meatus (see **Fig. 22.2**).
   a. The most prominent structure is the vaginal introitus. The urethral meatus lies immediately anterior (between the clitoris and the introitus).
   b. The meatus may be obscured by the introital fold. Gently push the fold down with a cotton-tipped applicator.
   c. If the meatus is not visible, the infant may have female hypospadias (the meatus is on the roof of the vagina, just inside the introitus). The urethra must then be catheterized blindly, which may require a curved-tip catheter or urologic assistance.
6. Gently insert the catheter only until urine appears in the tube. Do not insert extra tubing.
7. Follow steps 13 through 16 of technique for the male infant.

Female Infant in Prone Position (19)

This technique is useful in an infant who cannot be placed supine (e.g., one with a large meningomyelocele).

1. Position the infant prone on folded blankets so that the head and trunk are elevated about 3 in above the knees and lower legs. The hips should be flexed with knees abducted (**Fig. 22.3A**).
2. Place a gauze pad over the anus and secure with tape across the buttocks, to avoid contamination of the perineum from reflex bowel evacuation (**Fig. 22.3B**).

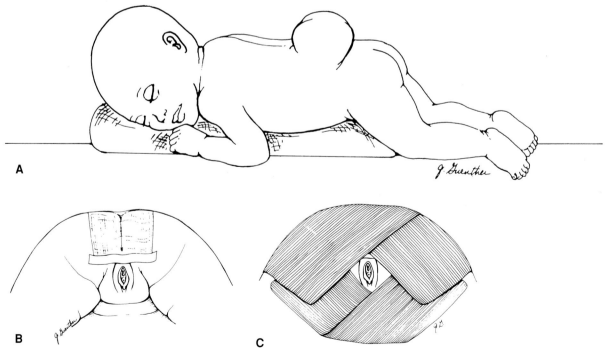

FIGURE 22.3 A: Position of infant for prone catheterization. **B:** Placement of gauze pad over anus. **C:** Placement of drapes. (Adapted with permission from Campbell J. Catheterizing prone female infants: How can you see what you're doing? *Am J Matern Child Nurs.* 1979;4(6):376–377. Based on drawing by N.L. Gahan.)

3. Place sterile drapes as shown in **Figure 22.3C**. Follow the procedure for female catheterization above.

F. Complications

1. Infection (20–24)
   a. Urethritis
   b. Epididymitis
   c. Cystitis
   d. Pyelonephritis
   e. Sepsis

   The most common complication of bladder catheterization is the introduction of bacteria into the urinary tract and potentially into the bloodstream. Catheterization is the leading cause of nosocomial urinary tract infection and gram-negative sepsis in adult patients (22). The risk of bacteriuria from straight ("in-and-out") catheterization is 1% to 5% in this population (21,22). The risk of infection is related directly to the duration of catheterization. In infants and children, approximately 50% to 75% of hospital-acquired urinary tract infections occur in catheterized patients, the highest rate being in neonates (23,24). Urinary tract infection developed in 10.8% of catheterized pediatric patients (23), and secondary bacteremia in 2.9% (24). Risk of infection is decreased by adhering to strict aseptic technique during catheter placement, maintaining a closed sterile collection system, and removing the catheter as soon as possible.

2. Trauma
   a. Hematuria
   b. Urethral erosion or tear (25)
   c. Urethral false passage (25,26)
   d. Perforation of the urethra or bladder (**Fig. 22.4**) (26–28)
   e. Tear of the fourchette (27)
   f. Meatal stenosis (17)
   g. Urethral stricture (29)
   h. Urinary retention secondary to urethral edema (27)

   The risk of trauma is reduced by using the smallest-diameter catheter with ample lubrication, advancing the catheter only as far as necessary to obtain urine, and never forcing a catheter through an obstruction. Erosion and perforation are associated with long-term indwelling catheters. This risk is reduced by removing the catheter as soon as possible.

3. Mechanical
   a. Catheter malposition (27)
   b. Catheter knot (30–33)

The risk of knotting is reduced by using the minimal length of catheter insertion. Standard insertion lengths of 6 cm for male and 5 cm for female term newborns have

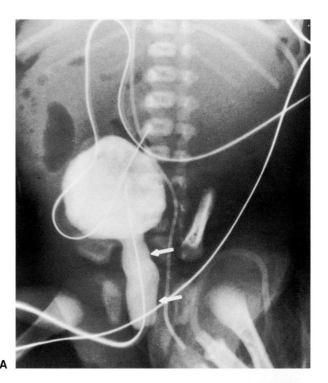

A

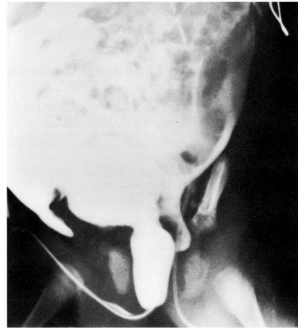

B

FIGURE 22.4 A: Cystogram shows dilated posterior urethra (*arrows*) secondary to posterior urethral valves. **B:** Subsequent film shows perforation of the bladder, with free contrast material in the peritoneal cavity.

been suggested (33). Shorter lengths would be appropriate for preterm infants. A more general standard is to insert the catheter only as far as needed to obtain urine. Using a feeding tube as a urinary catheter may also increase the risk of knotting, because these tubes are softer and more likely to coil.

References

1. Roberts KB; Subcommittee on Urinary Tract Infection, Steering Committee on Quality Improvement and Management. Urinary tract infection: clinical practice guideline for the diagnosis and management of the initial UTI in febrile infants and children 2 to 24 months. *Pediatrics.* 2011;128(3):595–610.

2. Bonadio W, Maida G. Urinary tract infection in outpatient febrile infants younger than 30 days of age: a 10-year evaluation. *Pediatr Infect Dis J.* 2014;33(4):342–344.

3. Karacan C, Erkek N, Senet S, et al. Evaluation of urine collection methods for the diagnosis of urinary tract infection in children. *Med Princ Pract.* 2010;19:188–191.

4. Ma JF, Shortliffe LM. Urinary tract infection in children: etiology and epidemiology. *Urol Clin NA.* 2004;31:517–526.

5. El-Naggar W, Yiu A, Mohamed A, et al. Comparison of pain during two methods of urine collection in preterm infants. *Pediatrics.* 2010;125:1224–1229.

6. Wingerter S, Bachur R. Risk factors for contamination of catheterized urine specimens in febrile children. *Pediatr Emerg Care.* 2011;27:1–4.

7. Phillips B. Towards evidence based medicine for paediatricians. Urethral catheter or suprapubic aspiration to reduce contamination of urine samples in young children? *Arch Dis Child.* 2009;94:736–739.

8. Pollack CV Jr, Pollack ES, Andrew ME. Suprapubic bladder aspiration versus urethral catheterization in ill infants: success, efficiency and complication rates. *Ann Emerg Med.* 1994;23:225–230.

9. Al-Orifi F, McGillivray D, Tange S, et al. Urine culture from bag specimens in young children: Are the risks too high? *J Pediatr.* 2000;137:221–226.

10. Tosif S, Baker A, Oakley E, et al. Contamination rates of different urine collection methods for the diagnosis of urinary tract infections in young children: an observational cohort study. *J Paediatr Child Health.* 2012;48(8):659–664.

11. Etoubleau C, Reveret M, Brouet D. Moving from bag to catheter for urine collection in non-toilet-trained children suspected of having urinary tract infection: paired comparison of urine cultures. *J Pediatr.* 2009;154:803–806.

12. Baskin LS, Kogan BA, Benard F. Treatment of infants with neurogenic bladder dysfunction using anticholinergic drugs and intermittent catheterisation. *Br J Urol.* 1990;66:532–534.

13. Shalaby-Rana E, Lowe LH, Blask AN, et al. Imaging in pediatric urology. *Pediatr Clin North Am.* 1997;44:1065–1089.

14. Milling TJ Jr, Van Amerongen R, Melville L, et al. Use of ultrasonography to identify infants in whom urinary catheterization will be unsuccessful because of insufficient urine volume: validation of the urinary bladder index. *Ann Emerg Med.* 2005;45:510–513.

15. Chen L, Hsiao AL, Moore CL, et al. Utility of bedside bladder ultrasound before urethral catheterization in young children. *Pediatrics.* 2005;115:108–111.

16. Robson WL, Leung AK, Thomason MA. Catheterization of the bladder in infants and children. *Clin Pediatr.* 2006;45:795–800.

17. Brown MR, Cartwright PC, Snow BW. Common office problems in pediatric urology and gynecology. *Pediatr Clin North Am.* 1997;44:1091–1115.

18. Redman JF. Techniques of genital examination and bladder catheterization in female children. *Urol Clin North Am.* 1990;17:1–4.

19. Campbell J. Catheterizing prone female infants: How can you see what you're doing? *MCN Am J Matern Child Nurs.* 1979;4:376–377.

20. Rosenthal VD, Al-Abdely HM, El-Kholy AA, et al. International nosocomial infection control consortium report, data summary of 50 countries for 2010–2015: device-associated module. *Am J Infect Control.* 2016;44(12):1495–1504.

21. Esteban E, Ferrer R, Urrea M, et al. The impact of a quality improvement intervention to reduce nosocomial infections in a PICU. *Pediatr Crit Care Med.* 2013;14(5):525–532.

22. Sedor J, Mulholland SG. Hospital-acquired urinary tract infections associated with the indwelling catheter. *Urol Clin North Am.* 1999;26:821–828.

23. Lohr JA, Downs SM, Dudley S, et al. Hospital-acquired urinary tract infections in the pediatric patient: a prospective study. *Pediatr Infect Dis J.* 1994;13:8–12.

24. Davies HD, Jones EL, Sheng RY, et al. Nosocomial urinary tract infections at a pediatric hospital. *Pediatr Infect Dis J.* 1992;11:349–354.

25. McAlister WH, Cacciarelli A, Shackelford GD. Complications associated with cystography in children. *Radiology.* 1974;111:167–172.

26. Basha M, Subhani M, Mersal A, et al. Urinary bladder perforation in a premature infant with Down syndrome. *Pediatr Nephrol.* 2003;18:1189–1190.

27. Koleilat N, Sidi AA, Gonzalez R. Urethral false passage as a complication of intermittent catheterization. *J Urol.* 1989;142:1216–1217.

28. Salama H, Al Ju Fairi M, Rejjal A, et al. Urinary bladder perforation in a very low birth weight infant. A case report. *J Perinat Med.* 2002;30:188–191.

29. Edwards LE, Lock R, Powell C, et al. Post-catheterisation urethral strictures. A clinical and experimental study. *Br J Urol.* 1983;55:53–56.

30. Pearson-Shaver AL, Anderson MH. Urethral catheter knots. *Pediatrics.* 1990;85(5):852–854.

31. Ozkan A, Okur M, Kaya M, et al. An easy technique for removal of knotted catheter in the bladder: percutaneous suprapubic cystoscopic intervention. *Int J Clin Exp Med.* 2013;6(7):603–605.

32. Lodha A, Ly L, Brindle M, et al. Intraurethral knot in a very-low-birth-weight infant: radiological recognition, surgical management and prevention. *Pediatr Radiol.* 2005;35:713–716.

33. Carlson D, Mowery BD. Standards to prevent complications of urinary catheterization in children: should and should-knots. *J Soc Pediatr Nurs.* 1997;2:37–41.

Tympanocentesis

Gregory J. Milmoe

Otitis media in neonates and infants under 6 months of age has been a confusing topic because of the overlap between acute otitis media and otitis media with effusion (1). The latter is most relevant for hearing issues while the former is an infection that a newborn might not handle as well as a toddler due to an immature immune system. The infection threat is compounded when a baby in intensive care has additional infections or has become debilitated by other comorbidities (2–5). In these circumstances, tympanocentesis can help in both the diagnosis and the treatment of the problem. Abnormal otoscopy may not be enough to distinguish among acute infection, chronic effusion, and nonresponding infection. Creating the opening in the ear drum will also allow some drainage for decompression and give a sample for culture that will help direct antibiotic therapy (1,6).

A. Indications

The situations in which tympanocentesis would be most helpful include:

1. Infection in severely immunocompromised infants
2. Infection in an infant already on antibiotics or not responding after 72 hours to chosen antibiotic
3. Infection with suppurative complications (e.g., mastoiditis, facial paralysis, sepsis)
4. Need to confirm the diagnosis when the clinical examination is not clear
5. Need to relieve severe otalgia

B. Contraindications

1. Difficulty in confirming ossicular landmarks. One must be able to identify the malleus and the annulus of the tympanic membrane (TM) (**Fig. 23.1**).
2. Suggestion of abnormal anatomy. This is more likely in patients with congenital malformation syndromes.

3. Suggestion of alternate pathology (e.g., cholesteatoma or neoplasm).

C. Precautions

1. Patient safety and comfort require proper restraint, adequate light, and appropriate instruments.
2. The kindest way is to be quick, and this means having the infant immobile.
3. Conscious sedation is feasible only if the infant is stable and has no issues with airway obstruction. It is not needed past the point of puncturing the TM; usually no medication is used.

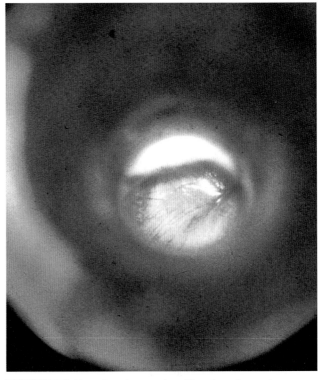

FIGURE 23.1 Normal newborn eardrum. View through speculum.

4. Good visualization is paramount. Sufficient cleaning must be done so the malleus and the anterior aspect of the annulus are clearly visible.
5. Avoid the posterior aspect of the TM. This is where the round window, stapes, and incus are located.

D. Technique (7)

1. Equipment includes otoscope with open operating head and proper-size speculum; an 18-gauge spinal needle with 1-mL syringe; blunt ear curette; 70% isopropyl alcohol in 3-mL syringe; 5-Fr Frazier ear suction; Culturettes with transport media.
2. Restrain infant (see Chapter 5).
3. Position the infant with the involved ear up. The assistant must keep the head still.
4. Rinse ear canal with alcohol solution. This will provide antisepsis and initiate cleaning.
5. Let fluid run out or use suction.
6. Use otoscope to visualize canal and remove debris with curette or suction.
7. Align speculum to get best view of TM landmarks. Pulling superiorly and laterally on the pinna will improve visibility (**Fig. 23.2**).

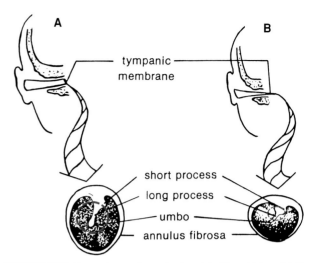

FIGURE 23.2 Tympanic membrane in the adult (**A**) and infant (**B**). The portion of the tympanic membrane that may be visualized through the speculum at one time is within the *dotted line.*

8. Attach spinal needle to 1-mL syringe, after bending it 45 to 60 degrees at the hub. This keeps the syringe out of the line of sight.
9. Hold the needle at the hub and introduce it through the otoscope. Puncture the drum anterior to the malleus at or below the umbo level (**Figs. 23.2** and **23.3**).

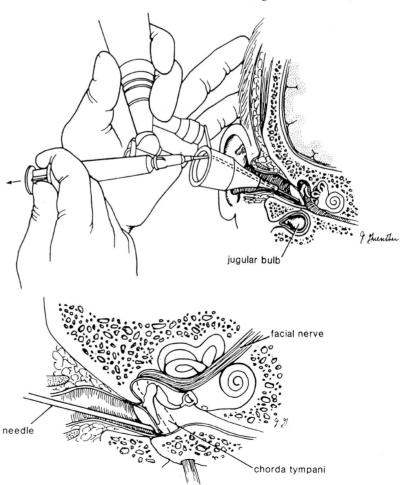

FIGURE 23.3 Tympanocentesis. Aspirating the middle ear using a 3-mL syringe. Needle is penetrating eardrum inferiorly.

10. Hold needle securely and have assistant draw back on the syringe to obtain sample.
11. Place sample in appropriate transport medium.
12. If more drainage is required, a myringotomy blade can be used to widen the opening. This will close in 48 to 72 hours.

E. Complications

1. Most common is bleeding from the canal wall. This usually will stop spontaneously but is preferably avoided.
2. TM perforation that persists. Initially, this may be helpful for additional drainage and ventilation of the middle ear.
3. Disruption of the ossicles from malpositioned needle (see B1 and C5).
4. Major bleeding from dehiscent jugular bulb or carotid artery—rare (8).

References

1. Coticchia J, Shah P, Sachdeva L, et al. Frequency of otitis media based on otoendoscopic evaluation in preterm infants. *Otolaryngol Head Neck Surg.* 2014;15(4):692–699.
2. Turner D, Leibovitz E, Aran A, et al. Acute otitis media in infants younger than two months of age: Microbiology, clinical presentation and therapeutic approach. *Pediatr Infect Dis J.* 2002;21(7):669–674.
3. Syggelou A, Fanos V, Iacovidou N. Acute otitis media in neonatal life: A review. *J Chemother.* 2011;23(3):123–126.
4. Ilia S, Galanakis E. Clinical features and outcome of acute otitis media in early infancy. *Int J Infect Dis.* 2013;17:e317–e320.
5. Sommerfleck P, González Macchi ME, Pellegrini S, et al. Acute otitis media in infants younger than three months not vaccinated against Streptococcus pneumonia. *Int J Pediatr Otorhinolaryngol.* 2013;77:976–980.
6. Block SL. Management of acute otitis media in afebrile neonates. *Pediatr Ann.* 2012;41:225.
7. Guarisco JL, Grundfast KM. A simple device for tympanocentesis in infants and children. *Laryngoscope.* 1988;98:244–246.
8. Hasebe S, Sando I, Orita Y. Proximity of carotid canal wall to tympanic membrane: A human temporal bone study. *Laryngoscope.* 2003;113:802–807.

CHAPTER

24

Bone Marrow Biopsy

Martha C. Sola-Visner, Lisa M. Rimsza, Tung T. Wynn, and Jolie S. Ramesar

A. Definitions

1. **Bone marrow aspirate:** Small amount of bone marrow fluid aspirated through a needle placed into a bone.
2. **Bone marrow biopsy:** Small sample of solid bone marrow tissue obtained using a specific needle.
3. **Bone marrow clot:** Bone marrow aspirate particles (and possible clot) placed in fixative, embedded in paraffin, and sectioned. This is commonly referred to as the "clot."

B. Indications

1. Evaluation of primary hematologic disorders (1,2)
   a. Suspected neonatal aplastic anemia (3,4)
   b. Suspected leukemia, when blood studies are insufficient to confirm the diagnosis (5–7)
   c. Neutropenia of unclear etiology, which is severe (absolute neutrophil count <500/mL) and persistent (8,9)
   d. Thrombocytopenia of unclear etiology, which is severe (platelets <50,000/mL) and persistent (3,10)
2. Evaluation of suspected metabolic/storage disorder (e.g., Niemann–Pick disease) (11)
3. Evaluation of suspected hemophagocytic syndrome or familial hemophagocytic lymphohistiocytosis (12,13)
4. Detection of infiltrating tumor cells, such as Hodgkin and non-Hodgkin lymphoma, neuroblastoma (14), rhabdomyosarcoma, Ewing sarcoma (15), or congenital systemic Langerhans cell histiocytosis
5. Microbiologic cultures (e.g., in disseminated tuberculosis or fungal disease)
6. Cytogenetic studies, for chromosomal analysis (7)
7. Evaluation of suspected osteopetrosis (16)

C. Contraindications

Bone marrow aspirations and biopsies have no absolute contraindications, but there may be relative contraindications based on the general condition of the patient, especially related to the risk of anesthesia or deep sedation.

Note the following considerations:

1. Sampling from the sternum is not recommended in any neonate because of danger of damage to intrathoracic and mediastinal organs
2. Risks/benefits should be considered carefully in the presence of coagulopathy or when administering anticoagulants or thrombolytics
3. Risks/benefits should be carefully considered in preterm infants with severe osteopenia of prematurity

D. Precautions

1. Correct any coagulopathy as much as possible prior to procedure (keep in mind that even in the setting of severe thrombocytopenia, a bone marrow aspirate can be performed safely).
2. Use a total of 0.2 to 0.4 mL of lidocaine.
3. Be aware that less pressure is required to insert the bone marrow needle in neonates (particularly in very low–birth-weight infants) than in older children.
4. When choosing the most appropriate site (tibia vs. iliac crest) and what needle to use (depending on the size and weight of the infant), the clinical stability, the ability to tolerate repositioning, and the personal preference of the person performing the procedure should be considered.
   a. The preferred site for obtaining bone marrow in older children is the posterior superior iliac crest for various reasons (it contains the most cellular marrow, there are no vital organs in close proximity, and it is a non–weight-bearing structure) (17).
   b. In children younger than 18 months of age, the anteromedial face of the tibia is the preferred site for bone marrow aspiration (17). However, this site may fail to yield adequate samples depending on the experience of the person performing it. There

is also the risk of fracturing the bone; this is only a risk for the tibial site, unless the child has a condition associated with bone fragility (i.e., osteogenesis imperfecta).

5. When performing a tibial bone marrow biopsy, be careful to enter the bone 1 to 2 cm below the tibial tuberosity (in smaller infants, this may be just below the tibial tuberosity) to minimize the risk of injuring the growth plate.

6. After the procedure, apply adequate pressure to control bleeding.

E. Equipment

1. **General**

   In general, a **bone marrow biopsy kit** will include all of the required items, with the exception of the needle to be used and the lidocaine. If a kit is not available, you will need the following:

   a. Sterile gloves

   b. Cup with antiseptic solution

   c. Gauze squares

   d. Sterile drapes

   e. 1% lidocaine without epinephrine in 1-mL syringe, with 27-gauge needle

   f. Cup containing 10% neutral buffered formalin or other appropriate fixative

2. **For tibial bone marrow biopsy**

   a. 19-gauge, 0.5-in Osgood bone marrow needle (Popper and Sons, New Hyde Park, New York) **(Fig. 24.1)**

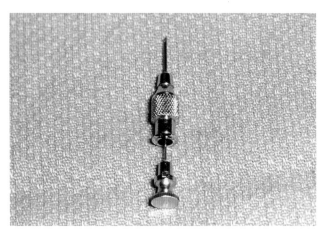

FIGURE 24.1 View of the 19-gauge, 0.5-in Osgood bone marrow needle. The trocar must be completely inserted in the Osgood needle prior to the procedure.

   b. 3-mL syringe without Luer-Lok

   c. 1- to 2-in needle to aid in removal of clot from the syringe

3. **For iliac crest bone marrow biopsy**

   a. 13-gauge, 2-in Jamshidi bone marrow biopsy needle

   b. 3-mL syringe without Luer-Lok

F. Procedure

1. **For tibial bone marrow biopsy**

   a. Place the infant in the supine position.

   b. Use the triangular area at the proximal end of the medial (flat) surface of the tibia, approximately 1 to 2 cm distal to the tibial tuberosity.

   c. Drape and clean creating a sterile field (see Chapter 6) (18).

   d. Infiltrate subcutaneous tissue with lidocaine as the needle is slowly advanced. Inject further small volume when the needle reaches the bone, making sure that the tip of the needle is inserted into the bone for subperiosteal injection.

   e. Remove the needle and wait 2 to 3 minutes.

   f. Use your nondominant hand to firmly stabilize the leg between your thumb and forefinger, providing support with your palm *directly opposite* the site of marrow puncture. To avoid bone fracture, be sure to apply counterpressure with your palm directly opposite the site of penetration. The hand stabilizing the leg cannot be reintroduced into the sterile field.

   g. Make sure that the trocar is completely inserted in the Osgood needle.

   h. Hold the needle between the thumb and forefinger of your dominant hand.

   i. Introduce the needle at a 90-degree angle, and advance it into the marrow cavity with a slow, twisting motion **(Fig. 24.2)**.

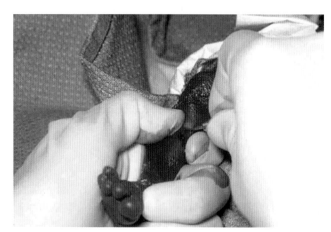

FIGURE 24.2 The Osgood needle is introduced into the tibial marrow cavity with a slow, twisting motion. Notice that the leg is firmly stabilized in the operator's nondominant hand.

   j. Continue to advance the needle until it is firmly fixed in bone (does not move when touched) **(Fig. 24.3)**.

   k. Remove the trocar from the needle and advance the hollow needle an additional 2 to 3 mm into the marrow space (this trephinates marrow spicules into the needle).

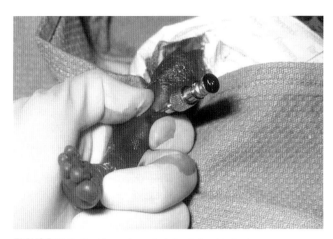

FIGURE 24.3 The Osgood needle is firmly fixed in the bone.

l. Attach a 3-mL syringe (without a Luer-Lok) firmly to the needle.

m. Withdraw the plunger forcefully until a small drop of marrow (~0.1 mL) appears in the syringe hub. Suction should be stopped as soon as the smallest amount of marrow is obtained, because excessive suction will dilute the sample with peripheral blood.

n. If no marrow is obtained initially, rotate, advance, or retract the needle and try again.

o. Remove the syringe as soon as bone marrow is obtained and withdraw the plunger (with marrow attached) to the bottom of the syringe. Allow the marrow to clot there.

p. Remove the needle and apply pressure over the site to achieve hemostasis.

q. After the marrow specimen has clotted, dislodge the clot gently with the use of a 1- or 2-in needle and place it into the fixative solution (**Fig. 24.4**).

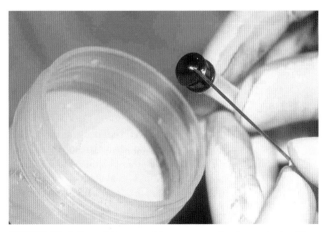

FIGURE 24.4 A small amount of bone marrow has been obtained in a 3-mL syringe and allowed to clot at the bottom of the syringe. The plunger has been removed, and the clot is now being gently dislodged from the plunger (with the use of a 1- or 2-in needle) and placed into the fixative solution.

r. Process the bone marrow clot in a manner identical to a typical bone marrow biopsy, except that decalcification is not required (**Fig. 24.5**).

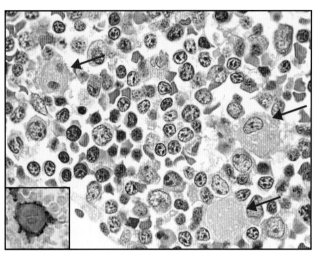

FIGURE 24.5 Photomicrograph of a bone marrow clot section obtained from a neutropenic neonate. The cellularity is 100%. There is a near absence of maturing myeloid precursors, many erythroid precursors, and three megakaryocytes (*arrows*), which show the characteristic small, hypolobated morphology seen in neonatal marrows. Hematoxylin and eosin; original magnification ×200. Insert: Special stains such as CD61 can be used to highlight the cytoplasm of the large cells, confirming their megakaryocytic lineage (10).

2. **For iliac crest bone marrow biopsy (Fig. 24.6)**

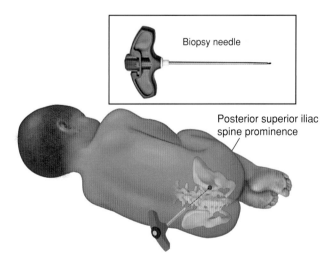

FIGURE 24.6 Iliac crest bone marrow biopsy site and approach. Insert shows the 13-gauge, 2-in Jamshidi bone marrow biopsy needle used in neonates and infants.

a. Place the infant in the prone or lateral decubitus position with the legs flexed at the hip.

b. Locate the spine of the posterior iliac crest and the medial prominence where the procedure is to be done.

c. Drape and clean creating a sterile field (see Chapter 6).

d. Infiltrate subcutaneous tissue with lidocaine as the needle is slowly advanced. Inject further small volume when the needle reaches the bone, making sure that the tip of the needle is inserted into the bone for subperiosteal injection.

e. Remove the needle and wait 2 to 3 minutes.

f. Make sure that the trocar is completely inserted in the Jamshidi needle.

g. Hold the needle between the thumb and forefinger of your dominant hand and introduce the needle at a 90-degree angle, and advance it into the marrow cavity with a slow, twisting motion. Make sure there is adequate pressure in order for the needle to advance.

h. Continue to advance the needle until it is firmly fixed in bone (does not move when touched).

i. To obtain a bone marrow aspirate, remove the trocar and attach a 3-mL syringe (without a Luer-Lok) firmly to the needle and withdraw the plunger forcefully until marrow appears in the syringe hub. Suction is stopped when a small amount of marrow is obtained. Be careful to obtain the aspirate quickly so a clot does not form.

j. If no marrow is obtained initially, rotate, advance, or retract the needle and try again.

k. If a bone marrow biopsy is to be obtained, the needle may be advanced an additional 0.5 to 1 cm without the trocar or the needle may be repositioned with the trocar replaced and advanced with the trocar removed again.

l. Gently rock the needle to dislodge a core within the needle and apply negative pressure by covering the opening of the needle with your thumb.

m. Carefully remove the needle, extract the core from the needle placing it into the fixative solution, and apply pressure over the site to achieve hemostasis.

G. Special Circumstances

1. In cases of suspected osteopetrosis, obtaining a posterior iliac crest bone marrow biopsy is preferable, because it allows quantification of osteoclasts and evaluation of marrow and bony changes consistent with osteopetrosis. In these cases, the tibial bone marrow biopsy technique usually yields only blood or no sample.

2. Consider that alternatives to the procedure may exist, such as observation in a child with Down syndrome with peripheral blasts or a child with stage IV neuroblastoma, or flow cytometry from peripheral blood to obtain diagnostic information for a suspected leukemia.

H. Complications[1]

1. Subperiosteal bleeding
2. Cellulitis or osteomyelitis
3. Limb fracture
4. Injury to blood vessels
5. Bone changes on x-ray film
   a. Lytic lesions
   b. Exostoses
   c. Subperiosteal calcification (secondary to hematoma)

Acknowledgment

This work was partially supported by National Institutes of Health grant HL69990.

References

1. Sreedharanunni S, Sachdeva MU, Kumar N, et al. Spectrum of diseases diagnosed on bone marrow examination of 285 infants in a single tertiary care center. *Hematology.* 2015;20(3):175–181.

2. Tadiotto E, Maines E, Degani D, et al. Bone marrow features in Pearson syndrome with neonatal onset: A case report and review of the literature. *Pediatr Blood Cancer.* 2018;65(4).

3. Stoddart MT, Connor P, Germeshausen M, et al. Congenital amegakaryocytic thrombocytopenia (CAMT) presenting as severe pancytopenia in the first month of life. *Pediatr Blood Cancer.* 2013;60(9):E94–E96.

4. Goldman FD, Gurel Z, Al-Zubeidi D, et al. Congenital pancytopenia and absence of B lymphocytes in a neonate with a mutation in the Ikaros gene. *Pediatr Blood Cancer.* 2012;58(4):591–597.

5. Tsujimoto H, Kounami S, Mitani Y, et al. Neonatal acute megakaryoblastic leukemia presenting with leukemia cutis and multiple intracranial lesions successfully treated with unrelated cord blood transplantation. *Case Rep Hematol.* 2015;2015:610581.

6. Ergin H, Ozdemir OM, Karaca A, et al. A newborn with congenital mixed phenotype acute leukemia after in vitro fertilization. *Pediatr Neonatol.* 2015;56(4):271–274.

7. Campos L, Nadal N, Flandrin-Gresta P, et al. Congenital acute leukemia with initial indolent presentation—a case report. *Cytometry B Clin Cytom.* 2011;80(2):130–133.

8. Del Vecchio A, Christensen RD. Neonatal neutropenia: What diagnostic evaluation is needed and when is treatment recommended? *Early Hum Dev.* 2012;88(Suppl 2):S19–S24.

9. Cosar H, Kahramaner Z, Erdemir A, et al. Reticular dysgenesis in a preterm infant: A case report. *Pediatr Hematol Oncol.* 2010;27(8):646–649.

10. Tighe P, Rimsza LM, Christensen RD, et al. Severe thrombocytopenia in a neonate with congenital HIV infection. *J Pediatr.* 2005;146(3):408–413.

---

[1]These complications refer to the bone marrow biopsy procedure in general.

11. Gumus E, Haliloglu G, Karhan AN, et al. Niemann-Pick disease type C in the newborn period: A single-center experience. *Eur J Pediatr.* 2017;176(12):1669–1676.

12. Fuwa K, Kubota M, Kanno M, et al. Mitochondrial disease as a cause of neonatal hemophagocytic lymphohistiocytosis. *Case Rep Pediatr.* 2016;2016:3932646.

13. Fukazawa M, Hoshina T, Nanishi E, et al. Neonatal hemophagocytic lymphohistiocytosis associated with a vertical transmission of coxsackievirus B1. *J Infect Chemother.* 2013;19(6):1210–1213.

14. van Wezel EM, Decarolis B, Stutterheim J, et al. Neuroblastoma messenger RNA is frequently detected in bone marrow at diagnosis of localised neuroblastoma patients. *Eur J Cancer.* 2016;54:149–158.

15. Esmaeili H, Azimpouran M. Congenital embryonal rhabdomyosarcoma; multiple lesions. *Int J Surg Case Rep.* 2017;31:47–50.

16. Almarzooqi S, Reed S, Fung B, et al. Infantile osteopetrosis and juvenile xanthogranuloma presenting together in a newborn: A case report and literature review. *Pediatr Dev Pathol.* 2011;14(4):307–312.

17. Riley RS, Hogan TF, Pavot DR, et al. A pathologist's perspective on bone marrow aspiration and biopsy: I. Performing a bone marrow examination. *J Clin Lab Anal.* 2004;18(2):70–90.

18. Sola MC, Rimsza LM, Christensen RD. A bone marrow biopsy technique suitable for use in neonates. *Br J Haematol.* 1999;107(2):458–460.

Punch Skin Biopsy

Maura Caufield and Cynthia M. C. DeKlotz

A. Definition

1. A small, full-thickness biopsy utilizing a cylindrical blade

B. Indications

1. Diagnosis of skin lesions (1–6) (**Fig. 25.1**)

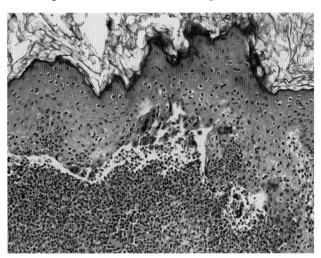

FIGURE 25.1 A neonatal skin biopsy demonstrating vesiculation, epidermal edema, inflammatory infiltrate, and viral cytopathic change in a case of congenital herpes simplex infection.

2. Electron and light microscopic identification of certain hereditary and metabolic disorders (7–10)
3. Genetic, enzymatic, or morphologic studies on established fibroblast strains (11,12)
4. Treatment of small skin lesions

C. Types of Skin Biopsy (13)

1. Punch skin biopsy is appropriate when epidermis, dermis, and, sometimes, subcutaneous fat is required.

It allows for pathologic evaluation and rapid diagnosis of certain conditions including cutaneous neoplasms and inflammatory disorders.
2. Shave biopsies are performed to obtain epidermis and superficial dermis.
3. Incisional biopsies are used predominantly for disorders of deep subcutaneous fat or fascia (e.g., erythema nodosum) and to remove part of a larger lesion for diagnostic purposes.
4. Excision of larger lesions by a trained dermatologist or surgeon is preferable when planning to remove an entire large lesion.

D. Contraindications

There are no absolute contraindications to skin biopsy.

1. Consider whether risks, for example, scarring, infection risk, or bleeding, outweighs benefit for the patient, particularly if certain underlying conditions, such as a bleeding disorder, are present.
2. Caution should be exercised in certain anatomic locations where nerves and arteries are more superficial.
3. Many cephalic and midline lesions may require radiologic examination prior to biopsy to rule out connection to the intracranial or intraspinal space (14,15).
4. Appropriate informed consent including risks/benefits should be obtained prior to proceeding with the biopsy.

E. Equipment

Punch skin biopsies are generally performed using a clean or modified sterile technique (16).

1. Sterile gloves
2. Towel or tray to form clean area
3. Isopropyl alcohol or other suitable antiseptic agent such as povidone-iodine

4. 4- × 4-in gauze squares
5. Sterile cotton-tip applicators
6. Lidocaine HCl 1% with or without epinephrine in 1-mL tuberculin syringe with 27- or 30-gauge needle
7. Blunt tissue forceps
8. Fine, curved scissors or no. 15 scalpel blade
9. Sharp 2- to 6-mm punch (**Fig. 25.2**). Disposable punches ranging from 2 to 8 mm are available

   Note: Specimens obtained with a 2-mm punch are very small and may not yield enough tissue for an accurate diagnosis. One recent study showed that accurate diagnoses were achieved in 79 out of 84 cases, when comparing 2-mm punch biopsies to excisional specimens (17). In most cases, a 3- to 4-mm punch is appropriate

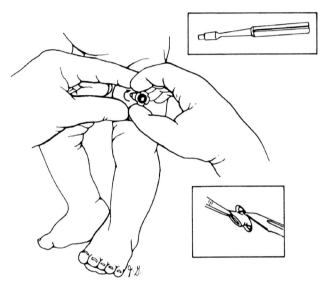

FIGURE 25.2 Punch skin biopsy. **Top (inset):** Disposable biopsy punch. **Bottom (inset):** Cutting the dermal pedicle.

10. 4-0, 5-0, or 6-0 nylon or polypropylene suture with small curved needle on needle holder, or Dermabond (Ethicon, Somerville, New Jersey)
11. Adhesive bandage with white petrolatum
12. Appropriate transport medium affixed with patient's information (**Table 25.1**)
13. Razor if necessary

F. Precautions

1. Avoid sites, if possible, where a small scar would potentially be cosmetically disfiguring
   a. Tip, bridge, and columella of nose
   b. Eyelids
   c. Lip margins
   d. Nipples
   e. Fingers or toes
   f. Areas overlying joints
   g. Lower leg below the knee

2. Avoid biopsy of midline lesion on head, neck, and spine and any lesion on head until appropriate evaluation and imaging (if indicated) is performed to rule out deeper connection (e.g., intracranial communication with aplasia cutis congenital associated with hair collar sign)
3. Avoid multiple procedures at one site
4. Be gentle, to avoid separating epidermis from dermis and crushing the specimen
5. Check biopsy site for signs of infection until healing occurs
6. Avoid freezing tissue for electron microscopy because cellular detail will then be destroyed (**Table 25.1**)

TABLE 25.1 Punch Biopsy Preservatives and Transport Media

TRANSPORT MEDIUM	INDICATIONS
Formalin 10%	Routine microscopic evaluation
Michel's medium or saline-soaked gauze	Blistering or autoimmune disorders (immunofluorescence)
Michel's medium or 2.5% glutaraldehyde (30)	Electron microscopy
Formalin 10%	Immunoperoxidase
DMEM high glucose media with 20% FBS (36)	Fibroblast culture

7. For specimens undergoing routine microscopic examination, avoid placing biopsy specimen in or on saline because artifactual hydropic degeneration of basal cells and subepidermal bullous formation may occur

G. Technique

See **Figure 25.2**.

1. Before performing the biopsy, we recommend photographs of the skin lesion to be biopsied to aid with clinical pathological diagnosis, if needed. Of course, informed consent would first need to be obtained.
2. Restrain and position patient. Infants may be held, or may require use of a wrapping technique or a papoose board in order to immobilize (18). From the experience of one author, infants when recently fed and swaddled, may actually sleep peacefully through the biopsy when distraction (e.g., gently rubbing/vibrating skin away from biopsy site either with hand or dedicated device such as Buzzy Bee) and comfort techniques (e.g., sugar solution coated pacifier) are used (19,20).

3. Choose site for biopsy (21–26).
   a. For suspected malignant lesions, choose the most atypical area if unable to excise completely.
   b. For most dermatoses, choose site of a fully developed, but not end-stage, lesion.
   c. Avoid lesions with secondary change, including excoriations and crust.
   d. For vesicular and bullous lesions, attempt to keep the blister roof attached with normal skin included at the edge. For suspected epidermolysis bullosa, it is ideal to biopsy freshly created vesicles/bullae that have been created with the eraser end of a pencil.
   e. When performing a biopsy for direct immunofluorescence (DIF), the site varies. DIF for autoimmune blistering diseases should be obtained from adjacent normal skin. For suspected vasculitis, DIF is obtained from an acute lesion (<24 hours old).
   f. For large lesions, obtain specimen from periphery, including some normal skin.
   g. For discrete small lesions, try to leave 1- to 2-mm margins of normal skin around the lesions.
   h. Skin biopsy has been performed on the fetus and may be done postmortem on stillborn or recently deceased infants to produce fibroblast cultures for karyotype (see Chapter 25). Under the latter circumstances, punch or excisional biopsy from the freshest-appearing, least-macerated skin area(s) is appropriate.
4. Shave or trim hairs, if needed. This step is not typically done by the author.
5. Prepare as for minor procedure (see Chapter 5).
6. Inject 0.25 to 1.0 mL of lidocaine intradermally beneath the lesion. The maximum dose of lidocaine to avoid toxicity is 4.5 mg/kg with epinephrine and 7.5 mg/kg without (27). Some techniques used to minimize pain include: use of a small-bore (30-gauge) needle, buffering anesthetic with sodium bicarbonate in a ratio of 1 mL sodium bicarbonate to 10 mL of lidocaine, pinching of the site during injection, and applying ice (28–30). Other distraction and comforting techniques are also recommended such as detailed above in section 2 of Technique.
7. Wait 5 minutes for maximal anesthesia. If using lidocaine with epinephrine, maximal vasoconstriction occurs at 15 minutes.
8. Stretch skin surrounding lesion taut, perpendicular to relaxed skin tension lines. This will allow for easier closure.
9. Carefully place punch over the lesion. Apply firm, downward pressure in a circular or back and forth motion until the subcutaneous fat is reached. Biopsy should include epidermis, full thickness of dermis, and some subcutaneous fat.
10. Remove punch.
11. Use blunt forceps in one hand to grasp the lateral edge of the biopsy specimen and elevate it, utilizing care to avoid crush artifact. Additionally, applying gentle pressure on the surrounding intact skin can help raise the biopsy specimen to allow easier removal.
12. Use curved scissors or a scalpel blade in the other hand to cut the punch specimen at its base, through the subcutaneous fat.
13. Place specimen in container with appropriate preservative or transport medium.
14. Label container with patient name, date, and exact site of biopsy.
15. Control bleeding at site of biopsy with gentle pressure using sterile 4- × 4-in gauze square.
16. Approximate wound margins and close the biopsy site. For best cosmetic result, this should be done with a simple interrupted suture using nylon or polypropylene, especially for lesions 4 mm or larger (31). For wounds 3 mm or less, healing via secondary intention and application of Dermabond or gelfoam are other options (13). With secondary intention, expect healing in 7 to 14 days, with a residual white area a few millimeters in diameter if the biopsy extended to the dermis–subcutaneous fat interface.
17. If suturing is performed, remove suture in 5 days for facial lesions and 10 to 14 days for lesions on the trunk, limbs, or scalp.
18. After the biopsy, apply white petrolatum followed by an adhesive bandage. Prevention of crust formation will help the wound to heal faster (32). A randomized control trial of patients undergoing ambulatory skin surgery showed an equally low infection rate with use of white petrolatum compared to Bacitracin ointment, as well as a lower risk for allergic contact dermatitis (33). Dressings should be changed every 24 hours.

H. Complications (13)

1. Infection
2. Unsightly scarring or keloid formation (rare)
3. Excessive bleeding (rare, except in patient with coagulation defect)
4. Pathologic uncertainty
5. Recurrence of lesion

References

1. Darby JB, Valentine G, Hillier K, et al. A 3-week-old with an isolated "blueberry muffin" rash. *Pediatrics*. 2017;140(1):pii: e20162598.
2. Leclerc-Mercier S, Bodemer C, Bourdon-Lanoy E, et al. Early skin biopsy is helpful for the diagnosis and management of neonatal and infantile erythrodermas. *J Cutan Pathol*. 2010; 37(2):249–255.

3. Lynch MC, Samson TD, Zaenglein AL, et al. Evolution of fibroblastic connective tissue nevus in an infant. *Am J Dermatopathol.* 2017;39(3):225–227.

4. Simons EA, Huang JT, Schmidt B. Congenital melanocytic nevi in young children: histopathologic features and clinical outcomes. *J Am Acad Dermatol.* 2017;76(5): 941–947.

5. Sina B, Kao GF, Deng AC, et al. Skin biopsy for inflammatory and common neoplastic skin diseases: optimum time, best location, and preferred techniques. A critical review. *J Cutan Pathol.* 2009;36(5):505–510.

6. Zelger BW, Sidoroff A, Orchard G, et al. Non-Langerhans cell histiocytoses. A new unifying concept. *Am J Dermatopathol.* 1996;18(5):490–504.

7. Alroy J, Ucci AA. Skin biopsy: a useful tool in the diagnosis of lysosomal storage diseases. *Ultrastruc Pathol.* 2006;30(6): 489–503.

8. Berk DR, Jazayeri L, Marinkovich MP, et al. Diagnosing epidermolysis bullosa type and subtype in infancy using immunofluorescence microscopy: the Stanford experience. *Pediatr Dermatol.* 2013;30(2):226–233.

9. Jaunzems AE, Woods AE, Staples A. Electron microscopy and morphometry enhances differentiation of epidermolysis bullosa subtypes. With normal values for 24 parameters in skin. *Arch Dermatol Res.* 1997;289(11):631–639.

10. Simonati A, Rizzuto N. Neuronal ceroid lipofuscinoses: pathological features of bioptic specimens from 28 patients. *Neurol Sci.* 2002;21(3):S63–S70.

11. Fuller M, Mellet N, Hein LK, et al. Absence of α-galactosidase cross-correction in Fabry heterozygote culture skin fibroblasts. *Mol Genet Metab.* 2015;114(2):268–273.

12. Vangipurum M, Ting D, Kim S, et al. Skin punch biopsy explants culture for derivation of primary human fibroblasts. *J Vis Exp.* 2013;77:e3779.

13. Alguire PC, Mathes BM. Skin biopsy techniques for the internist. *J Gen Intern Med.* 1998;13(1):46–54.

14. Kennard CD, Rasmussen JE. Congenital midline nasal masses: diagnosis and management. *J Dermatol Surg Oncol.* 1990;16: 1025–1036.

15. Baldwin HE, Berck CM, Lynfield YL. Subcutaneous nodules of the scalp: preoperative management. *J Am Acad Dermatol.* 1991;25:819–830.

16. Affleck GA, Colver G. Skin biopsy techniques. In: Robinson JK, ed. *Surgery of the Skin: Procedural Dermatology.* 2nd ed. Edinburgh: Mosby Elsevier; 2010:170–176.

17. Todd P, Garioch JJ, Humphreys S, et al. Evaluation of the 2-mm punch biopsy in dermatological diagnosis. *Clin Exp Dermatol.* 1996;21:11–13.

18. Bellet, JS. Diagnostic and therapeutic procedures. In: Eichenfield JF, ed. *Neonatal and Infant Dermatology.* 3rd ed. Philadelphia: Elsevier Saunders; 2015:57–64.

19. Eichenfield LF, Cunningham BB. Decreasing the pain of dermatologic procedures in children. *Curr Probl Dermatol.* 1999;11(1):3–34.

20. Moadad N, Kozman K, Shahine R, et al. Distraction using the BUZZY during an IV insertion. *J Pediatr Nurs.* 2016;31(1):64–72.

21. Ackerman AB. Biopsy: why, where, when, how? *J Dermatol Surg.* 1975;1:21–23.

22. Elston DM, Stratman EJ, Miller SJ. Skin biopsy: biopsy issues in specific diseases. *J Am Acad Dermatol.* 2016;74(1):1–16.

23. High WA, Tomasini CF, Argenziano G, et al. Basic principles of dermatology. In: Bolognia J, ed. *Dermatology.* 3rd ed. Philadelphia: Elsevier Saunders; 2012:12–16.

24. Golbus M, Sagebiel RW, Filly RA, et al. Prenatal diagnosis of ichthyosiform erythroderma (epidermolytic hyperkeratosis) by fetal skin biopsy. *N Engl J Med.* 1980;302:93–95.

25. Luu M, Cantatore-Francis JL, Glick SA. Prenatal diagnoses of genodermatoses: current scope and future capabilities. *Int J Dermatol.* 2010;49:353–361.

26. Intong LR, Murrell DF. How to take skin biopsies for epidermolysis bullosa. *Dermatol Clin.* 2010;28(2):197–200.

27. Heather MJ, Weinberger CH, Brodland DG. Local anesthetics. In: Wolverton SE. *Comprehensive Dermatologic Drug Therapy.* 3rd ed. Edinburgh: Elsevier Saunders; 2013:638.

28. Arndt KA, Burton C, Noe JM. Minimizing the pain of local anesthesia. *Plast Reconstr Surg.* 1983;72:676–679.

29. Stewart JH, Cole GW, Klein JA. Neutralized lidocaine with epinephrine for local anesthesia. *J Dermatol Surg Oncol.* 1989;15:1081–1083.

30. Kuwahara RT, Skinner RB. EMLA versus ice as a topical anesthetic. *Dermatol Surg.* 2001;27:495–496.

31. Christenson LJ, Phillips PK, Weaver AL, et al. Primary closure vs second-intention treatment of skin punch biopsy sites: a randomized trial. *Arch Dermatol.* 2005;141(9):1093–1099.

32. Telfer NR, Moy RL. Wound care after office procedures. *J Dermatol Surg Oncol.* 1993;19:722–731.

33. Smack DP, Harrington AC, Dunn C, et al. Infection and allergy incidence in ambulatory surgery patients using white petrolatum vs bacitracin ointment. A randomized control trial. *JAMA.* 1996;276(12):972–977.

Ophthalmic Specimen Collection

Jennifer A. Dunbar

A. Introduction

Neonatal conjunctivitis is considered an ocular emergency (1,2). Conjunctivitis may be the presenting sign of coexisting life-threatening systemic infection. Signs include diffuse conjunctival injection with mucoid, purulent, or watery ophthalmic discharge, and eyelid edema and erythema. Both bacterial and viral pathogens cause corneal ulceration and opacity, which may lead to blindness. *Neisseria gonorrhea*, *Klebsiella* species, or *Pseudomonas* species may rapidly perforate the globe (3).

B. Indications

1. To obtain specimen for testing to determine the cause of conjunctivitis (**Table 26.1**)
   a. The most common cause of neonatal conjunctivitis is chemical conjunctivitis, which presents in the first 24 hours of life as a reaction to prophylaxis and usually resolves within 48 hours.
   b. Infectious neonatal conjunctivitis may be bacterial or viral, and it is often associated with exposure in the birth canal or through spontaneous rupture of membranes. The classic causes include *Chlamydia*, *Streptococcus* spp., *Staphylococcus* spp., *Escherichia coli*, *Haemophilus* spp., *N. gonorrhea*, and herpes simplex (4).
   c. In addition to the classic causes of neonatal conjunctivitis above, methicillin-resistant *Staphylococcus aureus*, group B *Streptococcus*, and *N. meningitides* have been described in neonates (5–7).
   d. Hospital-acquired conjunctivitis affects 6% to 18% of infants in neonatal intensive care units (NICUs) and may occur in epidemics (8–11).
      (1) The eye may be contaminated by respiratory secretions, or gastrointestinal flora, with coagulase-negative *Staphylococcus*, *S. aureus*, and

Klebsiella sp. reported as the most common pathogens (6,12).
      (2) Hospitalized premature babies experience increased risk for infectious conjunctivitis due to gram-negative organisms, such as *Klebsiella*, *E. coli*, *Serratia*, and *Haemophilus influenzae*. This risk increases in neonates <1,500 g and 29 weeks' gestational age (13).
      (3) Epidemics of conjunctivitis have been associated with routine ophthalmic screening and ophthalmic procedures in the NICU. *Serratia marcescens*, *Klebsiella* sp., *Acinetobacter baumannii*, and adenovirus epidemics have been described (9,13–15).

C. Relative Contraindications

1. Corneal epithelial defect
   a. If fluorescein staining of the cornea reveals an epithelial staining defect, then corneal ulceration or infectious keratitis may be present. This requires referral to an ophthalmologist.

D. Special Considerations for Ophthalmic Specimen Management

1. Conjunctival scrapings are the specimen of choice because many pathogens are intraepithelial (1).
2. The ocular specimen size is small; requiring special care for specimen handling.
3. Direct placement of the conjunctival scrapings on slides for staining and direct plating onto culture medium at the bedside will maximize the yield.
4. Communication with laboratory personnel regarding specimen handling improves culture results (16).

TABLE 26.1 Analysis of Conjunctival Scrapings

TEST	ORGANISMS IDENTIFIED	FINDING
Stain		
Gram stain	*Neisseria gonorrhea*	Gram-negative diplococci
Giemsa stain	*Chlamydia trachomatis*	Intraepithelial intracytoplasmic inclusions
Papanicolaou stain	Herpes simplex virus	Multinucleate giant cells and inclusion-bearing cells
Direct Antigen Detection Techniques		
Immunofluorescent indicator system	*C. trachomatis*	
Immunosorbent assay (ELISA)	*C. trachomatis* Herpes simplex virus	
Fluorescein-labeled monoclonal antibodies (MicroTrak)	*C. trachomatis*	
Indirect fluorescence	Herpes simplex virus	
Culture		
Thayer–Martin	*N. gonorrhea*	
Aerobic	Gram-positive and gram-negative bacteria	
Anaerobic	Anaerobic bacteria	
Viral transport	Herpes simplex virus	
Chlamydia culture (McCoy culture)	*C. trachomatis*	

ELISA, enzyme-linked immunosorbent assay.

E. Materials

1. Equipment for staining the cornea to rule out epithelial defect
   a. Fluorescein dye or strips
   b. Wood lamp or other blue light source
2. Equipment for obtaining specimen
   a. Choose topical anesthetic:
      (1) 0.5% preservative-free tetracaine in unit-dose containers (Alcon Laboratories, Fort Worth, Texas).
      (2) 0.5% proparacaine hydrochloride ophthalmic solution (Akorn, Inc., Lake Forest, Illinois, USA).
      (3) Historically some physicians chose to perform the procedure without anesthetic because topical ophthalmic anesthetics, both containing preservatives and preservative-free may inhibit bacterial growth in culture. However, this is quite painful for the infant. Some anesthetics minimally inhibit bacterial growth (17,18).
   b. Sterile cotton swabs may be used to evert the eyelids but are not recommended for specimen collection (**Fig. 26.1**).

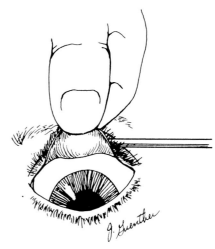

FIGURE 26.1 Everting the upper eyelid.

c. Choose instrument to obtain cultures.
   (1) Calcium alginate swabs
   (2) Sterile Dacron polyester-tipped applicator (Harwood Products Company, Guilford, Maine)

   Calcium alginate swabs have been shown to yield equal or better organism retrieval in cultures than spatulas or Dacron swabs (19,20). Moistening the swab with trypticase soy (Becton, Dickinson and Company, Franklin Lakes, New Jersey) broth or other culture medium enhances results. However, spatulas have been shown to provide better samples in smear than swabs. Spatulas preserve the conjunctival epithelial cells better, thus providing better opportunity for diagnosing pathogens with intracellular organisms or inclusions (21). Calcium alginate swabs may interfere with immunoassays.

   (3) ESwab (Copan Diagnostics, Inc., Murrieta, California, USA) is a simplified option for obtaining ophthalmic specimens if the above materials are not available (22).

d. Choose instrument for scraping the conjunctiva.
   (1) Kimura Platinum Spatula E1091 (Storz Ophthalmics, Division of Bausch & Lomb, Rochester, New York) (**Fig. 26.2**)

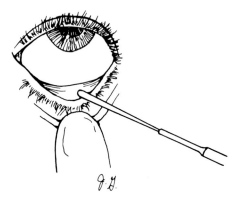

FIGURE 26.2 Using Kimura Platinum Spatula to take scraping from lower eyelid.

   (2) Nasopharyngeal swab with metal handle bent for scraping
   (3) No. 11 blade or no. 15 blade
   (4) Calcium alginate swabs

   If spatulas are not available, then swabs should be used vigorously on the tarsal conjunctival surface so as to débride epithelial cells.

e. Equipment for obtaining microscope slides
   (1) Frosted, etched glass slides
   (2) Microslide holders
   (3) Pencil or marker for labeling

F. Equipment for Identifying *Chlamydia* and Viral Agents

1. Equipment for nonculture chlamydial and viral studies
   a. Although McCoy culture was traditionally considered the "gold standard" for identification of *Chlamydia*, advances in polymerase chain reaction (PCR) elevate this test to the level of gold standard alongside culture (23). Real-time, or quantitative PCR (qPCR), shows quantification of the pathogen DNA in the original sample, and multiplex PCR allows for the detection of DNA from multiple organisms from a single sample. Results of PCR testing may be available within 24 hours while cultures may take several days to provide results. Specimens collected in the first few days of life may have less yield on culture because elementary bodies often take several days to form in neonates (24,25).
   b. Nonculture tests listed below, such as direct immunofluorescence, enzyme-linked immunosorbent assay, and PCR, all perform well for ocular specimens and provide a result more rapidly (26–30). PCR is the most sensitive nonculture test for *Chlamydia*, with the advantage of increased detection in mild disease (26–30). If PCR is not readily available, direct immunofluorescent monoclonal antibody stain may be the most sensitive and rapid option (31).
      (1) For chlamydial direct fluorescence antibody stain: MicroTrak *Chlamydia trachomatis* specimen collection kit (Trinity Biotech, Bray, County Wicklow, Ireland).
      (2) For enzyme-linked immunosorbent assay: Place specimen in media advised by the laboratory performing the study.
      (3) For chlamydial PCR: Place specimen in transport medium appropriate for the assay used. An example is M4 medium for the transport of viruses and *Chlamydia* (Remel, Lenexa, Kansas).
      (4) For adenovirus: AdenoPlus adenoviral point-of-care testing (RPS, Sarasota, Florida, USA) is available for rapid bedside diagnosis of adenovirus (32,33).

2. Media for culture
   Specimens should be plated onto culture medium at the bedside. Each laboratory will have specific media available for a particular type of organism. The following list is a suggestion of classic media used for each type of organism.
   a. Bacterial culture media
      (1) Trypticase soy broth
      (2) Blood agar plate
      (3) Chocolate agar plate for *H. influenzae, N. gonorrhea*
      (4) Thayer–Martin medium, if gonorrhea suspected

b. Virus-holding medium (i.e., M4 medium for the transport of viruses and *Chlamydia*) (Remel, Lenexa, Kansas)

c. *Chlamydia* culture transport medium (i.e., M4 medium for the transport of viruses and *Chlamydia*) (Remel, Lenexa, Kansas)

d. Sabouraud agar, if fungal conjunctivitis suspected

G. Technique

1. Method for staining the cornea for epithelial defect
   a. Instill a very small amount of fluorescein in the lower conjunctival fornix by lightly touching the tear film with a fluorescein strip. Flooding the eye with fluorescein may obscure a small corneal epithelial defect.
   b. Evaluate the cornea for staining with a Wood lamp or other blue light source.
   c. If a corneal epithelial defect is present, the cornea may be infected and an ophthalmologist should be consulted.
   d. Herpes virus may present in the neonate as a geographic-shaped epithelial defect rather than a dendrite.
2. Method for everting eyelids
   a. Upper lid (see **Fig. 26.1**)
      (1) Grasp lashes and border of lid between thumb and index finger of nondominant hand.
      (2) Draw lid downward and away from eyeball.
      (3) Indent upper lid, with handle of cotton-tipped applicator held in dominant hand and pull lid back and upward over applicator.
      (4) Remove applicator and hold lid in place with nondominant hand by gently pressing border of lid against superior orbital margin.
   b. Lower lid (see **Fig. 26.2**)
      (1) Place index finger of nondominant hand on margin of lower lid.
      (2) Pull downward.
3. Method for obtaining cultures

   Obtain cultures prior to conjunctival scraping. Take separate cultures from each eye with a separate sterile swab for each type of medium desired. Culture and label each eye separately, even if only one eye is symptomatic. The uninfected eye can serve as a control for indigenous flora (34).
   a. Moisten calcium alginate swabs with trypticase soy broth or other liquid culture medium.
   b. Evert eyelid.
   c. Apply swab to bulbar and palpebral conjunctiva of upper and lower fornices of eye.
   d. Apply swab directly to culture medium plates at the bedside with a single row of C-shaped inoculation streaks. Monitoring the growth of organisms along the shape of the inoculation streaks may help the laboratory in the diagnosis of the cultured pathogen.

e. Use a separate sterile swab for each culture plate or culture vial.

f. Label cultures meticulously with eye cultured (right or left) and part of eye cultured (conjunctiva, lid margin, etc.).

g. Incubate cultures immediately.

4. Method for obtaining conjunctival scrapings for smear and nonculture *Chlamydia* tests
   a. Evert eyelid as described above.
   b. Instill topical anesthetic into conjunctival fornix, if desired.
   c. Swab off excess discharge.
   d. Take scraping 2 mm from eye margin (normal keratinized epithelium from the lid margin may confound results of smear).
   e. Pass spatula or blade two to three times in the same direction, avoiding bleeding.
   f. Spread specimen from spatula or blade gently into a monolayer on a clean glass slide and label.
   g. Fix smears as required for proposed smears and nonculture *Chlamydia* tests.
   h. Repeat with separate sterile spatula or blade on second eye.

H. Interpretation of Conjunctival Cytology

1. Cellular reaction
   a. Polymorphonuclear reaction
      (1) Bacterial infections
      (2) Chlamydial infection
      (3) Very severe viral infection
   b. Mononuclear reactions: Viral infection
   c. Eosinophilia and basophilia: Allergic states
   d. Plasma cells: Chlamydial infection
2. Intraepithelial cell inclusions
   a. Chlamydial infection
      (1) Acidophilic inclusions in cytoplasm, capping epithelial cell nuclei
      (2) Basophilic "initial bodies" in cytoplasm
   b. Viral infection
      Giant, multinucleated epithelial cells may be seen (e.g., herpetic keratoconjunctivitis).

I. Complications of Scraping

1. Conjunctival bleeding
   a. Mild conjunctival bleeding, usually self-limiting, frequently occurs.
   b. Instill erythromycin ophthalmic ointment.
2. Corneal injury
   a. Keep the spatula or blade flat against the tarsal conjunctiva at all times to avoid trauma to the cornea.
   b. Corneal injury is confirmed by a staining defect on fluorescein staining.

   c. If corneal injury occurs, instill erythromycin ophthalmic ointment and contact an ophthalmologist.

3. Transfer of infection from infected to noninfected eye. This complication is avoided by using separate sterile instruments when taking samples from each eye.

4. Ocular irritation, pain, photophobia, lacrimation, swelling, and hyperemia. These problems are usually mild and self-limited.

References

1. Richards A, Guzman-Cottrill JA. Conjunctivitis. *Pediatr Rev.* 2010;31:196–208.

2. Teoh DL, Reynolds S. Diagnosis and management of pediatric conjunctivitis. *Pediatr Emerg Care.* 2003;19:48–55.

3. Aung T, Chan TK. Nosocomial Klebsiella pneumonia conjunctivitis resulting in infectious keratitis and bilateral corneal perforation. *Cornea.* 1998;17:558–561.

4. Wright KW. Pediatric conjunctivitis. In: Wright KW, Spiegel PH, eds. *Pediatric Ophthalmology and Strabismus.* 2nd ed. New York: Springer; 2003:335.

5. Sahu DN, Thomson S, Salam A, et al. Neonatal methicillin-resistant Staphylococcus aureus conjunctivitis. *Br J Ophthalmol.* 2006;90:794–795.

6. Kumar JB, Silverstein E, Wallace DK. Klebsiella pneumonia: an unusual cause of ophthalmia neonatorum in a healthy newborn. *J AAPOS.* 2015;19:564–566.

7. Pöschl JM, Hellstern G, Ruef P, et al. Ophthalmia neonatorum caused by group B Streptococcus. *Scand J Infect Dis.* 2002;34:921–922.

8. Haas J, Larson E, Ross B, et al. Epidemiology and diagnosis of hospital acquired conjunctivitis among neonatal intensive care unit patients. *Pediatr Infect Dis J.* 2005;24:586–589.

9. Faden H, Wynn RJ, Campagna L, et al. Outbreak of adenovirus type 30 in the neonatal intensive care unit. *J Pediatr.* 2005;146:523–527.

10. Couto RC, Carvalho EAA, Pedrosa TMG, et al. A 10-year prospective surveillance of nosocomial infections in neonatal intensive care units. *Am J Infect Control.* 2007;35:183–189.

11. Borer A, Livshiz-Riven I, Golan A, et al. Hospital-acquired conjunctivitis in a neonatal intensive care unit: bacterial etiology and susceptibility patterns. *Am J Infect Control.* 2010;38:650–652.

12. Chen CJ, Starr CE. Epidemiology of gram-negative conjunctivitis in neonatal intensive care unit patients. *Am J Ophthalmol.* 2008;145:966–970.

13. Casolari C, Pecorari M, Fabio G, et al. A simultaneous outbreak of Serratia marcescens and Klebsiella pneumoniae in a neonatal intensive care unit. *J Hosp Infect.* 2005;61:312–320.

14. Ersoy Y, Otlu B, Türkçüğlu P, et al. Outbreak of adenovirus serotype 8 conjunctivitis in preterm infants in a neonatal intensive care unit. *J Hosp Infect.* 2012;80:144–149.

15. McGrath EJ, Chopra T, Abdel-Haq N, et al. An outbreak of carbapenem-resistant Acinetobacter baumannii infection in a neonatal intensive care unit: investigation and control. *Infect Control Hosp Epidemiol.* 2011;32:34–41.

16. Miller JM, ed. *A Guide to Specimen Management in Clinical Microbiology.* 2nd ed. Washington, DC: American Society for Microbiology Press; 1999.

17. Mullin GS, Rubinfeld RS. The antibacterial activity of topical anesthetics. *Cornea.* 1997;16:662–665.

18. Pelosini L, Treffene S, Hollick EJ. Antibacterial activity of preservative-free topical anesthetic drops in current use in ophthalmology departments. *Cornea.* 2009;28:58–61.

19. Benson WH, Lanier JD. Comparison of techniques for culturing corneal ulcers. *Ophthalmology.* 1992;99:800–804.

20. Jacob P, Gopinathan U, Sharma S, et al. Calcium alginate swab versus Bard Parker blade in the diagnosis of microbial keratitis. *Cornea.* 1995;14:360–364.

21. Rapoza PA, Johnson S, Taylor HR. Platinum spatula vs Dacron swab in the preparation of conjunctival smears. *Am J Ophthalmol.* 1986;102:400–401.

22. Pakzad-Vaezi K, Levasseur SD, Schendel S, et al. The corneal ulcer one-touch study: a simplified microbiological specimen collection method. *Am J Ophthalmol.* 2015;159:37–43.

23. Taravati P, Lam D, Van Gelder RN. Role of molecular diagnostics in ocular microbiology. *Curr Ophthalmol Rep.* 2013;1(4).

24. Talley AR, Garcia-Ferrer F, Laycock KA, et al. Comparative diagnosis of neonatal chlamydial conjunctivitis by polymerase chain reaction and McCoy cell culture. *Am J Ophthalmol.* 1994;117:50–57.

25. Hammerschlag MR, Roblin PM, Gelling M, et al. Use of polymerase chain reaction for the detection of Chlamydia trachomatis in ocular and nasopharyngeal specimens from infants with conjunctivitis. *Pediatr Infect Dis J.* 1997;16:293–297.

26. Percivalle E, Sarasini A, Torsellini M, et al. A comparison of methods for detecting adenovirus type 8 keratoconjunctivitis during a nosocomial outbreak in a neonatal intensive care unit. *J Clin Virol.* 2003;28:257–264.

27. Thompson PP, Kowalski RP. A 13-year retrospective review of polymerase chain reaction testing for infectious agents from ocular samples. *Ophthalmology.* 2011;118:1449–1453.

28. Kowalski RP, Thompson PP, Kinchington PR, et al. Evaluation of the Smart Cycler II system for real-time detection of viruses and Chlamydia from ocular specimens. *Arch Ophthalmol.* 2006;124:1135–1139.

29. Chichili GR, Athmanathan S, Farhatullah S, et al. Multiplex polymerase chain reaction for the detection of herpes simplex virus, varicella-zoster virus and cytomegalovirus in ocular specimens. *Curr Eye Res.* 2003;27:85–90.

30. Yip PP, Chan WH, Yip KT, et al. The use of polymerase chain reaction assay versus conventional methods in detecting neonatal chlamydial conjunctivitis. *J Pediatr Ophthalmol Strabismus.* 2008;45:234–239.

31. Rapoza PA, Quinn TC, Kiessling LA, et al. Assessment of neonatal conjunctivitis with a direct immunofluorescent monoclonal antibody stain for Chlamydia. *JAMA.* 1986;24:3369–3373.

32. Sambursky R, Trattler W, Tauber S, et al. Sensitivity and specificity of the AdenoPlus test for diagnosing adenoviral conjunctivitis. *JAMA Ophthalmol.* 2013;131(1):17–22.

33. Kam KYR, Ong HS, Bunce C, et al. Sensitivity and specificity of the AdenoPlus point-of-care system in detecting adenovirus in conjunctivitis patients at an ophthalmic emergency department: a diagnostic accuracy study. *Br J Ophthalmol.* 2015;99:1186–1189.

34. Brito DV, Brito CS, Resende DS, et al. Nosocomial infections in a Brazilian neonatal intensive care unit: a 4-year surveillance study. *Rev Soc Bras Med Trop.* 2010;43:633–637.

27

Perimortem Sampling

Reem Saadeh-Haddad and Chahira Kozma

A. Background

1. Perimortem sampling may help to establish the diagnosis in infants who die before diagnostic evaluation is completed (1).

2. Approximately 25% of unexplained infant deaths in the 1st week of life are due to undiagnosed congenital anomalies. Infectious causes may account for a third of unexplained deaths (2,3). Unknown causes continue to play a significant role (4).

3. Inborn errors of metabolism are rare individually, but in the general population the incidence may be >1 in 1,000 live births (3).

4. Diagnostic testing for congenital and metabolic disorders can be time consuming, so some infants may go undiagnosed and even die before the exact cause is elucidated.

5. Whole exome sequencing has become a useful tool. Studies show that the yield of a diagnosis with whole exome sequencing is approximately 25%, thus supporting its use in cases where there is an unusual or nonspecific disease presentation (6).

6. The consideration of DNA banking should also be discussed with the family in hopes of obtaining a genetic diagnosis at a later date when all current testing is negative (7).

7. Autopsy is declining worldwide. Neonatal autopsy rates fell from 80% to 50% by the year 2000 (8). The decrease in autopsy rate is due to both more frequent refusal from parents and fewer proposals of the examination by medical staff (9).

8. Many parents today question the need for autopsy in an era of sophisticated diagnostic testing. For some families, cultural or religious traditions may be barriers to autopsy consent (10).

9. Even with autopsy, perimortem evaluation may be essential, as some tests have low yield when performed more than a few hours after death (11).

10. Neonatologists and pediatricians should be prepared to independently obtain any necessary samples for diagnosis and to counsel the family regarding options for postmortem evaluation.

11. Information gathered during this period can be very important for current and future generations (12).

12. If time allows, a genetics consult can be very useful in guiding testing. If an inborn error of metabolism or genetic disease is suspected, consultation before or immediately after death is vital.

13. The approach to investigate neonatal death varies widely and should be determined by the clinical team and guided by the infant's course, maternal and family history.

B. Indications (13,14)

1. Unknown cause of death
2. Suspected genetic disorder
3. Suspected inborn error of metabolism
4. Suspected undiagnosed infection
5. Hydropic infants
6. Severe growth retardation
7. Congenital infection
8. Suspected hypoxic ischemic encephalopathy (15)

C. Discussion With the Family

1. Families of dying infants are under great strain, particularly if diagnosis is uncertain. An in-depth conversation with the family can answer any questions they may have and create a plan for perimortem sampling and for possible autopsy.

2. This is also the time to discuss DNA banking for future genetic testing. Identification of a DNA banking laboratory and appropriate consent and financial forms

should be made available to the family. The purpose of DNA banking is to offer the family the possibility of future genetic diagnosis if one is not confirmed at the time of neonatal death (7).

3. Informed consent may be obtained at this time for any planned photographs or procedures.

D. Clinical Information

A detailed history and examination is important, particularly if a geneticist has been unable to see the infant (5).

1. History
   a. Maternal history: Ethnicity and medical history
   b. Previous pregnancy history: Stillbirths or pregnancy losses
   c. History of this pregnancy, including:
      (1) Exposure to teratogens
      (2) Amniotic fluid volume
      (3) Results of amniocentesis and ultrasound
      (4) Maternal illness
      (5) Fetal movements
      (6) Travel history
   d. Family history including three-generation pedigree (**Table 27.1**) (11)

TABLE 27.1 Key Elements of Family History

Gender of each individual using standard pedigree symbols
Male relatives on the maternal side when considering X-linked recessive disorder
Consanguinity
Miscarriage and stillbirths
Ethnic origin of family

   e. Infant history: Report medical course for the infant including diagnoses, treatments, and laboratory results
2. Physical examination
   a. Should be detailed and thorough. If a genetic disorder is suspected, it should be performed by a specialist in genetic metabolic disorders, if possible, to evaluate for major and minor malformations and anomalies.
   b. Important components include:
      (1) Growth parameters including head, chest, and abdominal circumference (16).
      (2) Hair pattern.
      (3) Facial features including eye and ear placement.
      (4) Abnormalities of hands and feet.
      (5) Genital and rectal examination.
      (6) Neurologic findings.
      (7) Skin abnormalities.

c. Further resources to guide physical examination are available online from the Wisconsin Stillbirth Service at http://www2.marshfieldclinic.org/wissp/ (17) and from the Perinatal Society of Australia and New Zealand at www.psanz.com.au/special-interest-groups/pnm.aspx (18).

E. Photographs

1. Digital photographs are the best; however, clinicians need to consider storage and privacy issues. Any image is better than none. Clinical photographs should be labeled, dated, and filed in the medical records. Consent should be obtained from parents.
2. Use of a blue background allows better definition of findings. Sterile towels or drapes can be used for this purpose.
3. Separate or duplicate copies of photographs should be obtained for diagnostic and bereavement purposes. Most parents support postmortem bereavement photographs (19).
4. Anterior and posterior view of the whole body, anterior and lateral side views of the face from the right and left (**Table 27.2**) (12,20).

TABLE 27.2 Photographic Format

Whole body
Face: Flat and profile, right and left
Right and left ear
Right and left hand: Dorsum and palm
Right and left foot: Dorsum and sole
Palate
Genitalia
Special view of any other abnormality

5. Every effort should be made to photograph any abnormalities seen on physical examination.

F. Examination of the Placenta

1. Ensure that the placenta is sent for pathology examination for all infants admitted to the neonatal intensive care unit. Examination of the placenta provides critical information in investigating neonatal deaths especially in cases of pregnancy-induced hypertension, placental dysfunction, and growth retardation (21,22).
2. Placental findings are positive in 30% to 60% of neonatal autopsies (23,24).

3. Evaluation of the placenta may reveal maternal or fetal vascular problems, in utero infections, inflammatory conditions, and some inborn errors of metabolism. Cultures for bacteria and fungus as well as viral polymerase chain reactions may be sent as applicable. A discussion with pathology can guide the evaluation (16). If congenital infection is suspected, maternal and infant serology, blood tests, antibody screen, and additional cultures are recommended.

G. Perimortem Sampling

1. General guidelines
   a. Sterile technique should be used for all procedures, even if they are performed postmortem. Contact the laboratory to discuss the tests being sent and volume of blood needed, to obtain appropriate containers and tubes, and to alert them to save any unused blood, fluid, or tissue samples (**Table 27.3** summarizes sample handling) (2,5,11,22).
   b. If a metabolic disorder is a possibility, tissue samples should be taken within 4 to 6 hours of death.
   c. Resources to guide molecular testing as indicated can be found at http://www.ncbi.nlm.nih.gov/sites/GeneTests/clinic (25), a voluntary listing of US and international genetics clinics providing genetic evaluation and genetic counseling.
   d. Remember to label all tubes and samples with patient name and date of birth.
2. Blood
   a. Draw percutaneously or directly from heart (after parental consent) if infant has expired. See **Table 27.3** for samples required (2,9).
   b. Be sure newborn screen sample has been sent (26). The number of conditions tested for varies from state to state. Remember to record which diseases are tested for in your state.
   c. Obtain additional dried blood spots on filter paper.
   d. If the family consents to DNA banking, obtain additional blood for this purpose.
   e. When ordering whole exome sequencing, include mitochondrial DNA testing. Most labs will require blood from the infant and both parents for analysis. Consultation with a geneticist can be helpful in determining the need for this type of test (6).
   f. Various labs will have a minimum amount of blood that they are able to process. Usually that amount is 1 to 2 mL. In **Table 27.3**, the ideal amount is listed but keep in mind if one is unable to obtain that amount, even less may be useful. Consult with the laboratory if necessary.
3. Urine
   a. 5 to 10 mL by catheterization or suprapubic tap (13).

4. Cerebrospinal fluid
   a. Obtain at least 1 mL of cerebrospinal fluid; may be obtained after death by needle insertion through anterior fontanelle. The sample must be free of RBC (22,27).
5. Skin sample
   a. Best collected within 4 to 12 hours of death. Skin biopsy up to 2 to 3 days postmortem may still provide a viable culture.
   b. Normal skin samples may be sent for fibroblast culture (28).
   c. Any skin lesions should also be biopsied.
   d. 3- × 3-mm punch or scalpel biopsies can be taken from forearm or anterior thigh (see Chapter 25) (29).
   e. Do not use iodine-containing preparations, since cell growth may be impaired.
   f. Place in viral transport media. If unavailable, may use normal saline or saline-soaked gauze.
   g. Samples may be kept at room temperature or refrigerated.
   h. Cells can be cultured and archived in liquid nitrogen for many years and still be successfully recovered for analysis.
6. Liver
   a. Obtain if hepatic disease was present or for suspected metabolic disease (30,31).
   b. Collect as soon as possible after death, preferably within 2 to 4 hours.
   c. Tissue may be obtained via open wedge biopsy or percutaneous needle biopsy.
      (1) Wedge biopsy: Locate the right costal margin (**Fig. 27.1**). Make a 2-cm incision just below and incise section of right lobe of liver. The sample should be cut into 5-mm cubes.

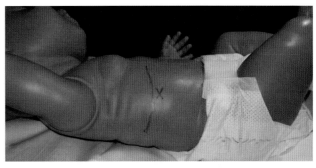

FIGURE 27.1 Landmark at the right costal margin for wedge biopsy.

      (2) Percutaneous biopsy (32). Several needles are available (16 or 18 gauge):
         (a) Aspiration or suction needles (Jamshidi, Klatskin, and Menghini)
         (b) Cutting-type needles (Tru-Cut and Vim-Silverman)
         (c) Spring-loaded devices

TABLE 27.3 Processing of Fluid and Tissue Samples Obtained by Perimortem Sampling

TISSUE TYPE	TESTING	SAMPLE COLLECTION AND HANDLING	STORAGE
Blood	Inborn errors of metabolism	Dried spots on filter paper/Newborn screen paper 2–3 cards for a total of 6–9 blood spots	Room temperature No plastic bag
	DNA extraction	5 mL in EDTA tube	Refrigerate at 4°C Do not freeze Can be stored for 48 hrs
	Chromosome analysis Microarray analysis	5 mL in sodium heparin tube	Keep cool or at room temperature Do not freeze
	Quantitative amino acids Fatty acids Carnitine Acylcarnitine profile	5 mL in sodium heparin tube, separate plasma within 20 min 1-mL red top for free fatty acids	Freeze and store at −80°C
	Whole exome sequencing with mitochondrial testing	2–5 mL in EDTA tube. If able send 2–5 mL parental blood as well	Keep cool or at room temperature
	DNA banking	5–10 mL in EDTA tube or ACD (yellow top) tube	
	Blood cultures	5–10 mL split between the aerobic and anaerobic blood culture tubes (minimum 1 mL per tube)	Keep at room temperature
Urine	Organic acids Amino acids Orotic acid Acylglycines	5–10 mL (minimum of 2 mL)	Freeze and store at −80°C
	Urine culture	Sterile container (at least 3 mL)	
CSF	Amino acids	1 mL in a sterile container Free of RBCs	Freeze and store at −80°C
	CSF for Gram stain, cell count, protein, glucose and aerobic culture	Sterile container (multiple if the volume allows)	Keep at room temperature
Skin	Fibroblast culture ■ Chromosome analysis ■ Genetic mutations ■ Enzyme analysis	Viral transport media The laboratory may have other options for sterile mediums enriched with antibiotics	Keep cool or at room temperature Do not freeze
Liver (3 pieces)	Histopathology Enzymology Electron microscopy	5-mm cube each sample, wrap each sample in foil and place into sterile container	Freeze and store at −80°C
Muscle (3 pieces)	Light microscopy	Wrap in moist saline-soaked gauze; do not immerse in saline	Keep cool (4°C) but do not freeze
	Enzyme analysis	Store in available container	Snap freeze in liquid nitrogen and store at −80°C
	Electron microscopy	Place in container with formalin or glutaraldehyde	Room temperature
Other as needed by infant's clinical presentation		Consult geneticist or pathologist	As instructed

EDTA, ethylenediaminetetraacetic acid.

d. Procedure
   (1) Make a small (0.25- to 0.5-cm) incision in the right anterior to midaxillary line at the 9th or 10th rib. See **Figure 27.2**.

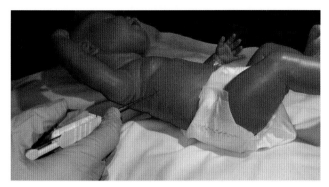

FIGURE 27.2 Percutaneous biopsy insertion site in the right anterior to midaxillary line at the 9th or 10th rib.

   (2) Flush the needle with saline.
   (3) Insert the needle parallel to the bed surface and advance toward the opposite shoulder.
   (4) Advance the needle 2 to 3 cm into the liver and apply suction, pulling a segment of liver into the needle. Spring-loaded needles do not need suction applied.
7. Muscle
   a. Collect if mitochondrial disorder or muscular dystrophy suspected (30,33). Surgeon or neurologist may be more adept at obtaining sample.
   b. Collect within 2 to 3 hours of death.
   c. Procedure
      (1) Make a 2- to 3-cm incision over mid-quadriceps.
      (2) Muscle clamps are not required but may be used for ease of sample removal.
      (3) Excise three 2- × 0.5-cm sections of muscle if possible.
      (4) Process the samples as indicated in **Table 27.3**.
      (5) If incisional biopsy is not possible, three cores of quadriceps muscle should be obtained using a percutaneous biopsy needle.
8. Other tissues may be sampled if specific related diagnoses are being considered. Some metabolic specialists have suggested collecting vitreous fluid for organic acids and bile for acylcarnitines. Conversation with a genetic or metabolic expert may guide collection of these fluids (11,13,31).

H. Imaging: May Be Used Alone or in Conjunction With Autopsy

1. X-rays
   a. Important, especially in diagnosing skeletal dysplasia. Placement of a radiopaque ruler adjacent to the body or extremities is helpful in measuring femur and humerus lengths (16).
   b. Include an anteroposterior and lateral view of skull, whole spine, long bones, pelvis, and images of hands and feet (34).
2. MRI
   a. Images of the neonatal brain are very useful and may provide information that is missed on autopsy in some cases (10,34).

I. Autopsy

1. Full autopsy (preferred)
   a. Provides the most complete picture of the infant and has been found to contribute useful information in 40% to 60% cases (3,34,35).
   b. Complete inspection of the neonatal brain requires 2 weeks' fixation prior to examination. This may mean that the burial is postponed or that the infant's body is buried without the brain.
2. Limited examination: If parents are reluctant to consent to a full autopsy, several choices exist.
   a. Full autopsy except examination of brain: This allows the brain to be buried with the body. Postmortem imaging of the brain with MRI may provide useful information on this organ.
   b. Limited autopsy: Examination is limited to certain organs or areas of the body. This can also be coupled with imaging for some families.
   c. Imaging only (MRI and/or x-rays): A wide range of sensitivities and specificities have been reported. Initial reports were promising with 90% to 100% sensitivity and specificity in diagnosis with whole body MRI. Recent studies have shown lower rates of concordance between MRI and autopsy of 30% to 60% (10,36).
   d. Peri- or postmortem sampling of body tissues and fluids only or in combination with any of the above (37).
3. Consult with pathologist before obtaining consent for limited autopsy so that examination is best directed at questions to be answered.

J. Postmortem Family Conference

1. After results are available from perimortem sampling evaluation and reports generated from autopsy and radiologic testing, a conference should be scheduled with the family.
2. The conference has many purposes (11,38):
   a. To give an overview of findings.
   b. Explain ramifications for future pregnancies and generations.

c. Allay feelings of guilt parents may have regarding the cause of death.

d. Answer questions regarding decisions made by the medical team.

e. Confirm or dispel allegations of abuse or neglect.

f. Provide emotional support to families.

3. The conference should be led by an experienced physician with great sensitivity and communication skills. He or she should be familiar with the case and have a complete understanding of case results and their implications. Nurses, therapists, social workers, and other physicians who are important to the infant's care team may also be present.

4. The meeting should be unhurried, with adequate time available for all the family's questions to be answered.

5. A written report summarizing the results of the meeting and written in language understandable to the family should be provided. A copy of the report should be sent to the family's primary care physician after obtaining appropriate consent from the family.

6. Bereavement photographs of the infant can be given at this time or at an earlier time if possible.

References

1. Nijkamp JW, Sebire NJ, Bouman K, et al. Perinatal death investigations: What is current practice? *Semin Fetal Neonatal Med.* 2017;22:167–175.

2. Christodoulou J, Wilcken B. Perimortem laboratory investigation of genetic metabolic disorders. *Semin Neonatol.* 2004;9:275–280.

3. Weber M, Ashworth M, Risdon RA. Sudden unexpected neonatal death in the first week of life: autopsy findings from a specialist center. *J Matern Fetal Neonatal Med.* 2009;22:398–404.

4. Basu MN, Johnsen IBG, Wehberg S, et al. Causes of death among full term stillbirths and early neonatal deaths in the region of Southern Denmark. *J Perinat Med.* 2018;46(2):197–202.

5. Champion MP. An approach to the diagnosis of inherited metabolic disease. *Arch Dis Child Educ Pract Ed.* 2010;95:40–46.

6. Yang Y, Muzny DM, Reid JG, et al. Clinical whole-exome sequencing for the diagnosis of mendelian disorders. *N Engl J Med.* 2013;369:1502–1511.

7. Godard B, Schmidtke J, Cassiman JJ, et al. Data storage and DNA banking for biomedical research. *Eur J Hum Genet.* 2003;(11)(Supp 2):S88–S122.

8. Laing I. Clinical aspects of neonatal death and autopsy. *Semin Neonatol.* 2004;9:247–254.

9. Jones F, Thibon P, Jeanne-Pasquier C, et al. Changes in fetal autopsy patterns over a 10-year period. *Arch Dis Child Fetal Neonatal Ed.* 2016;101:F481–F482.

10. Thayyil S. Less invasive autopsy: an evidenced based approach. *Arch Dis Child.* 2011;96:681–687.

11. Ernst L, Sondheimer N, Deardorff M, et al. The value of the metabolic autopsy in the pediatric hospital setting. *J Pediatr.* 2006;148:779–783.

12. Cernach MC, Patricio FR, Galera MF, et al. Evaluation of a protocol for postmortem examination of stillbirths and neonatal deaths with congenital anomalies. *Pediatr Dev Pathol.* 2004;7:335–341.

13. Olpin S. The metabolic investigation of sudden infant death. *Ann Clin Biochem.* 2004;41:282–293.

14. Chace D, Kalas T, Naylor E. Use of tandem mass spectrometry for multianalyte screening of dried blood specimens from newborns. *Clin Chem.* 2003;49:1797–1817.

15. Enns G. Inborn errors of metabolism masquerading as hypoxic-ischemic encephalopathy. *Neoreviews.* 2005;6:e549–e558.

16. Pinar H, Koch MA, Hawkins H, et al. The stillbirth collaborative research network postmortem examination protocol. *Am J Perinatol.* 2012;29(3):187–202.

17. The Wisconsin Stillbirth Service. http://www2.marshfieldclinic.org/wissp. Accessed October 16, 2016.

18. The Perinatal Society of Australia and New Zealand. https://www.psanz.com.au/. Accessed October 16, 2016.

19. Blood C, Cacciatore J. Best practice in bereavement photography after prenatal death: qualitative analysis with 104 parents. *BMC Psychol.* 2014;2(1):15.

20. Pitt DB, Bankier A, Skoroplas T, et al. The role of photography in syndrome identification. *J Clin Dysmorphol.* 1984;2:2.

21. Roberts DJ, Oliva E. Clinical significance of placental examination in perinatal medicine. *J Matern Fetal Neonatal Med.* 2006;19:255–264.

22. Frearson-Smith J, Dorling J. Guidelines for the collection of peri and post-mortem tissue samples on the neonatal unit. *Nottingham Neonatal Service-Clinical Guidelines.* Version 3. August 2015.

23. Wainwright HC. My approach to performing a perinatal or neonatal autopsy. *J Clin Pathol.* 2006;59:673–680.

24. Tellefsen CH, Vogt C. How important is placental examination in cases of perinatal deaths? *Pediatr Dev Pathol.* 2011;14:99–104.

25. The Genetic Testing Registry (GTR®). http://www.ncbi.nlm.nih.gov/sites/GeneTests/clinic. Accessed October 16, 2017.

26. Kayton A. Newborn screening: a literature review. *Neonatal Netw.* 2007;26:85–95.

27. Hoffmann GF, Surtees RAH, Wevers RA. Cerebrospinal fluid investigations for neurometabolic disorders. *Neuropediatrics.* 1998;29:59–71.

28. Lundemose JB, Kolvraa S, Gregerson N, et al. Fatty acid oxidation disorders as primary cause of sudden and unexpected death in infants and young children: an investigation performed on cultured fibroblasts from 79 children who died aged between 0–4 years. *J Clin Pathol: Mol Pathol.* 1997;50:212.

29. Alguire PC, Mathes BM. Skin biopsy techniques for the internist. *J Gen Intern Med.* 1998;13:46–54.

30. Wong LC, Scaglia F, Graham BH, et al. Current molecular diagnostic algorithm for mitochondrial disorders. *Mol Genet Metab.* 2010;100:111–117.

31. Rinaldo P, Yoon HR, Yu C, et al. Sudden and unexpected neonatal death: A protocol for the postmortem diagnosis of fatty acid oxidation disorders. *Semin Perinatol.* 1999;23:204–210.

32. Al Knawy B, Shiffman M. Percutaneous liver biopsy in clinical practice. *Liver Int.* 2007;27:1166–1173.

33. Kawashima H, Ishii C, Yamanaka G, et al. Myopathy and neurogenic muscular atrophy in unexpected cardiopulmonary arrest. *Pediatr Int.* 2011;53:159–161.

34. Pinar H. Postmortem findings in term neonates. *Semin Neonatol.* 2004;9:289–302.

35. Costa S, Rodrigues M, Centeno MJ. Diagnosis and cause of death in a neonatal intensive care unit—How important is autopsy? *J Matern Fetal Neonatal Med.* 2011;24:760–763.

36. Huisman T. Magnetic resonance imaging: An alternative to autopsy in neonatal death? *Semin Neonatol.* 2004;9: 347–353.

37. Putman MA. Perinatal, perimortem and postmortem examination, obligations and considerations for perinatal, neonatal and pediatric clinicians. *Adv Neonatal Care.* 2007;7:281–288.

38. McHaffie HE. Follow up care of bereaved parents after treatment withdrawal from newborns. *Arch Dis Child Fetal Neonat Ed.* 2001;84:F125–F128.

28

Abdominal Paracentesis

Kathryn M. Maselli, Megan E. Beck, Bavana Ketha, Anne S. Roberts, and A. Alfred Chahine

A. Definition

Paracentesis is the percutaneous drainage of ascites from the peritoneal cavity.

B. Indications

1. Therapeutic—to reduce intra-abdominal pressure in patients with massive ascites causing cardiorespiratory compromise.
2. Diagnostic—to aid in determining the etiology of neonatal ascites and/or peritonitis.
   a. Necrotizing enterocolitis with suspicion of gangrene or perforation: presence of fecal matter or bacteria and white blood cells on a smear (1–3)
   b. Hepatic ascites: comparison of serum and ascitic albumin levels, cell count, and culture in diagnosis of spontaneous bacterial peritonitis (4,5)
   c. Chylous ascites: testing for triglycerides, cholesterol, and lymphocytes on cell count of the fluid (3,6)
   d. Urinary ascites: test for creatinine content (7)
   e. Meconium peritonitis: gross appearance of ascites (8)
   f. Biliary ascites: test for bilirubin level (9)
   g. Pancreatic ascites: test for amylase, lipase levels (5,10)
   h. Congenital infections—cytomegalovirus (CMV), tuberculosis, toxoplasmosis, syphilis: test for inclusion bodies, treponemes (5,11)
   i. Inborn errors of metabolism—sialic acid storage disorders: test for vacuolated lymphocytes and free sialic acid (12)
   j. Iatrogenic ascites from extravasation of fluid from central venous catheters: test for glucose content

C. Contraindications

Coagulopathy is a relative contraindication; the procedure may be performed with concomitant treatment of thrombocytopenia or coagulopathy, though controversy exists over whether administration of blood products is necessary (4,13).

D. Equipment

1. 24- or 25-gauge catheter over a needle (e.g., Angiocath)
2. 5- or 10-mL syringe
3. Skin topical disinfectant (e.g., povidone-iodine, chlorhexidine)
4. Sterile towels
5. Sterile gloves
6. Extension tubing
7. 3-way stopcock
8. Collection tubes and specimen containers for fluid analysis
   a. Cell count and differential, culture, Gram stain, acid-fast bacillus smear, cytology, total protein, albumin, glucose, lactate dehydrogenase, amylase, bilirubin, creatinine, blood urea nitrogen, electrolytes, specific gravity, pH, cholesterol, triglycerides
9. Tuberculin syringe
10. Lidocaine (1%)
11. Dressing supplies

E. Technique (▶Video 28.1: Abdominal Paracentesis)

1. Obtain appropriate informed consent and time-out prior to procedure (Chapter 3). Patient should be on cardiorespiratory monitor and have appropriate temperature support (Chapter 4).
2. Place a soft support ("bump") under the supine neonate's left flank, to allow as much of the fluid to drain into a dependent position and allow the intestines to float away from the right lower quadrant (**Fig. 28.1**).

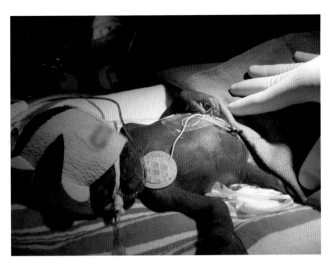

FIGURE 28.1 Appropriate position and disinfection of abdomen prior to performing paracentesis in preterm neonate.

3. Prepare the right lower quadrant with the disinfecting solution and drape with sterile towels.
4. Select a point between the umbilicus and the anterior superior iliac spine one-third of the way from the anterior superior iliac spine. Avoid the midline to minimize risk to the bladder and a patent umbilical vessel and avoid previous surgical scars to minimize risk of bowel injury. If not visible, transillumination of the abdominal wall will reveal the inferior epigastric vessels, which are to be avoided. An infraumbilical position avoids the liver and spleen.
5. Infiltrate the skin, muscles, and peritoneum with local anesthetic using the tuberculin syringe.
6. Connect the 10-mL syringe to the 24-gauge catheter and needle.
7. Direct the catheter toward the back at a 45-degree angle (**Fig. 28.2**). The nondominant hand may be used to

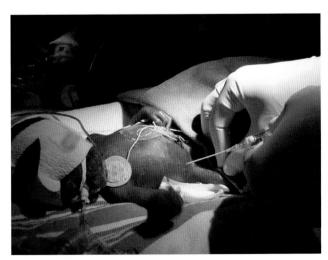

FIGURE 28.2 Entry site and direction of needle for abdominal paracentesis in preterm neonate.

retract the skin in a downward direction while advancing the needle to create a Z-track after removal of the needle and catheter.
8. Push the catheter and needle through the skin, muscles, and peritoneal surface while applying gentle suction on the syringe plunger.
9. When a sudden decrease in resistance is felt and peritoneal fluid is aspirated, advance the catheter further and withdraw the needle.
10. Connect an extension tube with a 3-way stopcock to the syringe and apply gentle, intermittent suction to aspirate as much fluid as possible.
11. If fluid is not free flowing, the catheter might be inside the intestinal lumen or in the retroperitoneum. Withdraw the catheter and repeat the maneuver with the catheter at a slightly different angle. Alternatively, reposition the patient carefully to maintain the catheter site in the dependent position to continue fluid aspiration.
12. When the fluid stops flowing, withdraw the catheter.
13. Distribute the fluid into the various tubes and cups for the appropriate studies.
14. Apply a bandage, holding pressure until leaking has stopped.

F. Complications

1. **Bleeding from the liver or intra-abdominal vessels:** may be severe enough to require a laparotomy.
2. **Intestinal perforation:** may lead to abdominal sepsis; however, it is more commonly inconsequential because the catheter and needle are of small diameter. Risk may be reduced with nasogastric or rectal tube decompression if intestinal distention is significant prior to the procedure.
3. **Hypotension:** may be due to sudden large fluid shifts during therapeutic paracentesis. Patients should be placed on a monitor during the procedure, and fluid withdrawn slowly. Large-volume paracentesis may require judicious administration of fluids to offset fluid shifts.
4. **Hematoma:** take care to avoid the inferior epigastric vessels, which can be transilluminated.
5. **Scrotal or labial edema:** due to tracking of fluid between layers of the abdominal wall.
6. **Persistent ascitic fluid leak:** may be prevented with Z-track technique, may require suture closure or bag drainage to prevent skin maceration.

References

1. Lee JS, Polin RA. Treatment and prevention of necrotizing enterocolitis. *Semin Neonatol.* 2003;8(6):449–459.
2. Rees CM, Eaton S, Pierro A. National prospective surveillance study of necrotizing enterocolitis in neonatal intensive care units. *J Pediatr Surg.* 2010;45:1391–1397.

3. Sabri M, Saps M, Peters JM. Pathophysiology and management of pediatric ascites. *Curr Gastroenterol Rep*. 2003;5:240–246.

4. Vieira SMG, Matte U, Kieling CO, et al. Infected and noninfected ascites in pediatric patients. *J Pediatr Gastroentrol Nutr*. 2005;40(3):289–294.

5. Aslam M, DeGrazia M, Gregory ML. Diagnostic evaluation of neonatal ascites. *Am J Perinatol*. 2007;24(10):603–609.

6. Herman TE, Siegel MJ. Congenital chylous ascites. *J Perinatol*. 2009;29(2):178–180.

7. Oei J, Garvey PA, Rosenberg AR. The diagnosis and management of neonatal urinary ascites. *J Paediatr Child Health*. 2001;37(5):513–515.

8. Shyu MK, Shih JC, Lee CN, et al. Correlation of prenatal ultrasound and postnatal outcome in meconium peritonitis. *Fetal Diagn Ther*. 2003;18(4):255–261.

9. Xanthakos SA, Yazigi NA, Ryckman FC, et al. Spontaneous perforation of the bile duct in infancy: A rare cause of irritability and abdominal distention. *J Pediatr Gastroenterol Nutr*. 2003;36(2):287–291.

10. Saps M, Slivka A, Khan S, et al. Pancreatic ascites in an infant: Lack of symptoms and normal amylase. *Dig Dis Sci*. 2003;48(9):1701–1704.

11. Nicol KK, Geisinger KR. Congenital toxoplasmosis: Diagnosis by exfoliative cytology. *Diagn Cytopathol*. 1998;18:357–361.

12. Lemyre E, Russo P, Melancon SB, et al. Clinical spectrum of infantile free sialic acid storage disease. *Am J Med Genet*. 1999;82:385–391.

13. Grabau CM, Crago SF, Hoff LK, et al. Performance standards for therapeutic abdominal paracentesis. *Hepatology*. 2004;40:484–488.

Vascular Access

CHAPTER

29

Peripheral Intravenous Line Placement

Ha-young Choi

A. Indication

1. Administration of intravenous (IV) medications, fluids, or parenteral nutrition when utilization of the gastrointestinal tract is not possible.

B. Equipment

Since the late 1960s, the variety of equipment available for peripheral vascular access has grown from metallic needles of limited size range and stiff polyethylene tubes to an array of plastic cannulas, single- and multilumen catheters of different sizes and materials, and totally implantable devices (ports). The safest and more effective vascular access is obtained by carefully matching the neonate's size, therapeutic needs, and the duration of required treatment with the most appropriate device and technique. Placement of peripheral IV lines is described in this chapter. Placement of central venous lines is described in Chapter 34.

Sterile Equipment (Fig. 29.1)

1. Povidone-iodine or other antiseptic swabs (see Chapter 6)
2. Appropriate needle (minimum 24 gauge for blood transfusion)
   a. 21- to 26-gauge IV catheter (preferably shielded for patient and operator safety)
3. Connection for cannula (i.e., T connector)
4. 2- × 2-in gauze squares
5. Isotonic saline in 2- or 3-mL syringe
6. Heparinized flush solution (heparin 0.5 to 1 U/mL normal saline) for heparin lock (optional); the use of heparinized saline to prolong patency of IV catheters remains controversial (1,2).

Nonsterile Clean Equipment

1. Tourniquet
2. Procedure light or transilluminator (3)
3. Materials for restraint (see Chapter 5)
4. Warm compress to warm limb, if necessary (infant heel warmer) (4)
5. Appropriate-sized armboard, if necessary
6. Cotton balls or other soft positioners to support IV catheter, if necessary
7. Scissors
8. Roll of 0.5- to 1-in porous adhesive tape, transparent tape, or semipermeable transparent dressings
   a. If using tape, use the minimum amount necessary on fragile premature skin, and consider using a pectin barrier (e.g., DuoDERM, ConvaTec/Bristol-Myers Squibb, Princeton, New Jersey; HolliHesive, Hollister, Libertyville, Illinois).
   b. Transparent tape or dressing will facilitate observation of IV site and semipermeable dressings allow

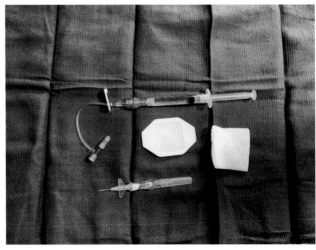

FIGURE 29.1 Sterile equipment necessary for peripheral IV line placement.

small amounts of fluid, such as sweat, under the dressing to evaporate to keep the area dry (e.g., Tegaderm, 3M Health Care, St. Paul, Minnesota).

   c. Precut self-adhesive taping devices are available (e.g., Veni-Gard Jr.—ConMed IV Site Care Products, Utica, New York).

9. Restraints and pain control, as appropriate for clinical situation

   a. Pacifier. Sucking releases endorphins, which decrease pain (5,6).

   b. Consider swaddling the baby, leaving the limb needed for IV placement exposed. In addition to serving to restrain the infant, swaddling is also a comfort measure (see Chapter 5).

   c. Oral sucrose is frequently used as a nonpharmacologic intervention for procedural pain relief in neonates (7,8).

   d. Some critically ill infants, such as those with persistent pulmonary hypertension, may require additional pain medication or sedatives, to prevent agitation and desaturation during painful procedures.

   e. Topical lidocaine cream preparations must be applied well before the start of the procedure, usually 30 to 60 minutes; follow manufacturer recommendations. Be sure to follow dosing recommendations, as it can be absorbed transcutaneously and cause methemoglobinemia (9).

C. Precautions

1. Avoid areas adjacent to superficial skin loss or infection.
2. Avoid vessels across joints, because immobilization is more difficult.
3. Take care to differentiate veins from arteries.

   a. Palpate for arterial pulsation.

   b. Note effect of vessel occlusion.

     (1) Limb vessel: Arteries collapse, veins fill

     (2) Scalp vessel: Arteries fill from below, veins fill from above

   c. Note color of blood obtained (arterial blood is bright red; venous blood is darker).

   d. Note pulsatility of flow once vessel is catheterized (arterial blood will have copious, pulsatile flow).

   e. Look for blanching of skin over vessel when fluid is infused (arterial spasm).

4. If limb requires warming prior to procedure, use an infant heel warmer (e.g., Fisherbrand Infant Heel Warmer, Prism Technologies, San Antonio, Texas; Heel Snuggler Infant Heel Warmer, Philips Children's Medical Ventures, Monroeville, Pennsylvania). "Homemade" compresses such as a diaper soaked in hot water can cause severe thermal injury or maceration. Heat levels appropriate for adults may cause severe burn injuries in the neonate (10).

5. Cut scalp hair using small scissors or trimmer to allow for stabilization of the IV. Do not shave the area, as this can cause abrasions in the skin (11).

6. Apply tourniquet prudently and correctly for quick release (see Fig. 16.3).

   a. Minimize time applied.

   b. Avoid use in areas with compromised circulation.

   c. Avoid use for scalp vessels.

7. When using scalp veins, avoid sites outside the hairline.

8. Be alert for signs of phlebitis or infiltration.

   a. Inspect site hourly.

   b. Discontinue IV immediately at any sign of local inflammation or cannula malfunction.

   c. Long plastic catheters are not recommended for use in neonates because their relative rigidity increases the risk of damage to the vascular endothelium, thus increasing the possibility of venous thrombosis.

   d. Arrange tape dressing at IV site to allow adequate inspection or use transparent sterile dressing over site of skin entry. Generally, no dressing change is required unless the dressing is unstable, soiled, or at time of catheter removal.

9. Consider using protective skin preparation in small premature infants to prevent skin trauma upon removal of tape or dressing. Cavilon No Sting Barrier Film, 3M Health Care, St. Paul, Minnesota is a non–alcohol-containing product that is available commercially; however, it, as well as other commercially available skin protectants, has not been tested on neonates.

   a. Forms a tough, protective coating that bonds to skin

   b. Does not require removal when changing dressing

10. The use of products to increase the adherence of tape should be limited, especially on the premature infant. These products create a tighter bond between the tape and the epidermis than the bond between the epidermis and the underlying dermis. This then causes stripping of the epidermis when the tape is removed.

11. Write date, time, and needle/cannula size on piece of tape secured to site.

12. Loop IV tubing and tape onto extremity to take tension off the IV device.

13. Limit to two to three placement attempts per person. Monitor carefully for clinical decompensation during placement, particularly in the very premature infant and in infants with cardiac or respiratory compromise.

14. If central venous access is anticipated, plan ahead so that veins are available for percutaneous central venous access. Ideally, the peripheral venous line should be placed in a different limb from the central line and the central line will likely require a large, straight vessel. See Chapter 34.

D. Technique

Prepare as for minor procedure (see Chapter 6). Ensure that neutral thermal environment is maintained and the infant is in an appropriate state for the procedure. If the infant has received a recent enteral feeding, consider delaying the procedure until before the next feeding.

1. Select vessel for cannulation.
   a. Use transillumination to visualize vessel, if needed (see Chapter 13). Other modalities such as ultrasonography or bedside near-infrared light devices may also be used for vein identification.
   b. Select straight segment of vein or confluence of two tributaries.
   c. It is recommended to begin with more distal sites and progress proximally, if needed. The following is the suggested order of preference (see **Fig. 29.1**):
      (1) Back of hand—dorsal venous plexus
      (2) Foot—dorsal venous plexus
      (3) Ankle—lesser saphenous, great saphenous veins
      (4) Forearm—median antebrachial, accessory cephalic veins
      (5) Antecubital fossa—basilic or cubital veins
      (6) Scalp veins—supratrochlear, superficial temporal, posterior auricular
2. Cut hair with small scissors close to scalp if using scalp vessels.
3. Warm limb with heel warmer for approximately 5 minutes, if necessary.

4. Apply tourniquet if anatomic site indicates.
   a. Place as close to venipuncture site as possible.
   b. Tighten until peripheral pulsation stops.
   c. Release partially until arterial pulse is fully palpable.
5. Prepare skin area with antiseptic. Allow to dry.

   In the United States, chlorhexidine, povidone-iodine solution, and isopropyl alcohol are the most commonly used skin disinfectant solutions. Chlorhexidine is often available in an alcohol-based preparation, which can cause damage to the immature skin of premature neonates (12). Povidone-iodine has been shown to have greater efficacy than isopropyl alcohol and, in addition, is less damaging to skin tissue. Povidone-iodine solution should be applied to the proposed insertion site and allowed to dry for at least 30 seconds. Excess povidone-iodine should be removed with sterile saline swab or sterile water, to prevent burns and absorption of iodine and hypothyroidism in premature infants caused by prolonged contact (13,14). See Chapter 6 for further details on antiseptics.
6. Grasp catheter between thumb and first finger. For winged Angiocaths, grasp the plastic wings (**Fig. 29.2A**).
7. Anchor vein with index finger of free hand and stretch skin overlying it. This maneuver may also be used to produce distention of scalp veins (**Fig. 29.2A**).
8. Hold needle parallel to vessel, in direction of blood flow (**Fig. 29.2A**).
9. Introduce needle through skin a few millimeters distal to point of entry into vessel (see Chapter 16) (**Fig. 29.2B**).

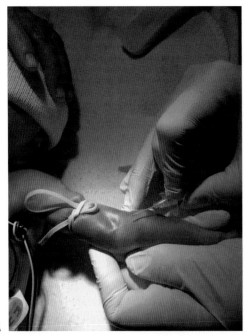
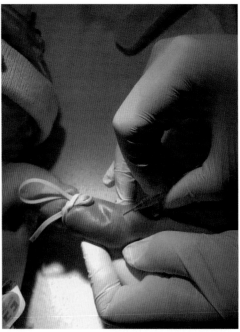

A   **B**

FIGURE 29.2 A: IV needle held in dominant hand, while index finger and thumb of nondominant hand are used to anchor vein and stretch overlying skin. Needle is parallel to vessel, with skin introduction point a few millimeters distal to point of entry of vessel. **B:** Needle is advanced until there is a "flash" of blood visible in the cannula. (*continued*)

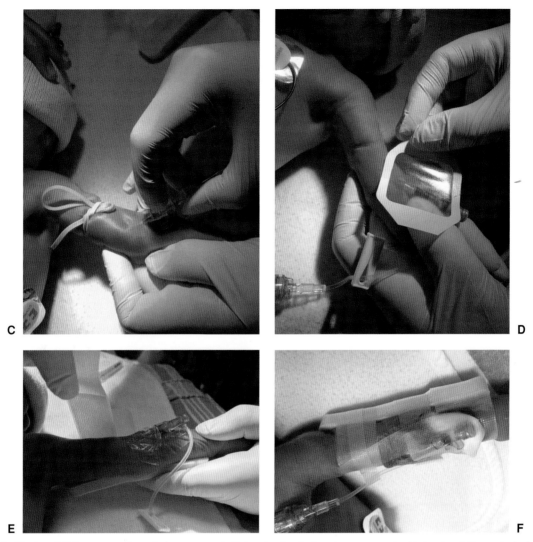

FIGURE 29.2 (*Continued*) **C:** Remove needle and advance cannula. **D:** Attach saline flush and secure cannula with dressing. **E:** If cannula site is over a major joint, consider immobilization of joint, such as with armboard. **F:** A cotton bud may be used to support the hub of the T connector to prevent pressure injury.

10. Introduce needle gently into vessel until blood appears in hub of needle or in cannula upon withdrawal of stylet (**Fig. 29.2B**). When using a very small vessel or in an infant with poor peripheral circulation, blood may not appear immediately in tubing. Wait. If in doubt, inject a small amount of saline after releasing tourniquet.
11. Remove stylet. Do not advance needle farther, because the back wall of the vessel may be pierced.
12. Advance cannula as far as possible (**Fig. 29.2C**). Injecting a small amount of blood or flush solution into the vein prior to advancing the cannula may assist cannulation.
13. Remove tourniquet.
14. Connect T connecter and syringe, and infuse small amount of saline gently to confirm intravascular position (**Fig. 29.2D**).
15. Anchor cannula (**Fig. 29.3**).

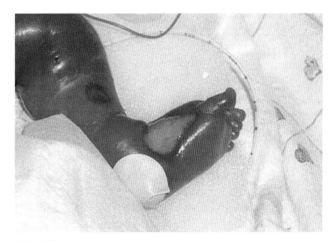

FIGURE 29.3 Result of infusion of lidocaine into subcutaneous tissues of lower limb.

16. Attach IV tubing and secure to skin.
17. If an armboard is necessary for securing site, place the affected extremity in an anatomically correct position before taping. Consider placing cotton or a 2- × 2-in gauze square beneath the hub of T connector to prevent a pressure injury (**Fig. 29.2E,F**).

CONVERSION OF PERIPHERAL IV LINE TO A SALINE LOCK

Technique

1. Wash hands and put on gloves.
2. Clean IV tubing and catheter connection with antiseptic solution.
3. Stop IV infusion and remove IV tubing from hub of IV needle or cannula.
4. Seal hub with a sterile plug or T-connector system (e.g., Argyle intermittent infusion plug [Consolidated Medical Equipment, Utica, New York; Sherwood Medical Co., St. Louis, Missouri] or spin-lock port extension set [B. Braun Medical Inc., Bethlehem, PA] that has been primed with the required quantity of saline). As an improvisation, a stopcock with two dead heads may be used. However, at least 3 mL of flush solution is necessary to flush all parts of a stopcock. This increases the margin for error, with possible fluid overload in very small premature infants.
5. Clean plug with antiseptic, and inject 0.4 to 0.8 mL of saline solution through plug to flush blood from needle or cannula.
6. Clean plug with antiseptic prior to every use.
7. Refill lock with flush solution after every IV infusion. (Flush routinely every 6 to 12 hours, depending on frequency of use.)

Complications

1. Hematoma: The most common but not usually significant complication. Hematomas can often be managed with gentle manual pressure.
2. Phlebitis is the most common significant complication associated with the use of peripheral venous catheters. When phlebitis does occur, the risk of local catheter–related infection may be increased (15). The catheter material, catheter size, and tonicity of the infusate also influence the incidence of phlebitis. When peripheral lines are used for parenteral nutrition, the co-infusion of a lipid solution with the hyperosmolar total parenteral nutrition solution prolongs the life of the vein (16,17).

3. Infiltration of subcutaneous tissue with IV solution. (For management of this complication, see Chapter 30.) Unfortunately, this is a common complication of peripheral IV infusion. Extreme vigilance and avoidance of hyperosmolar IV solutions will help to reduce the incidence to the minimum possible. Consequences of IV extravasation can include:
   a. Superficial blistering (**Fig. 29.3**).
   b. Deep slough, which may require skin graft (**Fig. 29.4**).
   c. Calcification of subcutaneous tissue due to infiltration of calcium-containing solution.

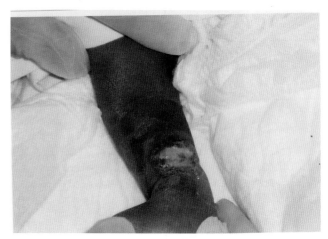

FIGURE 29.4 Extensive deep skin slough that required grafting, caused by IV infiltration.

4. Infection: There is an increase in the incidence of both phlebitis and infection when a catheter remains in place longer than 72 hours and is frequently manipulated. Manipulations of old catheters can lead to seeding of bacteria along a colonized catheter, so dressings should be changed only when visibly soiled (18). Frequent replacements of catheters have not been shown to decrease infection in adults and considering the difficulty of placement of peripheral venous catheters in neonates and children, general recommendations are to continue use until the line is not necessary or unusable (19).
5. Embolization of clot with forcible flushing.
6. Hypernatremia, fluid overload, or heparinization of the infant due to improper flushing technique or solution; also electrolyte derangements from IV fluid infused at an incorrect rate.
7. Accidental injection or infusion into artery, with arteriospasm and possible tissue necrosis (**Fig. 29.5**).
8. Burn from:
   a. Transilluminator (Fig. 27.8; also see Chapter 15)
   b. Compress used to warm limb prior to procedure
   c. Prolonged povidone-iodine, isopropyl alcohol, or chlorhexidine application to very premature skin
9. Air embolus.

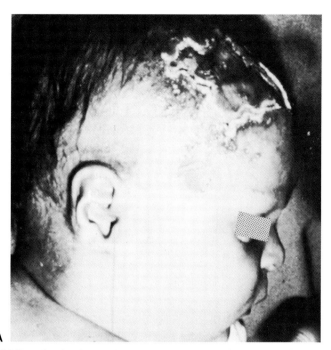 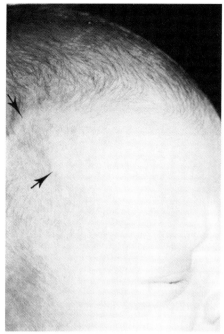

FIGURE 29.5 A: Skin slough on scalp caused by inadvertent infusion into the frontal branch of the temporal artery. **B:** This is indicated by *arrows*.

References

1. Shah PS, Ng E, Sinha AK. Heparin for prolonging peripheral intravenous catheter use in neonates. *Cochrane Database Syst Rev.* 2005;(4):CD002774.

2. Upadhyay A, Verma KK, Lal P, et al. Heparin for prolonging peripheral intravenous catheter use in neonates: A randomized controlled trial. *J Perinatol.* 2015;35(4):274–277.

3. Peterson KA, Phillips AL, Truemper E, et al. Does the use of an assistive device by nurses impact peripheral intravenous catheter insertion success in children? *J Pediatr Nurs.* 2012;27(2):134–143.

4. Biyik Bayram S, Caliskan N. Effects of local heat application before intravenous catheter insertion in chemotherapy patients. *J Clin Nurs.* 2016;25(11-12):1740–1747.

5. Naughton KA. The combined use of sucrose and nonnutritive sucking for procedural pain in both term and preterm neonates: An integrative review of the literature. *Adv Neonatal Care.* 2013;13(1):9–19.

6. Pillai Riddell RR, Racine NM, Gennis HG, et al. Non-pharmacological management of infant and young child procedural pain. *Cochrane Database Syst Rev.* 2015;(12):CD006275.

7. Taddio A, Shah V, Stephens D, et al. Effect of liposomal lidocaine and sucrose alone and in combination for venipuncture pain in newborns. *Pediatrics.* 2011;127(4):e940–e947.

8. Stevens B, Yamada J, Ohlsson A, et al. Sucrose for analgesia in newborn infants undergoing painful procedures. *Cochrane Database Syst Rev.* 2016;7:CD001069.

9. Kuiper-Prins E, Kerkhof GF, Reijnen CG, et al. A 12-day-old boy with methemoglobinemia after circumcision with local anesthesia (Lidocaine/Prilocaine). *Drug Saf Case Rep.* 2016;3(1):12.

10. Abboud L, Ghanimeh G. Thermal burn in a 30-minute-old newborn: Report on the youngest patient with iatrogenic burn injury. *Ann Burns Fire Disasters.* 2017;30(1):62–64.

11. Tanner J, Norrie P, Melen K. Preoperative hair removal to reduce surgical site infection. *Cochrane Database Syst Rev.* 2011;(11):CD004122.

12. Neri I, Ravaioli GM, Faldella G, et al. Chlorhexidine-induced chemical burns in very low birth weight infants. *J Pediatr.* 2017;191:262–265.

13. Chiang YC, Lin TS, Yeh MC. Povidone-iodine-related burn under the tourniquet of a child—a case report and literature review. *J Plast Reconstr Aesthet Surg.* 2011;64(3):412–415.

14. Aitken J, Williams FL. A systematic review of thyroid dysfunction in preterm neonates exposed to topical iodine. *Arch Dis Child Fetal Neonatal Ed.* 2014;99(1):F21–F28.

15. Mermel LA. Short-term peripheral venous catheter-related bloodstream infections: A systematic review. *Clin Infect Dis.* 2017;65(10):1757–1762.

16. Pineault M, Chessex P, Pledboeuf B, et al. Beneficial effect of coinfusing a lipid emulsion on venous patency. *J Parenter Enter Nutr.* 1989;13:637–640.

17. Phelps SJ, Lochrane EB. Effect of the continuous administration of fat emulsion on the infiltration rate of intravenous lines in infants receiving peripheral parenteral nutrition solutions. *J Parenter Enter Nutr.* 1989;13:628–632.

18. Zhang L, Cao S, Marsh N, et al. Infection risks associated with peripheral vascular catheters. *J Infect Prev.* 2016;17(5):207–213.

19. O'Grady NP, Alexander M, Dellinger EP, et al. Guidelines for the prevention of intravascular catheter-related infections. *Clin Infect Dis.* 2002;35:1281–1307.

Management of Extravasation Injuries

Aimee Vaughn and Ha-Young Choi

Introduction

Extravasation or inadvertent infiltration of intravenous (IV) administered solutions into subcutaneous tissue is a common adverse event in intensive care nurseries and may result in partial or complete skin loss, infection, and nerve and tendon damage, with the potential risk of cosmetic and functional impairment. Rates of IV infiltration are quoted to be as high as 57% to 70% in the NICU, with 11% to 23% being true extravasation injuries, that is, those infiltrative injuries that cause tissue damage and ischemic injury leading to tissue necrosis (1). Parenteral alimentation fluids, calcium, potassium, and sodium bicarbonate solutions, vasopressor agents, and antibiotics such as nafcillin, are often implicated.

An extravasation injury is an emergency that requires prompt identification and proper treatment, as early identification and appropriate management are vital to optimizing outcome (2).

A. Assessment

1. Early signs of IV infiltration: Fussiness, crying, or withdrawal of the limb when flushing the IV cannula. However, these early signs may be absent in an infant who is sedated or critically ill.
2. Late signs of injury: Blistering and discoloration of skin often portend at least partial skin loss, but visible skin changes do not always indicate the severity of underlying injury, which may evolve over several days (see Fig. 29.4, **Fig. 30.1**).
3. Staging of extravasations is recommended for objective evaluation to determine the degree of intervention required. Several staging systems are in use (1,3,4). **Table 30.1** outlines one that is commonly used.
4. Detailed descriptions, marking the area, or digital photographs provide better documentation of the extent of the wound and the healing process (3).

B. Management

The degree of intervention is determined by the stage of extravasation, the nature of the infiltrating solution, and the availability of specific antidotes. There is no consensus on

TABLE 30.1 **Staging of Extravasation Injury**

STAGE	CHARACTERISTICS
1	Pain at site—crying when IV cannula is flushed
	IV cannula flushes with difficulty
	No redness or swelling
2	Pain
	Redness and slight swelling at site
	Brisk capillary refill
3	Pain
	Moderate swelling
	Blanching of area
	Skin cool to touch
	Brisk capillary refill below site
	Good pulse below site
4	Pain
	Severe swelling around site
	Blanching of area
	Skin cool to touch
	Area of skin necrosis or blistering
	Prolonged capillary refill time (>4 sec)
	Decreased or absent pulse

Adapted from Restieaux M, Maw A, Broadbent R, et al. Neonatal extravasation injury: Prevention and management in Australia and New Zealand—a survey of current practice. *BMC Pediatr.* 2013;13(1):34.

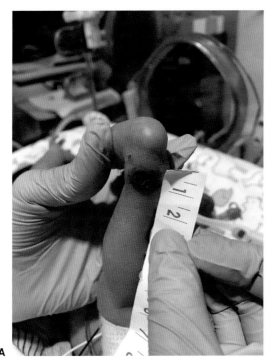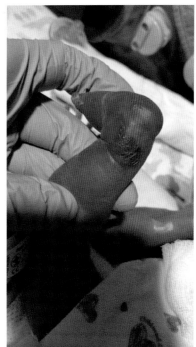

A   B

FIGURE 30.1 **A:** Stage IV extravasation injury with eschar formation. **B:** Same area 2 weeks later.

management of extravasation injuries. In the absence of randomized controlled trials, some institutions have established management protocols to guide therapy, based on local experience, case series, and anecdotal evidence (1–3,5,6).

1. In All Cases

a. Stop the IV infusion promptly.
b. Remove constricting bands that may act as tourniquets (e.g., armboard restraint).
c. Elevation of the limb may help to reduce edema (7).
d. The application of warm or cold packs is controversial and will depend on both the type of drug or fluid involved in the infiltration or extravasation as well as the unit preference (4). Warm packs may, by local vasodilation, help to reabsorb infiltrating solutions (1). However, warm moist packs may also cause maceration of the already compromised skin tissue.

2. Stage 1 or 2 Extravasation

a. Remove IV cannula, unless required for antidote.
b. Consider antidote (see Stage 3 or 4 Extravasation below).
c. Frequently assess site (6).

3. Stage 3 or 4 Extravasation

a. Leave the IV cannula in place and, using a 1-mL syringe, aspirate as much fluid as possible from the area (4,6). Usually, very little fluid can be aspirated.

b. Remove the cannula unless it is needed for administration of the antidote.

4. Antidotes and Treatments

a. Hyaluronidase (1,8,9)

Hyaluronidase is a dispersing agent, commonly used in extravasations involving calcium, parenteral alimentation fluids, antibiotics, sodium bicarbonate, etc. Although the FDA labeling states that hyaluronidase is not approved for treatment of vasopressor extravasation injury, there have been reports of successful treatment of such extravasations with a combination of hyaluronidase and saline irrigations, as described below.

1. *Mechanism of action:* Breakdown of hyaluronic acid, the ground substance or intercellular cement of tissues; minimizes tissue injury by enhancing dispersion and reabsorption of extravasated fluids.
2. *Formulations available:*
   a. *Animal derived:* Ovine-derived Vitrase (Alliance Medical Products, Irvine, California) or bovine-derived Amphadase (Amphastar Pharmaceuticals, Rancho Cucamonga, California). Amphadase contains small quantities of thimerosal, so it is not recommended in neonates.
   b. *Recombinant human hyaluronidase (rHuPH20) (Hylenex, Halozyme Therapeutics, San Diego, CA):* This product is reported to have up to 100 times greater enzymatic activity than the animal-derived

form, but there is little literature available on its effectiveness in extravasations.

3. *Timing*

Most effective within 1 hour; may be used for up to 12 hours after injury.

4. *Administration*

  a. Use a small needle, between 25 and 30 gauge, for administration.

  b. Protocols report use of concentrations from 15 to 150 units/mL. To dilute the drug, 0.1 mL of hyaluronidase (150 units/mL) can be mixed with 0.9 mL of normal saline to create hyaluronidase 15 units/mL.

  c. Total of 1 mL may be injected as five separate aliquots of 0.2 mL each, around the periphery of the extravasation site.

  If using recombinant human hyaluronidase, a single subcutaneous injection of 150 units may be equally effective (8).

5. *Adverse effects*

None reported in neonates, rare sensitivity reactions to the animal formulations of hyaluronidase report*ed in adults*. Potential side effects include tachycardia, hypotension, dizziness, chills, urticarial erythema, angioedema, nausea, vomiting, and injection site reactions.

b. Multiple Puncture Technique (10,11)

In infants who develop tense swelling of the site with blanching of the skin owing to infiltration, multiple punctures of the edematous area have been used to allow free drainage of the infiltrating solution.

1. Using strict aseptic technique and a sterile blood-drawing stylet, the area of greatest swelling is punctured multiple times.

2. Fluid is gently expressed out to decrease the swelling, and prevent necrosis.

3. The area may then be dressed with saline soaks or other wound dressing (see below, d. Wound Dressings) to aid drainage, draw out vesicant, and impede scab formation.

c. Saline Flush-Out Technique (12)

A technique of saline flushing of the subcutaneous tissue has been advocated by many authors for large-volume injury, but this has not been studied in randomized controlled trials (5,6,12–15).

1. Hyaluronidase may be injected subcutaneously to improve dispersion of fluid but does not necessarily improve outcomes compared to saline alone (15).

2. Four small stab incisions are made in the tissue plane with a scalpel blade at the periphery of the area.

3. Saline is injected through a blunt cannula inserted subcutaneously through one of the puncture sites and flushed through the other puncture sites.

4. Massaging the fluid toward the incisions facilitates removal of the extravasated material.

5. The affected area can then be treated with dressings and elevation, as appropriate.

d. Topical Nitroglycerine (16)

1. Effective in treating injury from vasoactive drugs, such as due to extravasation of dopamine

2. *Mechanism of action:* Vascular smooth muscle relaxant

3. *Administration*

  a. 2% nitroglycerine ointment, 4 mm/kg body weight, applied over the affected area, may be repeated every 8 hours if perfusion has not improved

4. *Precautions*

  a. Absorption through the skin may lead to hypotension; risk of methemoglobinemia

e. Phentolamine (1,17)

Effective in treating extravasations of vasopressors such as dopamine and epinephrine, which cause tissue damage by intense vasoconstriction and ischemia.

1. *Mechanism of action:* Competitive α-adrenergic blockade, leading to smooth muscle relaxation and hyperemia.

2. *Timing*: Effect should be seen almost immediately; most effective within 1 hour but may be used up to 12 hours. The biologic half-life of subcutaneous phentolamine is <20 minutes.

3. *Administration*: Doses have not been established for newborn infants. The exact dose is dependent on the size of the lesion and the size of the infant. Recommended doses range from 0.1 mg/kg per dose up to a maximum of 2.5 mg. Use 1 to 5 mL of 0.5-mg/mL solution or up to 2.5 mL of 1-mg/mL solution injected subcutaneously into infiltrated area, after removal of IV catheter.

4. *Precautions*: Hypotension, tachycardia, and dysrhythmias may occur; use with extreme caution in preterm infants; consider using repeated small doses.

5. Wound Management

a. Goal

The goal of wound management in neonates who have partial- or full-thickness skin loss is to achieve primary or secondary healing while avoiding scarring, contractures, and operative intervention.

There are several purposes for dressing wounds:

1. Maintain a moist pH-balanced environment to promote reepithelialization.

2. Manage exudates.

3. Decrease disruption of healing tissue.

4. Provide an antimicrobial barrier to prevent local and systemic infection.
5. Decrease pain.

b. Wound Care

Wound care regimens differ among experts and institutions (18,19). Consultation with a wound-ostomy-care nurse is often helpful (see Chapter 54).

1. Evaluate the wound: Size, depth, edges, wound bed, presence of exudate, necrotic tissue, eschar, margins, evaluation of skin around the wound for signs of inflammation or for maceration.
2. Evaluate wound healing every day. Time to heal ranges from 7 days to 3 months.
3. Dressing changes can be painful. Consider using comfort measures, sucrose, and analgesics, as needed.
4. Irrigate wound with sterile saline to remove exudate and debris. Use room temperature saline, and take care not to use excess pressure, which can damage healing tissue. A 35-mL syringe with a 19-gauge angiocatheter delivers about 8 to 12 psi, enough to remove debris (18).

c. Topical Agents

Topical agents may be used if the wound is colonized, infected, or at risk of being infected. Routine use of antiseptic solutions is not recommended because most solutions destroy granulation tissue.

1. Silver sulfadiazine cream is contraindicated in infants less than 30 days of age because the sulphonamides increase the risk of kernicterus. In addition, the cream can obscure the wound by forming a difficult-to-remove opaque layer.
2. Use of povidone-iodine is not recommended because absorption of iodine may suppress thyroid function.
3. Antibacterial creams and ointments have limited roles.

d. Wound Dressing

The selection of dressing material depends on the depth of the wound and the property of the wound bed (presence of granulation tissue, moist, dry, exudative) (18). Wet wounds require absorptive dressing, whereas dry wounds benefit from hydrating dressings.

1. Amorphous hydrogels consisting of carboxymethylcellulose polymer, propylene glycol, and water have been shown to keep the wound moist and facilitate wound healing (3,20). They are available in the form of gels or sheets, which may be applied directly to the wound surface and held in place by a secondary dressing. The gel is easily removed with saline and is generally changed every 3 days. More frequent dressing changes may be required if there is excessive exudation.
2. Silver-impregnated dressings are postulated to decrease wound infection, although concerns with silver toxicity have restricted its prolonged, routine use (21).
3. Alginate dressings are fibers derived from brown seaweed, and are useful for wounds with moderate to heavy exudates because of highly absorptive properties and for bleeding wounds because of hemostatic properties (18).
4. Polyurethane foams and hydrofibers are also useful for wounds with exudates because of their absorptive properties (18).
5. Medical grade honey has recently been used, largely due to its antimicrobial properties (22). The high osmolality may help to reduce skin edema. Medical grade honey and not food grade honey must be used, as medical grade is free of clostridial spores.

6. Consultations

a. If the scar involves a flexion crease, passive range-of-motion exercises with each diaper change may help to prevent contractures. Consider involving physical therapy (PT) and occupational therapy (OT), if they are available at your institution.
b. Plastic surgical consultation is recommended for all full-thickness and significant partial-thickness extravasation injuries. Enzymatic or surgical debridement or skin grafting may be required in cases involving deep necrosis. Surgical consultation is required when there is concern for compartment syndrome.

References

1. Beall V, Hall B, Mulholland JT, et al. Neonatal extravasation: an overview and algorithm for evidence-based treatment. *Newborn Infant Nurs Rev.* 2013;13(4):189–195.
2. Driscoll MC, Langer M, Burke S, et al. Improving detection of IV infiltrates in neonates. *BMJ Quality Improv Rep.* 2015;4(1): pii: u204253.w3874.
3. Leo AD, Leung BC, Giele H, et al. Management of extravasation injuries in preterm infants. *Surg Sci.* 2016;07(09):427–432.
4. Reynolds PM, Maclaren R, Mueller SW, et al. Management of extravasation injuries: a focused evaluation of noncytotoxic medications. *Pharmacotherapy.* 2014;34(6):617–632.
5. Restieaux M, Maw A, Broadbent R, et al. Neonatal extravasation injury: prevention and management in Australia and New Zealand—a survey of current practice. *BMC Pediatr.* 2013;13(1):34.
6. Ghanem AM, Mansour A, Exton R, et al. Childhood extravasation injuries: improved outcome following the introduction of hospital-wide guidelines. *J Plast Reconstr Aesthet Surg.* 2015;68(4):505–518.
7. Pantelides N, Shah A. Extravasation injury: a simple technique to maintain limb elevation within a neonatal intensive care unit. *J Neonatal Nurs.* 2013;19(5):243–245.

8. Beaulieu MJ. Hyaluronidase for extravasation management. *Neonatal Netw.* 2012;31(6):413–418.

9. Kuenstig LL. Treatment of intravenous infiltration in a neonate. *J Pediatr Health Care.* 2010;24:184–188.

10. Chandavasu O, Garrow E, Valda V, et al. A new method for the prevention of skin sloughs and necrosis secondary to intravenous infiltration. *Am J Perinatol.* 1986;3(1):4–5.

11. Sung KY, Lee SY. Nonoperative management of extravasation injuries associated with neonatal parenteral nutrition using multiple punctures and a hydrocolloid dressing. *Wounds.* 2016;28(5):145–151.

12. Gault DT. Extravasation injuries. *Br J Plast Surg.* 1993;46:91–96.

13. Kostogloudis N, Demiri E, Tsimponis A, et al. Severe extravasation injuries in neonates: a report of 34 cases. *Pediatr Dermatol.* 2015;32(6):830–835.

14. Ching DL, Wong KY, Milroy C. Paediatric extravasation injuries: a review of 69 consecutive patients. *Int J Surg.* 2014;12(10):1036–1037.

15. Gopalakrishnan PN, Goel N, Banerjee S. Saline irrigation for the management of skin extravasation injury in neonates. *Cochrane Database Syst Rev.* 2017;7:CD008404.

16. Samiee-Zafarghandy S, van den Anker JN, Ben Fadel N. Topical nitroglycerin in neonates with tissue injury: a case report and review of the literature. *Paediatr Child Health.* 2014;19(1):9–12.

17. Le A, Patel S. Extravasation of noncytotoxic drugs: a review of the literature. *Ann Pharmacother.* 2014;48(7):870–886.

18. Fox MD. Wound care in the neonatal intensive care unit. *Neonatal Netw.* 2011;30(5):291–303.

19. King A, Stellar JJ, Blevins A, et al. Dressings and products in pediatric wound care. *Adv Wound Care (New Rochelle).* 2014;3(4):324–334.

20. Cisler-Cahill L. A protocol for the use of amorphous hydrogel to support wound healing in neonatal patients: an adjunct to nursing care. *Neonatal Netw.* 2006;25(4):267–273.

21. Williams BC. Nanoscale silver for infection control. *Nursing.* 2014;44(5):68–69.

22. Mohr LD, Reyna R, Amaya R. Neonatal case studies using active leptospermum honey. *J Wound Ostomy Continence Nurs.* 2014;41(3):213–218.

CHAPTER

31

Umbilical Artery Catheterization

Suna Seo

Umbilical artery catheterization is performed in critically ill neonates, often soon after birth. The umbilical arteries are patent for 7 to 14 days, but are often accessible only in the first day or two after birth, after which vasoconstriction and clotting make access difficult.

A. Indications

Primary

1. Frequent or continuous (see Chapter 11) measurement of lower aortic blood gases for oxygen tension (PO_2) or oxygen content (percent saturation)
2. Continuous monitoring of arterial blood pressure
3. To provide a port for frequent blood sampling in the extremely low birth weight infant
4. Angiography
5. Resuscitation (use of umbilical venous catheter is the first choice)

Secondary

1. Umbilical arterial catheter is not usually recommended for infusion of maintenance glucose/electrolyte solutions or medications, but has been used for this purpose (1)
2. Exchange transfusion

B. Contraindications

1. Evidence of vascular compromise in lower limbs or buttock areas
2. Peritonitis
3. Necrotizing enterocolitis (2)
4. Omphalitis
5. Omphalocele
6. Gastroschisis
7. Acute abdomen etiology

C. Equipment

Sterile

1. Sterile gown and gloves
2. Cup with antiseptic solution
3. Surgical drape with central aperture
4. Catheter
   a. Single hole
      (1) Reduces surfaces for potential thrombus formation
      (2) Recorded pressure tracing will change when hole is occluded
   b. Made of flexible material that does not kink as it follows the curves of vessels
   c. Relatively rigid walls with frequency characteristics suitable for accurate measurement of intravascular pressure
   d. Small capacity (minimum volume of blood to be withdrawn to clear catheter prior to blood sampling)
   e. Radio-opaque: The need to visualize the catheter position on x-ray film outweighs the theoretical risk of increased thrombogenicity related to a radio-opaque strip (3)
   f. Smooth, rounded tip (4), nonthrombogenic material (5)
   g. 5-Fr gauge for infants weighing >1,200 g
   h. 3.5-Fr gauge for infants weighing <1,200 g
5. Three-way stopcock with Luer-Lock
6. 10-mL syringe
7. 0.45 to 0.9 normal saline (NS) flush solution (saline with heparin, 1 to 2 U/mL)
   a. In very small premature infants, particularly in the first week of life, hypernatremia may result from

receiving excess sodium in flush solutions. In these infants, 0.45 NS rather than more concentrated saline solutions is recommended

b. The use of hypotonic (0.25 NS) or dextrose solutions has been associated with hemolysis of red blood cells and should be avoided if possible (6)

c. Use of heparinized flush solution is common practice (7–11)

Heparin decreases the incidence of thrombotic complications (12), and a Cochrane Database Review found that the use of as little as 0.25 U/mL heparin in the infusate decreases the likelihood of line occlusion (13)

8. Tape measure
9. 20-cm narrow umbilical tie
10. No. 11 scalpel blade and holder
11. 4- × 4-in gauze sponges
12. Two curved mosquito hemostats
13. Toothed iris forceps
14. Two curved, nontoothed iris forceps
15. 2% lidocaine HCl without epinephrine
16. 3-mL syringe and needle to draw up lidocaine
17. Small needle holder
18. 4-0 silk suture on small, curved needle
19. Suture scissors

Nonsterile

1. Cap and mask

D. Precautions

1. Avoid use of feeding tubes as catheter (associated with higher incidence of thrombosis) (14)
2. Fold drapes so as not to obscure infant's face and upper chest, allowing access to airway and visual monitoring of infant's respiratory status during the procedure
3. Take time and care to dilate the lumen of the artery before attempting to insert catheter
4. Catheter should not be forced past an obstruction
5. Never advance catheter once placed and secured
6. Loosen umbilical tie slightly upon completion of procedure and obtain radiographic confirmation of position
7. Avoid covering the umbilicus with dressing. Dressing may delay recognition of bleeding or catheter displacement
8. Always obtain radiographic (including a lateral view) or ultrasound (15) confirmation of catheter position (16,17)
9. Be certain that catheter is secure, and examine frequently when infant is placed in prone position, because hemorrhage may go unrecognized
10. Take care not to allow air to enter the catheter. Always have catheter fluid filled and attached to a closed

stopcock prior to insertion. Check for air bubbles in catheter before flushing or starting infusion

11. When removing catheter, cut suture at skin, not on the catheter, to avoid catheter transection
12. Catheters should remain in place only as long as primary indications exist. Because of the risk of complications, catheters should usually not remain in place for more than 7 to 10 days

E. Technique (▶ Video 31.1: Umbilical Vein and Artery Catheterization)

Anatomic note: The umbilical arteries are the direct continuation of the internal iliac arteries (**Fig. 31.1**). Their diameters at their origins are 2 to 3 mm. As they approach the umbilicus, their lumina become small and the walls thicken significantly. A catheter introduced into the umbilical artery will usually pass into the aorta from the internal iliac artery. Occasionally, a catheter will pass into the femoral artery via the external iliac artery or into one of the gluteal arteries (see **Fig. 31.15D**). The latter two sites are unsuitable for sampling, pressure measurement, or infusion.

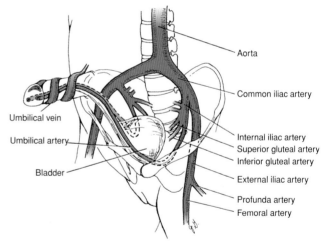

FIGURE 31.1 Anatomic relations of the umbilical arteries, showing relationships with major arteries supplying buttocks and lower limb.

1. Placement of UAC in high position should be used exclusively (18,19). In rare cases, if high position is not successful, a low position may be used (**Fig. 31.2**).
   a. **High position** (14,19): Level of thoracic vertebrae T6–T9 (**Fig. 31.3**); catheter tip above origin of celiac axis.
   b. **Low position** (14,19): Level of lumbar vertebrae L3–L4 (**Fig. 31.4**).
      (1) Catheter tip is below major aortic branches such as renal mesenteric arteries.
      (2) In most newborns, this position coincides with the aortic bifurcation at the upper end of the fourth vertebra.

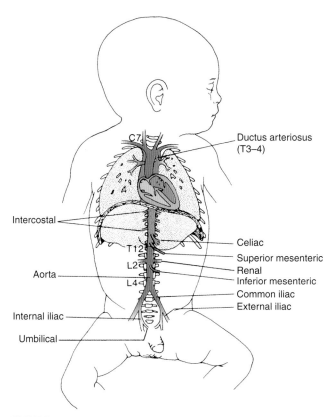

FIGURE 31.2 The aorta and branches.

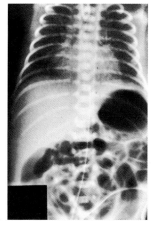
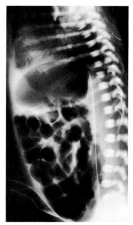

FIGURE 31.3 UAC in satisfactory high position at the level of the ninth thoracic vertebral body on anteroposterior (**A**) and lateral (**B**) projections.

2. Make external measurements as necessary to estimate length of catheter to be inserted (**Table 31.1**) (see **Fig. 31.5**) (20–26).

   a. There is no universal formula, measurement, or nomogram to accurately predict the UAC insertion length for infants of all birthweight and gestational ages (27,28).

      (1) Use Shukla (**Table 31.1**) for infants with birthweight >1,500 g (23).

      (2) Use Wright formula for infants with birthweight <1,500 g (24,26,28,29).

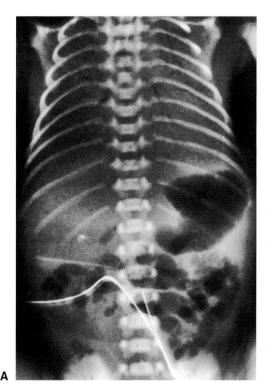
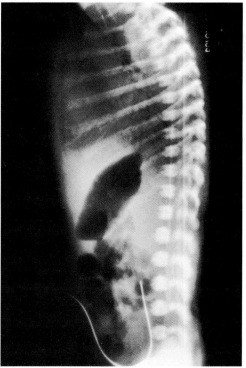

FIGURE 31.4 Anteroposterior (**A**) and lateral (**B**) radiographs showing satisfactory low position of a UAC. Catheter tip is at the level of the superior margin of the fourth lumbar vertebral body, which in newborns usually corresponds to the aortic bifurcation.

TABLE 31.1 Available Formulae to Estimate UAC Insertion Length (cm)

FORMULA AUTHOR (PUBLICATION YEAR)	CALCULATION OF UAC INSERTION LENGTH (cm) FROM ABDOMINAL WALL
Dunn (1966) (20)	Graph reference using shoulder–umbilicus distance (Fig. 31.5 (a))
Rosenfeld et al. (1980)(21,22)	Graph reference using total body length
Shukla and Ferrara (1986) (23)	[3 × weight (kg)] + 9
Wright et al. (2008) (24)	[4 × weight (kg)] + 7
Vali et al. (2010) (25)	1.1 × [xiphisternum to ASIS + ASIS to umbilicus] + 1.6
Gupta et al. (2015) (26)	(Umbilicus to nipple − 1) + (2 × umbilicus to symphysis pubis) (Fig. 31.5 (b and c))

UAC, umbilical arterial catheter; ASIS, anterior superior iliac spine.

(3) Published precision performance comparisons of the formulae are inconsistent and inconclusive (27,29,30).

(4) Morphometric measurement-based formulae may be more suitable for extremely preterm infants (25,26,31).

3. Prepare as for major procedure (see Chapters 5 and 6).

4. Attach stopcock to hub of catheter and fill system with flush solution (see Section C7). Turn stopcock to catheter "off."

5. Place sterile gauze around umbilical stump and elevate out of sterile field or have an assistant grasp the cord by the cord clamp or forceps and hold the cord vertically out of the sterile field.

6. Prepare cord and surrounding skin with antiseptic solution to radius of approximately 5 cm. The use of chlorhexidine in infants <2 months of age is not recommended (32,33).

7. Drape area surrounding cord.

8. Place umbilical tie around umbilicus and tie loosely with a single knot.

   a. Tighten only enough to prevent bleeding and, if possible, place around Wharton jelly rather than skin.

   b. It may be necessary to loosen the tie when inserting the catheter.

9. Cut cord horizontally at 1 to 1.5 cm from skin with scalpel (**Fig. 31.6**).

   (Note: Need longer length of umbilical cord for alternative technique—see Lateral Arteriotomy below.)

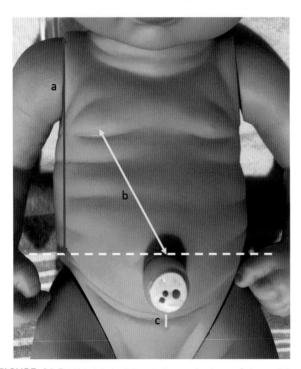

FIGURE 31.5 White dashed line indicates the base of the umbilicus. (*a*) Shoulder to umbilicus length measurement (20); (*b*) Umbilicus to nipple length measurement (26); (*c*) Umbilicus to symphysis pubis measurement (26).

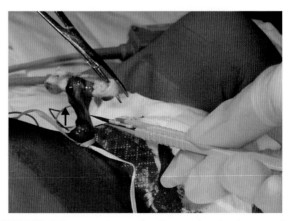

FIGURE 31.6 Traction is being placed on cord in the direction of the *arrow*. Operator is about to make a horizontal cut across cord.

10. Avoid tangential slice.
    Control bleeding by gentle tension on umbilical tape.
11. Blot surface of cord stump with gauze swab. Avoid rubbing, as this damages tissue and obscures anatomy.
12. Identify cord vessels (**Fig. 31.7**).

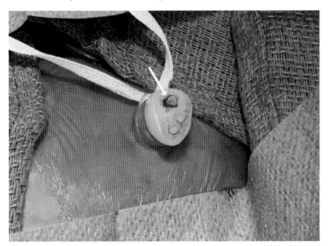

FIGURE 31.7 The vessels of the umbilical cord. Thin-walled umbilical vein at 12-o'clock position is indicated by a *white arrow*. The two umbilical arteries are directly below the vein at 4- and 6-o'clock positions.

a. Vein is easiest to identify as large, thin-walled, sometimes gaping vessel. It is most frequently situated at the 12-o'clock position at the base of the umbilical stump.
b. Arteries are smaller, thick-walled, and white and may protrude slightly from cut surface.
c. Omphalomesenteric duct is rarely present.
13. Grasp cord stump, using toothed forceps, at point close to (but not on) artery to be catheterized. If available, it may be helpful to have an assistant scrub and assist.
    a. Apply two curved mosquito hemostats to Wharton jelly on opposite sides of the cord, away from the vessel to be cannulated.
    b. Apply traction to stabilize cord stump.

14. Introduce one of the points of the curved iris forceps into the lumen of the artery and probe gently to a depth of 0.5 cm.
15. Remove forceps and bring points together before introducing them once more into the lumen.
16. Probe gently to a depth of 1 cm (up to the curved "shoulder" of the forceps), keeping the points together.
17. Allow the points to spring apart and maintain forceps in this position for 15 to 30 seconds to dilate vessel (**Fig. 31.8**). Time spent in ensuring dilatation prior to catheter insertion increases the likelihood of success.

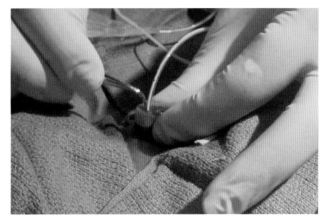

FIGURE 31.8 An iris forceps is pointed into the umbilical artery in order to dilate the lumen of the artery.

18. Release cord and set aside toothed forceps, while keeping curved forceps within artery.
19. Grasp catheter 1 cm from tip, between free thumb and forefinger or with curved iris forceps.
20. Insert catheter into lumen of artery, between prongs of dilating forceps (**Fig. 31.9**).

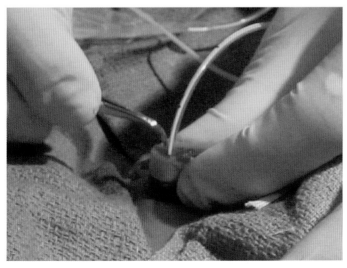
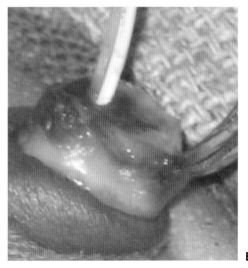

FIGURE 31.9 A: Inserting the catheter into the artery between the prongs of dilating forceps. Note that the umbilical tape has been tied around the skin of the umbilicus; this should be loosened once the catheter is secured in place. **B:** Close-up photo of the umbilical stump with the arterial catheter in place.

21. Remove curved forceps, having passed catheter approximately 2 cm into vessel with a firm, steady motion. Grasp cord again with toothed tissue forceps and pull gently toward head of infant. This mild traction will facilitate passage of catheter at an angle between the cord and the abdominal wall.
22. After passing the catheter approximately 5 cm, aspirate to verify intraluminal position. Clear blood in the catheter by injecting 0.5 mL of flush solution. Advance catheter to calculated appropriate length (see Section E2).
23. Take appropriate action if insertion is complicated (**Fig. 31.10**).
    a. Resistance before tip reaches abdominal wall (<3 cm from surface of abdominal stump).
       (1) Loosen umbilical tape.
       (2) Redilate artery.
    b. "Popping" sensation encountered rather than "relaxation."
       (1) Catheter may have exited lumen and created a false channel.

    (2) Remove and use second artery.
    (3) If unsuccessful, draw 0.5 mL of lidocaine from vial. Reinsert tip of catheter approximately 2 cm into UAC and drip lidocaine into vessel. Apply constant gentle pressure until vessel dilates.
    c. Backflow of blood, particularly around vessel.
       (1) Tighten the umbilical tape.
       (2) Catheter may be in false channel, with extravascular bleeding.
    d. Resistance is encountered at anterior abdominal wall or sharp turn in vessel as it angles around bladder toward internal iliac artery (approximately 6 to 8 cm from surface of umbilical stump in 2- to 4-kg neonate).
       (1) Apply gentle but steady pressure for 30 to 60 seconds.
       (2) Position infant on side with same side elevated as artery being catheterized. Flex hip.
       (3) Instill lidocaine as for E23b (3). Do not force catheter.

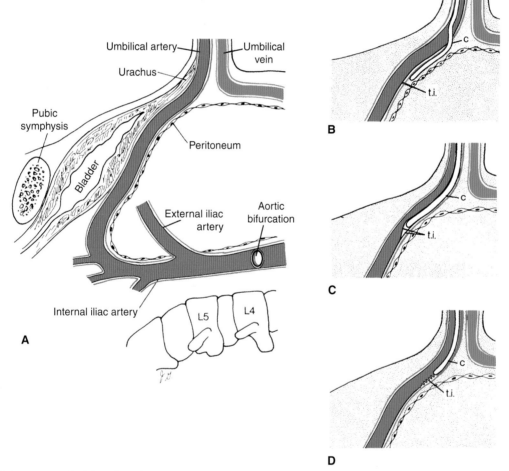

FIGURE 31.10 Some reasons for failure of umbilical artery catheterization. **A:** Sagittal midline section to show normal anatomy of umbilical artery. **B:** Catheter has perforated the umbilical artery within the anulus umbilicalis and is dissecting perivascularly and external to peritoneum. **C:** Catheter has ruptured through the tunica intima (*t.i.*) and dissected into subintimal space. **D:** Catheter invaginating the tunica intima after stripping it from a more distal point. (Adapted with permission from Clark JM, Jung AL. Umbilical artery catheterization by a cut down procedure. *Pediatrics*. 1977;59(6):1036–1040. Copyright © 1977 by the AAP.)

e. Easy insertion, but no blood return.
  (1) Catheter is outside vessel in false channel.
  (2) Remove and observe infant carefully for evidence of complication.
24. Place marker tape on catheter with base of tape flush with surface of cord so that displacement of the catheter may be readily recognized.

25. Place a suture around base of the cord (not through skin or vessels) (**Fig. 31.11A–C**). Secure the catheter to the stump by wrapping the tail of the suture snugly around the catheter and tying with a surgical instrument tie (**Fig. 31.11D**). Avoid multiple wraps around the catheter resembling a roman sandal lace appearance. Each loop around the catheter must be secured with a tied knot (**Fig. 31.11E**).

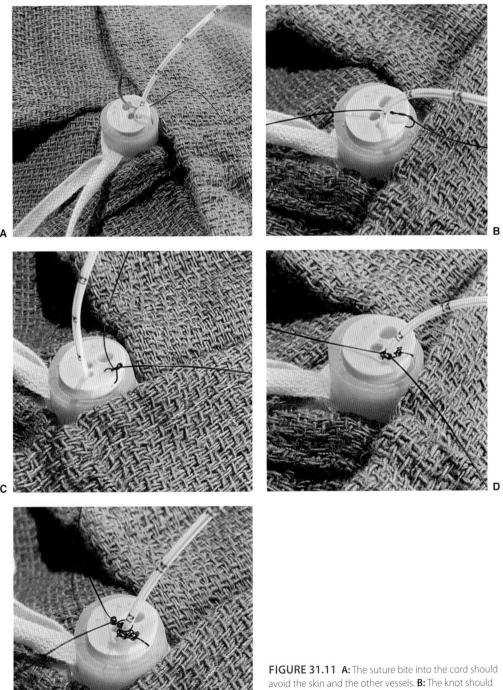

FIGURE 31.11 A: The suture bite into the cord should avoid the skin and the other vessels. **B:** The knot should lie flat without pursing the cord, and (**C**) be tight with a very small loop. **D:** Wrap the tail of the suture around the catheter and tie with a surgical instrument tie. **E:** Repeat the above step with each wrap around the tail ending with a knot.

26. Secure catheter temporarily by looping over upper abdomen and taping.
27. Obtain radiographs or ultrasound to check catheter position.

   The appropriate location of the tip of the UAC is between T7 to T9 thoracic vertebra on a chest x-ray. (Remember the pneumonic: "7 is heaven, 8 is great, 9 is fine.")

   a. Catheter tip above T6 or between T10 and L2.
      (1) Measure distance between actual and appropriate position on radiograph.
      (2) Withdraw equal length of catheter.
      (3) Repeat radiographic study.
      (4) Note procedure in chart.
   b. Catheter tip below L5.
      (1) Remove catheter.
      (2) Never advance catheter once in situ, because this will introduce a length of contaminated catheter into the vessel.
28. Once correct catheter tip placement is confirmed, secure the catheter per institutional protocol. Assemble tape bridge (**Fig. 31.12**), or secure catheter to abdominal wall with DuoDerm and Tegaderm (**Fig. 31.13**), or use a commercially available umbilical catheter bridge (34).

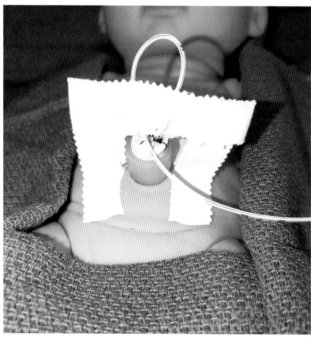

FIGURE 31.12 Tape bridge. Two vertical tape towers taped on either side of the umbilicus are connected by a bridge tape across securing a looped umbilical catheter.

29. Remove umbilical tape.
30. Continue routine cord care with 70% alcohol swab or other agent of choice.

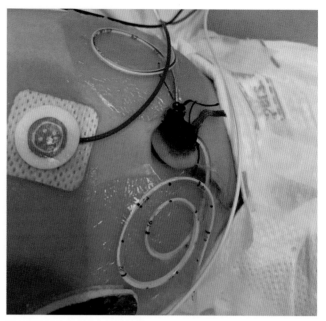

FIGURE 31.13 Umbilical catheters UVC (right) and UAC (left) secured on the abdomen with a DuoDerm affixed underneath and the Tegaderm affixed over the looped catheters.

F. Lateral Arteriotomy

An alternative approach to the umbilical artery catheterization is by means of a lateral arteriotomy. To perform this method, 3 to 4 cm of cord must be preserved because the cord must be rolled over a Kelly clamp 180 degrees (35–37).

1. Clamp across end of cord with a mosquito hemostat in the nondominant hand and pull firmly toward the infant's head.
2. Roll cord 180 degrees over hemostat toward abdominal wall.
3. Identify arteries in superior right and left lateral aspects of cord.
4. Approximately 1 cm from abdominal wall, incise Wharton jelly down to arterial wall, using a no. 11 scalpel blade.
5. Incise artery through half of circumference. If necessary, dilate lumen with iris forceps.
6. Insert catheter into lumen of artery, directed in a caudad direction, for predetermined distance.

G. Umbilical Artery Cutdown

This method is usually successful even after failed insertion through the umbilical stump, as there is less tendency for false tracts. The most frequent reason for failed umbilical artery cutdown is mistaking the urachus for a vessel. Because of the time and risks associated with the cutdown procedure, standard insertion should be attempted first.

Indications

1. Failed umbilical artery catheterization through conventional technique described earlier in this chapter

Contraindications

1. Same as for umbilical artery catheterization by conventional technique
2. Bleeding diathesis

Equipment

1. Same as for umbilical artery catheterization by conventional technique
2. 1% lidocaine HCl without epinephrine in 3-mL syringe with 25- to 27-gauge needle
3. No. 15 surgical blade and holder
4. Curved delicate dressing forceps, two pairs (1/4 or 1/2 curved)
5. Tissue forceps
6. Self-retaining retractor (such as eyelid retractor)
7. Absorbable suture, plain
8. Absorbable suture on small cutting needle
9. Nonabsorbable suture on a small, curved needle
10. Needle holder
11. Suture scissors
12. Skin-closure tapes

Precautions

1. Same as described earlier for conventional technique.
2. If possible, leave catheter from previously attempted standard procedure in place to aid in vessel identification.
3. Ensure that abdominal incision is on abdominal wall and not too close to umbilical stump.
4. Identify landmarks carefully to avoid cutting or catheterizing urachus.
5. When incising mesenchymal sheath, take care to avoid transecting vessel.
6. Secure the catheter with an internal ligature that is just tight enough to prevent accidental removal but loose enough for elective removal or reinsertion, in case the catheter becomes occluded by thrombus or precipitate.

Technique (38)

See **Figure 31.14**.

1. Insert an orogastric tube to keep the bowel as decompressed as possible.
2. Prepare infant and drape as for umbilical artery catheterization (see earlier in chapter).

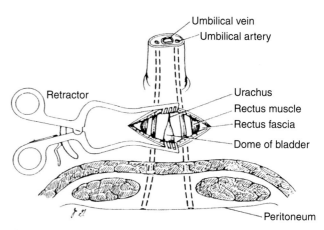

FIGURE 31.14 Sub-umbilical cutdown. Anatomic view through incision. (Redrawn from Sherman NJ. Umbilical artery cutdown. *J Pediatr Surg.* 1977;12(5):723–724. Copyright © 1997 Elsevier. With permission.)

3. If catheter has been left in place after previous attempt, include vessel and catheter in the preparation, leaving the catheter accessible for removal.
4. Anesthetize area of skin immediately below umbilicus, at umbilical stump–abdominal wall junction, with 0.5 mL of lidocaine.
5. Prepare UAC as for standard procedure, leaving catheter filled with flush solution. Estimate length for insertion based on patient size. Subtract 1 to 2 cm from that recommended for standard insertion, as cutdown catheter will enter vessel farther along course.
6. Make a smile-shaped incision from 4 to 8 o'clock through the skin of the abdominal wall at the junction with the umbilical stump.
7. Place self-retaining retractor to maintain exposure.
8. Using blunt dissection through the subcutaneous tissue with mosquito forceps, identify the fascia overlying the urachus and umbilical vessels.

   The mesenchymal sheath is composed of three layers of fascia and is from 1 to 3 mm thick. Although it is barely perceptible in extremely premature infants, in term infants it may be thick enough to require making an incision through the sheath prior to blunt dissection.
9. While elevating the fascia with two forceps, make a small incision between their tips. Enlarge incision with scissors to the same size as skin incision. In very immature infants, simple dissection should suffice.
10. With curved mosquito forceps, dissect in the midline and identify the urachus (**Fig. 31.14**).

    The urachus is a white, glistening, cordlike structure in the midline. Its position may be confirmed by traction cephalad, pulling the dome of the bladder into view. The umbilical arteries lie posterolaterally on either side but not touching the urachus.
11. Identify the umbilical arteries lying to either side of the urachus.

    The vessels with their surrounding tissues appear larger than expected. When elevated, there will be no caudal bulge, distinguishing them from the urachus. If a previously attempted catheter was left "in place," palpation of the area allows more ready identification of the vessel. Previously unsuccessful attempts, with failure to pass more than a few centimeters, are usually associated with perivascular hematoma formation from unrecognized perforation and dissection through a false tract. Visualization of a hematoma helps distinguish the vessel from the urachus.

12. Try to avoid entering the peritoneum. In infants with very little subcutaneous tissue, it may be impossible to avoid penetrating the peritoneum. Should this occur, replace any bowel that may protrude and carefully close the peritoneum with absorbable suture, taking extreme care not to include any bowel within the suture. Start antibiotics for peritonitis prophylaxis.

13. Insert the tip of the mosquito forceps under the vessel and pull a doubled strand of plain absorbable suture under the vessel. Position sutures 1 cm apart.

14. While elevating the sutures and with suture scissors directed cephalad, make a V-shaped incision through three fourths of the diameter of the vessel. Take care not to transect the vessel, but cut cleanly into the lumen.

    If the artery is accidentally transected and if the catheter insertion is unsuccessful, tie off the caudal end of the artery to prevent hemorrhage.

15. Use curved tissue forceps or a catheter introducer to dilate the artery.

16. Pass the catheter through the opening for the predetermined distance, checking for blood return after a few centimeters. The catheter should advance without resistance.

17. When the catheter is properly positioned, have an assistant check the perfusion in the lower extremities. If that is satisfactory, secure the catheter by tying the lower ligature firmly around the catheter.

18. Using absorbable suture, close the fascia and approximate the subcutaneous tissues.

    Hashimoto et al. (39) proposed an alternative technique that allows for catheter reinsertion in case of catheter thrombosis or occlusion. They use loose ligation around the artery once the catheter is in proper position. They then fix the artery by using the same sutures that close the fascia, thus creating an arteriocutaneous fistula, making it easy to find the insertion site and use it for reinsertion.

19. Close the skin with nonabsorbable suture or with skin-closure tape after cleaning the area.

20. The catheter may be further secured with a tape bridge **(Fig. 31.12)**.

Removal of Catheter

1. Remove any tape and withdraw catheter slowly, as described in Section J below.

2. If the internal ligature around a catheter is too tight to allow removal with reasonable traction, it may be necessary to dissect and cut the ligature, after sterile skin preparation.

3. Apply pressure for hemostasis.

4. Approximate wound edges with skin-closure tape.

Complications

1. Catheterization of urachus (40)
2. Vesicoumbilical fistula (40)
3. Transection of urachus with urinary ascites (41)
4. Perforation or rupture (42,43) of urinary bladder; the risk of bladder injury is minimal if bladder is emptied prior to procedure
5. Transection of umbilical artery with hemorrhage
6. Incision of peritoneum (with possible evisceration)
7. Bleeding from incision

H. Care of Dwelling Catheter

For setup and maintenance of arterial pressure transducer, see Chapter 10.

1. Keep catheter free of blood to prevent clot formation.
   a. Flush catheter with 0.5 mL of flush solution, slowly over at least 5 seconds, each time a blood sample is drawn.
   b. Between samples, infuse IV solution continuously through catheter to prevent retrograde flow.
   c. Note amounts of blood removed and IV fluid/flush solution infused, and add to fluid balance record.
2. Watch for indications of clot formation.
   a. Decrease in amplitude of pulse pressure on blood pressure tracing.
   b. Difficulty withdrawing blood samples.
3. Take appropriate action if clot forms.
   a. Do not attempt to flush clot forcibly.
      Remove catheter. Replace only if critical.
4. Enteral feeding in the presence of UACs remains controversial. Increased risk of mesenteric thromboembolism and its association with the development of necrotizing enterocolitis has been suggested (44). Other studies have shown no increased incidence of feeding problems or complications in infants fed with a UAC in situ (45,46).

I. Obtaining Blood Samples From Catheter

(With emphasis on aseptic technique and minimizing stress to the vessel)

Equipment

1. Gloves
2. Alcohol swabs
3. Rubber-tipped clamps or disposable IV tubing clamps
4. Syringe of 0.6 mL of flushing solution
5. Syringe for cleaning line
6. Syringe for blood sample
7. Ice, if necessary for sample preservation
8. Appropriate requisition slips and labels

Technique

1. Wash hands and put on sterile gloves.
2. Form sterile field.
3. Clean the connection site of the stopcock/catheter using an alcohol swab.
4. Clamp the umbilical catheter.
5. Connect the 3-mL syringe, release the clamp, and slowly draw back 2 to 3 mL of fluid over 1 minute to clear the line. Reclamp the catheter. Remove syringe and place on sterile field. Accurate measurements of electrolytes can be obtained after withdrawal of a minimum of 1.6 mL of blood (47). However, if blood glucose values are desired, a minimum of 3 mL from a 3.5-Fr and 4 mL from a 5-Fr catheter must be withdrawn.
6. It is important to draw back fluid/blood from the UAC slowly taking at least 30 to 40 seconds, in order to prevent decreases in cerebral oxygenation.
7. Attach sampling syringe. Release clamp and draw back specimen desired. Reclamp the catheter.
8. Reattach the syringe containing the fluid and blood cleared from the line.
   a. Clear the connection of air.
   b. Slowly replace the fluid and blood cleared from the line and remove the syringe.
9. Attach the syringe of flushing solution to the stopcock, clear air from the connection, and slowly flush the line.
10. Clean the stopcock connection with alcohol.
11. Record on infant's daily record sheet all blood removed and volume of flush used.

J. Removal of UAC

Indications

1. No further clinical indication
2. Need for less frequent direct PO_2 measurements
3. Sufficient stabilization of blood pressure to allow intermittent monitoring
4. Hypertension
5. Hematuria not due to other recognizable cause

6. Catheter-related sepsis and/or infections with *Staphylococcus aureus,* gram-negative bacilli, or *Candida* mandate removal of the catheter (48)
7. Catheter-related vascular compromise
8. Onset of platelet consumption coagulopathy
9. Peritonitis
10. Necrotizing enterocolitis
11. Omphalitis

Technique

1. Leave umbilical tie loose around cord stump as precaution against excessive bleeding.
2. Withdraw catheter slowly and evenly, until approximately 5 cm remains in vessel, tightening the umbilical tie.
3. Discontinue infusion.
4. Pull remainder of catheter out of the vessel at rate of 1 cm/min (to allow vasospasm). If there is bleeding, apply lateral pressure to the cord by compressing between thumb and first finger.

K. Complications (48–50)

Catheterization of the umbilical artery is probably always associated with some degree of reversible damage to the arterial intima (51).

1. Malpositioned catheter (**Figs. 31.15 to 31.17**)
   a. Vessel perforation (52)
   b. Refractory hypoglycemia with catheter tip opposite celiac axis (53)
   c. Peritoneal perforation (54)
   d. False aneurysm (55)
   e. Movement of catheter tip position because of changes in abdominal circumference
   f. Sciatic nerve palsy (56)
   g. Misdirection of catheter into internal or external iliac artery (see **Figs. 31.15D and 31.18**) (49)
      Double-arterial catheter technique may be used to correct this problem (57)
2. Vascular accident
   a. Thrombosis (**Fig. 31.19**) (58–61)
   b. Embolism/infarction (**Fig. 31.18** (17) seen days or weeks after line insertion (48)
   c. Vasospasm (17,48,62) is seen within minutes to a few hours after insertion.
   d. Loss of extremity (**Fig. 31.20**) (62,63)
   e. Hypertension (**Fig. 31.21**) (18,64)
   f. Abdominal aorta aneurysm (65)
   g. Paraplegia (66)
   h. Congestive heart failure (aortic thrombosis) (67)
   i. Air embolism (**Fig. 31.22**)
3. Equipment related
   a. Breaks in catheter and transection of catheter (68)
   b. Plasticizer in tissues (69,70)

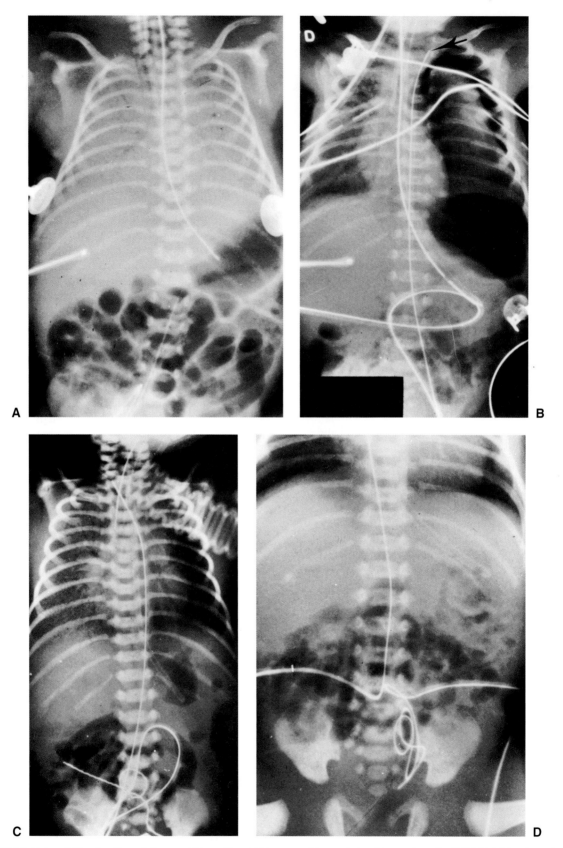

FIGURE 31.15 Various UAC malpositions. **A:** Unacceptable position at L2 because of the proximity of the renal arteries. **B:** UAC in left brachycephalic artery. **C:** UAC in right brachycephalic artery. **D:** UAC in pelvic artery.

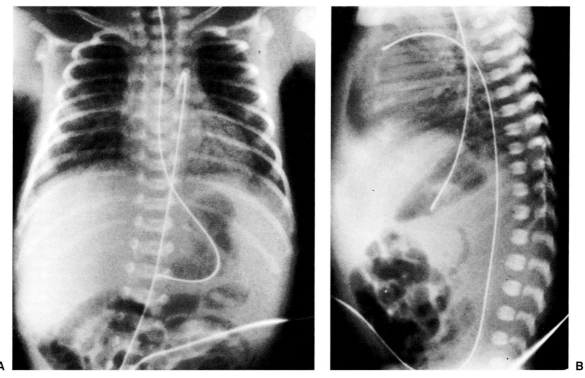

FIGURE 31.16 Anteroposterior (**A**) and lateral (**B**) radiographs demonstrating passage of a UAC into the pulmonary artery via a patent ductus arteriosus.

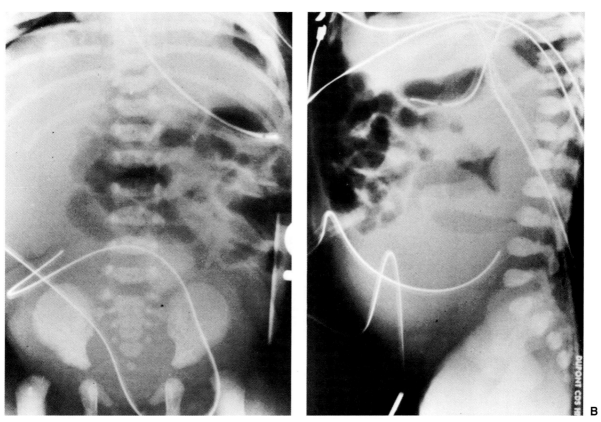

FIGURE 31.17 Effect of abdominal mass stimulating catheter misplacement. Anteroposterior (**A**) and lateral (**B**) films show remarkable displacement of a UAC by a giant hematocolpos in a 1-day-old infant.

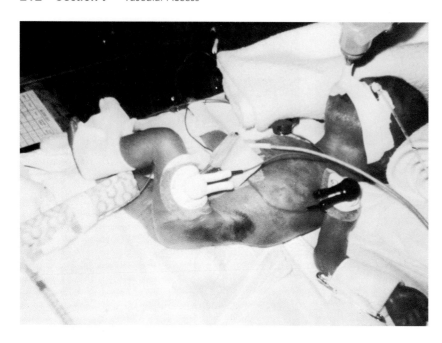

FIGURE 31.18 Vascular compromise in the left buttock and loin owing to a complication of a UAC displaced into the internal iliac artery. For vascular anatomy, see Figure 31.1.

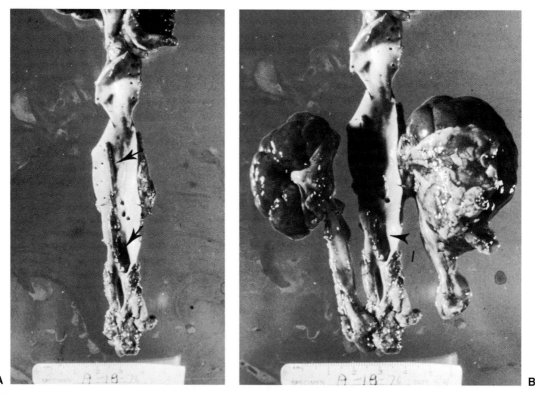

FIGURE 31.19 A: *Arrows* indicate mural thrombus in the abdominal aorta, which was associated with an umbilical arterial line. **B:** Upon further dissection of this autopsy specimen, the left renal artery was found to be occluded by thrombus. The left kidney is showing a degree of atrophy. Both kidneys showed scattered infarction.

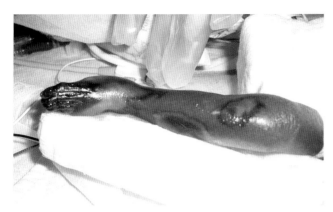

FIGURE 31.20 Vascular injury of the lower limb due to complication of a UAC.

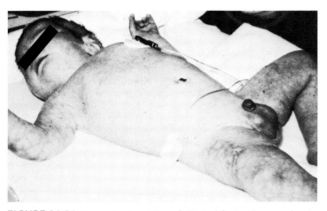

FIGURE 31.21 Generalized mottling of skin in infant with severe hypertension secondary to UAC-associated thrombus in renal artery.

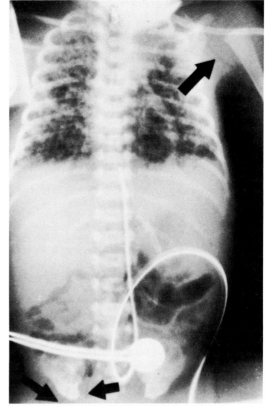

FIGURE 31.22 Anteroposterior roentgenogram demonstrating air embolism from a UAC in the left subclavian artery (*upper arrow*) and the femoral arteries (*lower arrows*).

   c. Electrical hazard
      (1) Improper grounding of electronic equipment
      (2) Conduction of current through fluid-filled catheter
   d. Intravascular knot in catheter (71)
  4. Other
   a. Hemorrhage (including that related to catheter loss or disconnection and overheparinization) (49,72,73)
   b. Infection (48)
   c. Necrotizing enterocolitis (44,62)
   d. Intestinal necrosis or perforation (74,75)
      (1) Vascular accident
      (2) Infusion of hypertonic solution (76)
   e. Transection of omphalocele **(Fig. 31.23)** (77)
   f. Herniation of appendix through umbilical ring (78)
   g. Cotton fiber embolus (79)
   h. Wharton jelly embolus (80)
   i. Hypernatremia
      (1) True
      (2) Factitious (70)
   j. Factitious hyperkalemia (70)
   k. Bladder injury (ascites) (41–43)

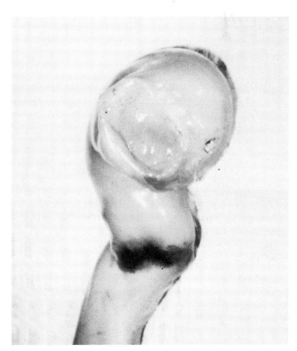

FIGURE 31.23 Small omphalocele. This gut-containing hernia was transected during placement of a UAC.

l. Curving back of the catheter on itself as a result of it catching in the intima (81)

m. Pseudocoarctation of the aorta (61)

n. Pseudomass in left atrium (82)

o. Displacement by thoracoabdominal abnormality (83)

References

1. Kanarek SK, Kuznicki MB, Blair RC. Infusion of total parenteral nutrition via the umbilical artery. *J Parenter Enter Nutr.* 1991;15:71–74.
2. Rand T, Weninger M, Kohlhauser C, et al. Effects of umbilical arterial catheterization on mesenteric hemodynamics. *Pediatr Radiol.* 1996;26:435–438.
3. Hecker JF, Scandrett LA. Roughness and thrombogenicity of the outer surfaces of intravascular catheters. *J Biomed Mater Res.* 1985;19(4):381–395.
4. Hecker JF. Thrombogenicity of tips of umbilical catheters. *Pediatrics.* 1981;67:467–471.
5. Boros SJ, Thompson TR, Reynolds JW, et al. Reduced thrombus formation with silicone elastomer (Silastic) umbilical artery catheters. *Pediatrics.* 1975;56:981–986.
6. Jackson JK, Derleth DP. Effects of various arterial infusion solutions on red blood cells in the newborn. *Arch Dis Child Fetal Neonatal Ed.* 2000;83:F130–F134.
7. Rajani K, Goetzman BW, Wennberg RP, et al. Effects of heparinization of fluids infused through an umbilical artery catheter on catheter patency and frequency of complications. *Pediatrics.* 1979;63:552–556.
8. Ankola PA, Atakent YS. Effect of adding heparin in very low concentration to the infusate to prolong the patency of umbilical artery catheters. *Am J Perinatol.* 1993;10:229–232.
9. Horgan MJ, Bartoletti A, Polansky S, et al. Effect of heparin infusates in umbilical arterial catheters on frequency of thrombotic complications. *J Pediatr.* 1987;111:774–778.
10. Butt W, Shann F, McDonnell G, et al. Effect of heparin concentration and infusion rate on the patency of arterial catheters. *Crit Care Med.* 1987;15:230–232.
11. Bosque E, Weaver L. Continuous versus intermittent heparin infusion of umbilical artery catheters in the newborn infant. *J Pediatr.* 1986;108:141–143.
12. Hentschel R, Weislock U, Von Lengerk C, et al. Coagulation-associated complications of indwelling arterial and central venous catheters during heparin prophylaxis: a prospective study. *Eur J Pediatr.* 1999;158:S126–S129.
13. Barrington KJ. Umbilical artery catheters in the newborn: effects of heparin. *Cochrane Database Syst Rev.* 2000;(2):CD000507.
14. Westrom G, Finstrom O, Stenport G. Umbilical artery catheterization in newborns: thrombosis in relation to catheter tip and position. *Acta Paediatr Scand.* 1979;68:575–581.
15. Sharma D, Farahbakhsh N, Tabatabaii SA. Role of ultrasound for central catheter tip localization in neonates: a review of the current evidence. *J Matern Fetal Neonatal Med.* 2019;32(14):2429–2437.
16. Baker DH, Berdon WE, James LS. Proper localization of umbilical arterial and venous catheters by lateral roentgenograms. *Pediatrics.* 1969;43:34–39.
17. Paster SB, Middleton P. Roentgenographic evaluation of umbilical artery and vein catheters. *JAMA.* 1975;231(7):742–746.
18. Mokrohisky ST, Levine RL, Blumhagen RD, et al. Low positioning of umbilical artery catheters increases associated complications in newborn infants. *N Engl J Med.* 1978;299:561–564.
19. Barrington KJ. Umbilical artery catheters in the newborn: effects of position of the catheter tip. *Cochrane Database Syst Rev.* 2000;(2):CD000505.
20. Dunn PM. Localization of the umbilical catheter by postmortem measurement. *Arch Dis Child.* 1966;41:69–75.
21. Rosenfeld W, Biagtan J, Schaeffer H, et al. A new graph for insertion of umbilical artery catheters. *J Pediatr.* 1980;96:735–737.
22. Rosenfeld W, Estrada R, Jhaveri R, et al. Evaluation of graphs for insertion of umbilical artery catheters below the diaphragm. *J Pediatr.* 1981;98:627–628.
23. Shukla H, Ferrara A. Rapid estimation of insertional length of umbilical catheters in newborns. *Am J Dis Child.* 1986;140:786–788.
24. Wright IM, Owers M, Wagner M. The umbilical arterial catheter: a formula for improved positioning in the very low birth weight infant. *Pediatr Crit Care Med.* 2008;9(5):498–501.
25. Vali P, Fleming SE, Kim JH. Determination of umbilical catheter placement using anatomic landmarks. *Neonatology.* 2010;98(4):381–386.
26. Gupta AO, Peesay MR, Ramasethu J. Simple measurements to place umbilical catheters using surface anatomy. *J Perinatol.* 2015;35(7):476–480.
27. Verheij GH, Te Pas AB, Witlox RS, et al. Poor accuracy of methods currently used to determine umbilical catheter insertion length. *Int J Pediatr.* 2010;2010:873167.
28. Kumar PP, Kumar CD, Nayak M, et al. Umbilical arterial catheter insertion length: in quest of a universal formula. *J Perinatol.* 2012;32(8):604–607.
29. Min SR, Lee HS. Comparison of Wright's formula and the Dunn method for measuring the umbilical arterial catheter insertion length. *Pediatr Neonatol.* 2015;56(2):120–125.
30. Kieran EA, Laffan EE, O'Donnell CP. Estimating umbilical catheter insertion depth in newborns using weight or body measurement: a randomised trial. *Arch Dis Child Fetal Neonatal Ed.* 2016;101(1):F10–F15.
31. Lean WL, Dawson JA, Davis PG, et al. Accuracy of 11 formulae to guide umbilical arterial catheter tip placement in newborn infants. *Arch Dis Child Fetal Neonatal Ed.* 2018;103(4):F364–F369.
32. Neri I, Ravaioli GM, Faldella G, et al. Chlorhexidine-induced chemical burns in very low birth weight infants. *J Pediatr.* 2017;191:262–265.e2.
33. Paternoster M, Niola M, Graziano V. Avoiding chlorhexidine burns in preterm infants. *J Obstet Gynecol Neonatal Nurs.* 2017;46(2):267–271.
34. Elser HE. Options for securing umbilical catheters. *Adv Neonatal Care.* 2013;13(6):426–429.
35. Bloom BT, Nelson RA, Dirksen HC. A new technique: umbilical arterial catheter placement. *J Perinatol.* 1986;6:174.
36. Gupta V, Kumar N, Jana AK, et al. A modified technique for umbilical arterial catheterization. *Indian Pediatr.* 2014;51(8):672.

37. Squire SJ, Hornung TL, Kirchhoff KT. Comparing two methods of umbilical artery catheter placement. *Am J Perinatol.* 1990;7:8–12.

38. Sherman NJ. Umbilical artery cutdown. *J Pediatr Surg.* 1977; 12:723–724.

39. Hashimoto T, Togari H, Yura J. Umbilical artery cutdown: an improved procedure for reinsertion. *Br J Surg.* 1985;72:194.

40. Waffarn F, Devaskar UP, Hodgman JE. Vesico-umbilical fistula: a complication of umbilical artery cutdown. *J Pediatr Surg.* 1980;15:211.

41. Mata JA, Livne PM, Gibbons MD. Urinary ascites: complication of umbilical artery catheterization. *Urology.* 1987;30:375–377.

42. Diamond DA, Ford C. Neonatal bladder rupture: a complication of umbilical artery catheterization. *J Urol.* 1989;142:1543–1544.

43. Nagarajan VP. Neonatal bladder injury after umbilical artery catheterization by cutdown. *JAMA.* 1984;252:765.

44. Lehmiller DJ, Kanto WP Jr. Relationships of mesenteric thromboembolism, oral feeding and necrotizing enterocolitis. *J Pediatr.* 1978;92:96–100.

45. Davey AM, Wagner CL, Cox C, et al. Feeding premature infants while low umbilical artery catheters are in place: a prospective, randomized trial. *J Pediatr.* 1994;124:795–799.

46. Havranek T, Johanboeke P, Madramootoo C, et al. Umbilical artery catheters do not affect intestinal blood flow responses to minimal enteral feedings. *J Perinatol.* 2007;27(6):375–379.

47. Davies MW, Mehr S, Morley CJ. The effect of draw-up volume on the accuracy of electrolyte measurements from neonatal arterial lines. *J Pediatr Child Health.* 2000;36:122–124.

48. Hermansen MC, Hermansen MG. Intravascular catheter complications in the neonatal intensive care unit. *Clin Perinatol.* 2005;32:141–156.

49. Miller D, Kirkpatrick BV, Kodroff M, et al. Pelvic exsanguination following umbilical artery catheterization in neonates. *J Pediatr Surg.* 1979;14:264–269.

50. Ramasethu J. Complications of vascular catheters in the neonatal intensive care unit. *Clin Perinatol.* 2008;35:199–222.

51. Chidi CC, King DR, Boles ET Jr. An ultrastructural study of intimal injury induced by an indwelling umbilical artery catheter. *J Pediatr Surg.* 1983;18:109–115.

52. Clark JM, Jung AL. Umbilical artery catheterization by a cut down procedure. *Pediatrics.* 1977;59:1036.

53. Carey BE, Zeilinger TC. Hypoglycemia due to high positioning of umbilical artery catheters. *J Perinatol.* 1989;9:407–410.

54. Van Leeuwen G, Patney M. Complications of umbilical artery catheterization: peritoneal perforation. *Pediatrics.* 1969;44:1028–1030.

55. Wyers MR, McAlister WH. Umbilical artery catheter use complicated by pseudoaneurysm of the aorta. *Pediatr Radiol.* 2002;32:199–201.

56. Giannakopoulou C, Korakaki E, Hatzidaki E, et al. Peroneal nerve palsy: a complication of umbilical artery catheterization in the full-term newborn of a mother with diabetes. *Pediatrics.* 2002;109:e66.

57. Schreiber MD, Perez CA, Kitterman JA. A double-catheter technique for caudally misdirected umbilical arterial catheters. *J Pediatr.* 1984;104:768–769.

58. Seibert JJ, Northington FJ, Miers JF, et al. Aortic thrombosis after umbilical artery catheterization in neonates: prevalence of complications on long-term follow-up. *AJR.* 1991;156:567–569.

59. Rizzi M, Goldenberg N, Bonduel M, et al. Catheter-related arterial thrombosis in neonates and children: a systematic review. *Thromb Haemost.* 2018;118(6):1058–1066.

60. Greenberg R, Waldman D, Brooks C, et al. Endovascular treatment of renal artery thrombosis caused by umbilical artery catheterization. *J Vasc Surg.* 1998;28:949–953.

61. Francis JV, Monagle P, Hope S, et al. Occlusive aortic arch thrombus in a preterm neonate. *Pediatr Crit Care Med.* 2010;11:e13–e15.

62. Gupta JM, Roberton NR, Wigglesworth JS. Umbilical artery catheterization in the newborn. *Arch Dis Child.* 1968;43:382–387.

63. Gallotti R, Cammock CE, Dixon N, et al. Neonatal ascending aortic thrombus: successful medical treatment. *Cardiol Young.* 2013;23(4):610–612.

64. Bauer SB, Feldman SM, Gellis SS, et al. Neonatal hypertension: a complication of umbilical artery catheterization. *N Engl J Med.* 1975;293:1032–1033.

65. Mendeloff J, Stallion A, Hutton M, et al. Aortic aneurysm resulting from umbilical artery catheterization: case report, literature review, and management algorithm. *J Vasc Surg.* 2001;33(2):419–424.

66. Muñoz ME, Roche C, Escribá R, et al. Flaccid paraplegia as complication of umbilical artery catheterization. *Pediatr Neurol.* 1993;9:401–403.

67. Henry CG, Gutierrez F, Joseph I, et al. Aortic thrombosis presenting as congestive heart failure: an umbilical artery catheter complication. *J Pediatr.* 1981;98:820–822.

68. Dilli D, Ozyazici E, Fettah N, et al. Rupture and displacement of umbilical arterial catheter: bilateral arterial occlusion in a very low birth weight preterm. *Arch Argent Pediatr.* 2015;113(5):e283–e285.

69. Hillman LS, Goodwin SL, Sherman WR. Identification of plasticizer in neonatal tissues after umbilical catheters and blood products. *N Engl J Med.* 1975;292:381–386.

70. Gaylord MS, Pittman PA, Bartness J, et al. Release of benzalkonium chloride from a heparin-bonded umbilical catheter with resultant factitious hypernatremia and hyperkalemia. *Pediatrics.* 1991;87:631–635.

71. Cochrane WD. Umbilical artery catheterization. In: *Iatrogenic Problems in Neonatal Intensive Care. Report of the 69th Ross Conference of Pediatric Research.* Columbus, OH: Ross Laboratories; 1976:28.

72. Johnson JF, Basilio FS, Pettett PG, et al. Hemoperitoneum secondary to umbilical artery catheterization in the newborn. *Radiology.* 1980;134:60.

73. Moncino MD, Kurtzberg J. Accidental heparinization in the newborn: a case report and brief review of the literature. *J Perinatol.* 1990;10:399–402.

74. Hwang H, Murphy JJ, Gow KW, et al. Are localized intestinal perforations distinct from necrotizing enterocolitis? *J Pediatr Surg.* 2003;38:763–767.

75. Hoekstra RE, Semba T, Fangman JJ, et al. Intestinal perforation following withdrawal of umbilical artery catheter. *J Pediatr.* 1977;90(2):290.

76. Book LS, Herbst JJ. Intraarterial infusions and intestinal necrosis in the rabbit: potential hazards of umbilical artery injections of ampicillin, glucose, and sodium bicarbonate. *Pediatrics.* 1980;65:1145–1149.

77. Simpson JS. Misdiagnosis complicating umbilical vessel catheterization. *Clin Pediatr.* 1977;16:569.

78. Biagtan J, Rosenfeld W, Salazard D, et al. Herniation of the appendix through the umbilical ring following umbilical artery catheterization. *J Pediatr Surg.* 1980;15:672–673.

79. Bavikatte K, Hillard J, Schreiner RL, et al. Systemic vascular cotton fiber emboli in the neonate. *J Pediatr.* 1979;95:614–616.

80. Abramowsky CR, Chrenka B, Fanaroff A. Wharton jelly embolism: an unusual complication of umbilical catheterization. *J Pediatr.* 1980;96:739–741.

81. McGravey VJ, Dabiri C, Bean MS. An unusual twist to umbilical artery catheterization. *Clin Pediatr (Phila).* 1983;22:587–588.

82. Crie JS, Hajar R, Folger G. Umbilical catheter masquerading at echocardiography as a left atrial mass. *Clin Cardiol.* 1989;12:728–730.

83. Sakurai M, Donnelly LF, Klosterman LA, et al. Congenital diaphragmatic hernia in neonates: variations in umbilical catheter and enteric tube position. *Radiology.* 2000;216:112–116.

CHAPTER
32

Umbilical Vein Catheterization

Suna Seo

A. Indications

1. Primary
   a. Emergency vascular access for fluid and medication infusion and for blood drawing
   b. Long-term central venous access in low-birth-weight infants
   c. Exchange transfusion
2. Secondary
   a. Central venous pressure monitoring (if catheter across ductus venosus) (1)
   b. Diagnosis of total anomalous pulmonary venous drainage below the diaphragm (2,3)

B. Contraindications

1. Omphalitis
2. Omphalocele
3. Necrotizing enterocolitis
4. Peritonitis

C. Equipment

1. Catheter—same as for umbilical artery catheterization, except:
   a. 3.5-Fr catheter for infants weighing <3.5 kg
   b. 5-Fr catheter for infants weighing >3.5 kg
   c. Double lumen umbilical venous catheters may be used in critically ill neonates to allow administration of inotropes or medications
   d. Catheters used for exchange transfusion (removed after procedure) should have side holes. This reduces risk of sucking the thin wall of inferior vena cava against catheter tip, with possible vascular perforation (4). Avoid double lumen catheters for exchange transfusions (see Chapter 49)

2. Other equipment as for umbilical artery catheter, but omit 2% lidocaine (see Chapter 31, C)

D. Precautions

1. If the line is to be used long term, particularly if parenteral nutrition is to be infused by this route, the same aseptic techniques must be used to prevent line-related sepsis as are used for any central venous line (see Chapter 34).
2. Keep catheter tip away from origin of hepatic vessels, portal vein, and foramen ovale. Ideally, the catheter tip should lie at the junction of the inferior vena cava and the right atrium. The tip should be at least well into the ductus venosus to protect the liver from receiving inappropriate infusions (5). Sometimes it will not be possible to advance the catheter through the ductus venosus. Vigorous attempts to advance are to be avoided. In an emergency, vital infusions (avoid very hypertonic solutions) may be given slowly after pulling catheter back into umbilical vein (approximately 2 cm) and checking blood return.
3. Check catheter position prior to exchange transfusion. Avoid performing exchange transfusion with catheter tip in portal system or intrahepatic venous branch (see **Fig. 32.1**).
4. Once secured, do not advance catheter into vein.
5. Avoid infusion of hypertonic solutions when catheter tip is not in the inferior vena cava.
6. Do not leave catheter open to atmosphere (danger of air embolus).
7. Avoid using a central venous pressure monitoring catheter for concomitant infusion of parenteral nutrition (risk of sepsis).
8. Be aware of potential inaccuracies of venous pressure measurements with the catheter tip in the inferior vena cava.

217

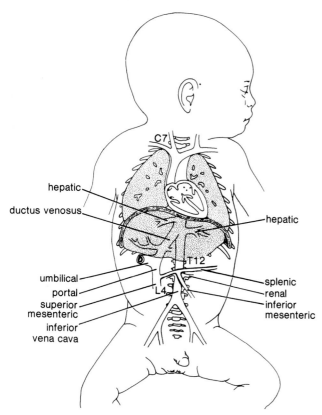

FIGURE 32.1 Anatomy of the umbilical and associated veins, with reference to external landmarks.

TABLE 32.1 Available Formulae to Estimate UVC Insertion Length (cm)

NAME	FORMULAE
Dunn (6)	Nomogram using shoulder–umbilicus length*
Shukla (7)	$\dfrac{3 \times \text{weight (kg)} + 9}{2} + 1$
Vali (8)	Measurement from the umbilicus to the mid-xiphoid-to-bed distance on the lateral aspect of the abdomen
Verheij (9)	$\dfrac{3 \times \text{weight (kg)} + 9}{2}$
Gupta (10)	Umbilicus to nipple length* – 1

*See Figure. 31.5.

consistent accuracy across infants of all birth-weight and gestational ages (11), and catheter tip placement must be verified (see 11 and 12 below).

2. Prepare for procedure as with umbilical artery catheter (see Chapter 31, E).
3. Identify thin-walled vein, close to periphery of umbilical stump (**Fig. 32.2**).

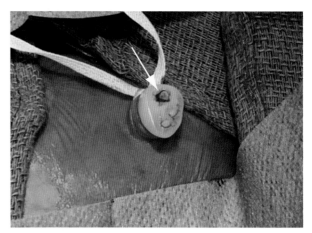

FIGURE 32.2 The umbilical stump. Vein is indicated with an *arrow*.

4. Grasp cord stump with toothed forceps.
5. Gently insert tips of iris forceps into lumen of vein and remove any clots.
6. Introduce fluid-filled catheter, attached to the stopcock and syringe, 2 to 3 cm into vein (measuring from anterior abdominal wall).
7. Apply gentle suction to syringe.
   a. If there is no easy blood return, the catheter may have a clot in the tip. Withdraw the catheter while maintaining gentle suction. Remove clot and reinsert catheter.

E. Technique (See ▶ Video 31.1: Umbilical Vein and Artery Catheterization)

Umbilical venous catheters may be placed within 5 to 7 days of birth, and occasionally up to 10 days after birth.

Anatomic note: In the full-term infant, the umbilical vein is 2 to 3 cm in length and 4 to 5 mm in diameter. From the umbilicus, it passes cephalad and slightly to the right, where it joins the portal sinus, a confluence of the umbilical vein with the right and left intrahepatic portal veins. The portal veins have intrahepatic branches that are distributed directly to the liver tissue. The ductus venosus becomes a continuation of the umbilical vein by arising from the left branch of the portal vein, directly opposite where the umbilical vein joins it. The ductus is located in a groove between the right and left lobes of the liver in the median sagittal plane of the body, at a level between the 9th and 10th thoracic vertebrae; it terminates in the inferior vena cava along with hepatic veins, as shown in **Figure 32.1**.

1. Make necessary measurements to determine length of catheter to be inserted, adding length of umbilical stump (6–10). Many formulas and measurements (**Table 32.1**) (see Chapter 31, Fig. 31.5) have been derived to predict the accurate placement of umbilical catheters; however, there is no universal formula, measurement, or nomogram that can be applied with

b. If there is smooth blood flow, continue to insert catheter for full estimated distance.

8. If catheter meets any obstruction prior to measured distance
   a. It has most commonly
      (1) Entered portal system, or
      (2) Wedged in an intrahepatic branch of portal vein
   b. Withdraw catheter 2 to 3 cm, gently rotate, and reinsert in an attempt to get tip through the ductus venosus.

9. If the catheter is in the portal circulation, some authors have recommended passing a new 3.5- or 5-Fr catheter into the same vessel, while leaving the misdirected catheter in its place. Once the new catheter is in a good position, remove the misdirected catheter. This procedure is reported to have a 50% success rate (12). No adverse events including perforation or internal bleeding were reported; however, in extremely low-birth-weight infants, inserting two catheters into small vessels concurrently could cause vessel damage.

10. The catheter tip position may be estimated by measurement of venous pressure (1–3) and observation of waveform. However, this is not routinely performed, with most centers performing radiographic or ultrasound confirmation of catheter position. The catheter has crossed the foramen ovale if the blood obtained is bright red (arterial in appearance). In this case, pull the catheter back. The ideal position is with the catheter tip at the junction of the inferior vena cava and the right atrium, although placement in ductus venosus is acceptable for purposes other than measurement of central venous pressure.

11. Obtain radiographic verification of catheter position. A lateral radiograph will aid in localization (**Fig. 32.3**) (13,14). The desired location is T9 to T10, just above the right diaphragm.

12. Other modalities to evaluate catheter placement include ultrasound (15–17) and echocardiography (18,19). These techniques may require fewer manipulations during catheter placement and reduce the number of x-rays a patient receives. Additionally, these types of imaging techniques may provide a more accurate assessment of catheter location.

13. Secure catheter as for umbilical artery catheter (see Chapter 31, E).

There may be more bleeding from the umbilical vein than from the umbilical artery because the vein is not a contractile vessel. Local pressure is usually sufficient to stop oozing. For care of an indwelling catheter, sampling techniques, and removal of a catheter, see Chapter 31.

F. Complications

1. Infections (20)
2. Thromboembolic (21)

Emboli from a venous catheter may be widely distributed. If the catheter tip lies in the portal system and the ductus venosus has closed, emboli will lodge in the liver. If the catheter has passed through ductus venosus, emboli will go to the lungs or, because of right-to-left shunting of blood through foramen ovale or ductus arteriosus in sick newborn infants, emboli may

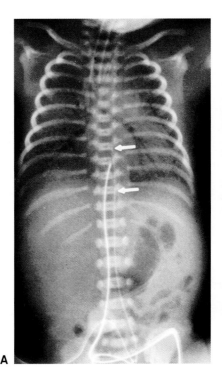
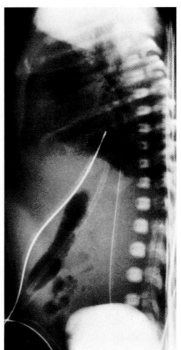

FIGURE 32.3 Anteroposterior (**A**) and lateral (**B**) radiographs demonstrating the normal course of an umbilical venous catheter, with an umbilical artery catheter (*arrows*) in position for comparison. Note how the venous catheter swings immediately superior from the umbilicus, slightly to the right as it traverses the ductus venosus into the inferior vena cava (IVC). The distal tip of this line is just superior to the right atrial–IVC junction, and it might optimally be pulled back slightly into the IVC. Note how the thinner umbilical artery catheter (*arrows*) heads inferiorly as it proceeds to the iliac artery and then ascends posteriorly and to the left until it reaches the level of T7.

A   B

be distributed throughout entire systemic circulation. These emboli may be infected and, therefore, may cause widespread abscesses.

3. Catheter malpositioned in heart and great vessels **(Fig. 32.4)**
   a. Pericardial effusion/cardiac tamponade (cardiac perforation) (5,18,22)
   b. Cardiac arrhythmias (23)
   c. Left atrial thrombus (18)
   d. Thrombotic endocarditis (24)
   e. Hemorrhagic infarction of lung (25)
   f. Hydrothorax (catheter lodged in or perforated pulmonary vein) (25)

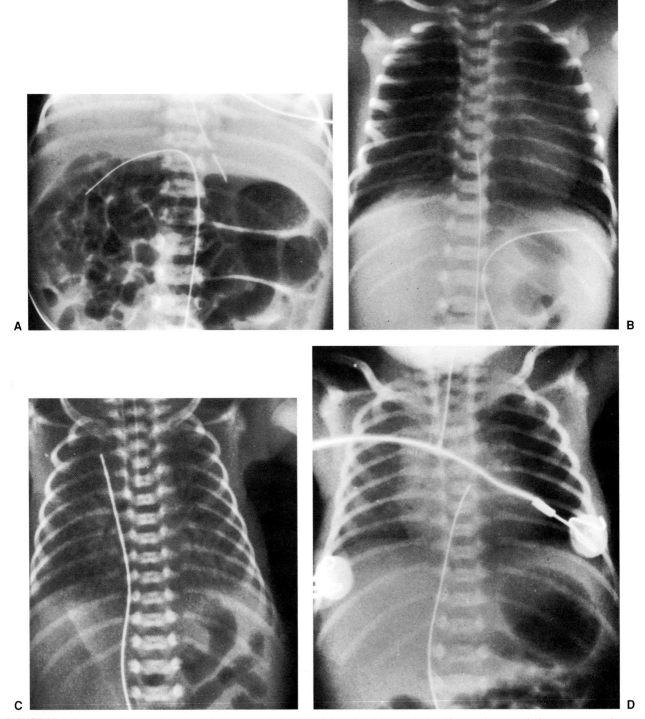

FIGURE 32.4 Spectrum of malpositions of umbilical venous catheters (UVCs). **A:** UVC in right portal vein with secondary air embolization into portal venous system. **B:** UVC in splenic vein. UAC catheter in good position with its tip at T7. **C:** UVC extending through heart into the superior vena cava. **D:** The anteroposterior film shows an indeterminate position of the UVC. The right atrium, the right ventricle, and the left atrium are all possibilities.

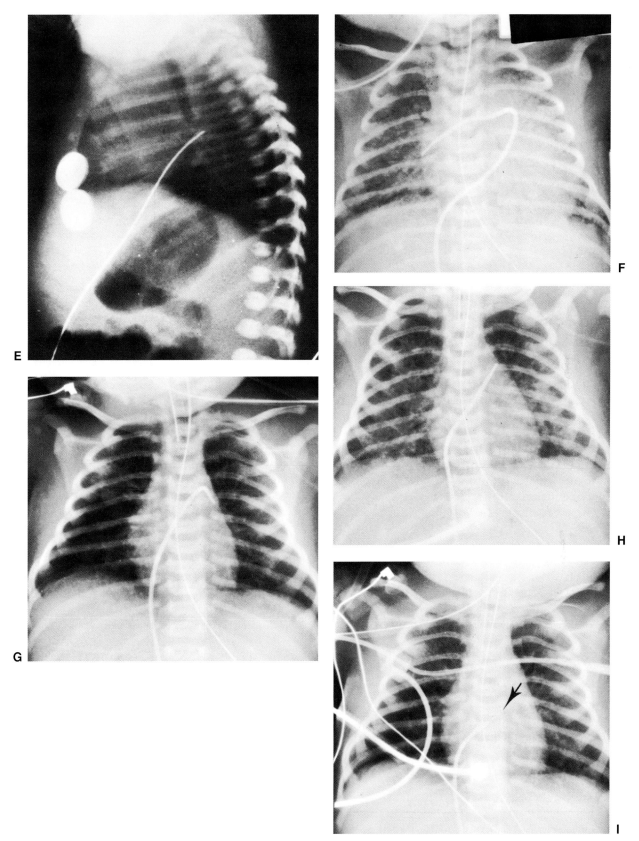

FIGURE 32.4 (*Continued*) **E:** The lateral film shows its posterior position, confirming its presence in the left atrium. The lateral film is particularly important in making this distinction. Measurement of the PO_2 in blood from the catheter will be diagnostic of misplacement, unless the infant has severe persistent pulmonary hypertension or other cause of severe intracardiac shunting. **F:** UVC in right pulmonary artery. **G:** UVC in left main pulmonary artery. **H:** UVC in main pulmonary artery. **I:** UVC (*arrow*) in right ventricle.

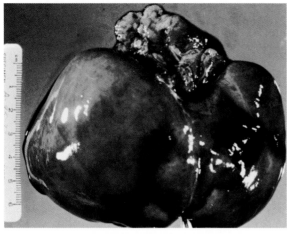
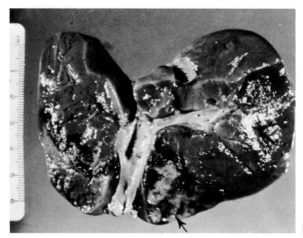

FIGURE 32.5 A: Hepatic infarction (darkened areas on anterior aspect of liver) related to umbilical vein catheter. **B:** Section through inferior aspect of liver to show internal appearance of infarcted areas (*arrow*).

4. Catheter malpositioned in portal system
   a. Hepatomegaly (26)
   b. Necrotizing enterocolitis (27)
   c. Perforation of colon (28)
   d. Hepatic necrosis (thrombosis of hepatic veins or infusion of hypertonic or vasospastic solutions into liver tissues) **(Fig. 32.5)** (26,29,30)
   e. Hepatic cyst (31)
   f. Hepatic abscess (32)
   g. Hepatic hematoma (33)
   h. Intra-abdominal hemorrhage (32)
   i. Ascites (secondary to extravasation of fluid through malpositioned catheter) (32,34)
   j. Hepatic laceration (17,35)
5. Other
   a. Perforation of peritoneum (36)
   b. Parenteral nutrition fluid extravasation (34)
   c. Obstruction of pulmonary venous return (in infant with anomalous pulmonary venous drainage) (2,3)
   d. Plasticizer in tissues (37)
   e. Portal hypertension (26,38)
   f. Electrical hazard (see Chapter 31, J3c) (4)
   g. Fungal mass in right atrium (39,40)
   h. Pseudomass in left atrium (41)
   i. Digital ischemia (42)
   j. Pneumopericardium (43)
   k. Catheter breakage and embolization (44)
   l. Hypothermia (45)

References

1. Trevor Inglis GD, Dunster KR, Davies MW. Establishing normal values of central venous pressure in very low birth weight infants. *Physiol Meas.* 2007;28(10):1283–1291.
2. Jones AJ, Zieba K, Starling L, et al. A clue to the diagnosis of TAPVD. *BMJ Case Rep.* 2012;2012:pii: bcr1220115400.
3. Rugolotto S, Beghini R, Padovani EM. Serendipitous diagnosis of infracardiac total anomalous pulmonary venous return by umbilical venous catheter blood gas samples. *J Perinatol.* 2004;24(5):315–316.
4. Kitterman JA, Phibbs RH, Tooley WH. Catheterization of umbilical vessels in newborn infants. *Pediatr Clin North Am.* 1970;17:895–912.
5. Oestreich AE. Umbilical vein catheterization—appropriate and inappropriate placement. *Pediatr Radiol.* 2010;40: 1941–1949.
6. Dunn P. Localization of the umbilical catheter by post-mortem measurement. *Arch Dis Child.* 1966;41:69–75.
7. Shukla H, Ferrara A. Rapid estimation of insertional length of umbilical catheters in newborns. *Am J Dis Child.* 1986; 140:786–788.
8. Vali P, Fleming SE, Kim JH. Determination of umbilical catheter placement using anatomic landmarks. *Neonatology.* 2010;98:381–386.
9. Verheij GH, te Pas AB, Smits-Wintjens VE, et al. Revised formula to determine the insertion length of umbilical vein catheters. *Eur J Pediatr.* 2013;172:1011–1015.
10. Gupta AO, Peesay MR, Ramasethu J. Simple measurements to place umbilical catheters using surface anatomy. *J Perinatol.* 2015;35(7):476–480.
11. Lean WL, Dawson JA, Davis PG, et al. Accuracy of five formulae to determine the insertion length of umbilical venous catheters. *Arch Dis Child Fetal Neonatal Ed.* 2019;104(2): F165–F169.
12. Mandel D, Mimouni FB, Littner Y, et al. Double catheter technique for misdirected umbilical vein catheter. *J Pediatr.* 2001;139:591–592.
13. Baker DH, Berdon WE, James LS. Proper localization of umbilical arterial and venous catheters by lateral roentgenograms. *Pediatrics.* 1969;43:34–39.
14. Hoellering AB, Koorts PJ, Cartwright DW, et al. Determination of umbilical venous catheter tip position with radiograph. *Pediatr Crit Care Med.* 2014;15(1):56–61.
15. Franta J, Harabor A, Soraisham AS. Ultrasound assessment of umbilical venous catheter migration in preterm infants: a prospective study. *Arch Dis Child Fetal Neonatal Ed.* 2017;102(3):F251–F255.

16. Selvam S, Humphrey T, Woodley H, et al. Sonographic features of umbilical catheter-related complications. *Pediatr Radiol*. 2018;48(13):1964–1970.

17. Derinkuyu BE, Boyunaga OL, Damar C, et al. Hepatic complications of umbilical venous catheters in the neonatal period: the ultrasound spectrum. *J Ultrasound Med*. 2018;37(6):1335–1344.

18. Abiramalatha T, Kumar M, Shabeer MP, et al. Advantages of being diligent: lessons learnt from umbilical venous catheterisation in neonates. *BMJ Case Rep*. 2016;2016:pii: bcr2015214073.

19. Plooij-Lusthusz AM, van Vreeswijk N, van Stuijvenberg M, et al. Migration of umbilical venous catheters [Epub ahead of print]. *Am J Perinatol*. 2019. doi: 10.1055/s-0038-1677016.

20. Gordon A, Greenhalgh M, McGuire W. Early planned removal of umbilical venous catheters to prevent infection in newborn infants. *Cochrane Database Syst Rev*. 2017;10:CD012142.

21. Raad II, Luna M, Kaliel SA, et al. The relationship between the thrombotic and infectious complications of central venous catheters. *JAMA*. 1994;271:1014–1016.

22. Chioukh FZ, Ameur KB, Hmida HB, et al. Pericardial effusion with cardiac tamponade caused by a central venous catheter in a very low birth weight infant. *Pan Afr Med J*. 2016;25:13.

23. Amer A, Broadbent RS, Edmonds L, et al. Central venous catheter-related tachycardia in the newborn: case report and literature review. *Case Rep Med*. 2016;2016:6206358.

24. Symchych PS, Krauss AN, Winchester P. Endocarditis following intracardiac placement of umbilical venous catheters in neonates. *J Pediatr*. 1977;90:287–289.

25. Bjorklund LJ, Malmgren N, Lindroth M. Pulmonary complications of umbilical venous catheters. *Pediatr Radiol*. 1995;25(2):149–152.

26. Grizelj R, Vukovic J, Bojanic K, et al. Severe liver injury while using umbilical venous catheter: case series and literature review. *Am J Perinatol*. 2014;31(11):965–974.

27. Sulemanji M, Vakili K, Zurakowski D, et al. Umbilical venous catheter malposition is associated with necrotizing enterocolitis in premature infants. *Neonatology*. 2017;111(4):337–343.

28. Friedman AB, Abellera RM, Lidsky I, et al. Perforation of the colon after exchange transfusion in the newborn. *N Engl J Med*. 1970;282:796.

29. Venkatavaman PS, Babcock DS, Tsang RC, et al. Hepatic injury: a possible complication of dopamine infusion through an inappropriately placed umbilical vein catheter. *Am J Perinatol*. 1984;1:351–354.

30. Hargitai B, Toldi G, Marton T, et al. Pathophysiological mechanism of extravasation via umbilical venous catheters. *Pediatr Dev Pathol*. 2019;22(4):340–343.

31. Hartley M, Ruppa Mohanram G, Ahmed I. TPNoma: an unusual complication of umbilical venous catheter malposition. *Arch Dis Child Fetal Neonatal Ed*. 2019;104(3):F326.

32. Bayhan C, Takci S, Ciftci TT, et al. Sterile hepatic abscess due to umbilical venous catheterization. *Turk J Pediatr*. 2012;54(6):671–673.

33. Fuchs EM, Sweeney AG, Schmidt JW. Umbilical venous catheter-induced hepatic hematoma in neonates. *J Neonatal Perinatal Med*. 2014;7(2):137–142.

34. Pegu S, Murthy P. Ascites with hepatic extravasation of total parenteral nutrition (TPN) secondary to umbilical venous catheter (UVC) malposition in an extremely preterm baby. *BMJ Case Rep*. 2018;2018:pii: bcr-2018-226377.

35. Pignotti MS, Monciotti F, Frati P, et al. Hepatic laceration due to umbilical venous catheter malpositioning. *Pediatr Neonatol*. 2017;58(4):386–387.

36. Kanto WP Jr, Parrish RA Jr. Perforation of the peritoneum and intraabdominal hemorrhage: a complication of umbilical vein catheterizations. *Am J Dis Child*. 1977;131:1102–1103.

37. Hillman LS, Goodwin SL, Sherwin WR. Identification and measurement of plasticizer in neonatal tissues after umbilical catheters and blood products. *N Engl J Med*. 1975;292:381–386.

38. Lauridsen UB, Enk B, Gammeltoft A. Oesophageal varices as a late complication of neonatal umbilical vein catheterization. *Acta Paediatr Scand*. 1978;67:633–636.

39. Johnson DE, Bass JL, Thomson TR, et al. Candida septicemia and right atrial mass secondary to umbilical vein catheterization. *Am J Dis Child*. 1981;135:275–277.

40. Shalabi M, Adel M, Yoon E, et al. Risk of infection using peripherally inserted central and umbilical catheters in preterm neonates. *Pediatrics*. 2015;136(6):1073–1079.

41. Crie JS, Hajar R, Folger G. Umbilical catheter masquerading at echocardiography as a left atrial mass. *Clin Cardiol*. 1989;12:728–730.

42. Welibae MA, Moore JH Jr. Digital ischemia in the neonate following intravenous therapy. *Pediatrics*. 1985;76:99–103.

43. Long WA. Pneumopericardium. In: Long WA, ed. *Fetal and Neonatal Cardiology*. Philadelphia, PA: WB Saunders; 1990:382.

44. Akin A, Bilici M, Demir F, et al. Percutaneous retrieval of umbilical vein catheter fragment in an infant two months after embolization. *Turk J Pediatr*. 2018;60(2):191–193.

45. Dubbink-Verheij GH, van Westerop TAJWM, Lopriore E, et al. Hypothermia during umbilical catheterization in preterm infants. *J Matern Fetal Neonatal Med*. 2019:1–6.

Peripheral Arterial Cannulation

Suhasini Kaushal and Jayashree Ramasethu

Arterial access is required for continuous hemodynamic monitoring and blood sampling when caring for a sick neonate. When it is not possible to catheterize the umbilical artery for either technical or clinical reasons, peripheral arterial cannulation may be required. As a rule, the most peripheral/distal artery should be used, to reduce potential sequelae from any associated vascular compromise or thromboembolic event.

Common sites for peripheral arterial cannulation include the radial, ulnar, and posterior tibial arteries (1–4). The dorsalis pedis artery is occasionally used (5). Although cannulation of the axillary (6) and brachial (7) arteries have been described, these sites are not recommended because of the limited collateral blood flow and high potential for ischemic complications. The temporal artery is also usually avoided because of the potential for neurologic sequelae (8,9).

A. Indications

1. Monitoring of arterial blood pressure
2. Frequent monitoring of blood gases or laboratory tests (e.g., critically ill ventilated neonates or extremely low–birth-weight premature infants)
3. When preductal monitoring is required (e.g., with persistent pulmonary hypertension) (right upper extremity cannulation)

B. Contraindications

1. Bleeding disorder that cannot be corrected
2. Pre-existing evidence of circulatory insufficiency in limb being used for cannulation
3. Evidence of inadequate collateral flow (i.e., occlusion of the vessel to be catheterized may compromise perfusion of extremity)
4. Local skin infection

5. Malformation of the extremity being used for cannulation
6. Previous surgery in the area (especially cut down)
7. Potential for adverse neurologic sequelae following cannulation

C. Equipment

Sterile

1. Gloves
2. Antiseptic solution (e.g., iodophor/povidone, chlorhexidine)
3. 4- × 4-in gauze squares
4. 0.5 to 0.95 normal saline (NS) with 1 to 2 U/mL heparin). Quarter NS (0.25 N saline) is often used in extremely preterm infants <24 weeks' gestational age, who are at risk for hypernatremia. Using heparinized saline has been shown to maintain line patency longer than hypotonic solutions such as heparinized 5% dextrose water or unheparinized NS (10,11)
5. 3- or 5-mL syringe
6. 20-gauge venipuncture needle (if using larger-sized 22-gauge cannula)
7. Appropriate-sized cannula: 22-gauge × 1-in (2.5 cm), 24-gauge × 0.75 in, or 24-gauge × 0.56 in tapered or nontapered cannula with stylet for larger to smaller neonates, respectively
8. Arterial pressure transducer and extension tubing (see Chapter 10)
9. T connector primed with heparinized flush solution
10. Transparent, semipermeable dressing

Non Sterile

1. Equipment for transillumination or Doppler ultrasound (12) (see Chapter 15)
2. 0.5 in, water-resistant adhesive tape

3. Materials for restraint of limb following arterial cannulation (see Chapter 5)
4. A constant-infusion pump capable of delivering flush solution at rate of 0.5 to 1 mL/hr against back pressure

Additional Equipment Required for Cut-Down Procedure

All equipment except mask must be sterile.

1. Gown and mask
2. 0.5% lidocaine hydrochloride in labeled 3-mL syringe
3. No. 11 scalpel and holder
4. Two curved mosquito hemostats
5. Nerve hook
6. 5-0 nylon suture

Anesthesia/Analgesia

Eutectic mixture of lidocaine–prilocaine (EMLA) cream 2.5% may be applied for local anesthesia prior to placing arterial line in addition to sedation in critical infants.

Ultrasound Guided Peripheral Arterial Cannulation

With the advent of point of care ultrasound at the bedside, linear probes have been used in the NICU to localize peripheral arteries for cannulation, particularly the radial and posterior tibial arteries, with improved success rates (12,13).

D. Precautions

1. When performing radial artery cannulation, check ulnar collateral circulation using the Allen test prior to undertaking the procedure. This test is recognized to have limitations regarding accuracy and interrater reliability (14), so careful observation for signs of impaired distal perfusion is still required during and after the procedure. Doppler ultrasound may also be useful in assessing collateral circulation.
2. When performing dorsalis pedis or posterior tibial cannulation, a modified Allen test can be performed by raising the foot, occluding the dorsalis pedis and posterior tibial arteries, releasing pressure over one, and monitoring for tissue perfusion within 10 seconds, although this technique is less reliable than testing in the hand (15).
3. When performing radial or ulnar cannulation, avoid excessive hyperextension of wrist, because this may result in occlusion of artery and a false-positive Allen

test (16) and has been associated with median nerve conduction block (17).
4. Never ligate artery.
5. Leave all fingertips/toes exposed so that circulatory status may be monitored. Examine limb frequently for changes in perfusion.
6. Inspect cannula insertion site at least daily.
   a. If signs of cellulitis are present, remove the cannula and send the cannula tip for culture. Also, send a wound culture if there is inflammation at the cut-down site.
   b. Obtain a blood culture from a peripheral site if signs of sepsis are present.
   c. Inspect the area distal and proximal to the insertion site for blanching, redness, cyanosis, or changes in temperature or capillary refill time.
7. Make sure that a continuous pressure waveform tracing is displayed on a monitor screen at all times after cannulation.
8. Take care not to introduce air bubbles into cannula while assembling infusion system or taking blood samples.
9. Use cannula for sampling only; no fluids other than heparinized saline flush solution should be administered via cannula.
10. Do not administer a rapid bolus injection of fluid via line. Flush infusion after sampling should be:
    a. Minimal volume (0.3 to 0.5 mL)
    b. Injected slowly
11. To reverse arteriospasm, see Chapter 36.
12. Remove cannula at first indication of clot formation or circulatory compromise (e.g., dampening of waveform on monitor). Do not flush to remove clots.
13. Remove cannula as soon as indications no longer exist.

E. Technique

Standard Technique for Percutaneous Arterial Cannulation

1. Choose a site for cannulation and secure the appropriate limb.
   a. **Radial artery:** This is the most common site for cannulation (1–3,18). The infant's forearm and hand can be transilluminated with the wrist in extension 45 to 60 degrees (**Fig. 33.1**), making sure that fingers are visible to monitor distal perfusion. The artery can be palpated proximal to the transverse crease on the palmar surface of the wrist, medial to the styloid process of the radius, and lateral to the flexor carpi radialis (19) (**Fig. 33.2**).
   b. **Ulnar artery:** In a small number of infants, the ulnar artery may be easier to locate than the radial artery (20). If an Allen test indicates that the collateral

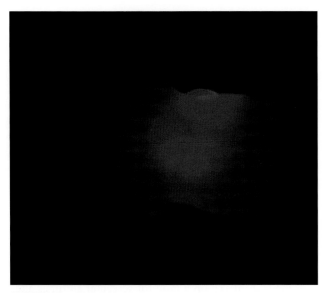

FIGURE 33.1 Transillumination of the radial artery.

blood supply is adequate, the ulnar artery may be cannulated using the same method as for a radial artery. The ulnar artery runs along the palmar margin of the flexor carpi ulnaris. Caution is necessary when cannulating the ulnar artery because it runs next to the ulnar nerve and is smaller in caliber than the radial artery (**Fig. 33.2**).

c. **Dorsalis pedis artery:** The dorsalis pedis artery can be found in the dorsal midfoot between the first and second toes with the foot held in plantar flexion (**Fig. 33.3**). It should be noted that the vascular anatomy of the foot is variable and the dorsalis pedis artery may be absent in some patients, whereas it may provide the main blood supply to the toes in others (21,22).

d. **Posterior tibial artery:** The posterior tibial artery runs posterior to the medial malleolus with the foot held in dorsiflexion (**Figs. 33.4** and **33.5**).

2. Identify artery by
   a. Palpation (see anatomic landmarks as described above or individual arterial sites)
   b. Transillumination (**Figs. 33.1** and **33.4** and Chapter 15)
   c. Doppler ultrasound, if available (Chapter 15)
3. Wash hands as for sterile procedure and wear sterile gloves.
4. If time permits, apply 0.5 to 1 g of EMLA cream to chosen arterial site and cover with occlusive dressing for 15 to 30 minutes. Remove occlusive dressing and wipe away cream just prior to cannulation.
5. Prepare skin over site with antiseptic (e.g., an iodophor).
6. Make small skin puncture with venipuncture needle over site (optional; to ease passage of cannula through skin and reduce chances of penetrating the posterior

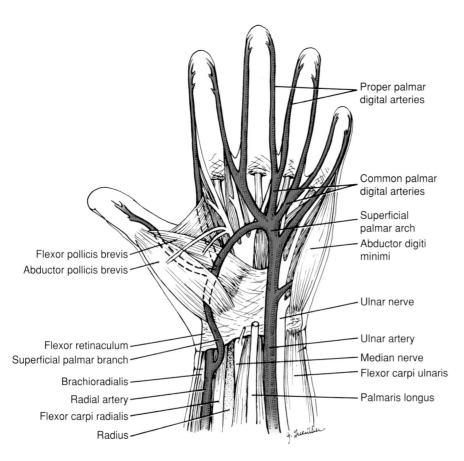

FIGURE 33.2 Anatomic relations of the major arteries of the wrist and hand.

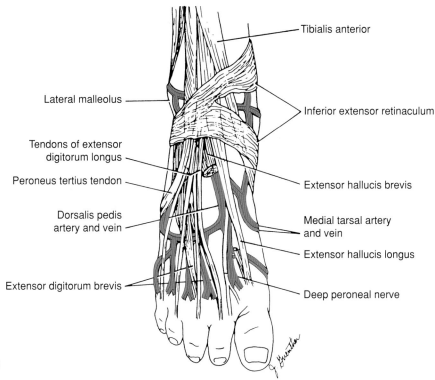

FIGURE 33.3 Anatomic relations of dorsalis pedis artery.

wall of the vessel, especially when using a larger-gauge cannula).

7. Accomplish cannulation of artery (**Figs. 33.6A,B** and **33.7**).

Method A (Preferred for Small Premature Neonates)

a. Puncture artery directly at an angle of 10 to 15 degrees to the skin, with the needle bevel down.

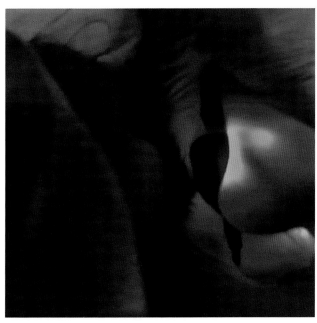

FIGURE 33.4 Transillumination of posterior tibial artery.

b. Advance slowly. There will be arteriospasm when the vessel is touched, and blood return may be delayed.

c. Withdraw needle stylet (blood should appear in the cannula) and advance cannula into artery as far as possible.

Method B (Fig. 33.6B)

a. Pass needle stylet (with bevel up) and cannula through artery at 30- to 40-degree angle to skin.

b. Remove stylet and withdraw cannula slowly until arterial flow is established.

c. Advance cannula into artery.

The inability to insert the cannula into the lumen usually indicates failure to puncture the artery centrally. This often results in laceration of the lateral wall of the artery with formation of a hematoma, which can be seen on transillumination.

8. Attach cannula firmly to T connector and gently flush with 0.5 mL of heparinized solution, observing for evidence of blanching or cyanosis.

9. Suture cannula to skin with 5-0 nylon suture if desired. This step may be omitted as long as cannula is securely taped (Fig. 27.4); use of sutures may produce a scar.

10. Secure cannula as done with peripheral IV line, as shown in Figure 27.4. Transparent semipermeable dressing may be used in place of tape to allow continuous visualization of skin entry site. Ensure that all digits are visible for frequent inspection (**Fig. 33.8**).

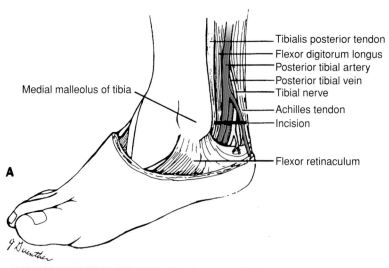

A

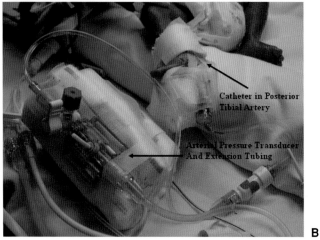

B

FIGURE 33.5 A: Anatomic relations of posterior tibial artery, showing site of incision for cut down. **B:** Cannulation of posterior tibial artery; cannula is attached to a transducer for continuous blood pressure monitoring.

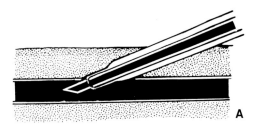

A

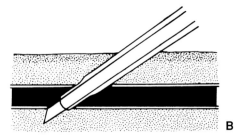

B

FIGURE 33.6 A: Cannulation of artery using Method A (see text). **B:** Cannulation of artery using Method B (see text). (Reprinted with permission from Filston HC, Johnson DG. Percutaneous venous cannulation in neonates and infants: A method for catheter insertion without "cut-down". *Pediatrics.* 1971;48(6):896–901. Copyright © 1971 by the AAP.)

11. Maintain patency by attaching T connector to extension tubing or arterial pressure line to run 1 mL/hr of heparinized flush solution by constant-infusion pump. Ensure that continuous infusion is started almost immediately after cannula is placed, to avoid clotting. An infusion rate of less than 1 mL/hr is often associated with blood backing into the T connector and clotting of the cannula.

12. Change IV tubing and flushing solution every 24 hours.

Guidewire-Assisted Radial Artery Cannulation (23)

1. Identify artery by palpation, transillumination, or ultrasound
2. Apply local anesthetic cream as above if time permits
3. Prepare area with antiseptic solution
4. Use 24-gauge ¾ in (0.7 mm × 3 cm) catheter over 24-gauge thin-walled needle
5. Insert needle at 45-degree angle to the skin toward the artery

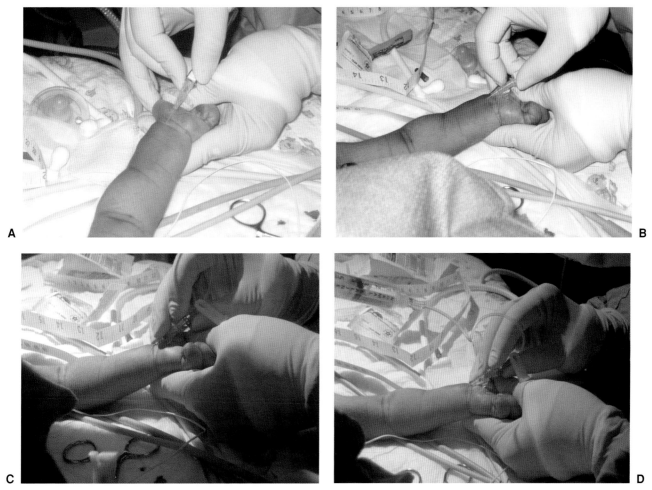

FIGURE 33.7 **A:** Puncture artery directly at angle of 10 to 15 degrees to skin, with needle bevel down. **B:** Advance slowly. **C:** Withdraw needle stylet, allow for blood return, and advance cannula into artery. **D:** Attach cannula firmly to T connector.

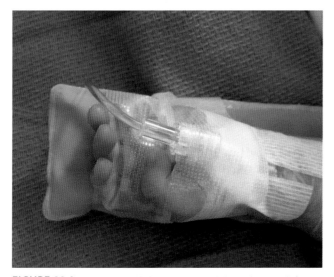

FIGURE 33.8 Radial artery catheter taped and dressed. Note all fingers and thumb are easily visible and not constricted by tape.

6. When flashback of blood is noted, advance guidewire into arterial lumen
7. Remove needle and advance catheter over the guidewire
8. Remove guidewire and connect T connector, flush with heparinized saline solution

Radial Artery Cut Down (24)

Cut-down technique may be required for the very small neonate, because trauma to the artery causes vasospasm, which makes percutaneous cannulation of a small vessel very difficult.

1. Technique I: Cut down at wrist
   The artery is initially exposed by cut down, and a catheter is inserted under direct vision.
   a. Prepare as for percutaneous procedure (Standard Technique, steps 1 to 3).
   b. Scrub and prepare as for major procedure (see Chapter 6).

c. Infiltrate site of incision (point of maximum pulsation just proximal to proximal wrist crease) with 0.5 to 1 mL of lidocaine.

d. Wait 5 minutes for anesthesia.

e. Make a 0.5-cm transverse skin incision.

f. Deepen incision into subcutaneous tissue by blunt longitudinal dissection with curved mosquito hemostat.

g. Use curved mosquito hemostat to dissect artery free.

    Be gentle, to avoid arteriospasm.

h. Elevate artery with hemostat or nerve hook.

i. Loop ligature (5-0 silk) around artery for traction purposes. Do not tie ligature.

j. Advance cannula stylet into artery with bevel down, until cannula is clearly within vessel lumen.

k. Remove stylet and advance cannula to hub.

l. Remove ligature.

m. See percutaneous method under E (Standard Technique, steps 7 to 11) for fixation and care of cannula.

    The incision can usually be kept small enough so that the hub of the cannula fills it and no closing suture is needed.

Posterior Tibial Artery Cannulation by a Cut-Down Procedure

1. Prepare as for percutaneous method.
2. Put on mask.
3. Tape foot to footboard in slightly dorsiflexed position (see Chapter 5).
4. Scrub and prepare as for major procedure (see Chapter 6).
5. Infiltrate incision site with 0.5 to 1 mL of 0.5% lidocaine (**Fig. 33.5**).
6. Wait 5 minutes for anesthesia.
7. Make transverse incision (0.5 cm) posteroinferior to medial malleolus (see **Fig. 33.5**).

    A vertical, rather than a transverse, incision is optional. The former has the advantage that it offers the opportunity to extend the incision cephalad, should the posterior wall of the vein be perforated on the initial attempt at cannulation. However, it has the disadvantage that it may be made too far lateral or medial to the artery.

8. Identify artery by longitudinal dissection with mosquito hemostat. The artery is usually found just anterior to the Achilles tendon and adjacent to the tibial nerve.
9. Place mosquito hemostat behind artery, and loop 5-0 nylon suture loosely around it.

    Be gentle, to avoid arteriospasm.

10. Elevate artery in wound with suture. Do not ligate artery.

11. While stabilizing artery with suture, insert needle and cannula, with bevel down.
12. Withdraw stylet and advance cannula to hub.
13. Remove nylon suture.
14. Close wound with 5-0 nylon suture (usually requires only one suture).
15. See percutaneous method under E (Standard Technique, steps 7 to 11) for fixation and care of cannula.

F. Obtaining Arterial Samples

Equipment

1. Gloves
2. Alcohol swabs
3. Sterile 2- × 2-in gauze squares (for three-drop method)
4. 25-gauge straight needle (for three-drop method)
5. Appropriate-sized syringe for sample (heparinized if sample is not processed on site)
6. Syringe with flush (for stopcock method)
7. Ice if necessary for sample preservation
8. Specimen labels and requisition slips

Technique I: Three-Drop Method

1. Wash hands and put on gloves.
2. Clean diaphragm of T connector with antiseptic solution and allow to dry.
3. Clamp T-connector tubing close to hub.
4. Place sterile gauze squares beneath hub.
5. Introduce 25-gauge needle through diaphragm and allow 3 to 4 drops of fluid/blood to drip onto gauze.
6. Attach syringe to needle and withdraw sample.
7. Remove needle from diaphragm.
8. Unclamp T connector and allow residual pump pressure to flush catheter.

Technique II: Stopcock Method (a Three-Way Stopcock Needs to Be Interposed Between the Patient and the Transducer)

1. Wash hands and put on gloves.
2. Clean hub of stopcock with antiseptic solution.
3. Attach syringe to stopcock.
4. Turn stopcock off to infusion pump.
5. Aspirate waste (volume depends on length of tubing).
6. Using second syringe, withdraw sample.
7. Flush cannula slowly, over 30 to 60 seconds, with 0.5 mL of flush solution.
8. Open stopcock to pump, to allow for continued infusion of heparinized saline.

G. Removal of the Cannula

Indications

1. Stabilization or resolution of the indications for cannulation of the artery
2. Cannula-related infection
3. Evidence of thrombosis or mechanical occlusion of the artery

Technique

1. Remove tape/dressing and cut stitch (if present) securing cannula to skin.
2. Remove cannula gently.
3. Apply local pressure for 5 to 10 minutes.

H. Complications of Peripheral Arterial Cannulation

1. Thromboembolism/vasospasm/thrombosis
   a. Blanching of hand, gangrene of fingertips, partial loss of digits (5,18,25,26). Topical nitroglycerine has been reported to restore perfusion in some cases (27,28). Warming of the contralateral limb, to produce reflex vasodilation, can also be used (29) (see Chapter 36)
   b. Necrosis of forearm and hand (**Fig. 33.9**) (26,28)
   c. Skin ulcers (30)
   d. Ischemia/necrosis of toes (**Fig. 33.10**) (31,32)
   e. Reversible occlusion of artery (33)
2. Infiltration of infusate (29)
3. Infection (34)
4. Hematoma (35)

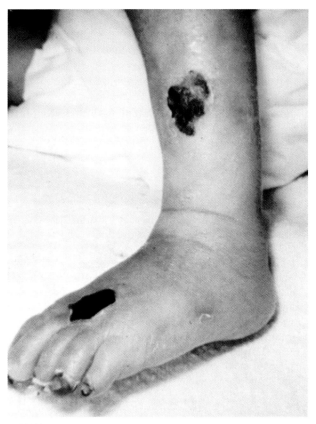

FIGURE 33.10 Complication of cannulation of dorsalis pedis artery. Healing areas of sloughed skin are seen at site of skin puncture on dorsum of foot and also on anterior aspect of lower leg. Tips of toes 1, 3, 4, and 5 are necrotic.

5. Damage to peripheral nerves
   a. Median nerve above medial epicondyle of humerus
   b. Median nerve at wrist
   c. Ulnar nerve at wrist
   d. Peripheral portion of deep peroneal nerve
   e. Posterior tibial nerve at medial malleolus

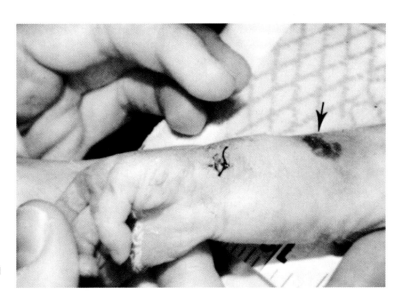

FIGURE 33.9 Complication of cannulation of the radial artery. *Arrow* indicates necrotic area on forearm.

6. False cortical thumbs (36)
7. Burns from transilluminator
8. Hemorrhage (including accidental dislodgement of cannula) (29)
9. Hypernatremia caused by heparinized saline infusion through cannula
10. Hypervolemia related to continuous flush device (37)
11. Air embolism (38)
12. Pseudoaneurysm (35)

References

1. Selldén H, Nilsson K, Larsson LE, et al. Radial arterial catheters in children and neonates: a prospective study. *Crit Care Med.* 1987;15(12):1106–1109.
2. Randel SN, Tsang BH, Wung JT, et al. Experience with percutaneous indwelling peripheral arterial catheterization in neonates. *Am J Dis Child.* 1987;141(8):848–851.
3. Karacalar S, Ture H, Baris S, et al. Ulnar artery versus radial artery approach for arterial cannulation: a prospective, comparative study. *J Clin Anesth.* 2007;19(3):209–213.
4. Kim EH, Lee JH, Song IK, et al. Posterior tibial artery as an alternative to the radial artery for arterial cannulation site in small children: a randomized controlled study. *Anesthesiology.* 2017;127(3):423–431.
5. Aldridge SA, Gupta JM. Peripheral artery cannulation in newborns. *J Singapore Paediatr Soc.* 1992;34:11–14.
6. Piotrowski A, Kawczynski P. Cannulation of the axillary artery in critically ill newborn infants. *Eur J Pediatr.* 1995;154:57–59.
7. Schindler E, Kowald B, Suess H, et al. Catheterization of the radial or brachial artery in neonates and infants. *Paediatr Anaesth.* 2005;15:677–682.
8. Bull MJ, Schreiner RL, Garg BP, et al. Neurologic complications following temporal artery catheterization. *J Pediatr.* 1980;96:1071–1073.
9. Bhaskar P, John J, Lone RA, et al. Selective use of superficial temporal artery cannulation in infants undergoing cardiac surgery. *Ann Card Anaesth.* 2015;18(4):606–608.
10. Rais-Bahrami K, Karna P, Dolanski EA. Effect of fluids on life span of peripheral arterial lines. *Am J Perinatol.* 1990;7:122–124.
11. Clifton GD, Branson P, Kelly HJ, et al. Comparison of normal saline and heparin solutions for maintenance of arterial catheter patency. *Heart Lung.* 1991;20:115–118.
12. White L, Halpin A, Turner M, et al. Ultrasound-guided radial artery cannulation in adult and paediatric populations: a systematic review and meta-analysis. *Br J Anaesth.* 2016;116(5):610–617.
13. Song IK, Choi JY, Lee JH, et al. Short-axis/out-of-plane or long-axis/in-plane ultrasound-guided arterial cannulation in children: a randomised controlled trial. *Eur J Anaesthesiol.* 2016;33(7):522–527.
14. Barone JE, Madlinger RV. Should an Allen test be performed before radial artery cannulation? *J Trauma.* 2006;61: 468–470.
15. Johnstone RE, Greenhow DE. Catheterization of the dorsalis pedis artery. *Anesthesiology.* 1973;39:654–655.
16. Greenhow DE. Incorrect performance of Allen's test: ulnar-artery flow erroneously presumed inadequate. *Anesthesiology.* 1972;37:356–357.

17. Chowet AL, Lopez JR, Brock-Utne JG, et al. Wrist hyperextension leads to median nerve conduction block: implications for intra-arterial catheter placement. *Anesthesiology.* 2004;100: 287–291.
18. Wallach SG. Cannulation injury of the radial artery: diagnosis and treatment algorithm. *Am J Crit Care.* 2004;13:315–319.
19. Brzezinski M, Luisetti T, London MJ. Radial artery cannulation: a comprehensive review of recent anatomic and physiologic investigations. *Anesth Analg.* 2009;109(6):1763–1781.
20. Kahler AC, Mirza F. Alternative arterial catheterization site using the ulnar artery in critically ill pediatric patients. *Pediatr Crit Care Med.* 2002;3:370–374.
21. Huber JF. The arterial network supplying the dorsum of the foot. *Anat Rec.* 1941;80:373–391.
22. Spoerel WE, Deimling P, Aitken R. Direct arterial pressure monitoring from the dorsalis pedis artery. *Can Anaesth Soc J.* 1975;22:91–99.
23. Yildirim V, Ozal E, Cosar A, et al. Direct versus guidewire-assisted pediatric radial artery cannulation technique. *J Cardiothorac Vasc Anesth.* 2006;20(1):48–50.
24. Pfenninger J, Bernasconi G, Sutter M. Radial artery catheterization by surgical exposure in infants. *Intensive Care Med.* 1982;8(3):139–141.
25. Brotschi B, Hug MI, Latal B, et al. Incidence and predictors of indwelling arterial catheter-related thrombosis in children. *J Thromb Haemost.* 2011;9(6):1157–1162.
26. Hack WW, Vos A, Okken A. Incidence of forearm and hand ischaemia related to radial artery cannulation in newborn infants. *Intensive Care Med.* 1990;16:50–53.
27. Vasquez P, Burd A, Mehta R, et al. Resolution of peripheral artery catheter-induced ischemic injury following prolonged treatment with topical nitroglycerin ointment in a newborn: a case report. *J Perinatol.* 2003;23:348–350.
28. Baserga MC, Puri A, Sola A. The use of topical nitroglycerin ointment to treat peripheral tissue ischemia secondary to arterial line complications in neonates. *J Perinatol.* 2002;22:416–419.
29. Detaille T, Pirotte T, Veyckemans F. Vascular access in the neonate. *Best Pract Res Clin Anaesthesiol.* 2010;24:403–418.
30. Wyatt R, Glaves I, Cooper DJ. Proximal skin necrosis after radial-artery cannulation. *Lancet.* 1974;1:1135–1138.
31. Spahr RC, MacDonald HM, Holzman IR. Catheterization of the posterior tibial artery in the neonate. *Am J Dis Child.* 1979;133:945–946.
32. Abrahamson EL, Scott RC, Jurges E, et al. Catheterization of posterior tibial artery leading to limb amputation. *Acta Paediatr.* 1993;82:618–619.
33. Hack WW, Vos A, van der Lei J, et al. Incidence and duration of total occlusion of the radial artery in newborn infants after catheter removal. *Eur J Pediatr.* 1990;149:275–277.
34. Adams JM, Speer ME, Rudolph AJ. Bacterial colonization of radial artery catheters. *Pediatrics.* 1980;65:94–97.
35. Vora S, Ibrahim T, Rajadurai VS. Radial artery pseudoaneurysm in a neonate with hemophilia A. *Indian Pediatr.* 2014; 51(11):921–923.
36. Skoglund RR, Giles EE. The false cortical thumb. *Am J Dis Child.* 1986;140:375–376.
37. Morray J, Todd S. A hazard of continuous flush systems for vascular pressure monitoring in infants. *Anesthesiology.* 1983;58:187–189.
38. Chang C, Dughi J, Shitabata P, et al. Air embolism and the radial arterial line. *Crit Care Med.* 1988;16:141–143.

Central Venous Catheterization

Ha-Young Choi, Angela Rivera, and A. Alfred Chahine

Central venous catheters provide stable intravenous (IV) access to sick or low–birth-weight infants who need long-term IV nutrition or medications (1).

A percutaneous central venous catheter, also known as a peripherally inserted central catheter (PICC), is a soft, flexible catheter that is inserted into a peripheral vein and threaded into the central venous system. Central venous catheters may be placed by percutaneous puncture or by surgical cutdown when peripheral percutaneous access is not possible. Totally implantable vascular access devices (ports) are rarely used in neonates and are thus not included in this chapter.

Regardless of the method employed to obtain secure and reliable venous access, the clinician should be familiar with the technique and anatomic considerations unique to the approach. Some form of analgesia and sedation is generally required, with general anesthesia being reserved for more complex access cases. The majority of venous access procedures in the critically ill neonate are performed at the bedside rather than in the operating room. Thus the practitioner should have familiarity with both the risks and benefits of the procedure and analgesia medications (see Chapter 7).

A. Indications

1. Total parenteral nutrition
2. Long-term IV medication administration
3. Administration of hyperosmolar IV fluids or irritating medications that cannot be administered through peripheral IV cannulas
4. Fluid resuscitation
5. Repetitive blood draws (catheters are not usually inserted primarily for this indication in neonates; only larger-lumen catheters may be used for blood draws without risk of clotting)

B. Relative Contraindications

There are no absolute contraindications, as the clinical situation dictates the need for venous access.

1. Skin infection or breakdown/loss of integrity at insertion site
2. Uncorrected bleeding diathesis (not a contraindication for percutaneous catheters inserted in distal peripheral venous sites)
3. Ongoing bacteremia or fungal infection (which may cause catheter colonization and infection)
4. The patient can be treated adequately with peripheral IV access. Central venous catheters have significant risks of complications (2) and must not be used when peripheral venous access is possible and adequate

C. General Considerations, Preparation, and Precautions

1. Plan ahead: Success with PICC placement is higher if the catheter is inserted electively before peripheral veins are "used up" by frequent cannulations.
2. Obtain informed consent prior to performing the procedure.
3. Infant should be on a cardiorespiratory monitor during the procedure.
4. Central venous catheterization must be performed by trained individuals.
5. Central line teams and the use of insertion and maintenance checklists and bundles have been shown to decrease the frequency of catheter-related infections (3–5).
6. Maintain strict aseptic technique for the insertion and care of central catheter. Hand hygiene (with soap and water or with alcohol-based hand rub) should be performed before and after palpating catheter insertion sites, as well as before and after inserting, replacing,

accessing, repairing, or dressing an intravascular catheter (3).

7. Never leave a catheter in a position where it does not easily and repeatedly withdraw blood during the insertion procedure, to ensure that the tip is not lodged against a blood vessel or cardiac wall as this may lead to infiltration, arrhythmia, and excessive pressure needed for fluid infusion.

8. Always confirm the position of the catheter tip by radiography (both AP and lateral radiographs are recommended) or echocardiography prior to using it.

9. Follow the manufacturer's instructions for catheter use.

10. Do not submerge the catheter or catheter site in water.

D. Vessels Amenable to Central Venous Access

Table 34.1 lists the sites usually used for central venous catheterization in the newborn.

TABLE 34.1 Vessels Amenable to Central Venous Access

BLOOD VESSEL	RECOMMENDED TECHNIQUE
Upper extremity: Cephalic, basilic, median cubital, or axillary vein	Percutaneous or surgical
Lower extremity: Saphenous vein or femoral vein	Percutaneous or surgical
Scalp vein	Percutaneous technique, amenable only to PICC lines
External jugular vein	Percutaneous or surgical
Internal jugular vein or common facial vein	Surgical technique

Vessels should be carefully assessed for optimal success in placement as well as decreased complications. Veins may be chosen by visual assessment, transilluminators, or ultrasound. Larger veins are easier to cannulate and are less likely to form a thrombus. Upper-extremity PICC may be associated with fewer complications in neonates than lower-extremity PICC, though reports are variable (6,7). However lower-extremity PICC is less likely to migrate, whereas the upper-extremity PICC tip location may be affected by arm position and movement (8,9). When deciding between upper-extremity veins, the basilic vein takes a straighter course to the superior vena cava (SVC) than the cephalic vein (9).

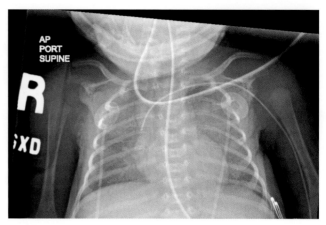

FIGURE 34.1 Chest radiograph with PICC tip in appropriate position, just above junction of superior vena cava and right atrium.

E. Position of Catheter Tip (Fig. 34.1)

1. The catheter should be placed in as large a vein as possible, ideally with the tip of the catheter outside the heart, and parallel with the long axis of the vein such that the tip does not abut the vein or heart wall. The recommendations for appropriate position of a central venous catheter tip vary, but there is general agreement that the tip should be located in a central vein but *not* within the right atrium (10). Noncentral, or "midline" PICCs have a shorter catheter life with higher risks of infiltration (11,12). Conversely when the catheter tip is in the right atrium, there is a risk of focal myocardial injury, leading to pericardial effusion and cardiac tamponade (13,14). However, one large retrospective audit of 2,186 catheters showed that catheters with their tips in the right atrium *and not coiled* were not associated with pericardial effusions (15).

    a. When inserted from the upper extremity, the catheter tip should be in the SVC, outside the cardiac reflection, or at the junction of the SVC and right atrium.

    b. When inserted from the lower extremity, the catheter tip should be above the L4–L5 vertebrae or the iliac crest, but not in the heart.

2. Confirmation of catheter tip placement.

    a. The tip of the radio-opaque catheter is usually seen on a routine chest radiograph **(Fig. 34.1)**.

    b. Two radiographic views (anteroposterior and lateral) help to confirm that the catheter is in a central vein. This is particularly important for catheters placed in a lower extremity, where the catheter may inadvertently be in an ascending lumbar vein and may appear to be in good position on an anteroposterior view (16).

    c. The use of radio-opaque contrast improves localization of the catheter tip, particularly when the catheter is difficult to see on a standard radiograph.

A 0.5-mL aliquot of 0.9% saline is instilled into the catheter to check patency, followed by 0.5 mL of iohexol. The radiograph is taken, and the line is flushed again with 0.5 mL of 0.9% saline. With this technique, there is no need to inject the contrast material while the radiograph is being taken (17).

d. Real-time bedside ultrasonography may also be useful in localizing the catheter tip, and decreases radiation exposure to the infant (18).

e. Chest radiographs obtained for any reason should be scrutinized for appropriate catheter position. Routine weekly radiographs taken for this purpose do not appear to reduce the risk of complications (19). The infant's arm position is important to assess, as there can be significant migration associated with arm movement.

F. Methods of Vascular Access

1. Percutaneous technique
   a. Advantages
      (1) Simpler to perform and relatively rapid procedure
      (2) Vessel is not ligated as in open cutdown methods
      (3) Decreased potential for wound infection/ dehiscence complications
   b. Disadvantages
      (1) Beyond the initial insertion into the peripheral vein, further passage of the catheter into its final position is essentially a blind technique, although there is increasing experience with ultrasound imaging during passage

      (2) A smaller-caliber catheter may preclude use for blood transfusions and blood draws
2. Cutdown or open surgical technique
   a. Advantages
      (1) Allows for insertion of larger silicone catheter (2.7 or 4.2 Fr)
      (2) If needed for prolonged periods, the catheters can be tunneled under the skin away from the venotomy site, so they can remain in place longer with a lower risk of infection
   b. Disadvantages
      (1) Requires general anesthesia or IV sedation
      (2) Requires surgical incision
      (3) Vein is often ligated, so it cannot be reused in the future
      (4) Potential for injury to adjacent anatomical structures
      (5) Increased potential for wound infection
      (6) An operating room is the ideal setting for the procedure, so risks of transport of critically ill neonates need to be taken into consideration

G. Types of Central Venous Catheters

1. Catheter materials: See **Table 34.2**
2. Types of catheters
   a. Percutaneous (PICC) catheters/introducers
      PICC catheters and kits are available commercially. PICCs are generally made of silicone or polyurethane. Sizes include 1.2, 1.9, 2, and 3 Fr. Larger sizes are generally not used in the neonatal

TABLE 34.2 **Catheter Materials**

TYPE OF CATHETER	ADVANTAGES	DISADVANTAGES
Silicone	Soft, pliable Lower risk of vessel perforation Reported to be thromboresistant	May be more difficult to insert percutaneously Thrombosis reported Fragile material: Less tolerance to pressure Poor tensile strength: Can tear or rupture May be less radio opaque
Polyurethane	Easier to insert percutaneously Stiffer on insertion but softens within body Some catheters are more radio opaque Tensile strength: More tolerant to pressure Reported to be thromboresistant	Increased risk of vessel perforation during insertion Thrombosis reported
Polyethylene	Easier to insert Very high tensile strength	High degree of stiffness may increase vessel perforation during insertion or throughout catheter dwell
Polyvinyl chloride (PVC)	Easier to insert percutaneously Stiff on insertion but softens within body	May leach plasticizers into body High incidence of thrombosis

population. Most catheters are single lumen. Double-lumen catheters can decrease the need for maintaining concurrent IV access when more than one site is required. PICC introducers/needles are available in 20 to 28 gauge.

b. Surgically placed central venous catheters

Surgically placed central venous catheters for neonates are available in sizes 2.5, 2.7, 3, 4.2, and 5 Fr. Catheters are usually silicone or polyurethane, with tissue ingrowth cuffs that adhere to the subcutaneous tract, anchoring the catheter. Recently, antimicrobial cuffs have become available. Most catheters are single lumen, but a few manufacturers make double-lumen catheters.

PERIPHERALLY INSERTED CENTRAL VENOUS CATHETERIZATION (▶ VIDEO 34.1)

A. Insertion Sites (Fig. 16.1, Table 34.1)

The veins used, in order of preference, are

1. Antecubital veins: Basilic and cephalic veins
2. Saphenous veins

3. Scalp veins: Temporal and posterior auricular veins
4. Axillary vein
5. External jugular vein

Right-sided and basilic veins are preferred because of the shorter and more direct route to the central vein. The cephalic vein may be more difficult to thread to the central position because of narrowing of the vessel as it enters the deltopectoral groove and the acute angle at which it joins the subclavian vein. The axillary and external jugular veins are the last choices because they are close to arteries and nerves.

B. Insertion Variations

1. Break-away needle: Needle is inserted into the vein. Next, the catheter is advanced through the needle. The needle is then retracted, split, and removed. There is a potential for shearing or severing the catheter if it is retracted while the needle is in the vein.
2. Peel-away introducer (**Figs. 34.2** and **34.3**): A needle introducer is used to place a small cannula or sheath into the vein. The needle is then removed and the catheter is threaded through the introducer cannula. The introducer cannula or sheath is then retracted from the vein, split or "peeled" apart, and removed from the catheter.

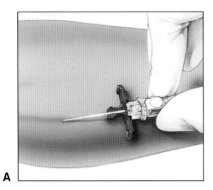
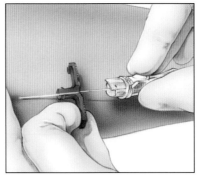
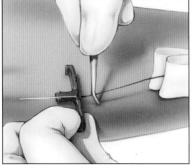
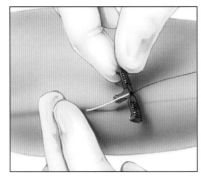
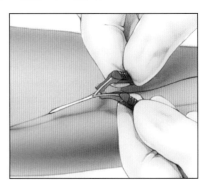

FIGURE 34.2 **A:** Cannulate the vein using the introducer and needle. **B:** Retract needle, leaving introducer in place in the vein. Apply pressure to the to vein proximal to the introducer to minimize blood loss. **C:** Insert the catheter into the introducer sheath to insert into the vein. **D:** After catheter has been introduced to desired depth, withdraw the introducer from the vein. **E:** Once introducer is completely outside of the skin, grasping both wings on either side of the introducer, split the introducer and peel it in half lengthwise. (Courtesy and © Becton, Dickinson and Company.)

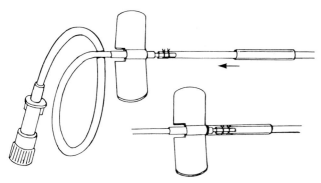

FIGURE 34.3 Use of a blunt scalp vein needle to form a hub for a silicone catheter. The plastic needle cover is used to stabilize the needle–catheter junction. A commercially available blunt needle adapter may be inserted and fixed in a similar manner.

3. Intact cannula (**Fig. 34.3**): This technique is now rarely used because most commercially available catheters have a hub and introducer needles. A regular IV cannula is used to obtain venous access. The needle is removed. The silicone catheter is threaded through the cannula to its final position. The cannula is then retracted and slipped off the end of the "hubless" catheter. A blunt needle with hub is connected to the end of the catheter. Disadvantage: The blunt needle attachment must be secured well, otherwise leakage can occur.

C. Placement of PICC

1. **Equipment** (Fig 34.4)

   All equipment used, except the mask, head cover, and tape measure, must be sterile. Commercial kits contain many of the necessary items. Assemble all supplies before starting procedure
   a. Radio-opaque central venous catheter
   b. Break-away or peel-away needle introducer
   c. Device for trimming the catheter (based on manufacturer recommendations)
   d. Tourniquet (optional)

e. Drapes
f. Smooth iris forceps
g. Gauze pads
h. Skin prep: 10% povidone–iodine or 0.5% chlorhexidine solution (per institutional policy)
i. Sterile saline or water (for cleaning skin prior to dressing placement)
j. Transparent dressing
k. Sterile tape strips
l. Sterile heparinized saline solution (0.5 to 1 U/mL heparin or per institutional policy)
m. 5- to 10-mL syringe with blunt needle
n. Connection cannula, or "t-connector"
o. Tape measure
p. Sterile surgical gown, sterile gloves, mask, and head cover

2. **Preparation**
   a. Obtain informed consent and perform "time-out" as per institutional regulations
   b. Although anesthesia is not required, nonpharmacologic comfort measures and pain medication should be provided as needed. A small dose of sedative or narcotic analgesic may be useful
   c. Gather supplies. Wash hands thoroughly
   d. Identify appropriate vein for insertion (see D)
   e. Position infant to facilitate insertion (**Table 34.3**). Restrain infant; provide comfort measures
   f. Measure approximate distance from the insertion site to the point where the catheter tip will be placed (**Table 34.3**)
   g. Don mask and head cover
   h. Set up/open sterile equipment tray
   i. Perform hand hygiene as for a major procedure and don sterile surgical gown and gloves
   j. Trim catheter to appropriate size (trimming is based on unit policy and manufacturer recommendations). The catheter is fragile and should be handled with care. Do not clamp, suture, stretch, or apply tension to catheter

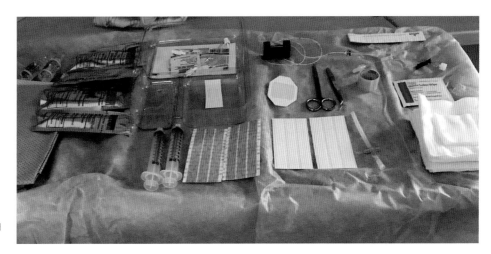

FIGURE 34.4 Sample PICC tray and sterile supplies.

TABLE 34.3 Patient Position and Measurement for PICC Insertion

SITE OF INSERTION	POSITION OF BABY	MEASUREMENT
Antecubital veins	Supine, abduct arm 90 degrees from trunk; turn head toward insertion site to prevent catheter from traveling cephalad through ipsilateral jugular vein	From planned insertion site, along venous pathway, to suprasternal notch, to third RICS
Saphenous or popliteal veins	Supine for greater saphenous vein, prone for small saphenous or popliteal; extend leg	From planned insertion site, along venous pathway, to xiphoid process
Scalp veins	Supine, turn head to side; may have to turn head to midline during procedure to assist advancement of catheter	Follow approximate venous pathway from planned insertion site near ear, to jugular vein, right SC joint, to third RICS
External jugular vein	Supine, turn head to side; place roll under neck to cause mild hyperextension	From planned insertion site, to right SC joint, to third RICS
Axillary vein	Supine, externally rotate and abduct arm 120 degrees, flex forearm and place baby's hand behind head; vein is found above artery between medial side of humeral head and small tuberosity of the humerus	From planned insertion site, to right SC joint, to third RICS

PICC, peripherally inserted central catheter; RICS, right intercostal space; SC, sternoclavicular.

k. Utilizing sterile technique and a 3-, 5-, or 10-mL syringe, flush catheter with heparinized saline solution, leaving syringe attached. A small-barreled syringe (such as a 1-mL syringe) may generate too much pressure, resulting in catheter rupture (21). Most PICC manufacturers will specify a minimum syringe size.

l. Prepare sterile field: Holding the extremity with sterile gauze prepare a large area at and around the insertion site, working outward in concentric circles. Allow the prep solution to dry. Repeat process with new gauze/prep solution. Place a *large* sterile drape under and above the extremity, leaving only the insertion site exposed. A large drape or multiple sterile towels should be used to cover an area well beyond the extremity to decrease the risk of accidental contamination (3).

3. **Catheter insertion using a break-away needle or a peel-away introducer (Figs. 34.2 and 34.3)**
   a. Apply tourniquet above insertion site on extremity (optional).
   b. Providing slight skin traction, insert needle about 0.5 to 1 cm below the intended vein, at a low angle (approximately 15 to 30 degrees).
   c. When a flashback is obtained, advance the needle about 5 to 6 mm at a lower angle to ensure that the whole bevel of the needle is within the vein. If a peel-away introducer with a needle is used, remove the needle at this time and advance the introducer sheath slightly. If the introducer (needle or sheath) is well within the vein, there will be continued blood flow through it.
   d. Remove the tourniquet.
   e. Using nontoothed iris forceps, gently grasp the catheter about 1 cm from its distal end and thread it slowly into the introducer, a few millimeters at a time.
      Caution: When using a break-away needle, never advance the needle or retract the catheter after inserting it into the needle; the catheter may be severed by this action.
   f. With small, gentle nudges, a few millimeters at a time, advance the catheter through the introducer to a distance of about 6 to 7 cm into the vein, or to the predetermined distance.
   g. Once the catheter is successfully advanced to about 6 or 7 cm, withdraw the introducer carefully (an alternative is to insert the catheter fully to the predetermined distance before withdrawing the introducer).
   h. To withdraw the introducer, stabilize the catheter by applying gentle pressure over the vein proximal to the introducer, and then remove it carefully from the insertion site. Break or peel away the introducer by splitting the wings, and then carefully peel it away from the catheter. Make certain the introducer is completely outside the insertion site prior to splitting the introducer, as splitting the introducer while it is still under the skin will tear the skin at the insertion site.

i. Continue to advance the catheter into the vein to the premeasured length, by nudging it farther, a few millimeters at a time, using the fine forceps.

j. Difficulties in advancing catheter: Gently massage the vein in the direction of blood flow, proximal to the insertion site, or gently flush the catheter intermittently with 0.5 to 1 mL of heparinized saline; repositioning the extremity or the head may help.

k. Aspirate to visualize blood return in the catheter, then flush with 0.5 to 1 mL of heparinized saline to clear the catheter.

l. Verify length of catheter inserted and adjust as necessary.

m. Attach sterile extension set as per unit protocol.

n. Apply gentle pressure on insertion site with gauze pad to stop any bleeding.

o. Secure catheter at skin insertion site with a small piece of sterile tape strip (avoid using tape that contains wire) and cover with sterile gauze until radiographic confirmation of position.

D. PICC Dressings (Figs. 34.5G and 34.6)

1. Iodine containing antimicrobial prep solutions should be removed from the skin with sterile water or saline and allowed to dry before dressing is placed. Do not use topical antibiotic ointments or creams on insertion sites (**Fig. 34.5**) (2).

2. To prevent migration of the catheter, secure it to the skin a few millimeters from the insertion site with a small piece of sterile tape. Avoid using tape that contains wire and ensure that the insertion site is visible.

3. If the catheter has not been trimmed, loosely coil the excess length of catheter close to the insertion site and secure to the skin with more sterile tape. Ensure that there is no kinking or stretching of the catheter under the dressing.

4. Apply a semipermeable transparent dressing over the area surrounding the insertion site.

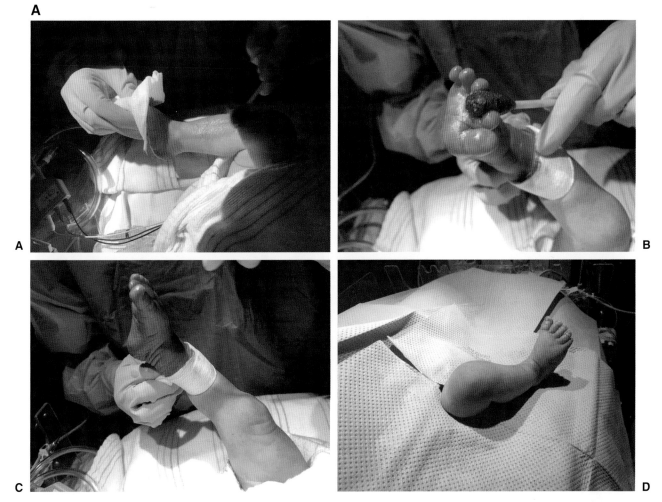

FIGURE 34.5 A: Demonstration of antisepsis of the extremity using Betadine. **A**) Note cleaning starts at distal end of limb, close to site of insertion, and moves proximally. **B**) Cleaning should include between fingers and toes. **C**) Note the use of a new sterile gauze to control the limb. **D**) After thorough cleaning the area should be draped to maintain a large sterile field. Be sure to allow for ready access to the infant's airway. Remove outer gloves that were used during the cleaning portion of the procedure. (*continued*)

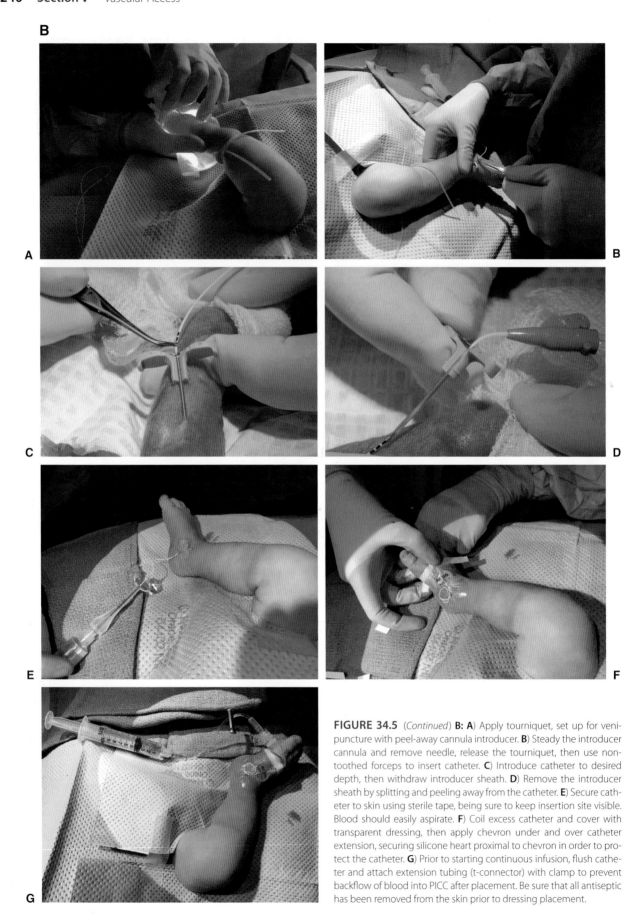

FIGURE 34.5 (*Continued*) **B: A**) Apply tourniquet, set up for venipuncture with peel-away cannula introducer. **B**) Steady the introducer cannula and remove needle, release the tourniquet, then use nontoothed forceps to insert catheter. **C**) Introduce catheter to desired depth, then withdraw introducer sheath. **D**) Remove the introducer sheath by splitting and peeling away from the catheter. **E**) Secure catheter to skin using sterile tape, being sure to keep insertion site visible. Blood should easily aspirate. **F**) Coil excess catheter and cover with transparent dressing, then apply chevron under and over catheter extension, securing silicone heart proximal to chevron in order to protect the catheter. **G**) Prior to starting continuous infusion, flush catheter and attach extension tubing (t-connector) with clamp to prevent backflow of blood into PICC after placement. Be sure that all antiseptic has been removed from the skin prior to dressing placement.

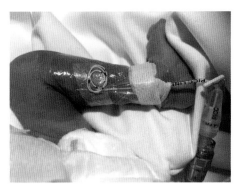

FIGURE 34.6 Secure, sterile PICC dressing: Note there is a small square of a skin-colored skin closure strip to prevent movement of the PICC line; this skin closure strip does not obscure visibility of the skin entry site of the PICC line. The excess external catheter is coiled in multiple "tension loops," which again do not obscure visibility of the skin entry site, but are also all contained under the sterile transparent dressing. The silicone hub of the PICC is anchored under the sterile transparent dressing and with adhesive strips of tape. Two pieces of anchoring tape should be used, one with use of a "chevron" technique to anchor the silicon hub, another piece of tape is crossed over on top of the first piece of anchoring tape, over the same distal portion of the silicon hub and over the edges of the transparent dressing. The anchoring tape is always over the silicone portion of the hub, not over the thin PICC line itself, containing the silicon hub under the transparent dressing. Especially in small infants care should be taken that these dressings are not circumferential around the limb.

5. Do not allow tapes or transparent dressing to extend circumferentially around the extremity. The dressing will form a constricting tourniquet as the infant grows or if there is venous congestion.
6. Place tape under the catheter hub and criss-cross it over the hub (chevron). Do not obscure visualization of the insertion site (**Fig. 34.6**).
7. To prevent skin breakdown, a skin barrier of hydrocolloid material or soft gauze can be placed under the hub.

E. Dressing Changes

1. Mild oozing of blood from the insertion site may occur for up to 24 hours. If oozing occurs, the initial dressing should be changed when it subsides. If oozing of blood is a problem, a small piece of thrombin foam can be applied over the insertion site and under the dressing for the first 24 hours after insertion.
2. The catheter site dressing should be replaced when it becomes damp, soiled, or loose.
3. Inspect catheter site carefully at each dressing change (**Table 34.4**).
4. If the catheter is too far in, as confirmed by radiography or echocardiography, it may be pulled back, prior to replacing dressing. Do not advance the catheter, as the risk of contamination is high.
5. Use sterile technique for dressing changes (mask, cap, and sterile gloves; sterile gown is optional). Ideally, dressing changes should be done with an assistant to

TABLE 34.4 Examination of the Catheter Site

ASSESSMENT	COMMENTS
Catheter: Note external catheter length	Catheter length should be clearly documented. If external length has changed, get radiograph(s) to assess where the catheter tip is located.
	If the catheter is pulled out, cover site with occlusive dressing and measure catheter length to assure that some of the catheter was not retained in the vessel.
Assess for kinks, tension, damage	Kinks and tension can damage catheter. It is recommended that damaged catheters be removed, but some manufacturers provide repair kits.
Insertion site/ surrounding skin: Erythema, drainage, bleeding, edema, phlebitis, skin breakdown	Mild erythema and/or phlebitis is common after the catheter is inserted. If condition is severe and/or is persistent, consider removing catheter.
	Mild oozing of blood should not persist longer than 24 hrs.
	Edema may be due to venous stasis from lack of extremity movement, constrictive dressings, thrombus, damage to internal structures, localized infection, or infiltration of infusion into soft tissue.
	Avoid skin breakdown by utilizing skin barriers underneath hub, removing dressing adhesives with care, minimizing tape, and removing antiseptics from skin before applying dressing.
Drainage/leaking	Purulent drainage may be due an infectious process. Consider obtaining blood cultures and/or removing the catheter.
	Clear drainage may be indicative of infusion leakage. This may be due to catheter occlusion, infiltration, or damage to catheter.

restrain the infant, keep the extremity immobile, and to assist as required.
6. Prepare sterile field: Place sterile towel/drape under extremity. Clean hands with alcohol hand sanitizer, and wearing clean gloves, remove old dressing, ensuring that the area under the dressing remains sterile. Remove gloves, clean hands with alcohol hand sanitizer again and wear sterile gloves. Utilizing antiseptic solution, prepare the skin at and around the insertion site, working outward in concentric circles. Allow the antiseptic solution to dry. Repeat process with antiseptic solution. Drape prepared area, leaving insertion site exposed.
7. Follow steps D1 through D7 to complete the PICC dressing change.

F. PICC Care and Maintenance

1. Evaluate appearance of the catheter and the tissue around the insertion site frequently.
2. Change IV tubing according to unit policy. Utilize aseptic technique when changing tubing.
3. To prevent contamination of the line, enter the PICC only when absolutely necessary.
    a. Avoid the use of stopcocks in the line.
    b. Always "scrub the hub" with alcohol pad (or similar product) prior to breaking a connection.
    c. If the catheter must be used to infuse medications, arrange the intermittent injection tubing so that it does not come in contact with the parenteral alimentation solution until the terminal infusion site. A dedicated "closed" medication administration system is recommended (20). Gently flush tubing prior to and after medication administration. Ensure that the flush and medication are compatible with the parenteral alimentation.
4. Prime volumes are usually <0.5 mL. Use a 5- to 10-mL syringe when needed to check catheter patency. Do not use force if resistance is encountered. A small-barreled syringe (such as a 1-mL syringe) may generate too much pressure, resulting in catheter rupture (21).
5. Administer a constant infusion of IV fluids at a rate of at least 1 mL/hr. Follow the manufacturer's recommendations for maximum flow rates.
6. The addition of heparin in small doses (0.5 units heparin/kg/hr or 0.5 units heparin/mL of IV fluids) reduces the risk of occlusion and prolongs catheter patency (22).
7. Do not utilize a small (less than 2 Fr) PICC for routine blood sampling.
8. Packed red blood cell transfusions should be given through a PICC only if absolutely necessary. Although there is no clinically significant hemolysis, there is a potential for occlusion of the catheter (23).
9. Monitor quality indicators to identify and solve problems. Infection rates, catheter dwell times, patient outcomes, and rates of complications should be monitored (2).
10. Remove catheter as soon as it is no longer medically necessary by slowly withdrawing it from insertion site. Clean insertion site with antiseptic prior to withdrawing catheter. Hold pressure over site if bleeding is a problem. Remove iodine containing antiseptic from skin. Place a clean gauze dressing over site. Document length removed.

PLACEMENT OF CENTRAL VENOUS CATHETERS BY SURGICAL CUTDOWN

A. Approach

If PICC access has been unsuccessful, surgical techniques can offer central access. Catheters can be placed into the internal jugular, subclavian, or femoral veins either percutaneously or via cutdown. Catheters can be placed in the facial, external jugular, and axillary veins via a cutdown approach. In general, for the tiny premature babies cutdown approaches are perceived to be safer and are more widely used in the NICU. If central access is needed for longer than about 2 weeks, catheters can be tunneled at the time of insertion to make them more stable (Broviac type catheters). These catheters are placed in a central vein, and the distal end is tunneled subcutaneously a short distance from the access site to an exit wound. The catheters usually have a single lumen with a Dacron cuff, which adheres to the subcutaneous tract, anchoring the catheter.

B. Types of Catheters

Silicone and polyurethane catheters are preferred because they are constructed of relatively inert materials, offer increased pliability, and are associated with lower rates of infection and thrombosis (24). Polyethylene catheters have a higher rate of infection and thrombolytic complications and are not recommended for long-term IV access.

C. Contraindications

In addition to the relative contraindications delineated earlier, the internal jugular vein should be avoided if the contralateral jugular vein has been catheterized previously, or if there is thrombosis of the jugular venous system on the opposite side.

D. Equipment

Sterile

1. Skin prep: Per institutional policy (e.g., 10% povidone–iodine, or 0.5% chlorhexidine solution). Chlorhexidine preps have been shown to decrease the infection rate of central venous catheters (25)
2. Gown and gloves
3. Cup with antiseptic solution
4. Sterile transparent aperture drape; four sterile towels to ensure a sterile operative field
5. Four 4- × 4-in gauze squares
6. Local anesthetic: 0.5% lidocaine HCl in labeled 3-mL syringe with 25-gauge venipuncture needle. Consider sedation and pain medication in addition to local anesthesia. Patients who are intubated may be given a sedative and muscle relaxant in addition to local anesthesia. When patients are taken to the operating room, general anesthesia is preferred
7. Catheter of choice
8. Heparinized 0.25 N saline flush solution (1 U/mL) in 3-mL syringe

9. 4-0 polyglactin suture (Vicryl; Ethicon, Somerville, New Jersey) and 5-0 nylon suture (black monofilament nylon) on cutting needles (see Appendix D)
10. T connector connected with a sterile 3-mL syringe filled with heparinized saline
11. No. 11 scalpel blade and holder
12. Two small tissue retractors or self-retaining retractor
13. Tissue forceps
14. Fine vascular forceps
15. Two small, curved mosquito hemostats
16. Dissecting scissors
17. 4-0 Vicryl suture on small, curved needle; 6-0 polypropylene on a tapered needle. This is used for a purse-string stitch as an alternative to ligation of the vessels
18. Needle holder
19. Suture scissors
20. Appropriate materials for occlusive dressing of choice

Nonsterile

1. Cap and mask
2. Roll of 4- × 4-in gauze
3. Tape measure
4. Adhesive tape

E. Techniques

In the neonate, the cervical veins are preferable to the lower-extremity veins. The cervical veins are easily accessible and are proportionately of larger size. When the lower extremities are used, the greater saphenous vein is often selected in pediatric patients because of its large size and consistent anatomy. It is not established whether femoral or jugular sites have fewer complications in neonates (26,27).

Catheter Placement Via Jugular Veins

1. Immobilize infant in position similar to that for percutaneous insertion of subclavian venous catheter. Make sure that the patient is in the Trendelenburg position to minimize the risk of an air embolism.
2. If right side is to be catheterized, turn head to left and extend neck. Care must be taken not to extend the head too much, as this may result in occlusion of the vein.
3. Estimate length of catheter to be inserted by measuring from a point midway between the nipple and the midpoint of the clavicle to a point over the sternocleidomastoid muscle at the junction of the middle and lower third of the neck (**Fig. 34.7**).
4. Put on cap and mask.
5. Clean hands as for major procedure and put on sterile gown and gloves.
6. Prepare neck and scalp area or right chest wall with antiseptic solution such as iodophor and drape out the sterile field.

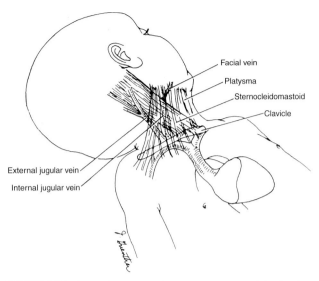

FIGURE 34.7 The jugular veins in relation to major anatomic landmarks.

7. Make small, transverse incision (1 to 2 cm) through skin and platysma muscle low in the neck for the external jugular and higher up for the facial vein.
8. Free external jugular or facial vein by blunt dissection with curved mosquito hemostat. If internal jugular vein is used, sternocleidomastoid muscle must be split to locate vein.
9. Pass curved mosquito hemostat behind the vein, and place proximal and distal ligatures of 4-0 absorbable suture loosely around vein (**Fig. 34.8**). Be careful not to twist the vessels as the suture is advanced.

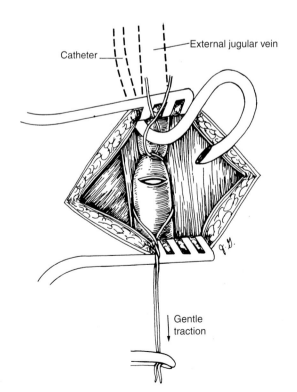

FIGURE 34.8 Catheterization of the external jugular vein; venotomy has been performed prior to inserting the catheter.

10. Using a blunt tunneler, create a subcutaneous tract from neck to exit on the chest wall medial to the right nipple. Make sure that the tunnel is far from the breast bud (**Figs. 34.9** and **34.10**). Introduce the cuff to within a centimeter from the exit site and make sure it sits comfortably in the subcutaneous space.

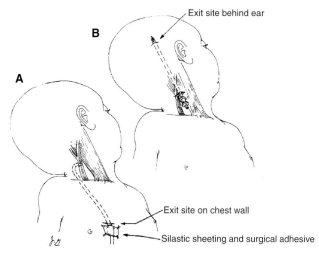

FIGURE 34.9 Formation of a subcutaneous tunnel with a Vim-Silverman needle. **A:** Tunnel on the anterior chest wall. **B:** Alternative route under the scalp.

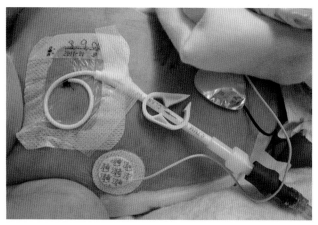

FIGURE 34.10 Broviac catheter with transparent dressing.

11. Thread the end of the catheter through the opening in the tunneler, and guide the catheter gently through the subcutaneous tract.
12. Fill the catheter system with heparinized flush solution.
13. Cut the catheter length to the premeasured distance between the neck incision and a point midway between the center of the nipple line and the suprasternal notch.
14. Perform transverse venotomy (**Fig. 34.8**).
    FOR EXTERNAL JUGULAR OR FACIAL VEIN
    (1) Tie cephalad-venous ligature, and exert traction on both ligatures in opposite directions with aid of appropriately prepared assistant.

(2) Make short, transverse incision in anterior wall of vein, and enlarge gently by inserting and spreading tips of fine vascular forceps.
    FOR INTERNAL JUGULAR VEIN
    (3) To avoid ligation of the vessel, use purse-string suture of 6-0 polypropylene, placed in vessel wall around point of catheter entrance.
    (4) Make incision in vessel as for external jugular vein.
15. Bevel intravascular end of catheter (optional).
16. Grasp catheter gently with blunt nontoothed tissue forceps, introduce catheter tip, and insert into the vein.
17. Leave loop of catheter in neck wound to dampen effect of head movement (**Fig. 34.11**).

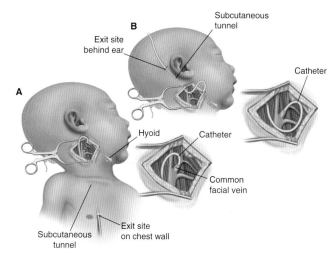

FIGURE 34.11 Insertion of a catheter into the common facial vein. Incision is below the angle of the mandible at the level of the hyoid bone. The facial vein is ligated at the junction of the anterior and posterior tributaries. Alternatively, the subcutaneous tunnel may be made with a catheter exit site on the anterior chest wall. *Inset:* The catheter is looped in the neck wound to "dampen" the effect of head movement. (Reproduced from Zumbro GL Jr, Mullin MJ, Nelson TG. Catheter placement in infants needing total parenteral nutrition utilizing common facial vein. *Arch Surg.* 1971;102:71, with permission of American Medical Association.)

18. Close wound with subcuticular 5-0 absorbable suture, taking care not to penetrate the catheter.
19. Secure the catheter to the skin with at least one nylon suture to hold it until the cuff has created enough tissue ingrowth.
20. Use selected method for fixation and dressing.

Proximal Saphenous Vein Cutdown

1. Clean hands and prepare as for major procedure.
2. Prepare as for cutdown on jugular vein. Make sure that the patient is in the reverse Trendelenburg position to minimize the risk of an air embolism.
    (1) Choose right or left groin area for insertion.
    (2) Prepare groin and abdomen on same side.

3. Make incision 1 cm long: 1 cm caudad and 1 cm lateral to pubic tubercle (**Fig. 34.12**).

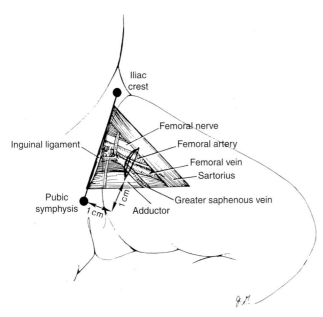

FIGURE 34.12 Anatomic view of the site of incision for proximal saphenous vein cutdown with underlying femoral triangle.

4. Spread incision into subcutaneous tissues, using curved mosquito hemostat.
   (1) Incise superficial fascia.
   (2) Identify saphenous vein lying medial and inferior to its junction with femoral vein at foramen ovale (Fig. 34.12).
   (3) Move 0.5 to 1 cm distally before passing curved mosquito hemostat behind vein. This avoids inadvertent damage to femoral vein.
   (4) Place two 4-0 absorbable suture ligatures loosely around vein.
5. Create a tunnel, using a small hemostat or tunneling instrument, in subcutaneous plane laterally onto abdomen, just above or lateral to umbilicus or on lateral thigh.
6. Flush catheter with heparinized saline and replace cap.
7. Pull catheter through tunnel into groin wound so that the Dacron cuff is just within the skin incision. Estimate the length of the catheter to be inserted so that the tip will be in inferior vena cava at junction with right atrium.
8. Cut catheter to appropriate length, and bevel intravascular end (optional).
9. Dissect saphenous vein to junction with common femoral vein.
   Visualizing the junction prevents inadvertent direction of catheter into lower extremity.
10. Apply traction to vein, using caudad suture. Lateral tension may also be applied by a scrubbed assistant, using fine nontoothed vascular forceps.

11. Make transverse venotomy.
12. Dilate vein, if necessary, with blunt dilatator.
13. Moisten catheter with saline to ease passage into vein.
14. Maintain back-traction on caudad suture to control bleeding.
15. Visualize catheter entering common femoral vein to ensure cephalad direction of catheter.
16. Obtain radiograph(s) to confirm position in inferior vena cava, once estimated length is inserted (radiographic contrast material may be required).
17. Ligate vessel with caudad suture, and tie down cephalad suture without occluding catheter.
18. Check for easy backflow of blood in catheter.
19. Flush catheter with 2.5 to 3 mL of heparinized saline. If catheter is capped, while infant is transferred from operating room to intensive care unit, clamp catheter while plunger of heparin syringe is moving forward to ensure positive pressure in line to prevent backflow and clotting of blood.
20. Close groin wound with subcuticular 5-0 absorbable suture, taking care not to penetrate catheter with needle.
21. Secure the catheter to the skin with at least one nylon suture to hold it until the cuff has created enough tissue ingrowth.
22. Cover with dressing of choice.

F. Sterile Dressing for Surgically Placed Central Venous Lines

Routine changing of central venous catheter dressings depends on the type of dressing. Transparent dressings should be changed at least every 7 days, and gauze dressings every 2 days. All dressings should be changed when damp, loose, or soiled (3).

Equipment

Strict sterile technique is used for all central line dressings.

1. Antiseptic skin prep solution: Per institutional policy (e.g., 10% povidone–iodine or 0.5% chlorhexidine solution)
2. Sterile gloves, mask, cap, and sterile gown (optional)
3. Scissors (optional)
4. Cotton-tipped applicator
5. 4- × 4-in sterile gauze square
6. Dressing of choice
   a. Semipermeable transparent dressing
   b. Sterile 2- × 2-in gauze squares or presplit 2- × 2-cm gauze dressing
7. Normal saline or sterile water
8. Adhesive tape (if sterile tape not available, use fresh unused roll)

Precautions

1. Procedure should be undertaken by trained personnel.
2. Ensure that all personnel wear masks if within 3 ft radius of sterile area.
3. Use strict aseptic technique.
4. Remove dressing with care, to avoid cutting or dislodging catheter.
5. If it is necessary to clamp the catheter, close the clamp on the catheter according to the manufacturer's directions. If the catheter does not have a clamp, use a rubber-shod clamp. Never place a clamp directly on the catheter.
6. Never advance a dislodged catheter into the patient.
7. Do not place adhesive tape on silicone tubing because this may occlude or damage the catheter.
8. Do not routinely apply prophylactic topical antimicrobial or antiseptic ointment at the insertion site because of the potential for promoting fungal infections and antimicrobial resistance (2).

Technique

When a subcutaneous tunnel is used, occlusive dressing should be applied to both the cutdown site and the catheter exit site. The dressing on the cutdown site can be removed after 48 hours if there is no oozing.

1. Restrain patient appropriately, utilizing nonpharmacologic comfort measures.
2. Put on head cover and mask.
3. Clean hands as for major procedure.
4. Put on gown and gloves.
5. Prepare sterile work area, using "no-touch" technique.
6. Remove old dressing and discard.
7. Inspect catheter site carefully (**Table 34.4**).
8. Culture site if there is drainage or it appears inflamed.
9. If area around catheter is contaminated with dried blood or drainage, clean with diluted hydrogen peroxide/sterile water solution (1:1).
10. Remove gloves. Don sterile gloves.
11. Cleanse area with antiseptic solution, starting at catheter site and working outward in circular motion for 2 to 4 cm. Repeat twice. Allow area to dry.
12. Remove antiseptic with sterile water or saline gauze and allow to dry.
13. Apply dressing of choice.
    a. Clear, adhesive, hypoallergenic, transparent dressing allows for continuous inspection of catheter insertion site, and is preferred (**Fig. 34.10**).
       (1) If necessary, cut dressing to desired size.
       (2) Anchor dressing to skin above catheter skin entry site so that the point of skin entry is at the center of the dressing.
       (3) Remove remainder of adhesive backing while applying dressing smoothly over site.
    b. Occlusive gauze dressing.
       (1) Cut gauze halfway across, or use presplit gauze. Place around catheter, as shown in **Figure 34.13**.

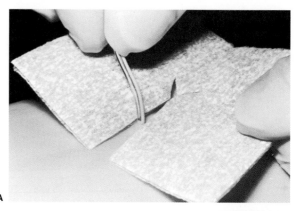

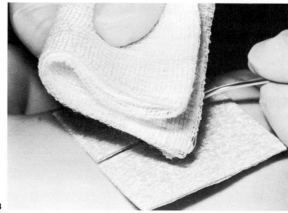

FIGURE 34.13 Occlusive dressing for a central venous line using presplit gauze. **A:** Placing split gauze over the skin entry site. **B:** Covering split gauze and the catheter with sterile gauze. Entire dressing is then covered with adhesive tape or clear dressing.

       (2) Cover remainder of external catheter length (not hub) with sterile gauze.
       (3) If sterile tape is not available, discard outer layer of tape on roll.
       (4) Cover gauze with tape.
       (5) Label dressing with initials and date.
       (6) Secure IV tubing with tape to prevent tension on the center (a stress loop can decrease tension on the catheter).

G. Care of the Catheter When Not in Use for Continuous Infusion

Indications

To maintain patency and prevent clotting of the catheter when the line is used intermittently. Only large-bore catheters (2.5 Fr or larger) may be kept patent by this technique. PICC lines that are 2 Fr or smaller tend to clot easily if continuous infusions are interrupted.

Equipment

1. 3 mL of heparin–saline solution (10 unit heparin/mL) in a 10-mL syringe (follow manufacturer's guidelines for syringe sizes)
2. Alcohol wipes
3. Catheter clamps (must have no teeth or be padded), or use clamp provided on catheter (**Fig. 34.10**)
4. Clean gloves
5. IV injection cap (needleless is recommended)

Technique

1. Converting to a heparin lock.
   a. Wash hands thoroughly.
   b. Don clean or sterile gloves.
   c. Prepare sterile work area.
   d. Using aseptic technique, open sterile injection cap package and prefill injection cap with heparinized saline.
   e. Clean the outside of the hub–IV tubing connection with an antiseptic such as alcohol wipes. Work outward in both directions. Allow to dry.
   f. Clamp catheter with padded hemostat, or close catheter clamp.
   g. Holding hub with alcohol swab, disconnect catheter hub from IV tubing.
   h. Connect preflushed injection cap into hub of catheter (gently flushing during connecting can prevent air from entering catheter).
   i. Release clamp and flush line with 1 to 3 mL of heparinized saline (depending on size of catheter).
   j. Reclamp catheter while plunger of heparin syringe is depressed to prevent blood from backing into catheter (positive pressure).
   k. Secure catheter and tape to chest or abdomen.
   l. Flush catheter with heparinized solution every 6 to 12 hours (per institution policy).
2. Flushing catheters.
   Equipment is same as for heparin lock.
   a. Wash hands thoroughly.
   b. Put on gloves and prepare sterile work area.
   c. Prepare IV injection cap with antiseptic solution. Allow to dry.
   d. If injection cap is part of a needleless system (recommended), connect flush syringe to cap. If the cap is not a needleless device, insert needle into IV catheter plug. Always use a 1-in or smaller needle. A longer needle can puncture the catheter.
   e. Unclamp catheter and slowly inject 1 to 2 mL of heparinized saline (depending on catheter size). Reclamp catheter while injecting solution to prevent blood from flowing back into catheter. Positive-pressure injection caps are available to prevent backflow.

f. Changing IV catheter injection cap: Most manufacturers recommend changing injection caps every 3 to 7 days, after blood product administration, or when they appear damaged (see specific manufacturer's instructions).

CATHETER REMOVAL

A. Indications

1. Patient's condition no longer necessitates use.
2. Occluded catheter.
3. Local infection/phlebitis.
4. Sepsis and/or positive blood cultures obtained through the catheter (catheter colonization). There are rare clinical circumstances when a catheter is left in place despite sepsis and antibiotic or antifungal therapy is administered through it in an attempt to clear the infection, but this may be associated with an increased risk of morbidity and mortality (28).

B. Technique

Surgically implanted central venous catheters should be removed by a physician or another person specifically trained to remove cuffed and/or tunneled catheters.

1. Remove dressing.
2. Make sure that the patient is in the Trendelenburg position (or reverse Trendelenburg position if the catheter is in the lower extremity) to minimize the risk of an air embolism.
3. Pull catheter from vessel slowly over 2 to 3 minutes. Avoid excessive traction if catheter is tethered, because the catheter may snap (see Complications).
4. Apply continuous pressure to the catheter insertion site for 5 to 10 minutes, until no bleeding is noted.
5. Inspect catheter (without contaminating tip) to ensure that entire length has been removed.
6. The cuff on the tunneled catheter should be dissected out under local anesthesia with IV sedation. If retained, they rarely cause more than a persistent subcutaneous lump, although they can extrude through the skin.
7. If desired, antibiotic ointment may be
8. Dress with small, self-adhesive bar and inspect daily until healing oc

COMPLICATIONS OF CATHETERS (2)

1. Damage to other ve
   a. Possible duri
      placement of

b. Complications include bleeding, pneumothorax, pneumomediastinum, hemothorax, arterial puncture, and brachial plexus injury.

2. Phlebitis.

   a. Mechanical phlebitis may occur in the first 24 hours after line placement as a normal response of the body to the irritation of the catheter in the vein.

   b. Management of mild phlebitis (mild erythema and/or edema): Apply moist, warm compress, and elevate extremity.

   c. Remove the catheter if symptoms do not improve, if phlebitis is severe (streak formation, palpable venous cord, and/or purulent drainage), or if there are signs of a catheter-related infection.

3. Catheter migration/malposition (**Fig. 34.14**).

   a. Catheter migration may occur at any point during the dwell time of the catheter; possibly as a consequence of poor catheter fixation at the skin surface

and movement of the joints (29). The catheter can enter a venous tributary during insertion or can reverse direction, causing it to loop back.

b. Sites of misplacement include the cardiac chambers, internal jugular vein, contralateral subclavian vein, ascending lumbar vein (which communicates with the vertebral venous plexus), superficial abdominal vein, renal vein, and others. Consequences include pericardial effusion or pleural effusion, cardiac arrhythmias, tissue extravasation/infiltration, neurological complications such as seizures or paraplegia, thrombosis, and death (2,11,13,14,16,19,30,31).

c. The decision to remove the catheter or attempt to correct the position is based on the location of the tip. Although PICCs are intended to be placed in central veins (see E, page 249), occasionally, the tip is in a noncentral location (e.g., in the subclavian vein). These noncentral PICCs may be used,

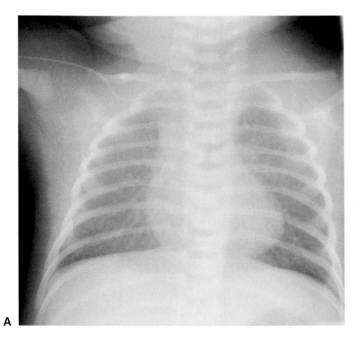

A

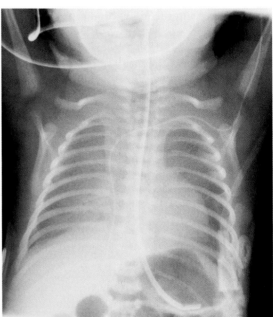

C

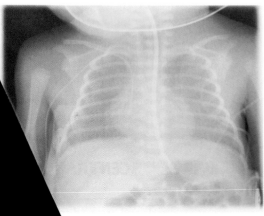

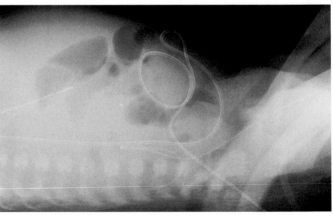

D

...rious venous malpositions of PICCs. **A:** Jugular. **B:** Tip in right atrium. **C:** PICC from left arm, through superior vena cava and right atrium, ... **D:** PICC from saphenous vein in leg entering vertebral venous plexus via ascending lumbar vein.

provided the fluids administered through them are isotonic, but the care of the catheters must be as stringent as for centrally placed catheters and they are at higher risk for complications (11,12).

   d. The catheter should be pulled back into an appropriate position if the tip is in the heart, as serious consequences such as cardiac arrhythmia, perforation, or pericardial effusion can occur (13,14).

   e. Catheters in the ascending lumbar vein or vertebral venous plexus must be removed, since the infusion of parenteral alimentation fluids in this area may lead to severe CNS damage, manifesting as seizures, paraplegia or death (Figs. 29.3 and 34.14D) (2,16,30).

   f. Spontaneous correction of malpositioned lines has been demonstrated in some cases (32). If the tip of the catheter is looped into the internal jugular or in the contralateral brachiocephalic vein, the catheter may be used temporarily (using isotonic fluids that are suitable for peripheral venous cannulae) and re-evaluated radiologically in 24 hours. If the catheter has not moved spontaneously into the desired location, it should be removed.

4. Infection.

   a. Infection is the most common complication of central venous catheters, with the smallest and most immature infants being at greatest risk. Other factors that increase the risk of infection include multiple attempts at placement, manipulation of the catheter, and contamination of the hub.

   b. Central line associated blood stream infection (CLABSI) rates range widely, but many centers have reported sustained reductions even to zero (4,5).

   c. The necessity of use of any indwelling catheter should be re-evaluated daily (33). Strict protocols for central line care and a methodology of surveillance with a data feedback mechanism are recommended to decrease CLABSI rates (3,33).

   d. Management (34).

     (1) Remove central venous line if possible.

     (2) Prompt removal of the line is recommended for *Staphylococcus aureus,* gram-negative, enterococcus, or *Candida* bacteremia.

     (3) Treatment with appropriate antibiotics without removal of the line may be attempted in infants with coagulase-negative *Staphylococcus* sepsis, but repeated positive cultures mandate removal of the line.

5. Catheter dysfunction.

   a. Obstruction of the catheter is characterized by increased pump pressures, or inability to infuse fluids or withdraw blood.

   b. Dysfunction may be due to malposition, fibrin thrombosis, precipitates caused by minerals or drugs, or lipid deposits (35).

   c. Management.

     (1) Check catheter position on chest radiograph.

     (2) If malposition is ruled out, review history of fluids and drugs administered through the catheter to determine probable cause of occlusion.

     (3) Remove the catheter if it is no longer medically critical.

     (4) Attempt clot dissolution only if maintenance of catheter is essential.

     (5) Equipment required: Face mask, sterile gloves and drape, antiseptic solution, sterile three-way stopcock, a 10-mL syringe, and a 3-mL syringe filled with 0.2 to 0.5 mL of agent for clot dissolution.

     (6) Agents for clot dissolution (35).

       (a) Hydrochloric acid 0.1 N, for calcium salt precipitates or drugs with pH < 7.

       (b) Sodium bicarbonate, 8.4%, 1 mEq/mL, for medications with pH > 7.

       (c) Ethanol, 70% concentration, for lipid deposits

       (d) Recombinant tissue plasminogen activator, 0.5 to 1 mg/mL, for fibrin or blood clot (36,37).

       (e) Recombinant urokinase, 2,000 to 5,000 IU/mL, for fibrin or blood clot.

     (7) Technique (38) (**Fig. 34.15**).

       (a) Use strict aseptic technique.

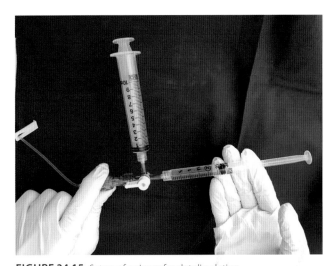

FIGURE 34.15 Set up of syringes for clot dissolution.

       (b) Remove IV tubing and cap to maintain sterility. After cleaning with prep, attach a three-way stopcock to catheter hub.

       (c) Attach an empty 10-mL syringe to the side port of the three-way stopcock and a pre-filled 3-mL syringe to the other port. Avoid use of 1-mL tuberculin syringe.

(d) Turn the stopcock off toward the pre-filled syringe and open toward the empty syringe.

(e) Aspirate on the empty syringe, creating negative pressure in the occluded catheter.

(f) While maintaining the negative pressure, turn the stopcock off to the empty syringe and open to the prefilled syringe. The negative pressure in the catheter will automatically cause the medication in the prefilled syringe to flow into the catheter toward the clot.

(g) Allow the medication to dwell in the catheter for 30 minutes to 2 hours.

(h) Aspirate after the dwell time to check for blood return, discard the aspirate, and flush the catheter with sterile normal saline. Resume catheter use.

(i) If the procedure is unsuccessful, it may be repeated once, or a different declotting agent may be tried.

(j) Do not use hydrochloric acid immediately before or after using sodium bicarbonate.

6. Thrombosis, thromboembolism.
   a. About 90% of venous thromboembolic events in neonates are associated with central venous catheters. They include deep venous thrombosis, SVC syndrome, intracardiac thrombus, pulmonary embolism, and renal vein thrombosis.
   b. The complications of venous thrombosis include loss of venous access, potential danger of injury to affected organ or limb, thrombus propagation, embolization to other areas, and infection.
   c. Management of thromboembolism in neonates is controversial, especially in infants under 32 weeks' gestational age. The severity of thrombosis and the potential risk to organs or limbs weighed against the degree of prematurity and risk of serious bleeding dictate the degree of intervention required, including the use of thrombolytic/anticoagulant therapy or surgical intervention (37) (see Chapter 36).

7. Extravascular collection of fluid.
   a. Pericardial effusion with or without cardiac tamponade **(Fig. 34.16)** (13,14,19). This serious complication presents as sudden cardiac collapse or unexplained cardiorespiratory instability. The cardiothoracic ratio is increased, and pulsus paradoxus may be noted (Fig. 39.1). Immediate pericardiocentesis may be life-saving (Chapter 42).
   b. Pleural effusion (39).
   c. Mediastinal extravasation.
   d. Hemothorax.
   e. Chylothorax (40).
   f. Ascites (41).

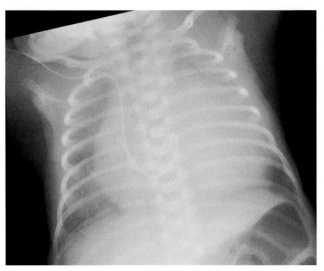

FIGURE 34.16 Pericardial effusion in preterm infant with PICC looped in right atrium.

8. Catheter breakage.
   a. Catheters may be severed by the introducer needle during insertion of a PICC, snap because of excessive tension on the external portion of the catheter, or rupture because of excessive pressure. Other common causes include external clamps, kinking of the catheter, constricting sutures, and poorly secured catheters. The intravascular portion of the broken catheter is at risk for embolization (42).
   b. In the event of catheter breakage, immediately grasp and secure the extravascular portion of the broken catheter to prevent migration.
   c. If the catheter is not visible outside the baby, apply pressure over the venous tract above the insertion site to prevent the catheter from advancing. Immobilize the infant, and obtain a radiograph immediately to localize the catheter.
   d. Surgical and/or cardiothoracic intervention may be required if the catheter is not visible externally (42).
   e. Damaged or broken catheters must be removed and replaced. Repaired catheters and catheter replacement over a guidewire place the patient at risk for infection or embolization. If no other options exist owing to limited venous access, the catheter can sometimes be repaired, utilizing meticulous aseptic technique. Repaired PICCs should be considered temporary, and a new catheter should be placed as soon as possible. Some manufacturers offer repair kits and instructions. A butterfly or blunt needle may be used in an emergency **(Fig. 34.17)** (43).

9. Tethered catheter.
   a. Difficulty in removing catheter may be due to the formation of a fibrin sheath.

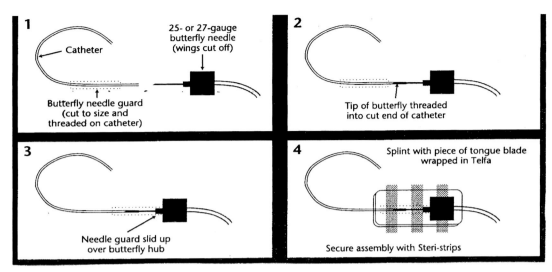

FIGURE 34.17 Emergency catheter repair using butterfly needle (43). (Reprinted with permission from Evans M, Lentsch D. Percutaneously inserted polyurethane central catheters in the NICU: One unit's experience. *Neonatal Netw.* 1999;18:37–46.)

b. Management.
   (1) Place warm compresses on skin along the vein.
   (2) Use gradual, gentle traction on the catheter.
   (3) Thrombolytic therapy (44).
   (4) Surgical removal through a peripheral incision.

References

1. Ainsworth S, McGuire W. Percutaneous central venous catheters versus peripheral cannulae for delivery of parenteral nutrition in neonates. *Cochrane Database Syst Rev.* 201510:CD004219.
2. Ramasethu J. Complications of vascular catheters in the neonatal intensive care unit. *Clin Perinatol.* 2008;35(1):199–222.
3. U.S. Department of Health and Human Services, Centers for Disease Control and Prevention. Guideline for prevention of intravascular catheter related infections; 2011:1. https://www.cdc.gov/infectioncontrol/guidelines/pdf/bsi/bsi-guidelines-H.pdf
4. Shepherd EG, Kelly TJ, Vinsel JA, et al. Significant reduction of central-line associated bloodstream infections in a network of diverse neonatal nurseries. *J Pediatr.* 2015;167(1):41–46.
5. Erdei C, McAvoy LL, Gupta M, et al. Is zero central line-associated bloodstream infection rate sustainable? A 5-year perspective. *Pediatrics.* 2015;135(6):e1485–e1493.
6. Panagiotounakou P, Antonogeorgos G, Gounari E, et al. Peripherally inserted central venous catheters: frequency of complications in premature newborn depends on the insertion site. *J Perinatology.* 2014;34(6):461–463.
7. Wrightson DD. Peripherally inserted central catheter complications in neonates with upper versus lower extremity insertion sites. *Adv Neonatal Care.* 2013;13(3):198–204.
8. Srinivasan HB, Tjin-A-Tam A, Galang R, et al. Migration patterns of peripherally inserted central venous catheters at 24 hours postinsertion in neonates. *Am J Perinatol.* 2013;30(10):871–874.
9. Braswell LE. Peripherally inserted central catheter placement in infants and children. *Tech Vasc Interv Radiol.* 2011;14(4):204–211.
10. Sneath N. Are supine chest and abdominal radiographs the best way to confirm PICC placement in neonates? *Neonatal Netw.* 2010;29(1):23–35.
11. Jain A, Deshpande P, Shah P. Peripherally inserted central catheter tip position and risk of associated complications in neonates. *J Perinatol.* 2013;33(4):307–312.
12. Goldwasser B, Baia C, Kim M, et al. Non-central peripherally inserted central catheters in neonatal intensive care: complication rates and longevity of catheters relative to tip position. *Pediatr Radiol.* 2017;47(12):1676–1681.
13. Nowlen TT, Rosenthal GL, Johnson GL, et al. Pericardial effusion and tamponade in infants with central catheters. *Pediatrics.* 2002;110:137–142.
14. Warren M, Thompson KS, Popek EJ, et al. Pericardial effusion and cardiac tamponade in neonates: sudden unexpected death associated with total parenteral nutrition via central venous catheterization. *Ann Clin Lab Sci.* 2013;43(2):163–171.
15. Cartwright DW. Central venous lines in neonates: a study of 2186 catheters. *Arch Dis Child Fetal Neonatal Ed.* 2004;89:F504–F508.
16. Coit AK, Kamitsuka MD; Pediatrix Medical Group. Peripherally inserted central catheter using the saphenous vein: importance of two-view radiographs to determine the tip location. *J Perinatol.* 2005;25:674–676.
17. Odd DE, Page B, Battin MR, et al. Does radio-opaque contrast improve radiographic localisation of percutaneous central venous lines? *Arch Dis Child Fetal Neonatal Ed.* 2004;89:F41–F43.
18. Sharma D, Farahbakhsh N, Tabatabaii SA. Role of ultrasound for central catheter tip localization in neonates: a review of the current evidence. *J Matern Fetal Neonatal Med.* 2019;32(14):2429–2437.
19. Pezzati M, Filippi L, Chiti G, et al. Central venous catheters and cardiac tamponade in preterm infants. *Intensive Care Med.* 2004;30:2253–2256.
20. Aly H, Herson V, Duncan A, et al. Is bloodstream infection preventable among premature infants? A tale of two cities. *Pediatrics.* 2005;115(6):1513–1518.
21. Smirk C, Soosay Raj T, Smith AL, et al. Neonatal percutaneous central venous lines: fit to burst. *Arch Dis Child Fetal Neonatal Ed.* 2009;94(4):F298–F300.

22. Shah PS, Shah VS. Continuous heparin infusion to prevent thrombosis and catheter occlusion in neonates with peripherally placed percutaneous central venous catheters. *Cochrane Database Syst Rev.* 2008;16:CD002772.

23. Repa A, Mayerhofer M, Worel N, et al. Blood transfusions using 27 gauge PICC lines: a retrospective clinical study on safety and feasibility. *Klin Padiatr.* 2014;226(1):3–7.

24. Seckold T, Walker S, Dwyer T. A comparison of silicone and polyurethane PICC lines and postinsertion complication rates: a systematic review. *J Vasc Access.* 2015;16(3):167–177.

25. Huang EY, Chen C, Abdullah F, et al. Strategies for the prevention of central venous catheter infections: an American Pediatric Surgical Association outcomes and clinical trials committee systematic review. *J Pediatr Surg.* 2011;46(10): 2000–2011.

26. Vegunta RK, Loethen P, Wallace LJ, et al. Differences in the outcome of surgically placed long-term central venous catheters in neonates: neck vs groin placement. *J Pediatr Surg.* 2005;40:47–51.

27. Murai DT. Are femoral Broviac catheters effective and safe? A prospective comparison of femoral and jugular venous Broviac catheters in newborn infants. *Chest.* 2002;121:1527–1530.

28. Vasudevan C, Oddie SJ, McGuire W. Early removal versus expectant management of central venous catheters in neonates with bloodstream infection. *Cochrane Database Syst Rev.* 2016;4:CD008436.

29. Gupta R, Drendel AL, Hoffmann RG, et al. Migration of central venous catheters in neonates: a radiographic assessment. *Am J Perinatol.* 2016;33(6):600–604.

30. Payne R, Sieg EP, Choudhary A, et al. Pneumorrhachis resulting in transient paresis after PICC line insertion into the ascending lumbar vein. *Cureus.* 2016;8(10):e833.

31. Wolfe DM. A previously undescribed etiology for oliguria in a premature infant with a peripherally inserted central catheter. *Adv Neonatal Care.* 2010;10(2):56–59.

32. Tawil KA, Eldemerdash A, Hathlol KA, et al. Peripherally inserted central venous catheters in newborn infants: malpositioning and spontaneous correction of catheter tips. *Am J Perinatol.* 2006;23(1):37–40.

33. The Joint Commission. Preventing central line–associated bloodstream infections: useful tools, an international perspective. Nov 20, 2013. http://www.jointcommission.org/CLABSIToolkit. Accessed March 2018.

34. Mermel LA, Allon M, Bouza E, et al. Clinical practice guidelines for the diagnosis and management of intravascular catheter-related infection: 2009 update by the Infectious Diseases Society of America. *Clin Infect Dis.* 2009;49:1–45.

35. Doellman D. Prevention, assessment and treatment of central venous catheter occlusions in neonatal and young pediatric patients. *J Infus Nurs.* 2011;34:251–258.

36. Soylu H, Brandao LR, Lee KS. Efficacy of local instillation of recombinant tissue plasminogen activator for restoring occluded central venous catheters in neonates. *J Pediatr.* 2010;156:197–201.

37. Monagle P, Chan AKC, Goldenberg NA, et al. Antithrombotic therapy for neonates and children: American College of Chest Physicians Evidence Based Clinical Practice Guidelines (9th Edition). *Chest.* 2012;141:737–801.

38. Hill J, Broadhurst D, Miller K, et al. Occlusion management guidelines for central venous access devices (CVADs). *Vascular Access.* 2013;7:1–36.

39. Bashir RA, Callejas AM, Osiovich HC, et al. Percutaneously inserted central catheter-related pleural effusion in a level III neonatal intensive care unit: a 5-year review (2008–2012). *JPEN J Parenter Enteral Nutr.* 2017;41(7):1234–1239.

40. Siu SL, Yang JY, Hui JP, et al. Chylothorax secondary to catheter related thrombosis successfully treated with heparin. *J Paediatr Child Health.* 2012;48(3):E105–E107.

41. Gupta A, Bhutada A, Yitayew M, et al. Extravasation of total parenteral nutrition into the liver from an upper extremity peripherally inserted central venous catheter. *J Neonatal Perinatal Med.* 2018;11(1):101–104.

42. Chiang MC, Chou YH, Chiang CC, et al. Successful removal of a ruptured silastic percutaneous central venous catheter in a tiny premature infant. *Chang Gung Med J.* 2006;29:603–606.

43. Evans M, Lentsch D. Percutaneously inserted polyurethane central catheters in the NICU: one unit's experience. *Neonatal Netw.* 1999;18:37–46.

44. Nguyen ST, Lund CH, Durand DJ. Thrombolytic therapy for adhesions of percutaneous central venous catheters to vein intima associated with Malassezia furfur infection. *J Perinatol.* 2001;21:331–333.

35

Extracorporeal Membrane Oxygenation Cannulation and Decannulation

M. Kabir Abubakar and Manuel B. Torres

Extracorporeal membrane oxygenation (ECMO) has now become the standard of care for patients with reversible pulmonary or cardiac insufficiency in whom optimized conventional treatments have failed. It is defined as the use of a modified heart–lung machine combined with an oxygenator to provide temporary cardiopulmonary support allowing time for recovery or as a bridge to organ transplant (1–7). As most causes of neonatal respiratory failure are self-limited, ECMO allows time for the lung to recover from the underlying disease process and for reversal of pulmonary hypertension, which frequently accompanies respiratory failure in the newborn.

VENOARTERIAL EXTRACORPOREAL MEMBRANE OXYGENATION— CANNULATION

A. Indications

Placement of carotid arterial and internal jugular venous catheters for use in venoarterial (VA) ECMO. VA ECMO should be used in patients with significant cardiovascular instability as it provides both respiratory and cardiac support.

B. Relative Contraindications for ECMO in the Neonatal Period (5,7)

1. Gestational age <34 weeks
2. Birthweight <2,000 g
3. Uncontrolled coagulopathy or bleeding disorders

4. Congenital heart disease without lung disease. Exception: Postoperative cardiac patients, a topic that will not be covered in this chapter
5. Irreversible lung pathology
6. Intracranial hemorrhage grade 3 or more
7. Major lethal congenital anomaly
8. Duration of maximum ventilatory support >10 to 14 days
9. Patients responding to ventilator management and/or inhaled nitric oxide

C. Precautions

1. Ensure that the patient is paralyzed before placing the venous catheter to prevent air embolus.
2. Recognize that
   a. Internal jugular lines placed for IV access prior to ECMO may cause clot formation, resulting in the need for thrombectomy before placement of the venous ECMO catheter.
   b. Excessive manipulation of the internal jugular vein may cause spasm and inability to place a catheter of appropriate gauge.
   c. A lacerated vessel may result in the need for a sternotomy for vessel retrieval.
      Appropriate instruments should be on the bedside tray or cart.
      A backup unit of blood should be available in the blood bank for immediate release.
   d. Blood loss sufficient to produce hypotension can occur during a difficult cannulation.
      Emergency blood should be available at the bedside (10 to 20 mL/kg).

e. The vagus nerve is located next to the neck vessels, and may be injured or manipulated during isolation of the vessels. Manipulation can cause bradycardia or other arrhythmias.

f. Vital signs and pulse oximetry values must be monitored at all times because clinical observation of the infant is prevented by the surgical drapes.

g. If the patient has been manually ventilated for stabilization with a self-inflating bag, do not place the bag on the bedside when surgical drapes are placed. The bag may entrap oxygen, which can result in a fire when electrocautery is used.

D. Personnel, Equipment, and Medications (8)

Personnel

1. Surgical team
   a. Experienced surgeon (pediatric, cardiovascular, or thoracic)
   b. Assistant surgeon (Fellow, resident, physician assistant, registered nurse first assistant)
   c. Surgical scrub nurse/tech
   d. Circulating nurse
2. Medical team
   a. A physician trained in management of ECMO patients and cannulation techniques, who will administer anesthetic agents and manage the infant medically during the procedure
   b. A bedside intensive care (neonatal or pediatric intensive care unit) nurse, who will monitor vital signs, record events, and draw up medications as needed by the ECMO physician
   c. A respiratory therapist, who will change ventilator settings as necessary
3. Circuit specialists
   a. A cardiovascular perfusionist, nurse, or respiratory therapist specially trained in this procedure, who will prime the pump
   b. A bedside ECMO specialist (nurse, respiratory therapist, or cardiovascular perfusionist with special training in ECMO management), who will manage the ECMO system after the patient is on ECMO

Equipment (Fig. 35.1)

Sterile

1. Arterial and venous catheters (9)
   a. Arterial
      (1) The size of the arterial catheter determines the resistance of the ECMO circuit because it is the part of the ECMO circuit with the

VENOARTERIAL ECMO CIRCUIT

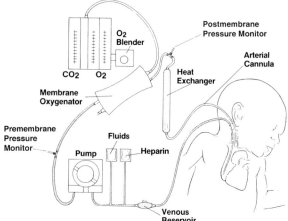

FIGURE 35.1 Schematic diagram of VA ECMO circuit, showing the drainage from the right atrium into the bladder of the circuit, with flow through the membrane lung, heat exchanger, and return flow to the arch of the aorta via the carotid artery catheter. (Reprinted from Polin RA, Fox WC, eds. *Fetal and Neonatal Physiology*. Vol. 1. Philadelphia, PA: WB Saunders; 1992:933. Copyright © 1992 Elsevier. With permission.)

smallest internal diameter and thus the highest resistance.

(2) This catheter should be as short as possible, with a thin wall and a large internal diameter (resistance is directly proportional to the length of the catheter and inversely proportional to the diameter). An example of a suitable catheter is the Bio-Medicus extracorporeal circulation cannula, 8 to 10 French (Fr) (Medtronic, Minneapolis, Minnesota).

b. Venous
   (1) Venous catheter with
      (a) As large an internal diameter as possible, to allow maximal blood flow (the patient's oxygenation is related directly to the rate of blood flow).
      (b) A thin wall/large internal diameter. An example of a suitable catheter is the Bio-Medicus extracorporeal circulation cannula, 8 to 14 Fr (Medtronic, Minneapolis, Minnesota).

2. Surgical instruments required are listed in **Tables 35.1** and **35.2**
3. Gowns and gloves
4. Saline for injection
5. Syringes (1 to 20 mL) and needles (19 to 26 gauge)
6. Povidone-iodine solution
7. Povidone-iodine ointment
8. Semipermeable transparent membrane–type dressing
9. Absorbable gelatin sponge, for example, Gelfoam (Upjohn, Kalamazoo, Michigan)
10. Surgical lubricant, bacteriostatic

TABLE 35.1 **Surgical Instruments for ECMO Cannulation**

NUMBER	ITEM	NUMBER	ITEM
Place in a 12- × 18-in Mayo tray with a Huck towel on the bottom of the tray.		String the following instruments from left to right on two 9-in sponge sticks or instrument stringer. Then place on top of a rolled Huck towel.	
2	Custard cup (place on inside of other cup with a 3- × 4-in sponge)	4	9-in sponge stick
1	Medicine cup (place inside of custard cup with a 3- × 4-in sponge)	1	Tonsil clamp (bleeder)
2	Straight bulldog clamps	1	6.5-in Crile
1	Sauer eye retractor	1	5.75-in Crile
1	Alm retractor	1	Baby right-angle clamp
1	Jansen Mastoid retractor	4	Straight mosquitoes
2	Vein retractors	6	Curved mosquitoes
2	Octagonal forceps	3	Fine curved mosquitoes
2	7-in Gerald forceps	2	Tubing clamp with guard
2	6-in DeBakey forceps	1	Ryder needle holder
1	Adson forceps, plain	1	Webster needle holder
2	Adson forceps with teeth	1	Straight Mayo scissor
2	No. 3 knife handles	1	5.75-in Metzenbaum scissor
1	Castroviejo needle holder	1	Curved Steven scissor
2	Right-angle retractors	1	Straight Iris scissor
2	Chops retractors	4	Small towel clips (nonpenetrating)
1	Set of Garrett dilators, nine pieces (sizes 1, 1.5, 2, 2.5, 3, 3.5, 4, 4.5, 5)	1	Baby Satinsky clamp
		1	Curved bulldog clamp
		1	Straight bulldog clamp
		1	Disposable ECMO tray (Table 35.2)

For information on suture material, see Appendix D.

ECMO, extracorporeal membrane oxygenation.

TABLE 35.2 Contents of Disposable ECMO Tray

NUMBER	ITEM
2	1-mL syringe
1	20-mL syringe
1	6-mL syringe
1	3-mL syringe
1	Needle adapter
3	Single-cavity tray
2	Gauze packages
1	Betadine ointment
1	Surgical blade no. 15 carbon
2	Semipermeable transparent dressings
1	Handle, suction Frazier, 8 Fr
1	Xylocaine insert
1	Mini yellow vessel loops
1	Hand-control cautery
1	Suture, 4-0 Vicryl/ monofilament
1	Suture, 2-0 silk
1	Suture, 6-0 Prolene
4	Forceps, sponge
1	25-gauge needle
1	NaCl, 5-mL amp
1	3-g foil package of Surgilube
1	Surgical blade, no. 11 carbon
2	Steri-Drapes
2	Connectors, straight 0.25 × 0.25 in
1	Xylocaine 1%
1	Suction tubing, 3/16 in × 10 feet
1	Package sterile towels (14)

Nonsterile

1. Surgical head covers and mask
2. Pulse oximeter
3. Surgical head light
4. Electrocautery
5. Wall suction
6. Shoulder roll, for example, a small blanket, to place under infant's shoulders
7. Tubing clamps

Medications

1. A long-acting paralyzing agent, for example, pancuronium bromide (0.1 mg/kg)
2. Fentanyl citrate (10 to 20 µg/kg)
3. Sodium heparin (50 to 150 U/kg)
4. Topical thrombin/Gelfoam
5. Lidocaine, 0.25%, with epinephrine
6. Lidocaine, 1%, plain (without epinephrine)
7. Cryoprecipitate, thawed, or commercially available fibrin sealant (optional)

E. Technique—Preparation for Cannulation

1. Place infant supine with head at the "foot" of the overhead warmer bed.
2. Place the x-ray cassette that is needed to quickly confirm catheter placement underneath the patient so as to avoid unnecessarily moving the patient and dislodging the cannulae during procedure.
3. Anesthetize the patient with fentanyl (10 to 20 µg/kg).
4. Paralyze the patient with pancuronium (0.1 mg/kg).
5. Hyperextend the patient's neck with a shoulder roll, and turn the head to the left (**Fig. 35.2**). Make sure that the Bovie ground pad is placed at this time. Ensure that

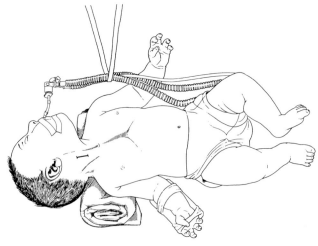

FIGURE 35.2 Infant positioned for cannulation with shoulder roll present and head extended to the left. Position of neck incision is indicated.

the endotracheal tube is positioned adequately so it does not kink under the drapes during the procedure and ensure access to infusion pumps, IVs, and arterial ports.

Observe closely for hypotension.

6. Monitor vital signs and give additional fentanyl and/or pancuronium as needed (see Chapter 7).
7. Clean a wide area of the right neck, chest, and ear with povidone-iodine solution.
8. Drape the infant and entire bed with sterile towels.
9. Use Steri-Drapes (3M Health Care, St. Paul, Minnesota) to secure the towels to the skin.
10. At the point of incision, infiltrate the skin with lidocaine (0.25%, with epinephrine) (see **Fig. 35.2**).
11. Wait at least 3 minutes for anesthesia to be effective.
12. Make a 2- to 3-cm cervical incision over the lower sternocleidomastoid muscle, 1 cm above the clavicle (**Fig. 35.3**).
13. Continue to use the electrocautery to cut through the platysma and subcutaneous tissue until the sternocleidomastoid muscle is reached.
14. Coagulate all visible bleeding sites.
15. Bluntly spread the sternal and clavicular heads of the sternocleidomastoid muscle apart with a hemostat and retract using self-retaining retractors (**Fig. 35.4**).
16. Open the carotid sheath, identify and isolate the common carotid artery, vagus nerve, and internal jugular vein.
17. Avoid excessive handling of the internal jugular vein. Some surgeons isolate the vein after cannulation of the carotid artery to avoid spasm.
18. Encircle the vessels with silicone vessel loops proximally and distally with 2-0 silk ties held with hemostat clamps but not tied. Avoid "sawing" the ties on the artery.

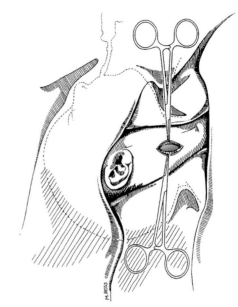

FIGURE 35.4 Split sternocleidomastoid and open carotid sheath.

19. Estimate the length of the cannula to be inserted.
    a. Identify the sternal notch and the xiphoid process.
    b. The arterial catheter is inserted approximately one-third of the distance between the sternal notch and the xiphoid process. This is typically between 3 and 4 cms.
    c. The venous catheter is inserted approximately one-half the distance between the sternal notch and the xiphoid process. This is typically between 7 and 7.5 cms.
    d. Mark these distances on the catheters with a 2-0 tie, or note the distance if the cannula is marked.
20. Heparinize the patient with a bolus of 50 to 150 U/kg of heparin, depending on the estimated risk of bleeding,

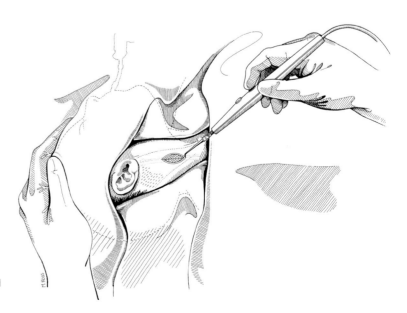

FIGURE 35.3 Landmarks over the sternocleidomastoid muscle for making the incision with electrocautery.

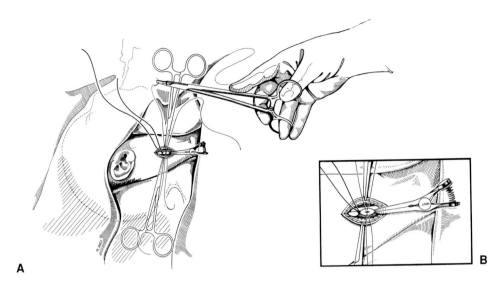

A

B

FIGURE 35.5 A: Carotid artery isolated with vessel clamp in place and with arteriotomy site showing the placement of the 6-0 Prolene traction sutures. **B (inset):** Magnified view of (**A**).

and wait 3 minutes to allow circulation before proceeding with cannulation.

21. During this time, you may irrigate both the common carotid artery and internal jugular vein with 1% plain lidocaine or papaverine to prevent vasospasm.

Arterial Cannulation

1. Tie the distal 2-0 silk ligature on the carotid artery, and place a bulldog clamp on the proximal portion of the artery.

   Allow blood to dilate the artery before placing the bulldog clamp.

2. Make a transverse arteriotomy using a no. 11 scalpel blade near the distal ligature, and place two

full-thickness traction sutures of 6-0 Prolene (Ethicon, Somerville, New Jersey) on the proximal side of the arteriotomy (**Fig. 35.5**).

Always use traction sutures to prevent subintimal dissection during cannula insertion.

3. If desired, lubricate Garrett dilators with sterile surgical lubricant and dilate the artery to the approximate size of the catheter.

4. Place a sterile tubing clamp on the catheter. Lubricate the catheter and insert the catheter into the vessel as the bulldog clamp is removed.

5. Secure the catheter with the proximal 2-0 silk ligature tied over a 0.5- to 1-cm cut piece of silastic vessel loop ("bootie") to protect the vessel from injury during decannulation (**Fig. 35.6**). Some surgeons place two ligatures proximally for added security.

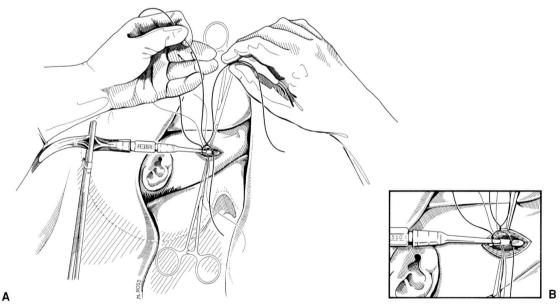

A

B

FIGURE 35.6 A: Securing the catheter with proximal and distal ties onto a "bootie." **B (inset):** Magnified view of (**A**).

6. Tie the distal tie around the catheter, and then tie the distal and proximal ties together.

7. Allow blood to back up into the catheter to remove air.

Venous Cannulation

1. Do not apply traction to the vein with the ties, to avoid spasm.

2. Place a bulldog clamp on the proximal end of the vein, allowing blood to distend it. Then tie the distal end of the vein with the 2-0 silk ligature.

3. Make a venotomy with a no. 11 scalpel blade; you may place two traction sutures of 6-0 Prolene, as for arterial cannulation but not routinely necessary.

4. Lubricate the venous catheter, place a sterile tubing clamp on the catheter, and dilate the venotomy.

5. Insert the catheter as surgical assistant places traction on the proximal tie, and apply pressure over the liver to increase the backflow of blood out of the catheter (to decrease the risk of an air embolus).

   There will be slight impedance to catheter advancement at the thoracic inlet—pushing against resistance will tear the vein. Use gentle downward and posterior pressure.

6. Secure the venous catheter in the same way as the arterial catheter (**Fig. 35.6**). Allow blood to back up into the catheter to remove air (may need to gently press on the liver).

7. If desired, pack the wound with absorbable gelatin sponge soaked in topical thrombin or commercially available topical fibrin sealant to assist in hemostasis.

   Cryoprecipitate and topical thrombin can be used to form a fibrin clot if dropped onto the field from separate syringes in a one-to-one concentration. Note: If they are mixed together in one syringe, they will form a solid clot in the syringe. A similar product is also commercially available as TISSEEL-HV fibrin sealant (Baxter Hyland Division, Glendale, California).

8. Confirm catheter placement by chest radiography and/or cardiac echocardiography, if the patient is stable (**Fig. 35.7**) (10,11). If the patient is unstable, he or she can be placed on ECMO and the radiograph taken when adequate oxygenation is achieved but prior to closing the surgical wound.

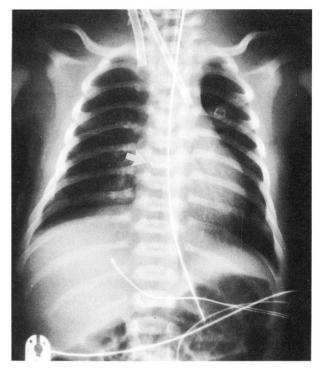

FIGURE 35.7 Radiograph at cannulation, showing proper placement of the arterial and venous catheters. Note the radio-opaque dot indicating the end of the Bio-Medicus venous extracorporeal membrane oxygenation catheter (*arrow*).

VENOVENOUS EXTRACORPOREAL MEMBRANE OXYGENATION— CANNULATION

More than 60% of neonatal ECMO patients reported in the ELSO registry have received treatment with VA bypass (12). In neonates with respiratory failure, VA ECMO is gradually being replaced by a venovenous (VV) technique, which uses a single double-lumen catheter (**Fig. 35.8**). The catheter is placed in the right atrium, where blood is drained and reinfused into the same chamber, thus requiring cannulation of only the right jugular vein, and sparing the carotid artery. The design of the original VV catheter resulted in significant recirculation, limiting its use when ECMO flows of >350 mL/min were required. Newer catheter designs have significantly

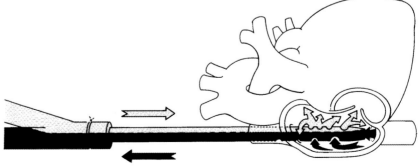

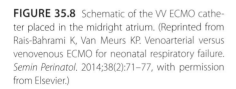

FIGURE 35.8 Schematic of the VV ECMO catheter placed in the midright atrium. (Reprinted from Rais-Bahrami K, Van Meurs KP. Venoarterial versus venovenous ECMO for neonatal respiratory failure. *Semin Perinatol.* 2014;38(2):71–77, with permission from Elsevier.)

lowered the degree of recirculation (13). The double-lumen catheter should be placed within the right atrium, directing the oxygenated blood from the return lumen through the tricuspid valve to minimize recirculation. This catheter design in 12-, 15-, and 18-Fr sizes allows the use of VV ECMO in a greater number of infants (14).

A. Double-Lumen VV Catheters

1. Kendall 14-Fr catheter (Kendall Health Care Products, Mansfield, Massachusetts)
2. OriGen 12-, 15-, and 18-Fr catheters (OriGen Biomedical, Austin, Texas)
3. Avalon Elite DLC, 13- to 31-Fr catheter (Getinge AB, Gothenburg, Sweden)

   Note: The Avalon catheter requires insertion under ultrasound or fluoroscopy guidance; refer to company recommendations at https://getinge.com

B. Advantages of VV Bypass

1. Provides excellent pulmonary support
2. Avoids carotid artery ligation
3. Maintains normal pulsatile blood flow
4. Oxygenated blood enters the pulmonary circulation.
5. Particles coming from the ECMO circuit enter the venous circulation instead of the arterial circulation

C. Disadvantages of VV Bypass

1. Lack of cardiac support
2. ECMO support is dependent on the patient's cardiac function
3. Catheter position and rotation are extremely critical
4. Amount of recirculation

D. Cannulation Technique

The cannulation technique for VV ECMO is essentially the same procedure as venous cannulation for VA ECMO, with the following exceptions.

1. Both internal jugular vein and carotid arteries are identified and dissected free, although the internal jugular vein is the only vessel cannulated with the double-lumen VV catheter. Both vessels are isolated in case a rapid conversion to VA bypass becomes necessary. A silastic loop may be tied loosely around the artery to facilitate potential conversion to VA flow.
2. The cannula is advanced with the lumen, which will carry oxygenated blood ("arterial side") upward and anterior to the venous side of the double lumen (see **Fig. 35.8**).

Caution: Avoid bending the catheter or creating a "crimp" in the catheter.

Correct positioning of the catheter helps direct the oxygenated blood return toward the tricuspid valve, thus minimizing the recirculation of the oxygenated blood back to the ECMO circuit.

3. The proximal end of the internal jugular vein is also cannulated for cephalad drainage, that is, a jugular bulb catheter. This catheter is connected to the venous tubing of the ECMO circuit via a Luer connector. For this, we use a custom-made Carmeda heparin-coated Bio-Medicus venous catheter (Medtronic, Minneapolis, MN), made specifically for use as a cephalad catheter.

   This allows additional venous drainage to the ECMO circuit, prevents venous congestion, and also allows for cephalic venous saturation measurement.
4. If using a jugular bulb catheter to measure cerebral saturations, care should be used when entering the circuit; air will draw into the venous side of the circuit rapidly if a stopcock is loose or is left open.

E. Placing Patient on the Extracorporeal Membrane Oxygenation Circuit

The circuit has been previously primed with packed cells/albumin. The priming procedure and the surgical placement of the ECMO catheters should be timed so that the two are completed at the same time. Priming of the circuit is beyond the scope of this chapter.

1. Fill catheters with sterile saline. Connect them to the ECMO circuit by inserting the 0.25- × 0.25-in connectors into the tubing as the assistant drips sterile saline into the ends of the circuit tubing and the catheter, to ensure that all residual air is eliminated prior to connection.
   a. Do not squeeze the tubing while attaching; air will enter when the tubing is released.
   b. If air is seen in the tubing, the catheters must be disconnected from the circuit. Prior to reconnection, air is removed, and the catheters are reconnected as described in E1.
2. Remove all sterile tubing clamps from the catheters, and have an assistant hold the catheters. Nonsterile tubing clamps remain in place on the arterial and venous sides of the circuit at this juncture.
3. Place the patient on ECMO by removing the arterial clamp, placing a clamp on the bridge (**Fig. 35.9A**), and removing the venous clamp. This will remove all nonsterile clamps from the circuit.

   Many centers are now using a "bloodless bridge" that has sterile heparinized saline with stopcock design; thus, a clamp on the bridge is not necessary. The bridge is left closed with the stopcock mechanism during cannulation so that only the clamps on the catheters need to be removed.

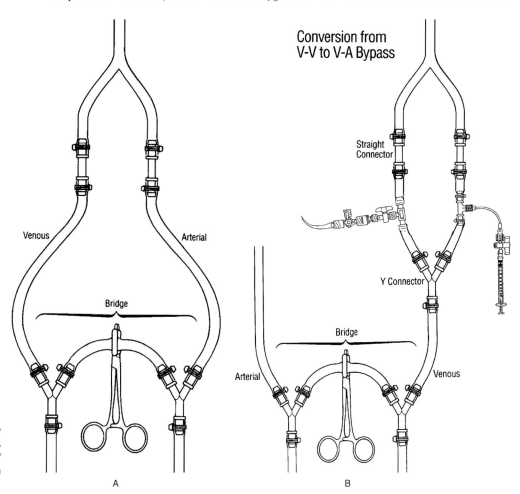

Conversion from V-V to V-A Bypass

FIGURE 35.9 Schematic view of converting from V-V (**A**) to V-A (**B**) ECMO. The double lumen VV catheter is "Yd" together to make a double lumen drainage catheter.

4. Increase ECMO flow in 50-mL increments over 20 to 30 minutes, until adequate oxygenation is achieved (usually at 120 mL/kg/min).

   Transfusion may be needed if hypotension occurs at this stage.

5. Decrease the ventilator settings and oxygen concentration gradually as the ECMO flows are increased.

   Typical resting ventilator settings for VA ECMO are at a rate of 10 to 15 breaths/min, a peak pressure limit of 15 to 20 cm H_2O, positive end-expiratory pressure (PEEP) of 8 to 10 cm H_2O (depending on lung expansion and underlying disease condition), and FiO_2 of 0.21 to 0.30. For VV ECMO, it is recommended to keep ventilator settings at a rate of 20 to 30 breaths/min, a peak inspiratory pressure of 20 to 25 cm H_2O, PEEP 8 to 10 cm H_2O, and FiO_2 of 0.30 to 0.35.

F. Closure of the Neck Wound

1. Obtain radiographic confirmation of appropriate catheter position and achievement of an adequate flow rate through the ECMO circuit prior to closure of the neck wound.
2. Cut and remove traction sutures.

3. Approximate the skin with a continuous monofilament suture on an atraumatic needle.
4. Use several 2-0 silk sutures on a noncutting needle to secure the catheters to the skin.
5. Dress the incision with povidone-iodine ointment, and cover the area with gauze and a semipermeable membrane dressing.
6. Affix the circuit tubing securely to the bed to reduce traction on the catheters.

G. Complications

1. Torn vessels, more commonly the vein.
   a. This risk is decreased if 6-0 Prolene stay sutures are always used.
   b. Do not attempt to use too large a catheter.
2. Aortic dissection associated with arterial cannulation (15).
3. Blood loss, particularly during the venous cannulation, when side holes in the catheter are outside the vein.
4. Venous spasm, resulting in inability to place a large enough venous catheter to meet the required ECMO flow to support the patient adequately.

The rate of blood flow is impeded by the small gauge of the catheter, requiring that a second venous catheter be placed in the femoral vein. The two catheters must be Y-connected together into the ECMO circuit.

5. Arrhythmias and/or bradycardia can occur, owing to stimulation of the vagus nerve.
6. Hypotension, due to an increase in the intravascular space when the patient is connected to the ECMO circuit.
7. Conversion to VA from VV ECMO. This will occur if
   a. The patient remains hypoxic despite adequate ECMO flow.
   b. The patient remains hypotensive despite vasopressor support.
   c. Cerebral venous saturations remain persistently <60% after adequate flows and ventilator management have been undertaken.
   Converting from VV to VA ECMO requires cannulation of carotid artery with a Bio-Medicus arterial catheter, and the double-lumen VV catheter must be "Y'd" in together to make a double-lumen venous drainage catheter (**Fig. 35.9**).

EXTRACORPOREAL MEMBRANE OXYGENATION—DECANNULATION

A. Indications

1. Removal from ECMO after lung recovery
2. Removal from ECMO because of a complication such as uncontrolled bleeding or failure of lung recovery

B. Contraindications

All intensive support is being withdrawn, and permission for autopsy is obtained. It is usually optimal to remove the catheters during the autopsy.

C. Precautions

1. The patient must be paralyzed during the removal of the venous catheter to avoid an air embolus.
2. The vessels are fragile and may tear. A backup unit of blood should be available at the bedside.
3. Delay removing catheter for 12 to 24 hours after taking the patient off bypass in cases in which there is a high risk of reoccurrence of pulmonary hypertension and thus need for second ECMO run (e.g., severe congenital diaphragmatic hernia). This procedure places a risk of development of right atrial clots from the venous catheter and, in some patients, has resulted in superior venocaval syndrome. Therefore, the time the catheters

are left in place after the patient has been taken off bypass (e.g., on idle) should be limited to no more than 24 hours.

D. Personnel, Equipment, and Medications

Personnel

Same as for cannulation, with the exception that the primer is not required

Equipment

Sterile

1. Surgical tray with towels and suture as for cannulation
2. Semipermeable transparent dressing
3. Povidone-iodine ointment
4. Syringes (1 to 20 mL) and needles (18 to 26 gauge)
5. Unit of blood
6. Absorbable gelatin sponge

Nonsterile

Same as for cannulation

Medications

1. Fentanyl (10 to 20 µg/kg)
2. Vecuronium bromide (0.2 mg/kg). A short-acting paralyzing agent is preferred because of the relatively short duration of the procedure. This allows the infant to breathe spontaneously as soon as possible after decannulation, which facilitates rapid weaning from ventilator support.
3. Lidocaine, 0.25%, with epinephrine
4. Topical thrombin
5. Protamine sulfate (1 mg only)

E. Technique

Postdecannulation vessel reconstruction is beyond the scope of this chapter.

1. Place the neck in an extended position, using the shoulder roll.
2. Give fentanyl for analgesia, prior to giving vecuronium.
   Because of the risk of air embolism during the removal of the venous catheter, the infant must *not* be allowed to breathe during decannulation. If two doses of vecuronium do not produce paralysis, give pancuronium.
3. Increase ventilator setting to a rate of 40 to 50 breaths/min, a peak inspiratory pressure of 20 to 25 cm H_2O

(depending on chest movement and tidal volume), and FiO_2 of 0.30 to 0.40 after paralytic agent is given.

4. Clean the neck, and drape as for cannulation.
5. Anesthetize with 0.25% lidocaine with epinephrine.
6. Cut and remove the continuous monofilament skin suture.
7. Remove absorbable gelatin sponge packing, exposing the catheters and vessels.

    If a jugular bulb catheter is in place, it is usually removed first to allow better visualization for removal of the VV ECMO catheter.

8. The jugular bulb catheter should be clamped off before removal, after the patient is taken off bypass. Be aware that removing the catheter while on bypass without a clamp in place will result in the introduction of air into the circuit.

    In case of VA ECMO, the venous catheter is usually removed first because it is most readily accessible.

9. Separate the catheter from surrounding tissue by blunt dissection.
10. Encircle the vein with a 2-0 silk tie, which is used for traction and hemostatic control.
11. Place a Satinsky clamp around the vein to stabilize the catheter (**Fig. 35.10**).

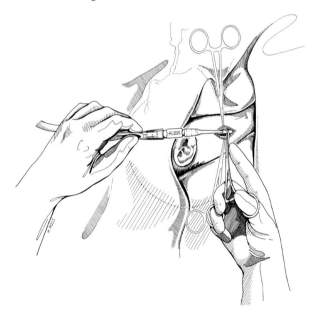

FIGURE 35.10 Placement of Satinsky vessel clamp prior to removal of ECMO catheter.

12. Place a 2-0 silk tie proximal to the clamp.
13. Cut the silk tie(s) securing the catheter in the vein with a no. 11 scalpel blade over the vessel loop ("bootie").
14. Ask the ECMO specialist to remove the patient from the ECMO circuit.
15. Monitor vital signs and oxygen saturation as an indication that ventilator settings are appropriate. Settings may have to be increased when the patient is removed from the circuit.

16. Provide an inspiratory "hold" on the ventilator while the surgeon removes the venous catheter. Failure to do this can result in air embolus.
17. Replace any significant blood loss.
18. Cut the 2-0 silk traction suture and tie the suture proximal to the Satinsky clamp. Remove the Satinsky clamp.
19. Isolate the arterial catheter, dissect free, and remove.

    The decannulation procedure is the same as for the venous catheter, with the exception of an inspiratory hold that is not required.

20. Give protamine (1 mg IV) after removal of both catheters.

    Administration of protamine is not mandatory if there is no significant bleeding.

21. Irrigate the wound with sterile saline and cauterize any bleeding sites.
22. If desired, pack the wound with a thrombin-soaked absorbable gelatin sponge and close the neck incision using interrupted absorbable sutures.
23. Remove the skin sutures holding the catheters.
24. Place povidone-iodine ointment over the incision and cover with gauze and semipermeable transparent dressing.

F. Complications

1. Vessel laceration, which may require a sternotomy for correction
2. Excessive blood loss
3. Venous air embolus

Acknowledgments

We gratefully acknowledge the important contributions of Khodayar Rais-Bahrami, Gary E. Hartman, and Billie Lou Short, who were the authors of this chapter in the previous editions of this book.

References

1. O'Rourke PP, Crone RK, Vacanti JP, et al. Extracorporeal membrane oxygenation and conventional medical therapy in neonates with persistent pulmonary hypertension of the newborn: a prospective randomized study. *Pediatrics.* 1989;84:957–963.
2. UK Collaborative ECMO Trail Group. UK collaborative randomised trial of neonatal extracorporeal membrane oxygenation. *Lancet.* 1996;348:75–82.
3. Mugford M, Elbourne D, Field D. Extracorporeal membrane oxygenation for severe respiratory failure in newborn infants. *Cochrane Database Syst Rev.* 2008;(3):CD001340.
4. Fortenberry JD, Lorusso R. The history and development of extracorporeal support. In: Brogan TV, Lequier L, Lorusso R, et al., eds. *Extracorporeal Life Support: The ELSO Red Book.* 5th ed. Ann Arbor, MI: Extracorporeal Life Support Organization; 2017:1.

5. Mahmood B, Newton D, Pallotto EK. Current trends in neonatal ECMO. *Semin Perinatol.* 2018;42(2):80–88.
6. Bartlett RH, Gattinoni L. Current status of extracorporeal life support (ECMO) for cardiopulmonary failure. *Minerva Anestesiol.* 2010;76(7):534–540.
7. Fletcher K, Chapman R, Keene S. An overview of medical ECMO for neonates. *Semin Perinatol.* 2018;42(2):68–79.
8. Sutton RG, Salatich A, Jegier B, et al. A 2007 survey of extracorporeal life support members: personnel and equipment. *J Extra Corpor Technol.* 2009;41:172–179.
9. Wang S, Palanzo D, Kunselman AR, et al. In vitro hemodynamic evaluation of five 6 Fr and 8 Fr arterial cannulae in simulated neonatal cardiopulmonary bypass circuits. *Artif Organs.* 2016;40(1):56–64.
10. Irish MS, O'Toole SJ, Kapur P, et al. Cervical ECMO cannula placement in infants and children: recommendations for assessment of adequate positioning and function. *J Pediatr Surg.* 1998;33:929–931.
11. Thomas TH, Price R, Ramaciotti C, et al. Echocardiography, not chest radiography, for evaluation of cannula placement during pediatric extracorporeal membrane oxygenation. *Pediatr Crit Care Med.* 2009;10:56–59.
12. *Neonatal ECMO Registry of the Extracorporeal Life Support Organization (ELSO).* Ann Arbor, MI: ELSO; 2018. https://www.elso.org/Registry.aspx
13. Rais-Bahrami K, Rivera O, Mikesell GT, et al. Improved oxygenation with reduced recirculation during venovenous extracorporeal membrane oxygenation: evaluation of a test catheter. *Crit Care Med.* 1995;23:1722–1725.
14. Rais-Bahrami K, Waltom DM, Sell JE, et al. Improved oxygenation with reduced recirculation during venovenous ECMO: comparison of two catheters. *Perfusion.* 2002;17:415–419.
15. Paul JJ, Desai H, Baumgart S, et al. Aortic dissection in a neonate associated with arterial cannulation for extracorporeal life support. *ASAIO J.* 1997;43:92–94.

36

Management of Vascular Spasm and Thrombosis

Matthew A. Saxonhouse and Ashley Hinson

A. Definitions

Within the pediatric population, neonates are at the highest risk for thrombosis. The combination of environmental and genetic prothrombotic risk factors significantly increases this risk. The use of arterial and central venous catheters represents the greatest risk for the development of thrombosis (1,2). Although thrombosis can occur at several sites, this chapter focuses on catheter-related thrombosis. Recommendations for treatment of neonatal thrombosis are based on expert opinion and data from case series/studies. Care for neonates with significant thromboses should occur at a tertiary referral center that has appropriate subspecialty and laboratory support.

1. Prothrombotic disorder is the inheritance of a genetic mutation that results in the absence or severe deficiency of an inhibitor of hemostasis, the production of an inhibitor of hemostasis that has inadequate function despite normal levels, or an overproduction of a procoagulant protein or cofactor.
2. Vascular spasm is transient, reversible arterial constriction, often triggered by intravascular catheterization or arterial blood sampling.
3. Thrombosis is the complete or partial obstruction of arteries or veins by blood clot(s).
4. Anticoagulation is the process of administering an agent that hinders the clotting of blood.
5. Thrombolysis refers to the process of providing an agent that destroys or dissolves an active blood clot.

B. Assessment

1. Clinical Diagnosis

a. Risk factors associated with the development of neonatal thrombosis are presented in **Table 36.1**.

b. Neonatal thromboses may occur in a variety of locations and may present with varying signs and symptoms (**Table 36.2**).
c. **Vascular spasm** of peripheral arteries is characterized by transient pallor, or cyanosis of the involved extremity with diminished pulses and perfusion. The clinical effects of vascular spasm usually last <4 hours from the onset, but the condition may be difficult to differentiate from more serious thrombosis. The diagnosis of vasospasm of arteries is usually made *retrospectively* after documentation of the transient nature of ischemic changes and complete recovery of circulation (**Figs. 36.1 and 36.2**) (3).

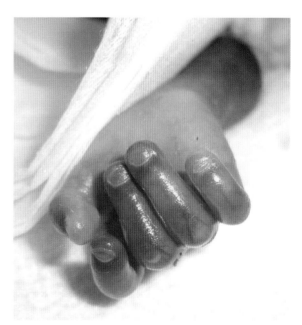

FIGURE 36.1 Vasospasm following attempted radial artery catheterization in extremely preterm infant.

TABLE 36.1 **Risk Factors for the Development of Neonatal Thromboses**

MATERNAL RISK FACTORS	DELIVERY RISK FACTORS	NEONATAL RISK FACTORS
Infertility Oligohydramnios Prothrombotic disorder Preeclampsia Diabetes Intrauterine growth restriction Chorioamnionitis Prolonged rupture of membranes Autoimmune disorders	Emergent cesarean section Fetal heart rate abnormalities Instrumentation Meconium-stained fluid	Central venous/arterial catheters[a] Congenital heart disease Sepsis Meningitis Birth asphyxia Respiratory distress syndrome Dehydration Congenital nephritic/nephrotic syndrome Necrotizing enterocolitis Polycythemia Pulmonary hypertension Surgery Extracorporeal membrane oxygenation Medications (steroids)

[a]Greatest risk factor for thrombosis.

From Saxonhouse MA, Manco-Johnson MJ. The evaluation and management of neonatal coagulation disorders. *Semin Perinatol.* 2009;33:56; and Data from (1,11,27–36).

TABLE 36.2 **Locations of Neonatal Thromboses and the Best Imaging Modalities to Diagnose Them**

VESSEL	TYPE OF THROMBOSES *(VESSELS POTENTIALLY INVOLVED)*	IMAGING MODALITY
Arterial	Perinatal arterial ischemic stroke *(left middle cerebral artery, anterior cerebral artery, posterior cerebral artery)*	Diffusion-weighted MRI/MRA
	Iatrogenic *(abdominal aorta, radial artery, renal artery, mesenteric artery, popliteal artery)*	Doppler ultrasound
	Spontaneous *(iliac artery, left pulmonary artery, aortic arch, descending aorta, renal artery)*	
Venous	Iatrogenic/spontaneous vessel occlusion *(SVC, IVC, hepatic vein, subclavian vein, abdominal veins, peripheral veins)*	
	Renal vein	
	Portal vein	
	Cerebral sinovenous *(superior sagittal sinus, transverse sinuses of the superficial venous system, straight sinus of the deep system)*	Diffusion-weighted MRI w/venography
	Congenital heart disease related *(right/left atria, right/left ventricle, superior vena cava, inferior vena cava)*	Echocardiography

Adapted from Saxonhouse MA. Management of neonatal thrombosis. *Clin Perinatol.* 2012;39:192–193; and Data from (4,35,37–40).

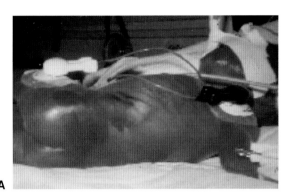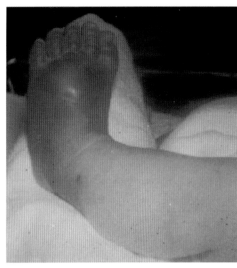

A

B

FIGURE 36.2 Skin necrosis associated with an umbilical artery catheter. Such lesions develop after vasospasm or embolism. **A:** Spinal injury may be present when ischemia involves this region. **B:** The distal part of an extremity is a common site for embolic arterial loss. The full extent of loss is unpredictable at this stage. (Reprinted with permission from Fletcher MA. *Physical Diagnosis in Neonatology.* 1st ed. Philadelphia, PA: Lippincott-Raven; 1998:127.)

d. Persistent bacteremia, thrombocytopenia, and/or central line dysfunction are nonspecific signs associated with vascular thrombosis at any site (4).

e. Clinical signs may be subtle or absent in many cases of thrombosis, which may be detected incidentally during ultrasonography for other indications.

2. Diagnostic Imaging

a. Optimal diagnostic modalities for diagnosing neonatal thromboses are presented in **Table 36.2**.

b. Contrast angiography: Gold standard; gives best definition of thrombosis but is difficult to perform in critically ill neonates; requires infusion of radiocontrast material that may be hypertonic or cause undesired increase in vascular volume (5).

c. Doppler ultrasonography: Portable, noninvasive monitors improve over time, but may give both false-positive and false-negative results compared with contrast angiography (6).

3. Additional Diagnostic Tests

a. Obtain detailed family history in all cases of vascular thrombosis.

b. Prothrombotic disorders increase a neonate's risk for developing pathologic thrombosis. It is recommended that neonates with significant thrombosis (other than asymptomatic central venous line thrombosis) be tested for genetic prothrombotic traits based on the presence of other risk factors (**Table 36.3**) (7).

c. Laboratory evaluation should take place at an experienced tertiary care center that has either self-laboratory

support or a reliable referral center. This approach can dramatically reduce the amount of blood required for this testing (2).

d. Due to many of the pro/anticoagulation protein levels being lower than adult values, the diagnosis of a prothrombotic disorder may be difficult to confirm in the immediate neonatal period. If abnormal values are obtained in the immediate neonatal period, these should be repeated at 3 to 6 months of age.

e. Lipoprotein(a) concentrations increase during the first year of life and should be repeated at 8 to 12 months of life if values obtained at 3 to 6 months are low, especially in Caucasian individuals.

f. DNA-based assays (see **Table 36.3**) are accurate during the neonatal period and may be obtained at any time.

g. The different evaluations presented (see **Table 36.3**) are based on the presence of acquired risk factors, type of thrombosis, severity of thrombosis, and treatment regimen.

h. Baseline complete blood count (CBC), prothrombin time (PT), activated partial thromboplastin time (aPTT), and fibrinogen levels should be obtained shortly after the acute event.

i. Placental pathology, especially in cases of ischemic perinatal stroke, should be requested (8).

C. Management of Arterial Vascular Spasm/Thromboses

1. Arterial Vascular Spasm

a. A stepwise approach to the management of vascular spasm is presented in **Figure 36.3**.

TABLE 36.3 Laboratory Evaluation for Prothrombotic Disorder

LABORATORY TESTING IF OTHER ACQUIRED RISK FACTORS PRESENT	LABORATORY TESTING IF OTHER ACQUIRED RISK FACTORS *NOT* PRESENT
■ Antiphospholipid antibody panel, anticardiolipin and lupus anticoagulant (IgG, IgM)[a]	■ Antiphospholipid antibody panel, anticardiolipin and lupus anticoagulant (IgG, IgM)[a]
■ Protein C activity[b]	■ Protein C activity[b]
■ Protein S activity[b]	■ Protein S activity[b]
■ Lipoprotein(a) (in Caucasian neonates)[b]	■ Antithrombin (activity assay)[b]
■ Plasminogen level[b] (if considering thrombolytic therapy)	■ Factor V Leiden[c]
■ Antithrombin III (AT-III) (activity assay)[b]	■ Prothrombin G[c]
■ Factor V Leiden[c]	■ PAI-1 4G/5G mutation[c]
■ Factor II G20210A (prothrombin G)[c]	■ Homocysteine[b] (if elevated, screen for methylenetetrahydrofolate reductase gene mutation)
	■ Lipoprotein(a)[b]
	■ Factor VIII activity[b]
	■ Factor XII activity[b]
	■ Plasminogen activity[b]
	■ Heparin cofactor II[b]

[a]May be performed from maternal serum during first few months of life.

[b]Protein-based assays are affected by the acute thrombosis and must be repeated at 3–6 months of life, before a definitive diagnosis may be made. Therefore, recommend that complete evaluation (excluding DNA-based assays) be performed at 3–6 months of life (21). If anticoagulation is being administered, then these assays should be obtained 14–30 days after discontinuing the anticoagulant. Lipoprotein(a) levels may need to be repeated at 8–12 months of life.

[c]DNA-based assays.

Adapted from Saxonhouse MA, Manco-Johnson MJ. The evaluation and management of neonatal coagulation disorders. *Semin Perinatol.* 2009;33:59; and Data from (16,27,28,32,41,42).

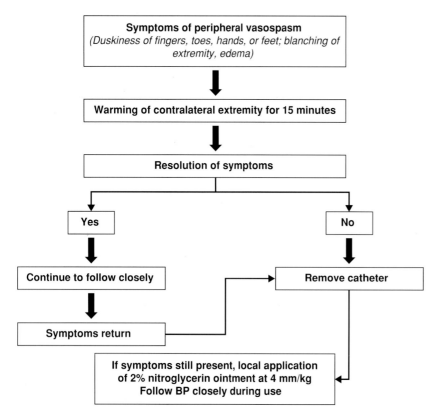

FIGURE 36.3 Management of peripheral vasospasm. The figure displayed represents current recommendations for the evaluation and management for neonates with peripheral vasospasm due to complications from PALs and UACs. Nitroglycerin dosing is provided. BP, blood pressure. (Adapted from Saxonhouse MA. Thrombosis in the neonatal intensive care unit. *Clin Perinatol.* 2015;42(3):651–673. Copyright © 2015 Elsevier. With permission.)

2. Arterial Thromboses (Catheter Related or Idiopathic) (12)

a. Remove catheter (9).
b. If non-life or limb threatening, anticoagulation should be started.
c. If there are life-, limb-, or organ-threatening signs, thrombolysis should be considered.
d. If there are contraindications to thrombolysis, surgical thrombectomy may be indicated.

D. Management of Venous Thromboses

1. Catheter-Related Thrombosis

a. General principles
(1) Thrombolysis to restore catheter patency for obstructed central venous catheters is described in Chapter 32.
(2) Management of venous thrombosis may involve one or more of the following: supportive care with continued close observation, anticoagulation, thrombolytic therapy, or surgical intervention (4).
(3) Treatment of catheter-related thrombosis in neonates is still evolving. Current published guidelines for treatment are based on common clinical practice, case studies, and extrapolation of principles of therapy from adult guidelines (2,4).
(4) Treatment is *highly individualized* and is determined by the site and extent of thrombosis, and the degree to which diminished perfusion to the affected extremity or organ affects function, and the potential risk of bleeding complications associated with anticoagulant or thrombolytic therapy (4,9).
(5) Expectant management or "watchful waiting"—close monitoring without anticoagulation or thrombolysis may be appropriate for some infants.
(6) Anticoagulation therapy is used for clinically significant thromboses with the goal of preventing clot extension or embolization (10).
(7) Thrombolysis is reserved for severe life-, organ-, or limb-threatening thrombosis (9).
(8) The International Children's Thrombophilia Network, which is based in Canada, is a free consultative service, maintained 24 hours a day, for physicians worldwide who are caring for children with thromboembolic disease. The toll free number in the North America is 1-800-NO-CLOTS; the number for physicians elsewhere is 1-905-573-4795 (Website http://www.1800noclots.ca/). The service provides current management protocols as well as links to the network and its services.

b. Management (4)
(1) Option no. 1
(a) Initiation of anticoagulation followed by removal of the catheter after 3 to 5 days of anticoagulation. Anticoagulation should continue until resolution of the thrombus has been documented. Treatment may last from 6 weeks to 3 months depending on the size, location, and symptoms from the thrombus.
(2) Option no. 2
(a) Supportive care only with removal of the catheter. Radiologic monitoring should continue monitoring for clot extension. If clot extension does occur, then anticoagulation should start and may last from 6 weeks to 3 months depending on the size, location, and symptoms from the thrombus.
(3) Thrombolytic therapy is not recommended for neonatal venous thrombosis unless major vessel occlusion is causing critical compromise of organs or limbs.

2. Renal Vein Thrombosis (RVT) (4,11,12)

a. Unilateral RVT
(1) Absence of renal impairment or extension into the inferior vena cava (IVC).
(a) Supportive care with monitoring of the RVT for extension. If extension occurs, then anticoagulation should be initiated for 6 weeks to 3 months.
(2) Extension into the IVC.
(a) Anticoagulation for 6 weeks to 3 months.
b. Bilateral RVT
(1) Absence of renal impairment or extension into IVC.
(a) Supportive care with monitoring of the RVT for extension. If extension occurs, then anticoagulation should be initiated for 6 weeks to 3 months.
(2) Extension into the IVC
(a) Anticoagulation for 6 weeks to 3 months.
(3) Renal failure
(a) Initial thrombolytic therapy with recombinant tissue plasminogen activator (rTPA), followed by anticoagulation for 6 weeks to 3 months.

3. Portal Venous Thrombosis (PVT) (13)

a. Infant clinically stable and no extension observed.
(1) No treatment needed and repeat ultrasound in 7 to 10 days.
b. Extension of the thrombus into the IVC, right atrium, and/or right ventricle but no end-organ compromise.
(1) Begin anticoagulation and repeat ultrasound in 10 days. If thrombus resolved, may stop therapy. If

still present, continue anticoagulation for 6 weeks to 3 months depending on follow-up imaging.

c. End-organ compromise with extension of the thrombus into the IVC, right atrium, and/or right ventricle.

(1) Initiate thrombolysis with daily ultrasounds. May stop thrombolysis when improvement noted but transition to anticoagulation for 6 weeks to 3 months.

E. Anticoagulant/Thrombolytic Therapy

1. General Principles

a. Most concerning complication associated with therapy in NICU is intracranial hemorrhage.
b. Clinician must consider potential for serious complications and assume that treatment's benefits outweigh its risks.
c. Treatment should include consultation with pediatric hematology.

2. Absolute Contraindications (1,4,14)

a. Central nervous system surgery or ischemia (including birth asphyxia) within the last 10 days.
b. Active or major bleeding.
c. Invasive procedure within the last 3 days.
d. Seizures within the last 48 hours.

3. Relative Contraindications[1] (1,4,14)

a. Platelet count <50 × 10^9/L (100 × 10^9/L, if neonate ill).
b. Fibrinogen concentration <100 mg/dL.
c. Severe coagulation deficiency.
d. Hypertension.

4. Precautions During Therapy

a. No arterial punctures.
b. No subcutaneous or intramuscular injections.
c. No urinary catheterizations.
d. Avoid aspirin or other antiplatelet drugs.
e. Monitor serial head ultrasound scans for intracranial hemorrhage.

5. Unfractionated Heparin (UFH)

a. Use recommended in neonates for asymptomatic or symptomatic thrombus but non-limb/life threatening.
b. Anticoagulant and antithrombotic effect limited by low plasma levels of antithrombin in neonates (15).

c. Check CBC, platelet count, aPTT, PT, and fibrinogen levels before starting UFH therapy.
d. Bolus dosing should ONLY be performed if there is significant risk or evidence of thrombus progression (10).
e. Dosing and monitoring provided in **Table 36.4**.
f. Check platelet counts daily for 2 to 3 days once therapeutic levels are achieved and at least twice weekly thereafter, while on UFH.
g. Monitor thrombus closely both during and following treatment.
h. Complications
(1) Bleeding: Discontinue UFH infusion; consider protamine sulfate if anti-factor Xa level is >0.8 U/mL and there is active bleeding. Dosage: 1 mg/100 U heparin received if the time since the last heparin dose is <30 minutes. Use protamine conservatively, starting with a smaller dose than calculated (16).
(2) Heparin-induced thrombocytopenia (rare in neonates) (17).

6. LMWH (16,17)

a. Use recommended in neonates for asymptomatic or symptomatic thrombus but non-limb/life threatening.
b. Enoxaparin is the LMWH most commonly used (18).
c. Dosing and monitoring provided in **Table 36.4**.
d. To discontinue anticoagulation, simply discontinue LMWH therapy. If an invasive procedure such as lumbar puncture is required, skip two doses of LMWH, and measure anti-factor Xa level prior to the procedure.
e. If an immediate antidote is required, protamine may be administered. The dose is usually a 1:1 ratio with LMWH; administration of the dose may be done in 2 to 3 aliquots with monitoring of anti-factor Xa levels (19).

7. Thrombolytic Agents

a. Consider in the presence of extensive or severe thrombosis when organ or limb viability is at risk (4,14,20).
b. Agent of choice is rTPA.
c. rTPA acts by converting fibrin-bound plasminogen to plasmin, which then proteolytically cleaves fibrin within the clot to fibrin degradation products. rTPA is nonantigenic and has a short half-life. Supplementation with plasminogen (10 mL/kg) in the form of fresh frozen plasma (FFP) enhances the thrombolytic effect and is recommended prior to starting therapy.
d. Thrombolysis does not inhibit clot propagation, so low-dose anticoagulation with UFH should be administered during thrombolytic therapy (10 U/kg/hr).
e. Dosing (20–22):
(1) Start at 0.03 mg/kg/hr.
(2) Dose titrations may be made every 12 to 24 hours and are as follows: 0.06 mg/kg/hr then 0.1 mg/kg/hr then 0.2 mg/kg/hr then 0.3 mg/kg/hr (max dose).

[1]Therapy may be provided after correction and/or resolution of these abnormalities.

TABLE 36.4 Recommended Dosing for UFH and LMWH Therapy in Neonates (4,21,22)

GESTATIONAL AGE[a]	UFH	LMWH
<32 wks	15 units/kg/hr	1.5 mg/kg SQ q 12 hrs
>32 wks	28 units/kg/hr	2 mg/kg SQ q 12 hrs
		Prophylactic dosing 0.75 mg/kg SQ q 12 hrs Goal for anti-factor Xa level of 0.1–0.3 U/mL
Dosage Monitoring for UFH and LMWH[b]		
UFH	Maintain anti-factor Xa level of 0.3–0.7 U/mL. Levels should be checked 4–6 hrs after initiating therapy. Anti-factor Xa levels should be checked daily during treatment. If provide loading dose, check level 4–6 hrs after loading dose. If need to make changes in dosing, check levels 4–6 hrs after each change in infusion rate.	
LMWH	Maintain anti-factor Xa level of 0.5–1.0 U/mL. Check level 4 hrs after third dose. If therapeutic, please repeat within 48 hrs. If remains therapeutic, then may check weekly.	

[a]Dosing applies also to postconceptional age (GA + weeks of life).

[b]Dosing adjustments for UFH and LMWH based on anti-factor Xa levels are published elsewhere (4).

Additional notes: Complete blood count, platelet count, and coagulation screening (including aPTT, PT, and fibrinogen) should be performed prior to starting anticoagulation. Bolus dosing for UFH should be performed only if there is a significant risk or evidence of thrombus progression (10). Otherwise, avoid bolus dosing in neonates. If bolus dosing is recommended: <32 wks 25 units/kg IV over 10 min; >32 wks 50 units/kg IV over 10 min. If infant with renal dysfunction, dosing should be discussed with pharmacist.

f. Imaging and dose adjustments during thrombolytic therapy:
   (1) Arterial thrombi should be reimaged at 6- to 8-hour intervals.
   (2) Venous thrombi should be reimaged at 12- to 24-hour intervals.
   (3) If repeat imaging reveals clot lysis <50%, increase infusion to next dosing level and repeat imaging in 12 to 24 hours.
   (4) If repeat imaging reveals clot lysis 51% to 94%, continue same dose infusion and repeat imaging in 12 to 24 hours.
   (5) If repeat imaging reveals clot lysis >95%, stop infusion and initiate anticoagulation.
   (6) If no clot dissolution occurs in 12 to 24 hours after starting infusion and/or d-dimers are not increasing, may give an additional 10 mL/kg of FFP to provide additional plasminogen to increase efficacy of rTPA.
g. Monitoring during therapy (**Table 36.5**).

8. Complications of Anticoagulation/ Fibrinolytic Therapy

a. Hemorrhagic complications
   (1) Intracerebral hemorrhage: Incidence approximately 1% in term neonates, 13% in preterm neonates, increasing to 25% in preterm infants treated in the first week of life. Data in preterm infants is confounded by the risk of "spontaneous" intraventricular hemorrhage (23)
   (2) Other major hemorrhage: Gastrointestinal, pulmonary
   (3) Bleeding from puncture sites and recent catheterization sites: Bleeding and hematoma at the site of the indwelling catheter for LMWH has been reported (24,25)
   (4) Hematuria
   (5) Embolization
      (a) Dislodgement of intracardiac thrombus, causing obstruction of cardiac valves or main vessels, or pulmonary or systemic embolization.

F. Surgical Intervention (26)

1. Use of microsurgical techniques and combined microsurgical/thrombolytic regimens has the potential to rapidly restore blood flow, avoiding tissue loss, without major bleeding complications, especially in patients with peripheral arterial occlusion (26).
2. Early consultation is recommended because surgical management may be required concomitantly, particularly for life- or limb-threatening emergencies.

TABLE 36.5 Monitoring Recommendations for Thrombolytic Therapy in Neonates

TESTING	WHEN PERFORMED	LEVELS DESIRED (IF APPLICABLE)
Imaging of thrombosis	Before initiation of treatment Every 12–24 hrs during treatment	
Fibrinogen level	Before initiation of treatment 4–6 hrs after starting treatment Every 12–24 hrs	Minimum of 100 mg/dL Supplement with cryoprecipitate
Platelet count	Before initiation of treatment 4–6 hrs after starting treatment Every 12–24 hrs	Minimum of 50–100 x 10⁴/microliter, dependent upon bleeding risk
Cranial imaging	Before initiation of treatment Daily during treatment	
Coagulation testing	Before initiation of treatment 4–6 hrs after starting treatment Every 12–24 hrs	
Plasminogen	Before initiation of treatment 4–6 hrs after starting treatment Every 12–24 hrs	Adequate to achieve thrombolysis Supplementation with plasminogen (FFP) prior to commencing therapy is recommended to ensure adequate thrombolysis
Line-associated or mucosal oozing	At all clinical assessments	Topical thrombin prn

Adapted from Saxonhouse MA. Management of neonatal thrombosis. *Clin Perinatol*. 2012;39:191–208; and Data from (18).

References

1. Beardsley DS. Venous thromboembolism in the neonatal period. *Semin Perinatol*. 2007;31:250–253.
2. Saxonhouse MA. Thrombosis in the neonatal intensive care unit. *Clin Perinatol*. 2015;42:651–673.
3. Haase R, Merkel N. Postnatal femoral artery spasm in a preterm infant. *J Pediatr*. 2008;153:871.
4. Monagle P, Chan AK, Goldenberg NA, et al. Antithrombotic therapy in neonates and children: Antithrombotic therapy and prevention of thrombosis, 9th ed: American college of chest physicians evidence-based clinical practice guidelines. *Chest*. 2012;141:e737S–e801S.
5. Greenway A, Massicotte MP, Monagle P. Neonatal thrombosis and its treatment. *Blood Rev*. 2004;18:75–84.
6. Albisetti M, Andrew M, Monagle P. Hemostatic abnormalities. In: de Alarcon PA, Werner EJ, eds. *Neonatal Hematology*. Cambridge: Cambridge University Press; 2005:310–348.
7. Manco-Johnson MJ, Grabowski EF, Hellgreen M, et al. Laboratory testing for thrombophilia in pediatric patients. On behalf of the subcommittee for perinatal and pediatric thrombosis of the scientific and standardization committee of the International Society of Thrombosis and Haemostasis (ISTH). *Thromb Haemost*. 2002;88:155–156.
8. Elbers J, Viero S, MacGregor D, et al. Placental pathology in neonatal stroke. *Pediatrics*. 2011;127:e722–e729.
9. Albisetti M. Thrombolytic therapy in children. *Thromb Res*. 2006;118:95–105.
10. Bhatt MD, Paes BA, Chan AK. How to use unfractionated heparin to treat neonatal thrombosis in clinical practice. *Blood Coagul Fibrinolysis*. 2016;27(6):605–614.
11. Lau KK, Stoffman JM, Williams S, et al. Neonatal renal vein thrombosis: review of the English-language literature between 1992 and 2006. *Pediatrics*. 2007;120:e1278–e1284.
12. Messinger Y, Sheaffer JW, Mrozek J, et al. Renal outcome of neonatal renal venous thrombosis: review of 28 patients and effectiveness of fibrinolytics and heparin in 10 patients. *Pediatrics*. 2006;118:e1478–e1484.
13. Williams S, Chan AK. Neonatal portal vein thrombosis: diagnosis and management. *Semin Fetal Neonatal Med*. 2011;16:329–339.
14. Manco-Johnson M. Controversies in neonatal thrombotic disorders. In: Ohls R, Yoder M, eds. *Hematology, Immunology and Infections Disease: Neonatology Questions and Controversies*. Philadelphia, PA: Saunders Elsevier; 2008:58–74.
15. Ignjatovic V, Straka E, Summerhayes R, et al. Age-specific differences in binding of heparin to plasma proteins. *J Thromb Haemost*. 2010;8:1290–1294.
16. Saxonhouse MA, Manco-Johnson MJ. The evaluation and management of neonatal coagulation disorders. *Semin Perinatol*. 2009;33:52–65.

17. Martchenke J, Boshkov L. Heparin-induced thrombocytopenia in neonates. *Neonatal Netw.* 2005;24:33–37.

18. Thornburg C, Pipe S. Neonatal thromboembolic emergencies. *Semin Fetal Neonatal Med.* 2006;11:198–206.

19. Wiernikowski JT, Chan A, Lo G. Reversal of anti-thrombin activity using protamine sulfate. Experience in a neonate with a 10-fold overdose of enoxaparin. *Thromb Res.* 2007;120:303–305.

20. Wang M, Hays T, Balasa V, et al. Low-dose tissue plasminogen activator thrombolysis in children. *J Pediatr Hematol Oncol.* 2003;25:379–386.

21. Manco-Johnson MJ. How I treat venous thrombosis in children. *Blood.* 2006;107:21–29.

22. Armstrong-Wells JL, Manco-Johnson MJ. Neonatal thrombosis. In: de Alarcon PA, Werner EJ, Christensen RD, eds. *Neonatal Hematology.* New York: Cambridge University Press; 2013:282.

23. Nowak-Gottl U, Auberger K, Halimeh S, et al. Thrombolysis in newborns and infants. *Thromb Haemost.* 1999;82(Suppl 1):112–116.

24. van Elteren HA, Veldt HS, Te Pas AB, et al. Management and outcome in 32 neonates with thrombotic events. *Int Jo Pediatr.* 2011;2011:217564.

25. van Elteren HA, Te Pas AB, Kollen WJ, et al. Severe hemorrhage after low-molecular-weight heparin treatment in a preterm neonate. *Neonatology.* 2011;99:247–249.

26. Coombs CJ, Richardson PW, Dowling GJ, et al. Brachial artery thrombosis in infants: an algorithm for limb salvage. *Plast Reconstr Surg.* 2006;117:1481–1488.

27. Alioglu B, Ozyurek E, Tarcan A, et al. Heterozygous methylenetetrahydrofolate reductase 677C-T gene mutation with mild hyperhomocysteinemia associated with intrauterine iliofemoral artery thrombosis. *Blood Coagul Fibrinolysis.* 2006;17:495–498.

28. Boffa MC, Lachassinne E. Infant perinatal thrombosis and antiphospholipid antibodies: a review. *Lupus.* 2007;16:634–641.

29. Kenet G, Nowak-Gottl U. Fetal and neonatal thrombophilia. *Obstet Gynecol Clin North Am.* 2006;33:457–466.

30. Kosch A, Kuwertz-Broking E, Heller C, et al. Renal venous thrombosis in neonates: prothrombotic risk factors and long-term follow-up. *Blood.* 2004;104:1356–1360.

31. Nagel K, Tuckuviene R, Paes B, et al. Neonatal aortic thrombosis: a comprehensive review. *Klin Padiatr.* 2010;222:134–139.

32. Sharathkumar AA, Lamear N, Pipe S, et al. Management of neonatal aortic arch thrombosis with low-molecular weight heparin: a case series. *J Pediatr Hematol Oncol.* 2009;31:516–521.

33. Tridapalli E, Stella M, Capretti MG, et al. Neonatal arterial iliac thrombosis in type-I protein C deficiency: a case report. *Ital J Pediatr.* 2010;36:23.

34. Rosendaal FR. Venous thrombosis: The role of genes, environment, and behavior. *Hematology Am Soc Hematol Educ Program.* 2005:1–12.

Respiratory Care

Bubble Nasal Continuous Positive Airway Pressure

Hany Aly and M.A. Mohamed

A. Definition

Continuous positive airway pressure (CPAP) is a noninvasive, continuous flow respiratory system that maintains positive pressure in the infant's airway during spontaneous breathing. CPAP was developed by George A. Gregory, in the late 1960s (1). Positive pressure was originally applied by placing the neonate's head into a semi-airtight "box" (the Gregory box) and, subsequently, by a fitted face mask covering the mouth and nose (2). A major problem with both these methods of application was the fact that it was difficult to feed the baby without discontinuing the CPAP; thus, the evolution to the current method of applying CPAP through bilateral nasal prongs (3). "Bubble CPAP" (b-CPAP) is a modern resurgence of the original method of supplying CPAP, wherein pressure is generated in the breathing circuit by immersing the distal end of the expiratory limb of the breathing circuit under water seal (**Fig. 37.1**) (4–6).

b-CPAP allows provision of CPAP without use of a ventilator, and is currently primarily used for early treatment of low-birthweight premature infants, with or at risk for, respiratory distress syndrome and/or with frequent apnea/bradycardia (7). In addition to cost considerations, there is early evidence that b-CPAP may be more effective in small premature babies than ventilator-derived CPAP (8).

CPAP Has the Following Physiologic Actions

- Prevents alveolar collapse and increases functional residual capacity
- Splints the airway and diaphragm
- Stimulates the act of breathing and decreases apnea

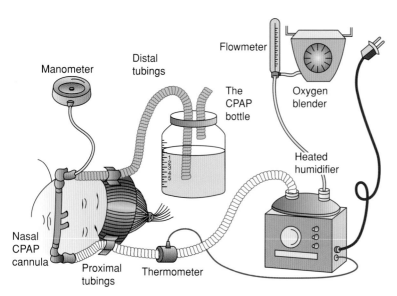

FIGURE 37.1 Bubble CPAP circuit. This simplified diagram demonstrates the components of the b-CPAP device that is either assembled at the bedside or commercially manufactured. Gas mixture flows to the infant from the wall source after it is warmed and humidified. The free expiratory limb of the tube is immersed under the surface of sterile water to produce the required CPAP (usually 5 cm H_2O). (Illustrations courtesy of Aser Kandel, MD.)

- Conserves surfactant via decreased inflammatory responses (9)
- Stimulates lung growth when applied for extended duration (10)

B. Indications

1. Premature infants with/at high risk for respiratory distress syndrome
2. Premature infants with frequent apnea and bradycardia of prematurity
3. Infants with transient tachypnea of the newborn
4. Infants who have weaned from mechanical ventilation
5. Infants with paralysis of the diaphragm and tracheomalacia

When to Start b-CPAP?

1. Premature infants with birthweight <1,200 g can be supported with b-CPAP starting in the delivery room, before any alveolar collapse occurs
2. Infants ≥1,200 g may benefit from b-CPAP in the following conditions:
   a. Respiratory rate >60/min
   b. Mild to moderate grunting
   c. Mild to moderate respiratory retraction
   d. Preductal oxygen saturation less than 93%
   e. Frequent apneas

C. Contraindications

1. Choanal atresia
2. Congenital diaphragmatic hernia
3. Conditions where b-CPAP is more than likely to fail in the delivery room such as:
   a. Extremely low gestational age of infants (≤24 weeks)
   b. Floppy infants with complete apnea due to maternal anesthesia
4. Relative contraindication: Infants with significant apnea of prematurity may require the introduction of nasal intermittent positive-pressure ventilation (NIPPV) via a variable flow device (11)

D. Equipment

b-CPAP System Consists of Two Components

1. A breathing circuit of light-weight corrugated tubing that has two limbs:
   a. Inspiratory limb to provide a continuous flow of heated and humidified gas

   b. Expiratory limb with its terminal end immersed in water (or 0.25% acetic acid) seal to create positive pressure
2. A device to safely connect the circuit to patient's nares that includes (**Fig. 37.2**):
   a. Short binasal prongs
   b. Hook and loop fastener; for example, Velcro (to make attachment circles and moustache for upper lip)
   c. Thin hydrocolloid dressing (to make nasal septum protective layer)
   d. CPAP head cap
   e. Adhesive tape

E. Technique (See ▶ Video 37.1)[1]

1. **Starting b-CPAP**
   a. Nonventilator-derived b-CPAP apparatus involves making a simple water seal device that can be put together in neonatal units.
      (1) It consists of a container of water through which the expiratory gas from the baby is bubbled at a measured level below the surface (e.g., 5 cm below the surface = 5 cm H_2O CPAP).
      (2) The lower the level of the tip of the expiratory tubing below the surface of the water, the higher the CPAP (see **Fig. 37.1**).
      (3) It is important to fix the water bottle to an IV pole at or below the level of the baby's chest in order to avoid any accidental displacement or water spills.
      (4) The commercially available, preassembled circuits rely on the same basic principle.
   b. *Before attaching the device to an infant:*
      (1) Position the infant with the head of the bed elevated 30 degrees.
      (2) *Gently* suction the mouth, nose, and pharynx.
         (a) Whenever possible, use size 8-Fr suction catheter. Smaller-size catheters are not as efficient.
      (3) Place a small roll under the infant's neck/shoulder. Allow slight neck extension to help maintaining the airway open.
      (4) Clean the infant's upper lip with water.
      (5) Put a thin hydrocolloid dressing over the upper lip. That should also cover the nasal columella and both sides of nasal apertures (see **Fig. 37.2**).
      (6) Cut a Velcro moustache and fix it over the thin hydrocolloid dressing.

---

[1]To view video associated with this chapter please refer to the eBook bundled with this text. eBook access instructions are located on the inside front cover.

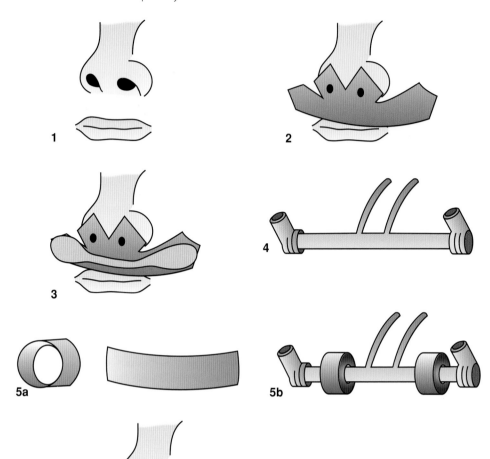

FIGURE 37.2 Components of the CPAP attachment device. (1) Infant's nose before applying b-CPAP. (2) Protective hydrocolloid dressing applied to upper lip and nose. (3) Thin Velcro—moustache piece: applied to upper lip on top of the protective hydrocolloid dressing with sharp edges not touching nose. (4) Nasal prongs (prongs are slightly curved to better fit within anatomy of nasal passages). (5) Thick Velcro—ring pieces: wrapped around both sides of the transverse arm. (6) Nasal prongs applied to baby—prongs inserted into nares with thick Velcro rings attached to thin Velcro moustache (allow a space between the transverse arm of the nasal prongs and nose to avoid damage to nasal columella/septum). (Illustrations courtesy of Aser Kandel, MD.)

(7) Cut two strips of soft Velcro (8-mm width) and wrap them around the transverse arm of the device, about 1 cm away, on each side, from the nasal prongs.

c. *Placing nasal prongs into infant's nostrils* (**Fig. 37.3**).

  (1) Use appropriate-sized CPAP prongs. The correct-sized nasal prongs should snugly fit the infant's nares without pinching the septum. If prongs are too small, they will increase airway resistance and allow air to leak around them, making it difficult to maintain appropriate pressure. If prongs are too large, they may cause mucosal and septal erosion.

  (2) Curve prongs gently down into the infant's nose.

  (3) Press gently on the prong device until the soft Velcro strips adhere to the moustache.

  (4) Make sure of the following points:

    (a) Nasal prongs are fitting completely in the nostrils.

    (b) Skin of nares is not stretched (indicated by blanching of the rim of the nostrils).

    (c) Corrugated tubes are not touching the infant's skin.

    (d) There is no lateral pressure on the nasal septum.

    (e) There is a small space between the nasal septum/columella and the bridge between the prongs.

    (f) Prongs are not resting on the philtrum.

d. *Fixing corrugated tubes in place.*

  (1) Use appropriate-sized hat and fold rim back 2 to 3 cm.

  (2) Place the hat on the infant's head so that rim is just over the top of the ears.

  (3) Hold the corrugated tubing to one side of the head.

  (4) Tape the tube to the hat at the side of the head.

  (5) Repeat the same procedure for the tubing on the other side of the head.

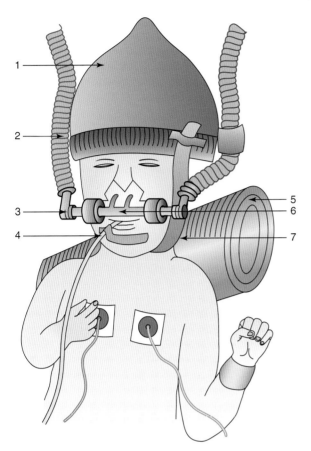

FIGURE 37.3 An infant with CPAP properly attached to the head. (1) Head cap (cap fit well on head covering down to eyebrows, almost entire ears, and back of head). (2) Breathing circuit tubes attached to side of hat while avoiding both eyes. (3) Three-way elbow at expiratory side allows the attachment of pressure manometer or could be capped to preserve pressure within circuit. (4) Orogastric tube attached to lower lip and chin with thin protective hydrocolloid dressing. (5) Neck roll allowing slight neck extension (sniff position). (6) Nasal prongs applied to baby—prongs inserted into nares allowing a space between the transverse arm of the nasal prongs and nose to avoid damage to nasal columella. (7) Supporting chin strip. (Illustrations courtesy of Aser Kandel, MD.)

  e. *Draining excess air from the stomach.*
   (1) Pass an orogastric tube and aspirate the stomach contents.
   (2) Fix tube at appropriate position.
   (3) Leave tube open to vent excess air from stomach.
  f. *Maintaining a good seal for CPAP pressure.*
   (1) Gently apply a chin strip to minimize air leak from the mouth.
2. **Maintenance of b-CPAP**
  a. Check the integrity of the entire CPAP system every 3 to 4 hours (12).
  b. Suction nasal cavities, mouth, pharynx, and stomach every 3 to 4 hours, and as needed.
  c. Keep CPAP prongs off nasal septum at all times.
  d. Change the infant's position every 4 to 6 hours, to allow postural drainage of lung secretions.

It is advisable to create a checklist and keep it at bedside to facilitate appropriate use of CPAP without missing any point (Appendix C) (13).

3. **Weaning off b-CPAP**
  a. A trial off CPAP should be given when the infant's weight is more than 1,200 g and he or she is breathing comfortably on b-CPAP without supplemental oxygen.
   (1) The nasal prongs should be separated from the corrugated tubing and removed from the infant's nose, keeping the tubing in place.
   (2) **Infant should be assessed during the trial for any tachypnea, retractions, oxygen desaturation, or apnea.**
   (3) If any of these signs are observed, the trial is considered as failed. Infant should be restarted immediately on CPAP, for at least 24 hours, before another trial is undertaken.
  b. There is no need to change the level of positive pressure during the weaning process. Infant is either on b-CPAP 5 cm H_2O or off CPAP.
  c. It is not advisable to alternate respiratory support between CPAP and nasal cannula. Therefore, at the time of weaning, infants are taken off CPAP straight to room air.
  d. Do not wean the infant off b-CPAP if there is any likelihood of respiratory compromise during the weaning process. It is wise to anticipate and prevent lung collapse, rather than risk having to manage collapsed lungs.
  e. Do not wean infants off b-CPAP if they require supplemental oxygen (14).
4. **Potential complications**
  a. *Nasal obstruction:* from secretions or improper positioning of b-CPAP prongs. To avoid obstruction, nares should be suctioned frequently and prongs checked for proper placement. Never use a nasal–pharyngeal tube to supply b-CPAP, because of significant risk of nasal airway obstruction.
  b. *Nasal septal erosion or necrosis:* due to pressure on the nasal septum. This can be avoided by maintaining a small space (use thin hydrocolloid dressing 2 to 3 mm) between the bridge of the prongs and the septum. Choosing the proper size snug-fitting nasal prongs, use of a Velcro mustache to secure the prongs in place, and avoiding pinching of the nasal septum, will minimize the risk of septal injury. Significant nasal septal erosion may require a consult with the ENT or plastic surgery team.
  c. *Gastric distention:* from swallowing air. Gastric distention is a benign finding and does not predispose the infant to necrotizing enterocolitis or bowel perforation (15). It is important to ensure patency of the indwelling orogastric tube, because secretions may block the tube and lead to distention.

d. *Pneumothorax:* during the first 2 days of life. Premature infants usually will require intubation, while full-term infants can manage on CPAP with a spontaneous nontension pneumothorax as long as they continue to be hemodynamically stable (16).

e. *Unintended increase/decrease in positive end pressure:* the tubing that is placed under water to provide positive end pressure must be firmly fixed in place, so that it cannot be displaced to produce unwanted pressure changes.

References

1. Gregory GA, Kitterman JA, Phibbs RH, et al. Treatment of the idiopathic respiratory distress syndrome with continuous positive airway pressure. *N Engl J Med.* 1971;384:1333–1340.

2. Gregory GA. Devices for applying continuous positive pressure. In: Thibeault DW, Gregory GA, eds. *Neonatal Pulmonary Care.* Menlo Park, CA: Addison-Wesley; 1979.

3. Katwinkel J, Fleming D, Cha CC, et al. A device for administration of continuous positive pressure by the nasal route. *Pediatrics.* 1973;52:131–134.

4. Wung JT. Continuous positive airway pressure. In: Wung JT, ed. *Respiratory care of the newborn: A practical approach.* New York: Columbia University Medical Center; 2009.

5. Aly HZ. Nasal prongs continuous positive airway pressure: a simple yet powerful tool. *Pediatrics.* 2001;108:759–761.

6. Aly HZ, Massaro AN, Patel K, et al. Is it safer to intubate premature infants in the delivery room? *Pediatrics.* 2005;115:1660–1665.

7. Nowadzky T, Pantoja A, Britton JR. Bubble continuous positive pressure, a potentially better practice, reducing the use of mechanical ventilation among very low birth weight infants with respiratory distress syndrome. *Pediatrics.* 2009;123:1534–1540.

8. Courtney SE, Kahn DJ, Singh R, et al. Bubble and ventilator-derived nasal continuous positive pressure in premature infants: work of breathing and gas exchange. *J Perinatol.* 2011;31:44.

9. Jobe AH, Kramer BW, Moss TJ, et al. Decreased indicators of lung injury with continuous positive expiratory pressure in preterm lambs. *Pediatr Res.* 2002;52:387–392.

10. Zhang S, Garbutt V, McBride JT. Strain-induced growth of the immature lung. *J Appl Physiol (1985).* 1996;81:1471–1476.

11. Lemyre B, Davis PG, dePaoli AG. Nasal intermittent positive pressure ventilation (NIPPV) versus nasal continuous positive airways pressure (NCPAP) for apnea of prematurity. *Cochrane Database Syst Rev.* 2002;1:CD002272.

12. Bonner KM, Mainous RO. The nursing care of the infant receiving bubble CPAP therapy. *Adv Neonatal Care.* 2008;8(2):78–95.

13. Aly H, Mohamed MA, Wung JT. Surfactant and continuous positive airway pressure for the prevention of chronic lung disease: history, reality, and new challenges. *Semin Fetal Neonatal Med.* 2017;22(5):348–353.

14. Abdel-Hady H, Shouman B, Aly H. Early weaning from CPAP to high flow nasal cannula in preterm infants is associated with prolonged oxygen requirement: a randomized controlled trial. *Early Hum Dev.* 2011;87:205–208.

15. Aly H, Massaro AN, Hammad TA, et al. Early nasal continuous positive airway pressure and necrotizing enterocolitis in preterm infants. *Pediatrics.* 2009;124:205–210.

16. Aly H, Massaro A, Acun C, et al. Pneumothorax in the newborn: clinical presentation, risk factors and outcomes. *J Matern Fetal Neonatal Med.* 2014;27:402–406.

38

Endotracheal Intubation

Anne Ades and Lindsay C. Johnston

Introduction

Endotracheal (ET) intubation is a life-saving procedure requiring background knowledge, psychomotor skills, effective communication, and coordinated teamwork to successfully and safely complete the procedure in a timely fashion. This chapter outlines the key steps and considerations for ET intubation of the neonate, laryngeal mask placement as well as other procedures related to the maintenance of endotracheal tube (ETT) patency.

A. Indications

1. For respiratory failure unresponsive to noninvasive ventilation
   a. Neonatal lung disease
   b. Cardiac disease with significant hypoxemia
   c. Upper airway obstruction
   d. Frequent apnea and bradycardia events
   e. Neuromuscular weakness
2. Surfactant administration
3. For maintenance of airway patency during procedures with moderate/deep sedation
4. When suctioning is required to clear an intratracheal obstruction or where airway clearance of secretions is impaired
5. When diaphragmatic hernia is prenatally diagnosed or suspected

B. Contraindications

There is no absolute contraindication to intubating a neonate who has one of the above-mentioned indications except in the patient with an advanced directive that specifies "Do Not Intubate." A relative contraindication is the patient who may be difficult to intubate based on history or physical examination findings. In these cases, if the patient is able to be transiently supported with noninvasive ventilation, consultation with anesthesia and otolaryngology should be considered. In older patients, the presence of cervical injuries is a contraindication to intubation with a laryngoscope; however, because the occurrence of cervical injuries/anomalies is infrequent in neonates, we consider that ET intubation is associated with less risk than performance of an emergency tracheotomy.

C. Considerations

1. Choice of blade size
   a. Miller (straight) blades are typically preferred for neonatal intubation, rather than Macintosh (curved) blades. Miller no. 1 blades are recommended for term infants, no. 0 blades are recommended for preterm infants, and no. 00 may be considered for extremely preterm infants (1).
   b. Adaptations to these guidelines may be needed in infants who are small or large for gestational age, who have limitations in opening their mouths, or have airway abnormalities.
   c. Alternate blade shapes and designs have been developed but their use is beyond the scope of this chapter.
2. Choice of ETT
   a. ETTs used for neonatal intubation should be of uniform internal and external diameter. Tubes that are tapered or cuffed are not typically recommended due to potential for increased risk of injury (2). The use of cuffed tubes is considered at some institutions for specific populations with small studies demonstrating no increase in adverse events (3). However, further research is needed before this can be recommended for broader use.
   b. ETT size is depicted by the internal diameter of the tube in millimeters. Optimal tube size selection is

important to avoid potential airway injury from a large tube or large air leak or obstruction by secretions with a small tube. Size may be selected using an infant's gestational age and/or weight (**Table 38.1**).

TABLE 38.1   Recommended Size of ETT Based on Patient Weight and Gestational Age

WEIGHT (g)	GESTATIONAL AGE (wk)	ENDOTRACHEAL TUBE SIZE (mm ID)
Below 1,000	Below 28	2.5
1,000–2,000	28–34	3.0
Greater than 2,000	Greater than 34	3.5

Data from Weiner GM, ed. *Textbook of Neonatal Resuscitation*. 7th ed. Elk Grove Village, IL: American Academy of Pediatrics; 2016.

3. Depth of insertion
    a. Ideal ETT position is in the midtrachea, approximately 1 to 2 cm below the vocal cords and above the carina and bronchi in most patients. Radiographic positioning of the end of the tube should lie between the first and second thoracic vertebral bodies (**Fig. 38.1**) (4).

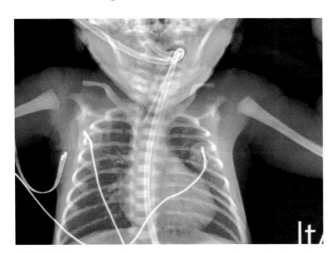

FIGURE 38.1 Chest radiography showing appropriate positioning of the ETT between thoracic vertebral bodies T1–T2.

    b. Methods of estimation of tube depth at infant's lip for orotracheal intubation
        (1) Gestational age and/or weight can be used to estimate appropriate depth of insertion. Cognitive aids are published and are available to providers. In general (5):
            (a) 25 to 26 weeks gestation infants: ET insertion depth 6 cm
            (b) 30 to 32 weeks gestation infants: ET insertion depth 7 cm
            (c) 35 to 37 weeks gestation infants: ET insertion depth 8 cm

        (d) >37 weeks gestation infants: ET insertion depth 9 cm
            Depth should be adjusted appropriately for patients who are extremely preterm, or small/large for gestational age.
        (2) Nasotragal length (NTL) is a measurement of the distance from the infant's nasal septum to their tragus in centimeters. This length +1 cm can be utilized to estimate depth of insertion (1).
        (3) Vocal cord guides on ETTs vary significantly between manufacturers, and may not provide an accurate estimate for depth of insertion, especially among extremely premature infants (6).
        (4) Other considerations that may affect depth of insertion:
            (a) Infants with congenital diaphragmatic hernia have been noted to have cephalad displacement of the carina upon antenatal MRI and confirmed on postnatal radiographs, which may increase risk for right-mainstem intubation. Recent authors have suggested modifying depth of insertion to 5.5 cm + infant weight in kg in this population (7).
            (b) In some cases, an anatomic defect (such as a tracheal fistula or subglottic/tracheal stenosis) may require a deeper position of the tube to allow for "bypassing" the level of the defect.
    c. Estimation of tube depth for nasotracheal intubation
        (1) For nasotracheal intubation, the tube depth should be approximately 2 cm more than the estimated depth for orotracheal intubation. A recent study of additional available formulas to calculate appropriate tube depth in pediatric patients found that there were high rates of inaccurate estimation, so clinical and radiographic assessment remain important (8).
    d. Confirmation of appropriate depth of insertion
        (1) As the above methods provide only an estimation of depth of insertion, providers should confirm appropriateness of depth using a number of methods:
            (a) Primary methods:
                i. Detection of exhaled CO_2
                    a. Colorimetric CO_2 detection: if CO_2 present, the indicator will change from purple to yellow (**Fig. 38.2**)
                    b. Capnographic CO_2 detectors: detect the concentration of CO_2 present, less commonly used in the delivery room setting
                ii. Improvement in heart rate
            (b) Secondary methods:
                i. Auscultation with bilateral equal breath sounds in axillae and absent over stomach
                ii. Symmetric chest rise with positive-pressure ventilation

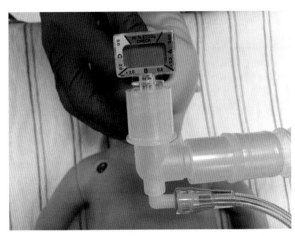 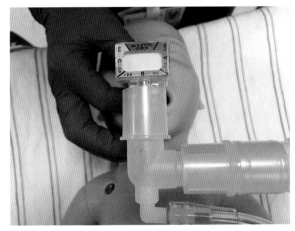

FIGURE 38.2 CO_2 detector. Note the indicator's change from purple to yellow upon CO_2 detection.

(c) Chest radiography can be used to confirm proper placement of the tube in the trachea. The chest x-ray (CXR) should be taken with the head in a midline position, the neck in a neutral position, and with the neonate supine. If the neck is in an extended position or if the infant is prone, the ETT will appear more cephalad (9,10). If the neck is flexed then the ETT will appear more caudad. In addition, with the head turned to the side, the ETT has been shown to appear more cephalad in children (11).

4. Premedication
   a. Use of premedication, including paralytics, for nonemergent intubation attempts in neonates has been shown to improve success rates; decrease risk of airway injury, pain and discomfort, and risk of intraventricular hemorrhage; and potentially positively impact neurodevelopmental outcomes (12–18). The American Academy of Pediatrics has issued a statement that endorses the use of premedication for neonatal intubation (19). A standardized premedication regimen has not been endorsed, but many providers choose to administer atropine (to decrease vagally mediated bradycardia and decrease oral secretions), a narcotic to decrease pain/discomfort, and a paralytic medication. Institutional guidelines should be developed. See **Table 38.2** for considerations for choice of premedications (19–21).

5. Length of attempt
   a. Intubation attempts should be limited to approximately 30 seconds, and should be discontinued earlier if significant hypoxia or bradycardia are present (1). The patient should receive positive-pressure ventilation via face mask or supraglottic device to stabilize their condition in between attempts.

6. Empty stomach
   a. Prior to intubation attempts, the infant's stomach should be emptied of any residual milk/formula. This recommendation is due to possible risk of emesis occurring with the administration of

positive-pressure ventilation or the induction of the gag reflex with insertion of the laryngoscope blade, which can increase the risk of aspiration.

7. Vallecular versus epiglottic holding
   a. It is generally recommended that, during neonatal intubation, the tip of the laryngoscope blade is advanced beyond the base of the tongue until it reaches the vallecula (**Figs. 38.3** (22) and **38.4**). When the blade is positioned in this manner, gently lifting the handle of the blade in the direction the

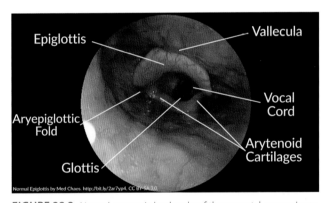

FIGURE 38.3 Normal anatomic landmarks of the neonatal upper airway. The glottis sits very close to the base of the tongue, so visualization is easiest without hyperextending the neck. (From Normal Epiglottis by Med Chaos. http://bit.ly/2ar7yp4. CC-BY-SA-3.0.)

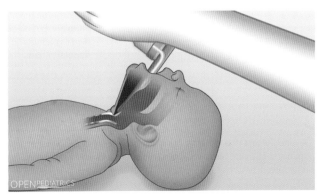

FIGURE 38.4 Positioning of blade in the vallecula. (Courtesy OPENPediatrics. Used with permission.)

TABLE 38.2 Premedication Considerations and Dosage Recommendations (19–21)

MEDICATION CATEGORY	PURPOSE	MECHANISM OF ACTION	TYPICAL MEDICATION,[a] RECOMMENDED DOSE, ONSET AND DURATION OF ACTION	NOTES
Vagolytic	Prevention of vagally mediated bradycardia; decrease in bronchial and salivary secretions	Antimuscarinic medication that competitively inhibits the postganglionic acetylcholine receptors and direct vagolytic action	**Atropine**[a] 0.02 mg/kg IV or IM Onset: 1–2 min Duration: 0.5–2 hrs	Side effects include tachycardia and dry, hot skin

Analgesic +/− sedative	Pain control; decrease level of consciousness; minimize adverse hemodynamic response to laryngoscopy	*Analgesic:*
		Acts at receptor sites in the central and peripheral nervous system to diminish perception of pain through modification of transmission of painful signals
		Sedative:
		Binds to receptor at GABA receptor–chloride ionophore complex in CNS, leading to membrane hyperpolarization and increase inhibitory effect of GABA in CNS, as well as interference with GABA reuptake
			Fentanyl[a]
			1–4 μg/kg IV or IM (only if IV access not available)
			Onset:
			  IV: almost immediate
			  IM: 7–15 min
			Duration:
			  IV: 30–60 min
			  IM: 1–2 hrs
			Midazolam
			0.05–0.1 mg/kg IV or IM
			Onset:
			  IV: 1–5 min
			  IM: 5–15 min
			Duration:
			  IV: 20–30 min
			  IM: 1–6 hrs
				Fentanyl preferable to morphine given more rapid onset of action; side effects include: apnea, hypotension, CNS depression, as well as chest wall rigidity; risk of the latter can be reduced using slow infusion, and can be treated with administration of naloxone (a competitive agonist at opioid receptors) or paralytic medication
				Midazolam is not recommended for preterm infants given concern for prolonged half-life and exposure to the preservative benzyl alcohol; use of sedative medication without analgesic agent should be avoided

Neuromuscular block	Improve conditions for intubation, and minimize chance of adverse events or need for multiple intubation attempts; decrease risk of increase in intracranial pressure during intubation	*Depolarizing:*
		Blocks neuromuscular transmission by binding acetylcholine receptors of muscle membrane and depolarizing it.
		Nondepolarizing[a]*:*
		Competes with acetylcholine for receptors on the motor endplate, but do not lead to membrane depolarization
			Succinylcholine 1–2 mg/kg IV; 2 mg/kg IM
			Onset:
			  IV: 30–60 sec
			  IM: 2–3 min
			Duration:
			  IV: 4–6 min
			  IM: 10–30 min
			Vecuronium[a]
			0.1 mg/kg IV
			Onset: 2–3 min
			Duration: 30–40 min
			Rocuronium[a]
			0.6–1.2 mg/kg IV
			Onset: 1–2 min
			Duration: 20–30 min
				Rare serious adverse events reported with use of succinylcholine in children include hyperkalemia, myoglobinemia, cardiac arrhythmia, and malignant hyperthermia; contraindicated in the setting of hyperkalemia or with a family history of malignant hyperthermia
				Nondepolarizing agents are typically preferred for neonates and infants. Both vecuronium and rocuronium may cause mild histamine release, hypertension/hypotension, arrhythmia, bronchospasm. Their effects can be reversed by administration of atropine and neostigmine

[a]Despite the fact that there are many options for premedication for intubation, a standardized regimen does not exist. A typical practice is to administer atropine (vagolytic), fentanyl (analgesic), and a nondepolarizing paralytic (such as vecuronium) prior to commencing with intubation procedure.

handle is pointing (45-degree angle with the warmer) will facilitate exposure of the glottis. In some situations, it may be preferable to utilize the tip of the laryngoscope blade to gently lift the tip of the epiglottis, compressing it against the base of the tongue (**Fig. 38.5**). Examples of these situations include extremely preterm infants, where the vallecula may be too small to accommodate the tip of the blade, or infants who have a large or floppy epiglottis.

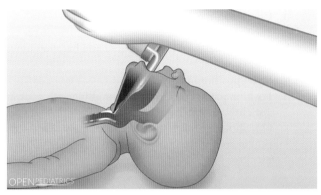

FIGURE 38.5 Positioning of blade lifting the epiglottis. (Courtesy OPEN-Pediatrics. Used with permission.)

8. Use of stylet
   a. A stylet may be used to make the ETT more rigid and introduce curvature to the tip that may facilitate intubation. If utilized, providers should ensure that the tip of the stylet is not protruding from the ETT's end or side hole, as this may lead to airway trauma. The stylet should also be secured to prevent its movement during the procedure. A recent study did not demonstrate a significant improvement in success rate when a stylet was used when compared to a control group in which a stylet was not used (**Fig. 38.6**) (23).

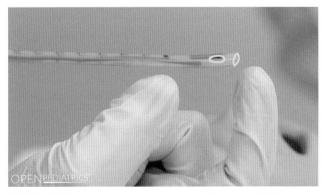

FIGURE 38.6 Appropriate position of stylet. (Courtesy OPENPediatrics. Used with permission.)

9. Videolaryngoscopic devices
   a. Videolaryngoscopes are devices that may be used to improve visualization of the airway through incorporation of a fiberoptic lens into the laryngoscope blade. The resultant image is projected to a monitor and presents a wider angle of visualization. There are a number of different classifications of videolaryngoscopes, including integrated channel laryngoscopes, laryngoscopes with video stylets, and laryngoscopes with rigid blades (i.e., C-MAC, GlideScope, Truview EVO2) (24). It is important to note that some videolaryngoscopes do not have blades that mimic the shape of traditional blades and may require different insertion techniques than described here. There has been great interest in assessing whether videolaryngoscopy is superior to direct laryngoscopy in improving success rates and minimizing adverse events. Previous studies performed in pediatric patients demonstrated improvement in airway visualization, but no difference was noted in number of attempts and the procedural duration was prolonged when videolaryngoscopy was utilized (25,26). Several single center trials have assessed neonatal intubation with videolaryngoscopy compared with direct laryngoscopy. Participants demonstrated improvement in per-attempt success rates and more rapid attainment of a predefined level of competency (27,28). Further research is required to clarify the potential benefits and drawbacks of videolaryngoscopy in neonatal intubation, but this technology may have great potential for improving intubation safety in the neonatal intensive care unit.

10. Tube change using tube exchanger versus "push–pull"
    a. In some instances, an existing ETT may need to be replaced due to inappropriate size or obstruction with secretions. Options to facilitate this change include removing the existing tube and replacing using direct laryngoscopy, using an ETT exchanger (ETTE), or using the "push–pull" method.
    b. The "push–pull" method of ETT exchange given below is beneficial because the patient's nonventilated time is extremely minimal.
    c. ETTEs are frequently utilized in pediatric or adult patients. These are long catheters that are placed through an existing ETT which is then removed and the new ETT is threaded over the ETTE catheter. Their use is limited in the neonatal population due to lack of exchangers that are of small-enough diameter to fit through neonatal-sized ETTs as well as safety concerns due to risk of tracheal perforation with their use. Decisions to use an ETTE in a neonate should be made on a case-by-case basis, and with respect to institutional guidelines.

D. Equipment

The following items should be available anywhere that neonates may require intubation such as the delivery room, neonatal intensive care unit, emergency room, operating room, or other locations where sedation of neonates is performed:

1. Gloves
2. 10-French (Fr) suction catheters
3. ETT stylet (optional)
4. ETTs with internal diameters of 2.5, 3, and 3.5 mm
5. Laryngoscope handle (with an extra set of batteries and extra bulb if nonfiberoptic device)
6. Laryngoscope blades—Miller no. 00, 0, 1
7. Scissors
8. Magill forceps for nasal intubation (optional)
9. Water-soluble lubricant (for lubrication of end of ETT when performing nasal intubation to ease passage through the nares and for oral intubation when there is difficulty passing tube through glottis/subglottic area due to possible stenosis)
10. Humidified oxygen/air source, blender, and analyzer
11. Resuscitation bag and mask or T-piece resuscitator
12. Monitoring equipment
    a. Cardiorespiratory monitor
    b. Pulse oximeter
13. End-tidal CO_2 detection device
    a. Colorimetric
    b. Quantitative
14. Stethoscope
15. Securement device/materials
    a. Commercially available device
    b. Adhesive tape

See ▶ *Videos 38.1 and 38.2 on Endotracheal Intubation for techniques/procedures.*

E. Procedure for Orotracheal Intubation (29)

1. Procedural planning:
   a. Review of patient history including identification of risk factors for difficult airway
   b. Equipment preparation
      (1) Ensure all equipment in above list is present for all intubations
      (2) For intubations where a difficult airway is suspected, alternative devices, such as oral airways, nasal airways, supraglottic devices, or other equipment for use by anesthesia/ENT/surgery such as fiberoptic scopes, tracheostomy trays, should be readily available
   c. Personnel:
      (1) Dedicated team lead who is not performing procedure (if available) to monitor patient stability and time elapsed

   (2) Person performing intubation
   (3) Respiratory therapist (if available)
   (4) Nurse
   d. Verification of informed consent if elective based on unit policy
   e. Time-out per unit policy
2. Procedure steps:
   a. Don appropriate personal protective equipment (may include eye protection based on patient characteristics)
   b. Perform equipment check
   c. Ensure light source functioning appropriately
   d. Check bag-mask ventilation device
   e. Suction oropharynx
   f. Appropriate-sized tube prepared and back-up tubes readily available
   g. Stylet positioning in ETT
   h. Position patient ensuring head midline with neck in a slightly extended position
      (1) Shoulder roll, to be used to maintain head/neck in appropriate position if needed (**Fig. 38.7**)

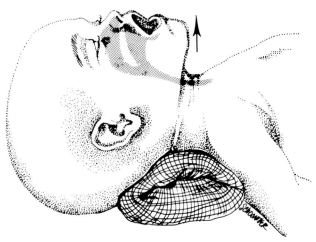

FIGURE 38.7 Appropriate sniff position for intubation. Note that the neck is not hyperextended; the roll provides stabilizing support.

   (2) Bed height adjusted to maintain patient head at level of upper abdomen of intubator
   (3) C-spine precautions, if appropriate
   i. Administration of premedication based on unit guidelines
   j. Preoxygenation based on unit guidelines/patient population
   k. Open mouth prior to inserting laryngoscope blade
   l. Hold laryngoscope handle with left hand (all laryngoscopes should be held in the left hand independent of handedness of operator)
   m. Insert blade with smooth motion into the mouth sliding over the tongue
   n. Advance blade until the tip of the blade is resting in the vallecula or lifting the epiglottis (see Considerations) (**Fig. 38.8**)
   o. Optimize glottis visualization using appropriate methods (**Fig. 38.9**). The laryngoscope blade should

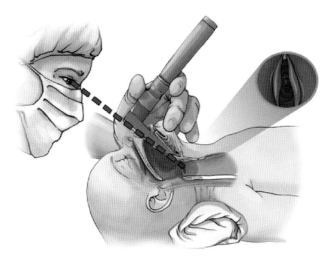

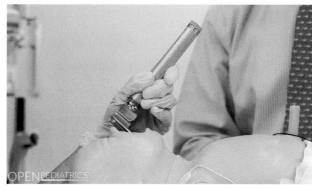

FIGURE 38.10 Inappropriate rocking of handle and blade. (Courtesy OPENPediatrics. Used with permission.)

FIGURE 38.8 With the laryngoscope at the proper depth, tilt the blade with the tongue as the fulcrum; at the same time, pull on the laryngoscope handle to move the tongue without extending the infant's neck. Use more traction than leverage.

be lifted in the direction the handle is pointing (approximately 45-degree angle with the warmer). Care should be taken to avoid a rocking motion **(Fig. 38.10)** which will obscure glottis visualization and apply excessive pressure to the alveolar ridge.

Problem	Landmarks	Corrective Action
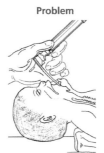	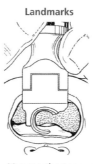	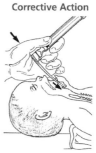
Laryngoscope not inserted far enough.	You see the tongue surrounding the blade.	Advance the blade farther.
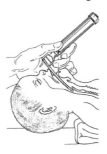	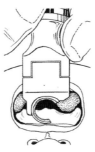	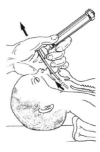
Laryngoscope inserted too far.	You see the walls of the esophagus surrounding the blade.	Withdraw the blade slowly until the epiglottis and glottis are seen.
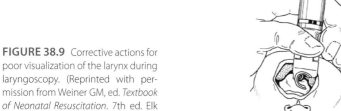		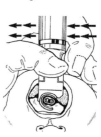
Laryngoscope inserted off to one side.	You see part of the glottis off to one side of the blade.	Gently move the blade back to the midline. Then advance or retreat according to landmarks seen.

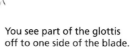

FIGURE 38.9 Corrective actions for poor visualization of the larynx during laryngoscopy. (Reprinted with permission from Weiner GM, ed. *Textbook of Neonatal Resuscitation*. 7th ed. Elk Grove Village, IL: American Academy of Pediatrics; 2016. Permission conveyed through Copyright Clearance Center, Inc.)

p. Hold ETT in right hand passing it down the right side of the mouth, outside the blade, while maintaining direct glottic visualization (**Fig. 38.11**)

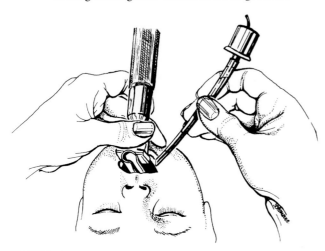

FIGURE 38.11 Visualize the glottis and pass the endotracheal tube into the oropharynx. Keep the tube outside the curve of the laryngoscope blade for better mobility.

q. Insert ETT through the vocal cords to the appropriate depth
r. Withdraw laryngoscope blade from mouth
s. Initiate positive-pressure ventilation
t. Confirm ETT position within the trachea using primary and secondary methods
3. Aftercare:
a. Secure the tube to the infant's face with either adhesive tape or commercially approved device (**Fig. 38.12**)
b. Place on ventilator
c. Obtain chest radiograph

F. Procedure for Nasotracheal Intubation

Some institutions use nasotracheal intubation as their primary intubation method. Others will transition from an oral approach to nasal based on age of patient, secretion burden–limiting ability to maintain security of tube taping, activity level of patient or in patients with oral pathology that limits or precludes an oral approach.

The initial procedural planning steps including equipment needs, procedural planning, steps through "j" above are identical to orotracheal intubation except for a stylet is not used for nasotracheal intubation. The aftercare is the same as for orotracheal intubation.

1. If orotracheal tube is already in place, release fixation and position at far left of the mouth, to allow continued ventilation during nasotracheal intubation (see procedure also for "push–pull" technique).
2. Lubricate end of ETT with water-soluble lubricant.
3. Insert tube through nostril following natural curve of nasopharynx.
4. Directly visualize oropharynx with laryngoscope as described previously, taking particular care not to hyperextend neck.
5. Insert Magill forceps into mouth and carefully grasp "new" tube between the middle and distal end, ensuring that pharyngeal tissue is not entrapped.
6. Advance laryngoscope blade to expose glottic opening.
7. Withdraw "old" orotracheal tube if present.
8. An assistant can advance "new" tube through nares while intubator guides the tip of tube to and through glottis. If no assistant is present, then forceps can be used to advance and guide tube through glottis.
9. Advance to desired depth.
10. Proceed with steps "r to t" of orotracheal intubation and aftercare.

G. Procedural Steps for "Push–Pull" Tube Exchange

1. Prepare equipment including everything that is necessary for the initial procedure.
2. Remove tape or device holding ETT in place, while the patient continues to receive positive-pressure ventilation through the existing ETT.

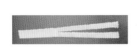
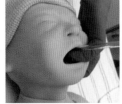
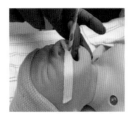
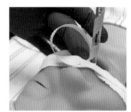
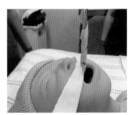

FIGURE 38.12 Y-Y-Y taping procedure to secure ETT. Step 1. Cut three pieces of adhesive tape in "Y" configuration. Step 2. Secure ETT by applying gentle yet firm pressure of ETT against palate with finger of helper. Step 3. Apply first piece of tape medial across the cheek, ensuring that the ear is not covered and that the ETT fits in the junction of the slit in the Y. The top thin piece is adhered across the philtrum to the opposite cheek. The lower piece is spiraled up the ETT. Step 4. The second piece of tape is adhered with the wide piece on the opposite cheek as the first. The top thin piece is still adhered across the philtrum. The junction of the slit in the tape should now be on the opposite side of the ETT as the first piece. The bottom thin piece of tape is then spiraled up the ETT in the other direction as the first piece. The helper at this time should be able to remove their finger from the patient's mouth. Step 5. The third piece tape is placed in the same fashion and direction as the first piece.

3. Move the existing ETT to the left side of the patient's mouth while maintaining the correct depth of insertion.
4. Insert the laryngoscope into the vallecula and visualize the airway.
5. Advance the new ETT until it is positioned just proximal to the glottis.
6. When the intubator is ready to advance the new ETT through the vocal cords, the assistant simultaneously removes the existing tube from the patient's airway.
7. Initiate positive-pressure ventilation through new ETT.
8. Secure the new ETT in place.

H. Selective Left Endobronchial Intubation

Severe unilateral lung disease (such as pulmonary interstitial emphysema, bullous emphysema, or persistent air leak) may lead a neonatal provider to consider selective intubation of a single bronchus (30–33). Due to the anatomy of the neonatal airway, an ETT that is deeply inserted will typically preferentially terminate in the right mainstem bronchus (34,35). Selective intubation of the left mainstem bronchus, however, is a more technically challenging procedure. In older patients, a balloon-tipped device can be used to obstruct one bronchus; however, this is not an option for neonatal providers in most situations (36).

Neonatal clinicians should consider performing selective left endobronchial intubation with guidance by direct bronchoscopy or fluoroscopy (33). If these resources are not available, this procedure can be approached using an alternate technique:

1. In a patient with an ETT in place, estimate the depth of the carina on a CXR. (If the patient is not intubated, prepare for ET intubation as described above.)
2. Rotate the ETT 180 degrees, until the concavity of the tube and the Murphy eye are directed to the patient's left (35).
3. Turn the patient's head to the right (35,37).
4. Insert the ETT and advance to a distance 0.5 to 1 cm below the predetermined depth of the carina.
5. Confirm that differential breath sounds are noted upon auscultation. If the left-sided breath sounds diminish, the ETT should be withdrawn until they return.
6. Position should be confirmed with a chest radiograph.
7. ETT should be secured, with final depth of insertion noted.
8. Previous modifications to this procedure include laterally tilting the patient's body 45 to 60 degrees to the right, but recent authors suggest that rotation of the ETT as described above makes this manipulation unnecessary (30,32,38).
9. Potential complications of this procedure include (39):
   a. Development of air leak in the ventilated lung
   b. Pneumonia in nonventilated lung
   c. ETT dislodgement from left mainstem bronchus
   d. Ventilatory insufficiency
   e. Severe left bronchomalacia

I. Tracheal Suctioning

When patients have an ETT in place, tracheal suctioning is frequently required to ensure maintenance of tube patency. The optimal frequency of tracheal suctioning is not known (40). However, in general, routine suctioning is not recommended but should be performed when clinically indicated.

1. Indications
   a. To clear tracheobronchial airway of secretions
2. Relative contraindications
   a. Recent surgery in the area
   b. Recent pulmonary hemorrhage
3. Considerations
   a. When feasible, use two people when suctioning the airway to minimize the risk of patient compromise and complications, as well as to shorten the procedure time. This is especially important for patients on high-frequency oscillator ventilators where interaction with the ventilator is needed to maintain mean airway pressure during the procedure.
   b. Attempt to limit the number of passes to retrieve secretions.
   c. Use of closed (in-line) suctioning may be beneficial in maintaining sterility and avoiding disruptions from mechanical ventilation compared to open suctioning with disconnection from the ventilator.
   d. Routine instillation of saline into the airway is not recommended during suctioning.
   e. Care should be taken to ensure that the suction catheter is not passed beyond the tip of the ETT due to the risk of trauma to the trachea.
   f. If there is a concern for an obstruction that is below the ETT and is not relieved with suctioning using the closed or open technique, using a meconium aspirator might be useful.
   g. Medications administered through an ETT used to "loosen" secretions have not been well evaluated, especially in emergency situations.
4. Equipment
   a. Sterile normal saline for flushing of catheter
   b. Gloves
   c. Sterile suction catheters if in-line suction catheter not available (Table 38.3)
   d. Meconium aspirator (optional)
   e. Adjustable vacuum source and attachments
5. Procedure for intubated patients
   a. Ensure equipment available
   b. Monitor heart rate and oxygen saturation continuously during suctioning

TABLE 38.3 Recommended Size of Suction Catheter Based on ETT Size

ENDOTRACHEAL TUBE SIZE (mm ID)	CATHETER SIZE (Fr)
2.5	5 or 6
3.0	6 or 8
3.5	8

Data from Weiner GM, ed. *Textbook of Neonatal Resuscitation.* 7th ed. Elk Grove Village, IL: American Academy of Pediatrics; 2016.

c. If using open suctioning, determine length of ETT plus adapter and note on suction catheter as limit of depth of insertion. For closed suctioning devices, follow manufacturer guidelines for determining appropriate depth

d. Set suction pressure at 80 to 100 mm Hg

e. Perform hand hygiene and use appropriate personal protective equipment. If using an open suctioning technique, eye goggles should also be considered

f. Pass catheter down airway to predetermined depth. Do not apply vacuum during insertion (i.e., keep suction control port open or avoid depression of valve if using in-line suctioning)

g. Close proximal suction control port or depress valve and withdraw catheter

h. Limit time for insertion and removal to 10 seconds

i. Clear catheter with sterile saline or water

j. Reestablish ventilation and then repeat as needed to clear secretions ensuring patient is allowed to recover between attempts. If using in-line suctioning, ensure valve is in locked position when suctioning is complete.

J. Intubation Procedural Complications

Adverse events are not infrequently associated with procedure of neonatal intubation. The most frequent complications include severe desaturation and esophageal intubation (41).

1. Dysrhythmia (including bradycardia)
2. Hypoxemia
3. Main stem bronchial intubation
4. Esophageal intubation
5. Emesis with and without aspiration
6. Hypotension
7. Hypertension (including increased intracranial pressure)
8. Epistaxis
9. Gum, lip, or dental trauma
10. Laryngospasm
11. Medication error
12. Airway trauma
    a. Perforation of hypopharynx or trachea
    b. Hemorrhage
    c. Laryngeal edema
    d. Vocal cord injury
    e. Dislocation of arytenoid
13. Cardiac arrest
14. Death
15. Other complications that can occur with long duration of orotracheal intubation include palatal and alveolar ridge deformities. Prolonged nasal intubation can lead to nasal passage stenosis and nasal deformities. Prolonged intubation can also lead to subglottic stenosis

K. Planned Extubation

Prior to performing a planned extubation, it is essential to be prepared to perform bag-mask ventilation and to replace the ETT quickly if the patient does not tolerate the procedure. Thus intubation equipment and personnel qualified to perform reintubation should be nearby if not at the bedside. In addition, it is important to have available the appropriate respiratory support desired to support the patient after the extubation, such as nasal cannula or nasal prongs for continuous positive airway pressure administration. Dexamethasone has been shown to likely be beneficial to prevent extubation failure from presumed laryngeal edema in patients with specific risk factors (42,43). Given the known adverse effects of dexamethasone, routine use is not recommended, especially in the preterm population.

1. Ensure appropriate personnel and equipment at the bedside.
2. Perform suction prior to extubation.
3. Release all fixation devices while holding tube in place. Ensure cuff is fully deflated if cuffed ETT is in place.
4. Using manual ventilation, provide the infant a sigh breath, and then withdraw tube during exhalation. Avoid suctioning during tube withdrawal, unless specifically utilizing the tube to remove thick foreign material from trachea.
5. Place the neonate on the predetermined noninvasive respiratory support.
6. Allow recovery time before suctioning oropharynx.

L. Placement of Supraglottic/Laryngeal Mask Device

1. Laryngeal mask (supraglottic) devices are useful in situations where a neonate needs more than noninvasive respiratory support but mask ventilation and/or ET intubation is not feasible.

2. Indications:
   a. Patients with craniofacial abnormalities that preclude adequate mask ventilation due to inability to achieve appropriate seal.
   b. Patients who cannot be intubated due to inadequate visualization.
3. Several studies have suggested that laryngeal masks are superior to bag-mask ventilation in the delivery room when positive pressure is needed and can help avoid intubation in cases where bag-mask ventilation has failed (44).
4. Considerations:
   a. Size 1 devices are appropriate for neonates less than 5 kg and size 1.5 for infants 5 to 10 kg. There is very limited data on use of a laryngeal mask in neonates <1.5 kg (44).
   b. Evidence is limited on the use of supraglottic devices during cardiac compressions and for administration of surfactant or intratracheal epinephrine (45).
   c. Several devices are available and have different designs that may slightly affect the procedure for placement.
   d. Premedication: Passage of the device can cause vagally mediated bradycardia thus some providers will give atropine prior to placement if time allows.
   e. Oral/naso-gastric catheter placement: If the device does not have an integrated channel for an oral gastric catheter, a naso-gastric tube should be inserted prior to insertion of the supraglottic device.
5. Equipment needed:
   a. Laryngeal mask device
   b. Syringe if cuff present on device
   c. Water-soluble lubricant
   d. Gloves and other personal protective equipment as indicated
   e. Humidified oxygen/air source, blender, and analyzer
   f. Monitoring equipment
      (1) Cardiorespiratory monitor
      (2) Pulse oximeter
   g. Resuscitation bag and mask
   h. End-tidal CO_2 detection device
      (1) Colorimetric
      (2) Quantitative
   i. Stethoscope
   j. Adhesive tape for securing device
6. Procedural steps for laryngeal mask placement:
   a. Don appropriate personal protective equipment (may include eye protection based on patient characteristics).
   b. Perform equipment check. If a device with a cuff is used, ensure the cuff on the device is intact by filling with attached air through attached pilot balloon. The supraglottic device can be inserted with the cuff deflated or partially or mostly inflated depending on institution/provider preference.

c. Lubricate device along the posterior surface using water-soluble lubricant.
   d. Perform time-out (if not in an emergency situation).
   e. Give premedication if indicated.
   f. Stand at head of bed with infant's head in sniffing position.
   g. Open infant's mouth using nondominant hand and insert device passing it along the hard palate and into the hypopharynx until resistance is felt. The thumb of the nondominant hand may need to be used to depress and hold the tongue in place to prevent retrodisplacement of tongue.
   h. If a cuff is present, inflate the cuff with air until a slight rise is seen, ensuring not to exceed the maximum recommended volume of air per the manufacturer of the device. The device should not be held while inflating the cuff.
   i. Proceed with providing ventilation and confirming adequate positioning with use of end-tidal CO_2 device as well as chest rise, breath sounds, and vital sign response.
   j. Secure device with adhesive. Taping techniques that work with an ETT will work with supraglottic devices.

M. Management Considerations for the Patient With an Anticipated Difficult Airway

Patients with obvious craniofacial malformations, macroglossia, or neck masses may be difficult to intubate with routine techniques due to inability to visualize the glottis. Intubation attempts should be minimized due to increasing airway trauma and increased risk of severe complications with multiple attempts (46,47). In the nonemergent setting, if there is concern for the inability to provide effective noninvasive ventilation whether with a mask or a supraglottic device, premedication beyond atropine should not be utilized for the intubation attempt due to suppression of the patient's respiratory drive. Ideally, these patients should be transferred to locations where a surgical airway could potentially be established in a timely fashion before the nonemergent intubation is attempted. In the emergency setting, if the patient with an anticipated difficult airway has a failed intubation using routine laryngoscopy, alternative intubation techniques could be considered depending on the resources available in terms of equipment and skilled personnel. These techniques include:

1. Fiberoptic intubation: This requires the prerequisite skill to use the fiberoptic scope and appropriate-sized equipment to fit the appropriate-sized ETT over the scope to introduce once the scope is advanced through the glottis.

2. Intubation through a supraglottic device: This can be done with or without fiberoptic assistance, that is, advancing the fiberoptic scope through the supraglottic device, advancing the ETT over the fiberoptic device through the supraglottic airway and then removing the fiberoptic scope while maintaining, with forceps or other means, the ETT in place. Then the supraglottic device is removed from the mouth after confirmation that the ETT is still in place with usual confirmation techniques. There are commercially available supraglottic devices that are designed to enhance the ability to insert an ETT without the use of a fiberoptic scope, though many of these are not sized appropriately for a neonate and overall success without the use of a fiberoptic scope is decreased (48). Some supraglottic devices have either webs at the glottic interface or pronounced curvature that would preclude the advancement of an ETT through them. Note that to do this successfully, the connector of the ETT needs to be removed to facilitate removal of the supraglottic device. Thus, this procedure has increased risk if care is not made to ensure the ETT is not displaced down the trachea where it may not be retrievable.

3. Videolaryngoscopy: Several videolaryngoscopic devices exist. Those with a blade configuration similar to traditional laryngoscopes may not confer significant added benefit in patients with difficult airways. Other devices such as the GlideScope, may offer benefit but require different psychomotor techniques, and thus require personnel to be trained specifically for use.

4. Digital intubation: In this technique, there is no visualization of the airway. The intubator stands at the side or at the feet of the patient. He/she introduces the index finger of a nondominant hand over the midline of the tongue until the glottis is identified by palpation. The ETT is then introduced and guided through the glottis by the index finger. There are reports of improved success and decreased time of procedure with the digital technique; however, it has not been well studied especially in the population of neonates with concern for difficult airways (49). In an emergency, if there are no other alternatives for ventilation or intubation, it may be reasonable to try a digital intubation.

References

1. Weiner G. *Textbook of Neonatal Resuscitation (NRP)*. 7th ed. Elk Grove Village, IL: American Academy of Pediatrics and American Heart Association; 2016.
2. Wei JL, Bond J. Management and prevention of endotracheal intubation injury in neonates. *Curr Opin Otolaryngol Head Neck Surg.* 2011;19:474–477.
3. Thomas R, Rao S, Minutillo C, et al. Cuffed endotracheal tubes in infants less than 3 kg: A retrospective cohort study. *Pediatr Anaesth.* 2018;28:204–209.
4. Blayney M, Logan D. First thoracic vertebral body as reference for endotracheal tube placement. *Arch Dis Child Fetal Neonatal Ed.* 1994;71:F32–F35.
5. Kempley S, Moreira J, Petrone F. Endotracheal tube length for neonatal intubation. *Resuscitation.* 2008;77:369–373.
6. Gill I, Stafford A, Murphy M, et al. Randomised trial of estimating oral endotracheal tube insertion depth in newborns using weight or vocal cord guide. *Arch Dis Child Fetal Neonatal Ed.* 2018;103:F312–F316.
7. Gien J, Meyers ML, Kinsella JP. Assessment of carina position antenatally and postnatally in infants with congenital diaphragmatic hernia. *J Pediatr.* 2018;192:93–98.
8. Kemper M, Dullenkopf A, Schmidt A, et al. Nasotracheal intubation depth in paediatric patients. *Br J Anaesth.* 2014;113:840–846.
9. Rost J, Frush D, Auten R. Effect of neck position on endotracheal tube location in low birth weight infants. *Pediatr Pulmonol.* 1999;27:199–202.
10. Marcano B, Silver P, Mayer S. Cephalad movement of endotracheal tubes caused by prone positioning in pediatric patients with acute respiratory distress syndrome. *Pediatr Crit Care Med.* 2003;4:186–189.
11. Kim J, Kim H, Ahn W, et al. Head rotation, flexion and extension alter endotracheal tube position in adults and children. *Can J Anesth.* 2009;56:751–756.
12. Roberts K, Leone T, Edwards W, et al. Premedication for nonemergent neonatal intubations: a randomized, controlled trial comparing atropine and fentanyl to atropine, fentanyl and mivacurium. *Pediatrics.* 2006;118:1583–1591.
13. Lemyre B, Cheng R, Gaboury I. Atropine, fentanyl and succinylcholine for non-urgent intubations in newborns. *Arch Dis Child Fetal Neonatal Ed.* 2009;94:F349–F442.
14. Le C, Garey D, Leone T, et al. Impact of premedication on neonatal intubations by pediatric and neonatal trainees. *J Perinatol.* 2014;34(6):458–460.
15. Feltman D, Weiss M, Nicoski P, et al. Rocuronium for nonemergent intubation of term and preterm infants. *J Perinatol.* 2011;31:38–43.
16. Caldwell C, Watterberg K. Effect of premedication regimen on infant pain and stress response to endotracheal intubation. *J Perinatol.* 2015;35(6):415–418.
17. Friesen R, Honda A, Thieme R. Changes in anterior fontanel pressure in preterm neonates during tracheal intubation. *Anesth Analg.* 1987;66:874–878.
18. Wallenstein B, Birnie K, Arain Y, et al. Failed endotracheal intubation and adverse outcomes among extremely low birth weight infants. *J Perinatol.* 2016;36:112–115.
19. Kumar P, Denson SE, Mancuso TJ; Committee on Fetus and Newborn. Premedication for nonemergency endotracheal intubation in the neonate. *Pediatrics.* 2010;125:608–615.
20. McLendon K, Preuss CV. Atropine. [Updated November 23, 2018]. In: *StatPearls [Internet]*. Treasure Island, FL: StatPearls Publishing; 2018. https://www.ncbi.nlm.nih.gov/books/NBK470551/.
21. National Center for Biotechnology Information. PubChem Compound Database; CID = 4192. https://pubchem.ncbi.nlm.nih.gov/compound/4192. Accessed January 8, 2019.
22. Normal Epiglottis by Med Chaos. http://bit.ly/2ar7yp4. CC-BY-SA-3.0.

23. Kamlin C, O'Connell L, Morley C, et al. A randomized trial of stylets for intubation newborn infants. *Pediatrics.* 2013;131:e198–e205.

24. Healy D, Maties O, Hovord D, et al. A systematic review of the role of videolaryngoscopy in successful orotracheal intubation. *BMC Anesthesiology.* 2012;12:32.

25. Fiadjoe J, Gurnaney H, Dalesio N, et al. A prospective randomized equivalence trial of the GlideScope Cobalt video laryngoscope to traditional direct laryngoscopy in neonates and infants. *Anesthesiology.* 2012;116:622–628.

26. Vlatten A, Aucoin S, Litz S, et al. A comparison of the STORZ video laryngoscope and standard direct laryngoscopy for intubation in the Pediatric airway—a randomized clinical trial. *Paediatr Anaesth.* 2009;19:1102–1107.

27. Moussa A, Luangxay Y, Tremblay S, et al. Videolaryngoscope for teaching neonatal endotracheal intubation: a randomized controlled trial. *Pediatrics.* 2016;137:1–8.

28. O'Shea J, Thio M, Kamlin C, et al. Videolaryngoscopy to teach neonatal intubation. *Pediatrics.* 2015;136:912–919.

29. Johnston L, Auerbach M, Nagler J, et al. *Neonatal Tracheal Intubation.* 2016. https://www.openpediatrics.org/assets/video/neonatal-tracheal-intubation.

30. Chalak L, Kaiser J, Arrington R. Resolution of pulmonary interstitial emphysema following selective left main stem intubation in a premature newborn: an old procedure revisited. *Paediatr Anaesth.* 2007;17:183–186.

31. Jakob A, Bender C, Henschen M, et al. Selective unilateral lung ventilation in preterm infants with acquired bullous emphysema: a series of nine cases. *Pediatr Pulmonol.* 2013;48:9–14.

32. Joseph L, Bromiker R, Toker O, et al. Unilateral lung intubation for pulmonary air leak syndrome in neonates: a case series and a review of the literature. *Am J Perinatol.* 2011;28:151–156.

33. Van Dorn C, Sittig S, Koch C, et al. Selective fiberoptic left mainstem intubation to treat bronchial laceration in an extremely low birthweight neonate. *Int J Pediatr Otorhinolaryngol.* 2019;74:707–710.

34. Ryan S, Curran J. Embryology and anatomy of the neonatal chest. In: Donoghue V, ed. *Radiological Imaging of the Neonatal Chest.* Berlin Heidelberg GmbH: Springer-Verlag; 2002:1–9.

35. Kubota H, Kubota Y, Toyada Y, et al. Selective blind endobronchial intubation in children and adults. *Anesthesiology.* 1987;67:587–589.

36. Jishi N, Kyer D, Sharief N, et al. Selective bronchial occlusion for treatment of bullous interstitial emphysema and bronchopleural fistula. *J Pediatr Surg.* 1994;29:1545–1547.

37. Sivasubramanian K. Technique of selective intubation of the left bronchus in newborn infants. *J Pediatr.* 1979;94:479–480.

38. Ho AMH, Flavin MP, Fleming ML, et al. Selective left mainstem bronchial intubation in the neonatal intensive care unit. *Rev Bras Anestesiol.* 2018;68:318–321.

39. Glenski JA, Thibeault DW, Hall FK, et al. Selective bronchial intubation in infants with lobar emphysema: indications, complications, and long-term outcome. *Am J Perinatol.* 1986;3:199–204.

40. Bruschettini M, Zappettini S, Moja L, et al. Frequency of endotracheal suctioning for the prevention of respiratory morbidity in ventilated newborns. *Cochrane Database Syst Rev.* 2016;3:CD011493.

41. Foglia E, Ades A, Napolitano N, et al. Factors associated with adverse events during tracheal intubation in the NICU. *Neonatology.* 2015;108:23–29.

42. Davis P, Henderson-Smart D. Intravenous dexamethasone for extubation of newborn infants. *Cochrane Data Syst Rev.* 2001;(4):CD000308.

43. Veldhoen E, Smulders C, Kappen T, et al. Post-extubation stridor in respiratory syncytial virus bronchiolitis: Is there a role for prophylactic dexamethasone? *PLoS ONE.* 2017;12:e0172096.

44. Qureshi M, Kumaj M. Laryngeal mask airway versus bag-mask ventilation or endotracheal intubation for neonatal resuscitation. *Cochrane Database Syst Rev.* 2018;3:CD003314.

45. Bansal S, Caoci S, Dempsey E, et al. The laryngeal mask airway and its use in neonatal resuscitation: a critical review of where we are in 2017/2018. *Neonatology.* 2018;113:152–161.

46. Fiadjoe J, Nishisaki A, Jagannathan N, et al. Airway management complications in children with difficult tracheal intubation from the pediatric difficult intubation (PeDI) registry: a prospective cohort analysis. *Lancet Respir Med.* 2016;4:37–48.

47. Foglia E, Ades A, Sawyer T, et al. Neonatal intubation practice and outcomes: an international registry study. *Pediatrics.* 2019;143(1):e20180902.

48. Naik L, Bhardwaj N, Sen IM, et al. Intubation success through I-Gel® and Intubating Laryngeal Mask Airway® using flexible silicone tubes: a randomised noninferiority trial. *Anesthesiol Res Pract.* 2016;2016:7318595.

49. Moura J, Da Silvia G. Neonatal laryngoscope intubation and the digital method: a randomized controlled trial. *J Pediatr.* 2006;148:840–841.

CHAPTER

39

Surfactant Administration via Thin Catheter

Peter A. Dargaville and Harley Mason

A. Definitions

Respiratory distress syndrome (RDS): The clinical manifestation of surfactant deficiency in the preterm lung, cardinal features being tachypnea, retractions, grunting, and need for oxygen.

Thin catheter: A catheter of external diameter ~1.3 to 1.7 mm (4 to 5 FG) used for the purpose of surfactant instillation.

B. Purpose

To administer exogenous surfactant by thin catheter to a preterm infant with RDS receiving noninvasive respiratory support, most usually nasal continuous positive airway pressure (CPAP).

C. Background

Exogenous surfactant has been a mainstay of therapy for the preterm infant with RDS for over 30 years, delivered via an endotracheal tube with dose repetition as necessary. Nowadays, however, many preterm infants are managed from the outset on noninvasive respiratory support, in particular nasal CPAP, and thus lack the usual conduit by which surfactant is administered. Amongst infants on CPAP, many of those with RDS are adequately supported with CPAP alone, with gradual improvement in surfactant status and thus lung function. Some infants continue to exhibit features of RDS, including significant oxygen requirements, raising the dilemma of whether to continue with CPAP or to intubate for the purpose of giving surfactant.

Whilst the obvious resolution of the CPAP–surfactant dilemma is to briefly intubate for surfactant delivery, several recent randomized controlled trials have not shown a major benefit of this approach, mostly related to difficulty with extubation (1,2). For this reason, a number of different techniques of delivering surfactant in a nonintubated spontaneously breathing infant have been pursued (3,4). There is now wide experience of surfactant administration via a thin catheter briefly placed in the trachea (5–7), and enthusiasm for this method is burgeoning. A number of randomized controlled trials have suggested that this approach is a more effective means of delivering surfactant than standard intubation (8,9), most likely related to a positive effect of spontaneous breathing on surfactant distribution.

Two main methods of thin catheter placement for surfactant delivery have emerged, both of which are performed with the aid of direct laryngoscopy.

1. The **Cologne method**, in which the tip of a flexible feeding tube is directed through the vocal cords with Magill forceps (10)
2. The **Hobart method**, where the tip of a semirigid catheter (e.g., a vascular catheter) is guided into the trachea without Magill forceps (11)

Numerous variations on these methods now exist.

D. Indications

The indications for surfactant therapy via thin catheter are yet to be fully resolved. Nevertheless, based on the results of nonrandomized studies and clinical trials (12), the following gestation-specific thresholds for therapy can be provided.

1. **All gestations:**
    Respiratory insufficiency thought to be related to RDS and managed with noninvasive respiratory support, most usually CPAP or a form of noninvasive positive pressure ventilation.

2. **23 to 25 weeks' gestation**
   a. CPAP level ≥ 6 cm H_2O.
   b. Any requirement for oxygen to maintain SpO_2 in the local target range.
   c. Age <6 hours, and preferably <2 hours.
3. **26 to 28 weeks' gestation**
   a. CPAP level ≥ 6 cm H_2O.
   b. $FiO_2 \geq 0.30$ to maintain SpO_2 in the local target range.
   c. Age <24 hours, with an emphasis on early recognition and treatment at an age <6 to 12 hours.
4. **Beyond 28 weeks' gestation**
   a. CPAP level ≥ 6 cm H_2O, or nasal high flow ≥ 7 L/min.
   b. $FiO_2 \geq 0.30$ to 0.35 to maintain SpO_2 in the local target range.
   c. Age <24 hours.

E. Contraindications

1. **Absolute contraindications**
   a. Severe RDS with high oxygen requirements and/or severe respiratory acidosis, along with prominent atelectasis radiographically, such that ongoing ventilatory support will be necessary after surfactant therapy. The suggested FiO_2 thresholds above which intubation for surfactant should be considered for surfactant delivery are >0.40 to 0.50 at gestations <30 weeks, and FiO_2 >0.60 for more mature infants.
   b. An alternative cause for respiratory distress (e.g., congenital pneumonia or pulmonary hypoplasia).
   c. Maxillofacial, tracheal, or known pulmonary malformations.
   d. No experienced personnel available to perform the tracheal catheterization.

2. **Relative contraindications**
   a. Infant <26 weeks' gestation—the procedure can be technically challenging and destabilizing in inexperienced hands.
   b. Pneumothorax requiring drainage.
   c. Prominent apnoea despite caffeine administration.

F. Precautions

1. Performing direct laryngoscopy in a spontaneously breathing preterm infant for the purpose of tracheal catheterization requires considerable skill, and should not be performed by clinicians unfamiliar and/or untrained in the technique. Practice on a realistic resuscitation mannequin is essential before attempting the method in human infants.
2. All reports to date of surfactant delivery to preterm infants via thin catheter involve the use of a catheter used "off-label," for a purpose other than that for which it was intended. A purpose-built semirigid catheter is now available (LISAcath, Chiesi Farmaceutici, Parma, Italy), and appears to have favorable design characteristics compared with a vascular catheter (13).

G. Equipment (Fig. 39.1)

1. *Cologne method*
   a. Flexible end-hole catheter with rounded tip, preferably with depth markings. Options include a 5 Fr feeding tube or 3.5 to 5 Fr umbilical catheter.
   b. Magill forceps (appropriate size for infant).

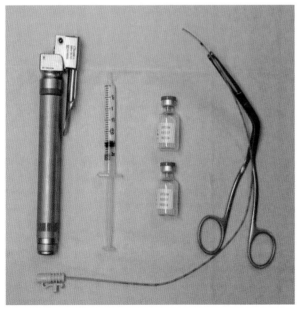
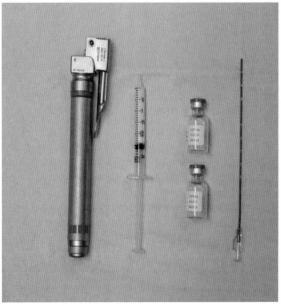

FIGURE 39.1 Equipment. **A:** Equipment for Cologne method. **B:** Equipment for Hobart method. The catheter depicted is the LISAcath; if not available a 16G vascular catheter (Angiocath) is a satisfactory alternative.

c. Prepare the catheter for insertion by grasping it with Magill forceps at an angle of 120 degrees, around 2 cm from the tip.

2. *Hobart method*

   a. Semirigid catheter, including a vascular catheter (16G Angiocath) or, if available, a purpose-built catheter (LISAcath, Chiesi Farmaceutici).

3. *Both methods*

   a. Laryngoscope with Miller 00 blade (<28 to 30 weeks), otherwise Miller 0 or Macintosh 1 blade.

   b. *If necessary:* Wax pencil to place depth mark near catheter tip (1.5 cm for <27 weeks' gestation, otherwise 2 cm). A pencil mark or silk tie can also be placed further up the catheter shaft to indicate an appropriate depth at the lip (same depth as for oral intubation).

   c. Surfactant, dose 100 to 200 mg/kg, in a syringe with an additional 0.5 mL air.

H. Technique

A video of the Hobart method is shown in ▶ Video 39.1. Video footage of the Cologne method is available at https://www.youtube.com/watch?v=OUvgJ57FQR8.

The infant should be swaddled and placed in a position to facilitate laryngoscopy, with a neck roll in place.

1. CPAP should be maintained throughout the procedure, with an interface that permits direct laryngoscopy to be performed. Some CPAP interfaces have a high profile on the face, precluding direct laryngoscopy.

2. Monitoring of heart rate and SpO_2 should be maintained throughout.

3. Premedication with caffeine is recommended for infants <1,250 gm (and for larger infants at the discretion of the proceduralist).

4. Use of nonpharmacologic means of minimizing discomfort is encouraged (e.g., 25% sucrose), along with peripheral tactile stimulation during and after surfactant administration to encourage spontaneous breathing.

5. Use of sedating premedication for surfactant delivery via thin catheter remains controversial. Fentanyl, propofol, and ketamine have been used in this setting; none is without risk, including depression of spontaneous respiration, along with concern for an effect on neuronal development. Use of sedating premedication appears to be associated with greater need for positive pressure ventilation during and after the procedure, and higher rates of subsequent intubation.

Method

Both Methods

1. Consider preoxygenation with an increase in FiO_2 by 0.05 to 0.10 for 1 to 2 minutes.

2. Perform laryngoscopy with CPAP support maintained. Bring vocal cords into view with a combination of anterior pressure on the pharynx and cricoid pressure, performed by the proceduralist with the fifth finger.

3. Suction secretions as necessary.

Cologne Method

1. Using the Magill forceps, pass the catheter tip through the vocal cords.

Hobart Method

1. Using a three-finger hold (**Fig. 39.2**), pass the catheter tip through the vocal cords.

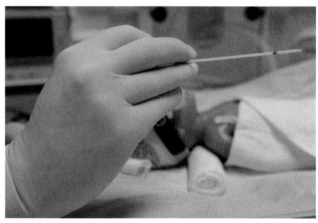

FIGURE 39.2 Catheter hold (Hobart method). Three-finger grasp of the semirigid catheter, allowing the fourth finger to be used to guide catheter tip anteriorly.

Both Methods

1. Troubleshooting: If cord adduction precludes catheter insertion, withdraw catheter tip slightly and await opening of the larynx.

2. Troubleshooting: If a view of the cords is not obtained, or the catheter cannot be inserted, or the infant has persistent bradycardia during laryngoscopy, temporarily halt the procedure, remove the laryngoscope, and provide CPAP support with the mouth closed.

3. Insert catheter to the desired depth beyond the cords: 1.5 cm <27 weeks' gestation, 2 cm otherwise (**Fig. 39.3**).

4. Pinch-hold the catheter at the lip, and note and maintain depth at lip (**Fig. 39.4**).

5. Remove the laryngoscope, close the mouth to optimize CPAP support. There is no need to continue laryngoscopy as the surfactant is being instilled.

6. Connect preloaded syringe to the catheter and administer surfactant over 30 seconds to 3 minutes according to local preference. The surfactant should not be given as an infusion, but rather as repeated small bolus injections (3 to 5 boluses depending on volume and infant size).

7. Troubleshooting: Slow the rate of administration if surfactant reflux is seen or breathing is irregular. For

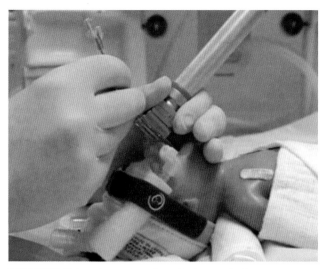

FIGURE 39.3 Introducing the catheter (Hobart method).

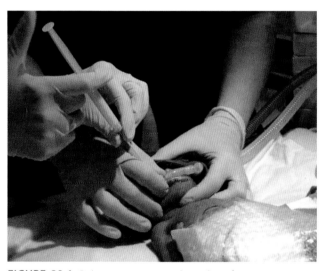

FIGURE 39.4 Catheter in position at lip with surfactant syringe connected.

pronounced reflux, stop surfactant administration, hold the mouth closed, and encourage spontaneous breathing with the aid of CPAP to redirect the surfactant back into the lung. Only apply suction if there are persistent signs of airway obstruction.

8. Once all surfactant is administered, evacuate surfactant from catheter with air from the syringe, and remove the catheter.

9. Encourage spontaneous breathing during surfactant instillation by consistent application of CPAP and gentle stimulation if necessary.

10. Increase FiO_2 if SpO_2 is persistently low at any time.

11. Use positive pressure ventilation only if the infant is apnoeic or has prolonged hypoxaemia/bradycardia.

12. Reduce FiO_2 soon after the procedure according to SpO_2. The oxygenation response after surfactant instillation should be almost immediate.

I. Special Circumstances

Surfactant Therapy in the Delivery Room

Administration of exogenous surfactant via endotracheal tube to unselected preterm infants in the delivery room does not appear to confer advantages over early selective surfactant therapy in the NICU, especially where CPAP is used in the transition (14). This finding may also apply to surfactant therapy via thin catheter, but remains largely untested. Current evidence would suggest that, other than perhaps for the most immature infants <26 weeks' gestation, surfactant delivery via thin catheter can and should be deferred until the infant is in the NICU environment, stable on CPAP and on cardiorespiratory monitoring.

Surfactant Therapy at Gestational Age >32 Weeks

Recommendations regarding thin catheter surfactant administration are still emerging for the understudied subgroup of infants beyond 32 weeks' gestation, where considerations of procedural tolerance and possible need for analgesic premedication come to the fore. For this group, there appears to be a benefit of thin catheter surfactant delivery (with fentanyl premedication) over continuation of CPAP once an FiO_2 threshold of 0.35 is reached (15), but studies directly comparing thin catheter and endotracheal tube administration are lacking.

J. Complications

1. **Need for multiple catheterization attempts**
   The rate of successful tracheal catheterization at first attempt is around 70%. Failure of catheterization on repeated attempts occurs with a frequency of <5%.

2. **Hypoxic and/or bradycardic episodes**
   Episodes of hypoxia and bradycardia are commonly reported during tracheal catheterization for surfactant delivery. Hypoxic events with SpO_2 <80% occur in around 40% to 60% of catheterization attempts, and bradycardia with a heart rate <100 bpm is seen in around 10% to 20% of cases. Such events are more likely to occur (i) if laryngoscopy is prolonged or unduly forceful, (ii) if no CPAP/supplemental oxygen is applied during the procedure, and (iii) after administration of a large bolus of surfactant into the trachea. Frequency of use of PPV to aid recovery from these events is relatively low, and PPV can be avoided in most instances by skilled proceduralists. Intubation during or after the procedure is rarely needed.

3. **Surfactant reflux**
   The appearance of some surfactant in the mouth or at the lips during instillation via the intratracheal

catheter is noted in around one-third of reported cases. Closure of the mouth and promotion of spontaneous breathing may aid in returning the surfactant to the lung. PPV and suction are rarely needed in this circumstance.

4. **Surfactant maldistribution**

As for surfactant administration via an endotracheal tube, if the installation catheter is inserted too deeply, the bulk of the delivered surfactant will be deposited in the right lung, with resultant difference in compliance and aeration between the two lungs. Vigilance in achieving and maintaining the correct position of the catheter tip is crucial.

5. **Failure of surfactant delivery**

Malposition of the catheter in the esophagus and thus failure of delivery of surfactant to the lung undoubtedly occurs with the thin catheter technique, and will manifest as a failure to induce the usual improvement in FiO_2 after the procedure. At present, confirmation that the catheter tip has passed through the vocal cords relies solely on the observations of the proceduralist. Videolaryngoscopy certainly offers a partial solution, allowing other observers to visualize the path of the catheter.

References

1. Sandri F, Plavka R, Ancora G, et al. Prophylactic or early selective surfactant combined with nCPAP in very preterm infants. *Pediatrics*. 2010;125:e1402–e1409.
2. Dunn MS, Kaempf J, de Klerk A, et al. Randomized trial comparing 3 approaches to the initial respiratory management of preterm neonates. *Pediatrics*. 2011;128:e1069–e1076.
3. Dargaville PA. Innovation in surfactant therapy I: surfactant lavage and surfactant administration by fluid bolus using minimally invasive techniques. *Neonatology*. 2012;101:326–336.
4. Kribs A. Minimally invasive surfactant therapy and noninvasive respiratory support. *Clin Perinatol*. 2016;43:755–771.
5. Dargaville PA, Aiyappan A, De Paoli AG, et al. Minimally-invasive surfactant therapy in preterm infants on continuous positive airway pressure. *Arch Dis Child Fetal Neonatal Ed*. 2013;98:F122–F126.
6. Klebermass-Schrehof K, Wald M, Schwindt J, et al. Less invasive surfactant administration in extremely preterm infants: impact on mortality and morbidity. *Neonatology*. 2013;103:252–258.
7. Göpel W, Kribs A, Hartel C, et al. Less invasive surfactant administration is associated with improved pulmonary outcomes in spontaneously breathing preterm infants. *Acta Paediatr*. 2015;104:241–246.
8. Kanmaz HG, Erdeve O, Canpolat FE, et al. Surfactant administration via thin catheter during spontaneous breathing: randomized controlled trial. *Pediatrics*. 2013;131:e502–e509.
9. Kribs A, Roll C, Gopel W, et al. Nonintubated surfactant application vs conventional therapy in extremely preterm infants: a randomized clinical trial. *JAMA Pediatr*. 2015;169:723–730.
10. Kribs A, Pillekamp F, Hunseler C, et al. Early administration of surfactant in spontaneous breathing with nCPAP: feasibility and outcome in extremely premature infants (postmenstrual age </ = 27 weeks). *Paediatr Anaesth*. 2007;17:364–369.
11. Dargaville PA, Aiyappan A, Cornelius A, et al. Preliminary evaluation of a new technique of minimally invasive surfactant therapy. *Arch Dis Child Fetal Neonatal Ed*. 2011;96:F243–F248.
12. Dargaville PA. Newer strategies for surfactant delivery. In: Bancalari E, Keszler M, Davis PG, eds. *The Newborn Lung*, 3rd ed. Philadelphia, PA: Elsevier; 2019:221–238.
13. Fabbri L, Klebermass-Schrehof K, Aguar M, et al. Five-country manikin study found that neonatologists preferred using the LISAcath rather than the Angiocath for less invasive surfactant administration. *Acta Paediatr*. 2018;107:780–783.
14. Rojas-Reyes MX, Morley CJ, Soll R. Prophylactic versus selective use of surfactant in preventing morbidity and mortality in preterm infants. *Cochrane Database Syst Rev*. 2012;3:CD000510.
15. Olivier F, Nadeau S, Belanger S, et al. Efficacy of minimally invasive surfactant therapy in moderate and late preterm infants: a multicentre randomized control trial. *Paediatr Child Health*. 2017;22:120–124.

Tube Placement and Care

Tracheostomy and Tracheostomy Care

Margaret Mary Kuczkowski and Gregory J. Milmoe

Infants with airway obstruction or need for prolonged ventilatory support are often considered for tracheostomy as an alternative to endotracheal intubation. The timing and sequelae have long been debated (1–5). Emphasis on ongoing care aims to improve management and safety (3). Early involvement of the family helps to allay fears, and promote safety for home care.

A. Indications

1. Prolonged ventilator support—for pulmonary, neurologic, or neuromuscular reasons
2. Congenital airway anomalies, craniofacial or laryngotracheal
3. Acquired subglottic or tracheal stenosis

B. Contraindications

1. Unstable physiology
   a. Sepsis
   b. Pneumonia not yet controlled
   c. Pulmonary instability requiring high inspiratory pressures or need for high-frequency ventilation
   d. Cardiovascular instability—shunting, arrhythmia, or hypotension
   e. Evolving neurologic or renal injuries
2. Distal obstruction not relieved by tracheostomy—mediastinal mass or severe stenosis at carina

C. Precautions

1. Patient should be stable but this is always relative
2. This procedure should be done only in facilities where there is appropriate support for postoperative management
3. Anticipate anomalies that make trachea relatively inaccessible

   a. Massive cervical hemangioma—bleeding issues
   b. Massive cervical lymphangioma—severe distortion of neck anatomy
   c. Massive goiter—might be manageable medically
   d. Chest syndromes with severe kyphoscoliosis or tracheal distortion
4. Anticipate need for increased pulmonary support afterward to counter atelectasis and increased secretions immediately postop. Tracheostomy tubes allow for air leak through the stoma and larynx (even with cuff). In contrast, an endotracheal tube fits more snugly at the cricoids, creating a more closed system for ventilation.
5. Neonates are less able to tolerate bacteremia. Use perioperative antibiotic to cover skin flora.
6. If the patient is not currently intubated, have endoscopy equipment available and discuss intubation options with the anesthesiologist.
7. The infant larynx differs from that of the adult and older child (Fig. 40.1)
   a. More pliable and mobile
   b. Relatively higher in the neck
   c. Thymus and innominate artery can override the trachea in the surgical field

D. Procedure

1. Obtain informed consent and perform "time-out" procedure as per institutional guidelines (see Chapter 3).
2. Equipment check done for instruments, sutures, endoscopy backup and available trach tubes. Tubes are selected based on needed caliber and length.
3. Anesthesia team will apply monitors, check IV line, and confirm satisfactory ventilation through the endotracheal tube before administering anesthetic agents.
4. Remove nasogastric tube to avoid confusion when palpating the trachea. Do not place an esophageal stethoscope.

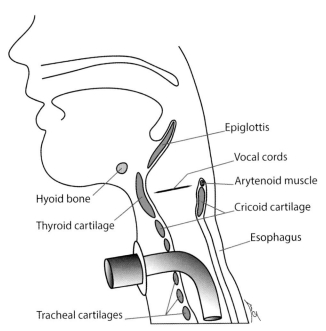

FIGURE 40.1 Side-profile anatomy of upper airway and location of tracheostomy tube. (Courtesy of Dr. Marko Culjat, MD, PhD, MedStar Georgetown University Hospital.)

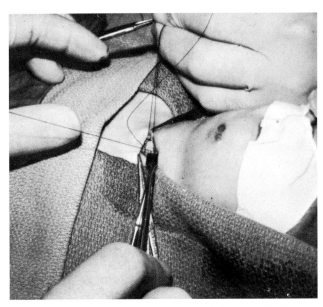

FIGURE 40.2 Placement of stay sutures through the tracheal wall.

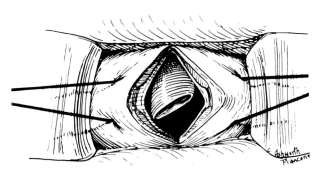

FIGURE 40.3 Artistic conception of view through tracheal incision with the tip of the endotracheal tube visible. Stay sutures hold cartilages open.

5. Position patient with neck extended, using shoulder roll. Prep the surgical site from above the chin to below the clavicles. Then drape the patient, allowing the anesthesiologist access to the endotracheal tube and the securing tape.

6. Inject the skin and deeper tissues with local anesthetic (0.5 to 1 mL of 1% lidocaine with 1:100,000 epinephrine).

7. Identify the following landmarks: Suprasternal notch, chin, midline, trachea, and cricoid. In small neonates the cricoid may be difficult to palpate.

8. Make the skin incision vertically in the midline. This allows easier retraction and avoids excessive lateral dissection.

9. Dissect in the midline down to the tracheal wall, identifying strap muscles, thyroid gland, trachea, thyroid cartilage, and cricoid ring.

10. Place Senn or Ragnell retractors on either side of the trachea for optimal visibility. If the thyroid gland cannot be displaced by blunt dissection, then divide the isthmus and ligate with silk sutures.

11. Place vertical stay sutures on either side of the planned tracheal incision (usually the third and fourth rings). These sutures are the infant's lifeline should the tube become dislodged or need urgent replacement in the first week before the wound matures (**Fig. 40.2**).

12. Incise the trachea vertically for two or three rings depending on the size of the tube needed. The anesthesiologist will loosen the tape and withdraw the endotracheal tube until the tip is just visible (**Fig. 40.3**). The tracheostomy tube is then placed in the airway.

13. Ventilation is then confirmed by end-tidal carbon dioxide measure and oxygen saturation, as well as auscultation of both lung fields.

14. Secure the tube with twill tape or Velcro ties. Either way, only one finger should fit between the tape and the neck when the baby's neck is in neutral position. At most centers the flange itself will be sutured to the neck until the first tube change.

15. Secure the tracheal stay sutures to the neck with tape labeled as to the correct side (**Fig. 40.4**).

16. Transport the patient back to the intensive care unit with a backup endotracheal tube and laryngoscope available. Upon arrival obtain chest radiograph to check tube position and lung status. If needed, replace NG tube before x-ray.

E. Immediate Postoperative Care (Day 0 Until First Trach Change)

Note: The first tracheostomy tube change is to be performed by the surgical team and the timing is at the discretion of

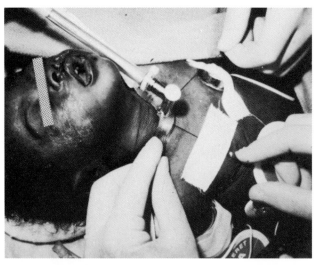

FIGURE 40.4 Fixation of stay sutures. As soon as the position of the tracheostomy tube is confirmed and stomal ventilation is started, the tube may be fixed. Equal tension is kept on the stay sutures during taping. Right suture is marked to avoid confusion in future placement.

the surgeon (varies between postop days 3 and 7, majority between days 5 and 7) (4).

1. Provide bedside nursing and respiratory therapy care in intensive care setting with nurses and therapists who are trained and competent in the care of infants with upper airway disorders and tracheostomies. These nurses and respiratory therapists need to be skilled in respiratory assessment, routine tracheostomy management, and can anticipate and manage tracheostomy emergencies (6).

2. Keep spare tracheostomy tubes at bedside at all times (one of the same size and one size smaller) (4,6–8).

3. Airway information sheet at bedside needs to include: Tracheostomy brand and tube size, suction catheter size, suction depth including any adapter **(Fig. 40.5)** (7,8).

My trach tube is: (<u>brand and size</u>)

_____

Suction Catheter Size:

_____

Suction Catheter Depth:

_____

FIGURE 40.5 Figure representing an Emergency Airway Information Sheet for the bedside.

4. Airway management
   a. Humidification: Provide adequate humidification via assisted ventilation or heated humidification tracheostomy collar.
      (1) Rationale: Normally the nasal airway warms and humidifies air that enters the body;

however, a tracheostomy bypasses the nasal airway allowing less humidified air to enter. Air that is not humidified can thicken secretions and increase the risk of mucus plugging.
      (2) Precaution: Condensation from the water vapor can collect on the tubing walls and in the tubing and can be a potential source of bacterial growth (7).
   b. Ventilation: Wean ventilator setting with a goal of tracheostomy collar unless patient is chemically paralyzed (see Chapter 7)
      (1) Keep head of bed (HOB) elevated 20 to 30 degrees (4).
      (2) Precaution: Correct tracheostomy tube placement is essential. Continually monitor respiratory status, including vital signs and clinical appearance of adequate oxygenation and ventilation. Infants can exhibit diminished breath sounds, changes in color, increased peak pressures, increased work of breathing, and change in mental status and increase in agitation if the tube becomes dislodged, blocked, or misplaced (8).
   c. Suctioning: Suction every 4 hours and as needed (4).
      (1) Indication: Suctioning may be required if the patient exhibits increased work of breathing, respiratory distress, desaturation, increased restlessness, visible secretions, audible respirations, tachypnea (7).
      (2) Precaution: Careful suctioning practices must be followed to avoid complications, including hypoxemia, bronchospasm, hypo- or hypertension, laryngospasm, atelectasis, decreased lung compliance, airway trauma, and increased intracranial pressure (4,7).
      (3) Sterile technique is recommended in a hospital setting: Including good handwashing, sterile gloves, disposable sterile catheters.
      (4) The diameter of the suction catheter (6 or 8 Fr) should be selected so that the catheter is easy to insert and is less than 70% of the internal diameter of the tracheostomy tube (6,8). A larger catheter removes more secretions than a smaller catheter (6).
      (5) Measure appropriate suction length according to the brand of tracheostomy tube. Care must be taken to correctly measure no more than 0.5 cm beyond the end of the tracheotomy tube to avoid trauma to the tracheal wall or carina (6–8).
      (6) Utilize a multiholed suction catheter with holes close to the distal end to remove secretions from a greater surface area (6).
      (7) Instillation of a normal saline bolus directly into the infant's tracheostomy tube was previously utilized to thin, loosen, and mobilize secretions. However, research shows that

it increases risk of infection, can cause an increase in pain and anxiety, and does not aid in thinning or loosening secretions. Therefore, humidification, nebulized saline, vibration vests, prescription respiratory medications, and cough-assistive devices can be utilized for secretion mobilization if necessary (6,8). In the case of an acute mucus plug, sterile normal saline bolus may be utilized.

- (8) Suction pressure recommendation: Neonates: 60 to 80 mm Hg; Infants and children: 80 to 100 mm Hg (6–8).
- (9) Rapid catheter insertion, suction, and withdrawal of the suction catheter (no more than 5 seconds total). Twirling the catheter between the thumb and fingers will maximize contact with the tube and secretions and minimize friction (6,7). Do not apply suction until ready to withdraw catheter.

5. Sedation management
   a. Establish pain and sedation goal with multidisciplinary team prior to surgery and reassess daily and PRN.
      (1) Individualized sedation plan is necessary for young patients with a critical airway especially in the immediate postop period.
      (2) Utilize Pain/Sedation scores (i.e., N-PASS) or State Behavioral Scales (SBS)—see Chapter 7.
   b. Provide adequate sedation to minimize shearing effect as well as enforce goal of transitioning to trach collar.

6. Skin management
   a. Maintain proper head position—midline/sniffing position (**Fig. 40.6**).

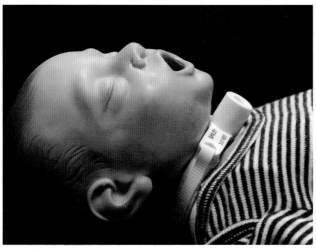

FIGURE 40.6 Tracheostomy tube in baby manikin.

   b. If moving patient, keep nose, chin, and sternum aligned.

   c. Careful attention should be made to ensure that stay sutures are aligned on the correct side, labeled, secured, and frequently assessed. These sutures come out with the first trach change but are essential for maintaining the airway in the immediate postop period (4).
   d. Assess skin surrounding the stoma and the entire circumference of the infant's neck every 4 hours and PRN for signs and symptoms of skin breakdown or infection (4,6,8).
   e. Prevent tension or pulling on the tracheostomy tube from the ventilator tubing or trach collar (7).
   f. Clean stoma twice a day and PRN to maintain skin integrity and prevent infection.
      (1) Use cotton-tipped applicators or gauze. Caution: Avoid products that are made of small fibers that could inadvertently enter the airway/stoma when cleaning (7).
      (2) Normal saline or ¼ strength of 3% hydrogen peroxide to moisten the cotton-tipped applicators (4,7,8).
      (3) Start at the stoma and wipe away or outward to ensure no dried secretions or particles enter the airway/stoma (7).
      (4) Clean the infant's neck with soap and water, rinse, and pat dry (4,7,8).
         (a) Contact surgical team if dressing needs to be changed or if the tracheostomy ties are too tight or too loose (4).

7. Nutrition management—Good nutrition promotes good wound and pulmonary healing as well as overall growth of the infant.
   a. Consider parenteral nutrition if patient is unable to be fed enterally.
   b. Consider trophic feeds and parenteral nutrition if patient must be NPO.
   c. Proceed with individualized nutrition plan, based on patient's tolerance of progression of enteral feeds.
   d. If patient is able to feed orally, collaborate with speech therapy team to begin assessment of swallow and introduction of oral feedings (4).
      (1) Rationale: Oral motor problems are common in neonatal patients who require tracheotomy placement. Oral aversion is a frequent problem due to noxious stimulation such as prolonged endotracheal intubation and suctioning.
      (2) Interventions: Different nipples to control flow of milk, frequent burping, smaller bolus feedings, thickening of milk, warming milk (7,9). One-way valves during feeding can be helpful once it is proven safe by a speech therapist or member of the surgical team. Adequate airflow superiorly to the trach site must be sufficient otherwise there is a risk of pneumothorax (7).

F. Intermediate Postop Care (From First Trach Change Until Transitioned to Home Care)

1. Continue intensive bedside nursing and respiratory therapy care.
2. Airway management
   a. Tracheostomy change
      (1) First tracheostomy change should be performed by the surgical team.
      (2) Subsequent tracheostomy changes occur according to patient's needs and physician preferences.
      (3) Tracheostomy ties secure the tube in place and should be tight enough to allow only one finger between the tie and infant's neck. The infant should be in flexion when checking the fit.
      (4) Trach ties should be changed every time a tracheostomy tube is replaced. There are a variety of devices used to secure the trach in place including the cotton/polyester twill tape that comes in the package with a new tracheostomy tube. Velcro ties are convenient, easy to secure, and come in a variety of sizes for infants and children (7).
      (5) Equipment including proper lighting, proper positioning with a shoulder roll, emergency equipment (replacement and one size smaller tracheostomy tube), suction, ambu-bag with adapter, and appropriate-sized mask. Flexible tracheoscopy, if desired (7,8).
      (6) Two-person technique: One removes the old tube and one inserts the clean tube using a downward curving motion (8).
      (7) The new clean tracheostomy tube should have an obturator in place before insertion. An obturator is a rigid curved piece that fits inside the tracheostomy tube and helps to maintain the appropriate curve of the trach tube for insertion. The obturator also has a rounded end to decrease the risk of tissue damage and irritation during insertion **(Fig. 40.7)**. The obturator must be removed carefully and immediately after the trach tube is inserted into the infant.
   b. Humidification—see above—Airway Management in Immediate Postoperative Care
      (1) Consider a heat moisture exchanges (HMEs)—also known as "artificial noses." HMEs contain hydrophilic material that allows the infant to retain their own exhaled heat and moisture. The device is simple to use, inexpensive, and allows for more portability of the infant. Caution:

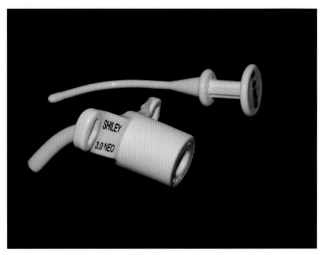

FIGURE 40.7 Tracheostomy tube and obturator.

   Airway obstruction can occur if secretions clog the device (7).
   c. Ventilation—see above—Ventilation in Immediate Postoperative Care.
   d. Suctioning—every 4 hours and as needed—see above—Suctioning in Immediate Postoperative Care.
3. Sedation management
   a. Reassess sedation goal as a multidisciplinary team.
   b. Provide adequate sedation (see Chapter 7)—consider wean and transition to enteral agents as necessary.
4. Skin management
   a. Change tracheostomy ties every 24 hours and PRN when wet or soiled. This should be done in coordination with the tracheostomy tube change when appropriate.
   b. Routinely check under the tracheostomy ties along the full circumference of the infant's neck for signs of skin irritation, rash, and/or breakdown (4).
   c. Clean stoma twice a day and as needed to maintain skin integrity and prevent infection—see above—Skin Management in Immediate Postoperative Care.
5. Nutrition management—see above—Nutrition in Immediate Postoperative Care

G. Transitioning to Home Care

1. Family education
   a. Begins PRIOR to surgery
      (1) Family must understand need for the surgery
      (2) Family must be educated and demonstrate understanding of the anatomy of the airway and tube location, including how their child

will look after the surgery (7). Meeting other families who have experience with tracheostomy tubes is a great resource.

   (3) Family must be educated and demonstrate understanding of signs of breathing difficulties and how to manage routine care.

   (4) Family must be educated and demonstrate understanding of how to assess for emergencies and how to respond (6,7).

  b. CPR training

   (1) Family must be taught the differences due to tracheostomy tube

   (2) Establishing a patent airway—trach tube change, mouth to mouth and nose if upper airway is patent, or mouth to stoma (7).

  c. Community resources

   (1) Support groups

   (2) Internet resources

2. Family participation

  a. Bedside care providers should foster positive interactions and active participation in the care of the patient and education of the family members. Families need to verbalize their fears and anxieties to overcome them (7).

  b. Variety of teaching techniques

   (1) Written material with pictures

   (2) Audiovisuals—videotapes, supplies

   (3) Hands-on with a lifelike manikin or doll and progressing to hands-on with the infant

3. Coordination of care

  a. Supplies for home—including tracheostomy tubes, tracheostomy ties, skin/stoma cleaning supplies, suctioning supplies including portable suction machine (with internal battery) and DeLee suction trap (Cascade Health Care Products, Inc., Portland, Oregon), humidification supplies, ambu-bag (with appropriate-sized masks), and oxygen supplies (if needed).

  b. Emergency box or backpack of supplies (including suction device/machine) should be with the infant at all times, including car trips, doctor appointments, outdoor walks.

  c. Home health nurses—must be trained in respiratory assessment and tracheostomy management (both routine and emergency response); prior pediatric experience should be required (6).

  d. Coordination of complex medical care is essential for the safe transition of the infant into the family environment (7).

H. Complications

The effort to minimize adverse events will always be a challenge in medicine. Tracheostomy in infants is no exception

(10,11). Tables 40.1 and 40.2 group the complications in a temporal fashion but with some overlap.

TABLE 40.1 Early Complications

1. Bleeding—thyroid, venous, arterial
2. Tube displacement—stay sutures are child's lifeline back to the trachea
3. Plugging of tube with secretions (Fig. 40.8)—needs constant attention early on
4. Air leaks
  a. Pneumothorax—may need chest tube
  b. Pneumomediastinum—observe with serial films
  c. Cervical subcutaneous emphysema (usually limited)—avoid occlusive dressings
5. Infection wound—minimize risk by attentive local care
6. Infection pneumonia—minimize risk by managing secretions and atelectasis

TABLE 40.2 Late Complications

1. Obstruction and decannulation
2. Granulation
  a. Stomal
  b. Proximal tracheal
  c. Distal tracheal
3. Stenosis
4. Tracheocutaneous fistula

1. Early complications

  a. Bleeding

   (1) The risk for bleeding is increased by anticoagulant therapy, thrombocytopenia, liver failure, previous neck surgery (e.g., ECMO) and anatomic status (e.g., thyromegaly, venous distension, high riding innominate artery).

   (2) For intraoperative bleeding either ligation or cautery is done but for diffuse oozing topical measures have been used (e.g., Surgicel, spray thrombin).

   (3) Delayed bleeding can be intratracheal from suctioning, acute tracheitis, unrelated pulmonary hemorrhage, or trachea-innominate artery fistula (rare). The first two are moderate issues but the latter two are catastrophes.

   (4) Bleeding from the stoma itself is generally related to granulation tissue formation and is managed with topical care of the wound.

  b. Tube displacement

   (1) Tube displacement is an emergency whenever it occurs.

   (2) It can produce complete airway obstruction, pneumothorax, or progressive neck swelling—

especially if the patient is aggressively hand ventilated without confirming tube position.

(3) Before the first tube change the sutures placed either side of the tracheal opening serve as the child's lifeline by ensuring access to the trachea.

c. Plugging of the tube (**Fig. 40.8**)

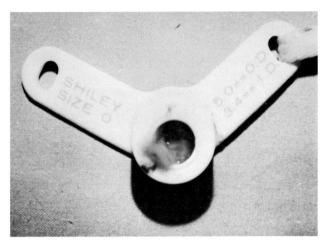

FIGURE 40.8 Total obstruction of tracheostomy tubes. Mucus plug incompletely suctioned.

(1) Needs careful monitoring in the immediate postop period.

(2) Also needs careful monitoring during periods of increased secretions from infection or other inflammation.

2. Late complications

a. Granulation

(1) Granulation is a product of mucosal injury, perichondrial inflammation, and infection.

(2) Intratracheal granulation can be proximal or distal to the tube.

(3) If proximal, that is, between the vocal cords and the tube, ventilation through the tube is unaffected but the patient can be aphonic and does not have an alternate airway.

(4) If distal, then there is direct impact on ventilation and frequently has associated bleeding with suctioning.

(5) Distal granulation requires surgical intervention promptly while proximal cases are more elective.

b. Stenosis

(1) Stenosis is a product of mucosal injury, perichondrial inflammation, and infection.

(2) Stenosis results from ongoing perichondritis and can give either intraluminal cicatrix or collapse from loss of tracheal ring support. Collapse may not be apparent until efforts are made for planned removal of the tube.

(3) Eventual reconstruction may be required.

c. Tracheocutaneous fistula

(1) Is not uncommon after removal of the tracheostomy tube.

(2) Closure is often delayed until time shows that the trachea remains adequate for ventilation. This is both a matter of caliber and secretion clearance.

References

1. Isaiah A, Moyer K, Periera KD. Current trends in neonatal tracheostomy. *JAMA Otolaryngology Head Neck Surg.* 2016;142:738–742.

2. Mahida JB, Asti L, Boss E, Shah RK, et al. Tracheostomy placement in children younger than two years. *JAMA Otolaryngology Head Neck Surg.* 2016;142:241–246.

3. Lee JH, Smith PB, Quek M, et al. Risk factors and in-hospital outcomes following tracheostomy in infants. *J Pediatr.* 2016;173:39–44.

4. Strychowsky J, Albert D, Chan K, et al. International Pediatric Otolaryngology Group (IPOG) consensus recommendations: routine peri-operative pediatric tracheostomy care. *Int J Pediatr Otorhinolaryngol.* 2016;86:250–255.

5. DeMauro S, D'Agostino J, Bann C, et al. Developmental outcomes of very preterm infants with tracheostomies. *J Pediatr.* 2014;164:1303–1310.

6. Boroughs DS, Dougherty JM. Pediatric tracheostomy care: what home care nurses need to know. *Am Nurse Today.* 2015;10(3);8–10.

7. Fiske E. Effective strategies to prepare infants and families for home tracheostomy care. *Adv Neonatal Care.* 2004;4(1);42–53.

8. Perry AG, Potter PA. *Clinical Nursing Skills and Techniques.* 9th ed. St. Louis, MO: Mosby/Elsevier; 2017.

9. Joseph RA, Evitts P, Bayley EW, et al. Oral feeding outcomes in infants with tracheostomy. *J Pediatr Nurs.* 2017;33:70–75.

10. Dong Y, Dunn WF. Accidental decannulation: systems thinking, patient protection, and affordable care. *Respir Care.* 2012;57:2133–2135.

11. White AC, Purcell E, Urquhart MB, et al. Accidental decannulation following placement of a tracheostomy tube. *Resp Care.* 2012;57:2019–2025.

Thoracostomy

Ashish O. Gupta and Daniel R. Dirnberger

Pneumothorax is a serious and potentially life-threatening complication in neonates. Although advances in mechanical ventilation have reduced the incidence of pneumothorax in infants, it remains a significant problem. Management of pneumothorax is an emergency and often necessitates needle thoracentesis and insertion of a chest tube drain. Appropriate training and competence in the procedure increases the provider's skill and comfort, and reduces the incidence of complications (1,2). This chapter reviews current indications for chest tube placement, insertion techniques, and equipment. Guidelines for chest tube maintenance and discontinuation are discussed as well.

Note: In the figures in this chapter, the sterile drapes have been excluded in order to show the procedure steps clearly.

A. Diagnosis of Pneumothorax

1. Clinical diagnosis
   a. Desaturation, signs of respiratory distress, decreased or absent air entry on the affected side, increased oxygen requirement. A large or tension pneumo-

thorax may be associated with hypotension or bradycardia.

2. Transillumination
   a. Darken the room and dim the ambient light. Place a flexible fiberoptic light probe with a transilluminating light source on the anterior and lateral chest wall of the affected side.
   b. A pneumothorax appears as a translucent area in the chest cavity. Illumination follows the shape of the thoracic cavity not just the corona of light source. With a large pneumothorax, the entire hemithorax lights up (Fig. 41.1).
   c. Transillumination can be falsely positive in cases of subcutaneous emphysema and severe pulmonary interstitial emphysema, and falsely negative in the event of too much ambient light, thick chest wall, darkly pigmented skin, or weak fiberoptic light (3,4).

3. Imaging
   a. Chest x-ray: Anteroposterior and lateral views can reveal even a small amount of air in the interpleural space. In a tension pneumothorax, chest x-ray shows a mediastinal shift to the opposite side, compressed

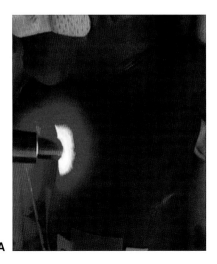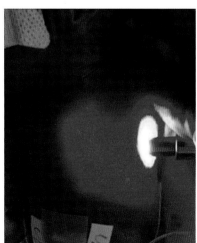

FIGURE 41.1 A: Negative transillumination test showing the illumination only around the corona of the light source. **B:** Positive transillumination test showing the illumination of the entire left hemithorax.

A

B

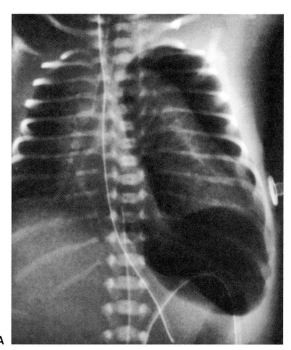 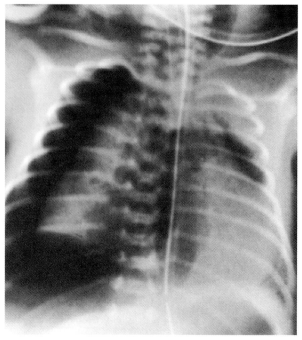

FIGURE 41.2 **A:** Anteroposterior chest radiograph demonstrating a left-sided tension pneumothorax. **B:** Anteroposterior chest radiograph demonstrating a right-sided tension pneumothorax.

opaque lung, and collection of air between the visceral pleura (lung edge), and the chest wall with no pulmonary vascular markings **(Fig. 41.2)**.

  b. Ultrasound: Positive sonographic signs of pneumothorax include the presence of "A-lines," the lung point sign, and the "barcode sign" on M-mode. More specifically, pneumothorax can be identified by the absence of the otherwise normal sonographic features of "lung sliding," "B-lines," or comet tail artifacts, and the "seashore sign" on M-mode (5,6).

NEEDLE EVACUATION OF AIR LEAKS (NEEDLE THORACENTESIS)

Emergency evacuation of air leaks is recommended for life-threatening air accumulations (tension pneumothorax). This provides *temporary* relief to the patient while preparing for thoracostomy tube placement. On occasion, needle evacuation may prove definitive for a nontension pneumothorax, especially in infants not receiving positive pressure ventilation (7). The following techniques using modified equipment are less traumatic than using straight needles or scalp vein sets. We suggest using an anterior approach for emergency evacuation, because this position will not interfere with the preparation of the lateral chest site for an indwelling chest tube. Use emergency pneumothorax evacuation only if the patient is critically compromised. If emergency evacuation is performed with the intent to subsequently place a thoracostomy tube, remove air only until vital signs stabilize, rather than attempting to completely evacuate the pneumothorax.

This will retain an interpleural air pocket for safer insertion of the thoracostomy tube.

A. Equipment (Fig. 41.3)

1. Sterile gloves
2. Antiseptic solution (8)
   0.1% chlorhexidine gluconate or 0.5% chlorhexidine in 70% isopropyl alcohol. Allow 60 seconds to dry. Chlorhexidine is not recommended in preterm neonates <32 weeks due to the risk of chemical burn and absorption through the thin skin. Use 10% povidone iodine solution in preterm infants but remove residual solution from the skin with sterile saline or water after the procedure
3. 20- or 22-gauge angiocatheter (percutaneous catheter over needle device) (9)
4. IV extension tubing (T-connector)
5. Three-way stopcock
6. 10- and 20-mL syringe

B. Technique (▶Video 41.1: Emergency Needle Aspiration)

1. Connect a syringe to a three-way stopcock, attached to IV extension tubing. *Ensure the three-way stopcock is open to the patient* and to the syringe **(Fig. 41.3)**.
2. Prepare skin of affected hemithorax with antiseptic solution.

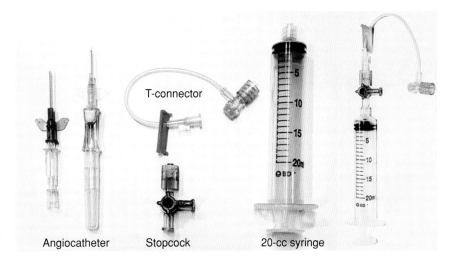

FIGURE 41.3 Equipment for emergency thoracentesis.

Angiocatheter   Stopcock   20-cc syringe

3. Identify landmarks: Second intercostal space in the midclavicular line, or fourth intercostal space in the anterior axillary line. Avoid the breast bud.
4. Create a "Z-track" by lateral traction on the skin over the insertion site. Insert angiocatheter perpendicular to the skin just over the lower rib to avoid trauma to the neurovascular bundle (**Fig. 41.4A**).
5. Advance the angiocatheter slowly. Once it enters the pleural space (noted by lack of resistance, humidity in catheter, or gush of air), slide the catheter in and remove the needle.
6. Attach the IV extension tubing–stopcock apparatus to the catheter and evacuate air with the syringe (**Fig. 41.4B**). Using the syringe rather than leaving the catheter open to air (a) ensures controlled evacuation of the pneumothorax and (b) avoids air entrainment in a spontaneously breathing infant.

    Continue evacuation as the patient's condition warrants, while preparing for definitive tube placement.

7. Allow some air to remain within pleural space as protective buffer between the lung and chest wall (10).
8. Cover the insertion site with petroleum gauze and a small occlusive dressing after the procedure.
9. Remove residual povidone iodine or chlorhexidine with sterile saline after the procedure.

    Angiocatheter can be secured and left in place for a short time while awaiting chest tube placement.

C. Complications

1. Lung penetration
2. Trauma to blood vessel or viscera in the path of the needle
3. Creation of air leak
4. Infection

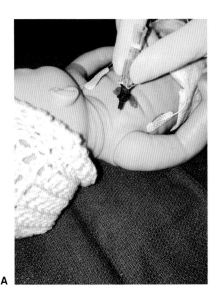
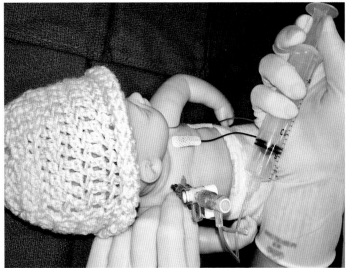

A   **B**

FIGURE 41.4 A: Insertion of angiocatheter perpendicular to the skin in second intercostal space, midclavicular line. **B:** Evacuation of air using stopcock-connecting tube–syringe apparatus.

THORACOSTOMY TUBE PLACEMENT

See ▶ *Video 41.2: Thoracostomy Tubes.*

A. Indications

1. Evacuation of pneumothorax
   a. Tension pneumothorax
   b. Persistent pneumothorax at risk of tension physiology
   c. Bronchopleural fistula
2. Evacuation of large pleural fluid collections
   a. Significant pleural effusion
   b. Postoperative hemothorax
   c. Empyema
   d. Chylothorax
   e. Extravasated fluid from a central venous catheter
3. Extrapleural drainage after tracheal or esophageal surgery (e.g., repair of esophageal atresia, tracheoesophageal fistula)

B. Relative Contraindications

1. Small air or fluid collection without significant hemodynamic symptoms
2. Spontaneous pneumothorax that, in the absence of lung disease, is likely to resolve with noninvasive management (11,12)

C. Equipment

Sterile

1. Gloves
2. Marking pen
3. Antiseptic solution
4. 1% lidocaine, syringe and small gauge needle (25 or 26 gauge)
5. Intravenous narcotic analgesic for pain relief (use caution if infant is not intubated)
6. Surgical drapes
7. Probe cover for tip of transillumination device
8. Evacuation device: Chest tube drainage device
9. Male–male adapter (two-way adapter)
10. Semipermeable transparent dressing
11. Petroleum gauze
12. Thoracostomy tube: There are several pleural drainage devices available. We will discuss the most commonly used techniques using the following variety of thoracostomy tubes
    a. **Pigtail catheter with suture lock**
       (1) Product examples:
          (i) NAVARRE Universal drainage catheter with Nitinol (Bard Access System, Salt Lake City, UT, USA): 6–12 Fr

(ii) All-purpose drainage catheter locking pigtail (Argon medical, Athens, TX, USA): 6 and 8.
    (2) Advantages: Simpler technique, does not require experience with Seldinger technique
       (a) Quick procedure, requires less equipment
       (b) More secure, mitigates accidental dislodgment due to suture locked pigtail; may be advantageous for transport
       (c) Requires smaller or no skin incision, minimal scar, and no suturing
    (3) Disadvantages: No immediate feedback to indicate that the tip has entered the air pocket
       (a) Increased risk for lung trauma, compared to Seldinger technique or chest tube with color indicator
 b. **Pigtail catheter with natural coil, nonlocking** (modified Seldinger technique)
    (1) For example, Fuhrman pleural/pneumopericardial drainage set (Cook medical, Bloomington, IN, USA): 6 and 8.5 Fr
    (2) Advantages
       (a) Provides immediate feedback upon entering the air pocket by collection of air in the syringe: Advantageous in the event of smaller air pocket or smaller patient
       (b) Minimal risk of puncturing the lung
       (c) Requires smaller or no skin incision, minimal scar, and no suturing
       (d) Enters the chest least traumatically
       (e) Effective with coil position lateral to aerated lung, less risk of secondary lung trauma
    (3) Disadvantages
       (a) Increased risk of dislodgment compared to locking pigtail
       (b) Requires proficiency with the Seldinger technique
 c. **Chest tube with safety color change indicator**
    (1) Product examples: Argyle Turkel safety thoracentesis system [Covidien, Mansfield, MA, USA]: 8 Fr
    (2) Advantages: Provides feedback upon entering the air pocket by a color indicator
       (a) Decreased risk of lung puncture upon chest entry
       (b) Quick and simple procedure, does not require proficiency with Seldinger technique
    (3) Disadvantages
       (a) Increased risk of dislodgment compared to pigtail catheters
       (b) Straight tube requires anterior or posterior placement to avoid secondary lung trauma
 d. **Straight chest tube**
    (1) For example, Argyle trocar catheter (Covidien, Mansfield, MA, USA): 8–12 Fr or Thal-Quick chest tube set (Cook medical, Bloomington, IN, USA)

(2) Advantages: Larger chest tube could be advantageous in the event of pleural effusion or hemothorax

(3) Disadvantages: Increased risk of complications including lung puncture and false tracking during placement

(a) Most traumatic technique compared to pigtail catheters or Turkel

(b) Greater risk of injury to lung, ribs, and other tissues

(c) Increased risk of dislodgement

(d) Requires anterior or posterior placement to avoid secondary lung trauma

(e) Requires skin incision, suture closure, resulting in larger scar

Nonsterile

1. 0.5-in adhesive surgical tape
2. Transillumination device
3. Towel roll

TECHNIQUE INSERTION OF ANTERIOR TUBE FOR PNEUMOTHORAX

A. Common Steps

1. Determine the location of the air collection
   a. Auscultation: Decreased air entry on the affected side, a shift of point of maximum impulse toward the other side
   b. Transillumination (**Fig. 41.1**)

c. Chest radiograph (**Fig. 41.2**)
d. Ultrasound
2. Provide ventilator support as needed
3. Monitor cardiorespiratory status and vital signs. Move any electrode from the operative site to alternative sites
4. Position the infant with the affected side elevated 45 to 60 degrees with a towel roll. Secure the arm above the head, with shoulder internally rotated and abducted (**Fig. 41.5A**)
5. Locate essential landmarks (**Fig. 41.5B**)
   a. Nipple and fourth or fifth intercostal space
   b. Anterior and midaxillary lines
   c. The skin insertion site is slightly anterior to the midaxillary line, in the fourth or fifth intercostal space. A horizontal line from the nipple is a good landmark for identifying the fourth intercostal space
6. Prepare the skin with an antiseptic solution over the entire lateral portion of the chest to the midclavicular line, and allow skin to dry
7. Mark the chest tube insertion site with a sterile marking pen
8. Drape surgical area from third to eighth ribs, and from latissimus dorsi muscle to midclavicular line. Using a transparent drape allows for visualization of landmarks
9. Infiltrate the skin at the insertion site with approximately 0.5 to 1 mL of 1% lidocaine

   Note: Maximum recommended lidocaine dose for local anesthetic is 3 mg/kg (0.3 mL/kg of 1% lidocaine solution). Consider a dose of intravenous fentanyl at 1 µg/kg to provide additional pain relief. Use with caution if patient is not on a ventilator.

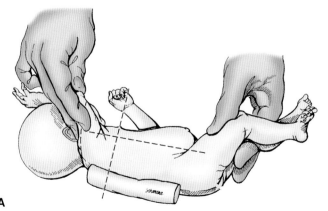

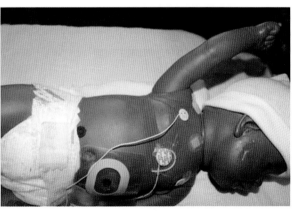

A   B

FIGURE 41.5 **A:** Position the baby with affected side elevated 45 to 60 degrees with a towel roll. Secure the arm above the head, with shoulder internally rotated and abducted. Note the midaxillary line and the line through the nipple through the fourth intercostal space. **B:** Landmarks for chest tube placement: Anterior and midaxillary line, nipple, and fourth intercostal space.

TECHNIQUE 1: PIGTAIL, PERCUTANEOUS DRAINAGE SYSTEM WITH SUTURE LOCK (BARD)

A. Equipment (Fig. 41.6)

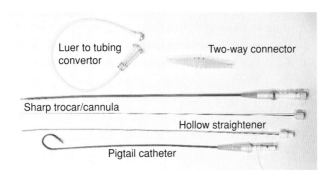

Luer to tubing convertor

Two-way connector

Sharp trocar/cannula

Hollow straightener

Pigtail catheter

FIGURE 41.6 Pigtail catheter with suture lock.

1. Pigtail drainage catheter with suture lock: Size 6 or 8 Fr (<28 weeks), 8 Fr (>28 weeks)
2. Metal straightener (hollow)
3. Trocar cannula/stylet
4. Two-way adapter
5. Connecting tube

B. Procedure

1. Follow **Common Steps 1–9**.
2. Uncoil the catheter pigtail once by hand to loosen the locking suture. Insert the metal straightener through the catheter to straighten the pigtail; lock at the hub.
3. Insert the trocar/stylet through the hollow straightener; lock at the hub. The tip of the stylet will protrude slightly out of the catheter (**Fig. 41.6**).
4. Insert the pigtail with stylet into fourth intercostal space between anterior and midaxillary lines, above the upper margin of the fifth rib (**Fig. 41.7A**).
5. Advance the pigtail with stylet until you feel the lack of resistance or "give." Typically, a small amount of fluid or bubbling will also be visible through the side holes of the catheter.
6. Unlock the metal straightener and stylet together from the catheter (**Fig. 41.7B**).
7. Maintaining stability of the distal stylet and straightener, advance the catheter into the pleural space (anteriorly and cranially toward the second intercostal space and midclavicular line). Advance until all the side holes of the catheter AND the locking suture exit hole are inside the chest wall. A small loop of locking suture may remain outside the chest temporarily, until the pigtail is locked (**Fig. 41.7C**).
8. Pull the distal end of the locking suture to tighten the pigtail inside the chest. Wrap the suture at the hub of the

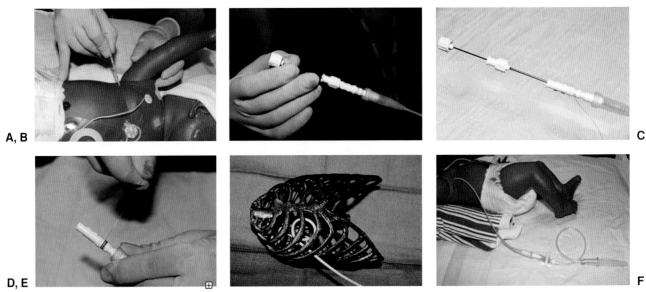

A, B

C

D, E

F

FIGURE 41.7 Percutaneous pigtail catheter placement with a suture lock. **A:** Insert the catheter with stylet in the fourth intercostal space and advance until you feel lack of resistance **B:** Unlock the metal straightener and stylet. **C:** Remove the metal straightener and stylet together from the catheter while advancing the catheter into the pleural space. Advance until all the side holes and the suture exit hole are inside the chest cavity. **D:** Pull the suture tight and wrap it around the distal end of the catheter; slide the plastic cover over it. **E:** After locking the suture, the catheter will coil in a pigtail inside the pleural cavity. **F:** Attach the catheter to the suction drainage device via connecting tube and two-way adapter.

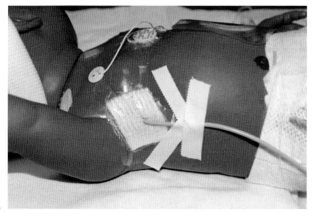
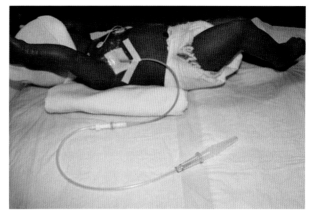

FIGURE 41.8 Dressing the chest tube. **A:** Apply a pre-cut 2- × 2-in sterile gauze at the chest tube site, cover it with semitransparent dressing. **B:** Secure the tube with a surgical tape to prevent tube dislodgement.

tube and fasten it by either sliding the plastic cover over it (Bard) or locking it at the hub (Argon) **(Fig. 41.7D)**.

9. Attach the connecting tube (luer-to-tubing adapter) to the external end of the catheter and connect it to the suction apparatus with two-way adapter **(Fig. 41.7F)**.
10. Secure the chest tube with a semipermeable transparent dressing and surgical tape **(Fig. 41.8)**.
11. Suturing the catheter in place is optional but typically not necessary, as there is no skin incision to close, the skin and tissue tract will be snug against the catheter, and the locking mechanism ensures that the catheter will not inadvertently back out.

TECHNIQUE 2: PIGTAIL, PERCUTANEOUS DRAINAGE SYSTEM WITHOUT LOCKING DEVICE (COOK): MODIFIED SELDINGER TECHNIQUE

A. Equipment (Fig. 41.9)

1. Pigtail catheter (natural coil): Size 6 or 8 Fr (<28 weeks), 8 Fr (>28 weeks)
2. Introducer and J-shaped guidewire (inserted in a sleeve)
3. Needle (20 gauge) with syringe
4. Dilator
5. Adaptor for external end of the catheter to connect to suction apparatus

B. Procedure

1. Follow **Common Steps 1–9**.
2. Mount the finder needle to the syringe. Insert the tip of the needle into the skin in fourth intercostal space between anterior and midaxillary lines above the upper border of the fifth rib **(Fig. 41.10A)**.

3. Advance the finder needle slowly, simultaneously applying negative pressure to the syringe. The needle should be advanced perpendicular to the chest wall, generally in the direction of the opposite shoulder.
4. Advance the needle until you feel the lack of resistance or "give," and air enters the syringe. Do not evacuate more than 1 to 2 mL of air.
5. While stabilizing the needle with one hand, remove the syringe and insert the guidewire through the finder needle. Advance the guidewire until the depth marking at 10 cm reaches the hub of the needle **(Fig. 41.10B)**.
6. Maintaining stability of the wire, remove the finder needle.
7. Feed the dilator over the wire and insert in a slow twisting motion to dilate the tract. Advance the dilator only far enough to dilate the skin tract and parietal pleura. This is normally about 1 cm in the preterm and 2 cm in the term infant **(Fig. 41.10C)**.

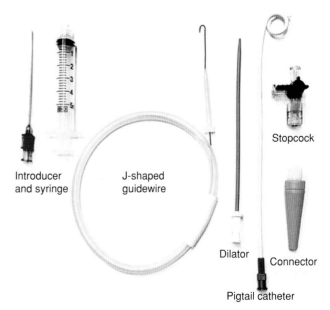

FIGURE 41.9 Pigtail catheter for pleural drainage (Fuhrman pleural drainage set). (Illustration provided by Cook Critical Care, Bloomington, IN.)

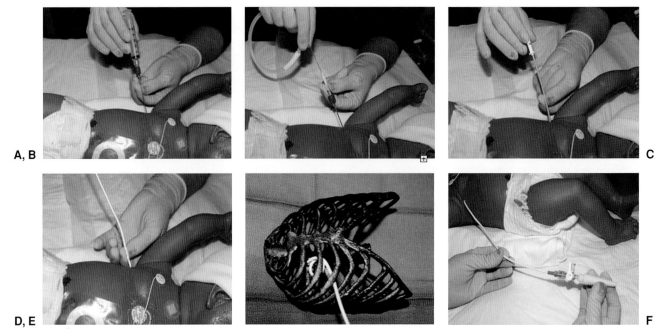

A, B

C

D, E

F

FIGURE 41.10 Percutaneous pigtail catheter placement without locking device (modified Seldinger technique). **A:** Insert the tip of the finder needle on syringe in the fourth intercostal space directing toward the opposite shoulder. Advance the needle until you feel lack of resistance and see air return in the syringe. **B:** Remove the syringe and feed the guidewire through introducer. Advance the guidewire until 10 cm mark at the needle hub. **C:** Remove the introducer and finder needle while holding the guidewire steady, and insert dilator over the guidewire. Dilate the insertion site with a slow twisting motion. **D:** Remove the dilator and insert the chest tube catheter over the guidewire until all the side holes are in the chest. **E:** Maintain the stability of the catheter and remove the guidewire. Catheter will coil into a pigtail loop inside the pleural space. **F:** Attach the catheter to the suction drainage device via luer adapter.

8. Maintaining stability of the wire, remove the dilator.
9. Insert the pigtail catheter over the wire and advance it into the chest wall toward the apex of the lung (anteriorly and cranially toward the second intercostal space and midclavicular line) until all the side holes of the catheter are inside the chest wall. This requires uncoiling and holding the pigtail straight with one hand while advancing it onto the wire **(Fig. 41.10D)**.
10. Maintaining stability of the catheter, remove the guidewire. The catheter will spontaneously coil into a pigtail loop inside the pleural space **(Fig. 41.10E)**.
11. Attach the luer adaptor at the external end of the catheter and connect it to the suction apparatus tubing **(Fig. 41.10F)**.
12. Secure the chest tube with a semipermeable transparent dressing and surgical tape **(Fig. 41.8)**.
13. Suturing the catheter in place is optional but typically not necessary, as there is no skin incision to close and the skin and tract will be snug against the catheter. Additionally, it is easy to inadvertently compress the catheter with suture if secured too tightly.

TECHNIQUE 3: CHEST TUBE WITH SAFETY COLOR INDICATOR (TURKEL)

The Turkel chest tube is a polyurethane catheter with a blunt safety cannula housed within a sharp beveled hollow safety needle, with a color-coded safety indicator. As the needle

and blunt cannula penetrate the chest, the blunt cannula is forced into the shaft of the needle. When the tip of the needle encounters low resistance, such as the pneumothorax within the pleural cavity, the spring-loaded cannula extends automatically beyond the bevel, thus protecting underlying tissue (such as the lungs) from inadvertent penetration.

A. Equipment

1. Chest tube assembly: Polyurethane catheter with a blunt safety cannula housed within a sharp beveled hollow needle with a color-coded safety indicator
2. Connecting tube
3. Syringe

B. Procedure

1. Follow **Common Steps 1–9**.
2. Confirm that the safety introducer needle assembly is functioning properly. Confirm the locked out status of the obturator by gently exerting downward pressure on the distal tip of the needle assembly. The color change indicator should display safe (green).
3. Gently load the safety introducer needle assembly into the catheter. Confirm the blunt obturator and needle cannula extend beyond the tip of the catheter. Check

the unlock status of the blunted obturator by gently exerting a downward pressure on the needle assembly. The color change indicator should change from safe (green) to caution (red).

4. The catheter assembly floats freely on the needle assembly. Hold the catheter firmly near the insertion site to avoid inadvertent catheter movement or uncoupling.

5. Insert the chest tube assembly into the fourth intercostal space between the anterior and midaxillary lines, while holding the catheter firmly near the insertion site.

6. When the blunt obturator comes in contact with an anatomical structure (e.g., skin and subcutaneous tissue), the spring-loaded obturator will recede into the needle, exposing the sharp needle tip; this is indicated by change of the color indicator from green to red. When the distal end of the device clears the tissue resistance and enters the pleural space, the spring-loaded blunt obturator will automatically advance forward to prevent lung penetration. This is indicated by change of the color indicator from red to green.

7. Confirm proper placement by aspirating no more than 1 to 2 mL of air with a syringe.

8. Once confirmed, without further advancing the needle, slide the catheter off the needle assembly to the desired depth inside the pleural space.

9. Maintaining stability of the catheter, remove the cannula and needle assembly.

10. Attach the connecting tube to the external end of the catheter and connect it to the suction apparatus.

11. Secure the chest tube with a semipermeable transparent dressing and surgical tape.

12. Suturing the catheter in place is optional but typically not necessary, as there is no skin incision to close and the skin and tract will be snug against the catheter.

TECHNIQUE 4: POLYVINYL CHLORIDE (PVC) STRAIGHT CHEST TUBE WITH OR WITHOUT TROCAR

A. Equipment

1. Straight chest tube with trocar
2. Scalpel (no. 15 or no. 11 blade is recommended)
3. Curved hemostat
4. Nonabsorbable suture on small cutting needle, 4.0 silk
5. Two-way connector
6. Petroleum gauze

B. Procedure

1. Follow **Common Steps 1–9**.
2. Remove the trocar from the tube.
   Note: Using a trocar during tube insertion is not recommended due to the risk of lung perforation. Blunt dissection to the pleura is preferred, with puncture of the pleura by the tip of the closed forceps.
3. With the scalpel, make a 0.5- to 1-cm skin incision overlying the rib **(Fig. 41.11B)**. With the curved hemostat, bluntly dissect cephalad to the fourth intercostal space.

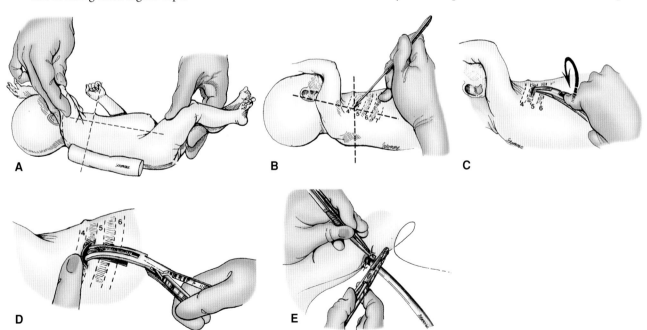

FIGURE 41.11 Straight chest tube procedure. **A:** Position the infant with affected side elevated. **B:** Incision in the fourth intercostal space between anterior and midaxillary lines. **C:** Turning the hemostat to puncture the pleura in the fourth intercostal space. **D:** Open the hemostat to allow the chest tube to pass through to the pleural space. **E:** Close the end of the skin incision with a suture to make an airtight seal with the chest tube. Use the free ends of the suture to secure the tube, taking care not to compress and impinge the tube.

4. Puncture the pleura immediately above the fifth rib by applying pressure on the tip of the closed forceps with the index finger (**Fig. 41.11C**).
   a. Place the forefinger as shown in **Figure 41.11C** and not further forward than the curvature of the hemostat, to prevent the tip from plunging too deep into the pleural space.
   b. A definite "give" will be felt as the forceps tip penetrates the pleura; there may also be an audible rush of air and visible fluid leakage.
   c. After puncturing the pleura, open the hemostat just wide enough to admit the chest tube.
5. Leaving the hemostat in place, thread the tube between the open tips to the predetermined depth (approximately 2 to 3 cm in preterm infants and 3 to 4 cm in term infants) (**Fig. 41.11D**).
   a. Direct the chest tube cephalad and anterior, toward the apex of the thorax (midclavicle), and advance the tip to the midclavicular line, ensuring that all side holes are within the pleural space.
   b. Observe for humidity or bubbling in the chest tube, to verify interpleural location.
6. Connect the tube to vacuum drainage system and observe fluctuations of the meniscus and pattern of bubbling. Avoid tension on the tube while connecting to the drainage device.
7. Secure the chest tube to the skin with suture (**Fig. 41.11E**).
   a. Use one suture to close the end of the skin incision and make an airtight seal with the chest tube. Use the free ends of the suture to secure the tube, taking care not to compress and impinge the tube.
   b. Do not use a purse string suture, which may result in a puckered scar.
8. Apply petroleum gauze around the skin incision. Cover with a small semipermeable transparent dressing.

ADDITIONAL TECHNIQUES AND STEPS

A. Insertion of Posterior Tube for Fluid Accumulation

The technique is similar to that for an anteriorly positioned tube, with the following differences.

1. Position the infant supine, elevating the affected side by 15 to 30 degrees from the table. Secure the arm over the head.
2. Prepare the skin over lateral portion of the hemithorax from anterior to posterior axillary lines.
3. Penetrate the pleura posteriorly while following the other steps as described for an anterior chest tube. Insert the chest tube within the following landmarks (**Fig. 41.12**).
   a. Fourth or fifth space for high posterior tube tip.
   b. Sixth space for low posterior tube tip.
4. Advance the tube posteriorly, only deep enough to place all side holes within the pleural space.

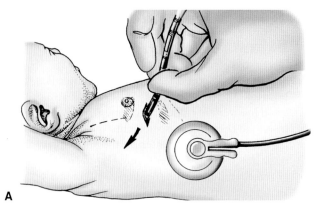

A

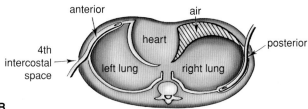

B

FIGURE 41.12 Posterior chest tube. **A:** Insertion of posterior chest tube. Incision is in or just below the anterior axillary line, with the tube entry into the pleura more posteriorly. **B:** Anterior versus posterior position of chest tube for drainage of air and fluid, respectively.

5. Collect drainage material for culture, chemical analysis, and therapeutic evacuation.
6. Connect to an underwater seal drainage system that includes a specimen trap.
7. Strip the tube regularly as needed while holding the chest tube firmly at the skin insertion site.

B. Post Thoracostomy Tube Placement Steps

1. Secure the chest tube with semipermeable transparent dressing and surgical tape (**Fig. 41.8**).
2. Verify the correct position of the chest tube.
   a. Anteroposterior and lateral radiographs (**Fig. 41.13**): Both views are recommended to confirm the anterior course of the tube. See **Tables 41.1** and **41.2** for

TABLE 41.1 Clues to Recognize Thoracostomy Tube Perforation of the Lung (14)

1. Bleeding from endotracheal tube
2. Continuous bubbling in underwater seal
3. Hemothorax
4. Blood return from chest tube
5. Increased density around tip of tube on radiograph
6. Persistent pneumothorax despite satisfactory position on frontal view
7. Tube lying neither anterior nor posterior to lung on lateral view
8. Tube positioned in fissure

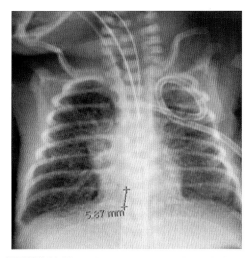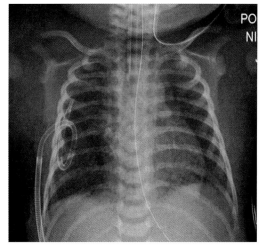

FIGURE 41.13 Anteroposterior chest radiograph demonstrating a correctly placed pigtail chest tube in pleural space.

TABLE 41.2   Clues to Thoracostomy Tube Positioned in Fissure (15)

1. Major interlobar fissure
   (a) Frontal view: Upper medial hemithorax
   (b) Lateral view: Oblique course posterior and upward
2. Minor fissure (on right)
   (a) Horizontal course toward medial side of lung

radiographic clues to malposition. A malpositioned tube tip results in an increased risk of complications and/or poor air evacuation. A chest radiograph should confirm that the side holes are within the chest cavity.
  b. Pattern of bubbling.
  c. Sonogram.
3. "Strip" the tube if the meniscus stops fluctuating or as air evacuation decreases. Take extreme care not to dislodge the tube by holding the tube firmly with one hand close to the chest wall.
4. Modify positive pressure ventilator settings by decreasing peak and mean airway pressure and I-time to mitigate the risk of further air leak (13).

EVACUATION (16)

A. Preparations

1. Prepare the chest drainage system at the beginning of thoracostomy procedure. Drainage device contains three chambers (Fig. 41.14).
   a. Suction control chamber: Fill this chamber with water to the desired negative pressure or amount of suction, which is controlled by the level of water in the chamber. 10 to 15 cm H_2O is appropriate for most ventilated infants. Excessive suction pressure

may draw tissue into the side holes of the chest tube and could be potentially harmful by changing intrapulmonary airflow in the presence of a smaller pleural leak.
   b. Water seal chamber: Fill with water using a funnel device to the "2-cm" mark. The presence of ongoing air leak is monitored in this chamber, which also prevents air from moving back to the patient.
   c. Collection chamber: Pleural fluid is collected in this chamber.
2. After filling the suction control chamber and the water seal chamber to the desired level, connect the patient connector to the chest tube catheter. Connect the suction source to the suction connector on the drainage device.
3. Note: In the transport environment, if a suction device is not available, the chest tube should be attached to a one-way valve (e.g., Heimlich valve) to prevent air entrainment.

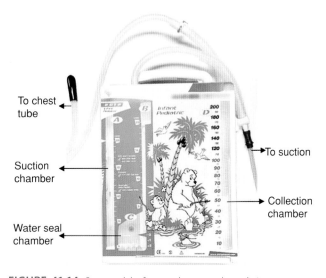

FIGURE 41.14 One model of an underwater chest drainage system, demonstrating the three necessary chambers.

B. Factors Influencing Efficiency of Air Evacuation

1. Contiguity of air to chest tube portals; they must be patent
   a. In the supine infant, air accumulates in the medial, anterior, or inferior hemithorax, making a low anterior location for the chest tube tip ideal for evacuation
   b. If the head of the bed is elevated, air accumulates in the anterior, superior hemithorax, making a high anterior location ideal for evacuation
2. Rate of air accumulation is proportional to
   a. Airway flow and pressure
   b. Size of fistula or tear
   c. Infant position: The dependent placement of the affected lung allows reduction of both the alveolar size and alveolar-to-pleural pressure difference in the region surrounding the leak, thereby reducing and possibly stopping pneumothorax accumulation (17)

C. Removal of Thoracostomy Tube

1. Ascertain that the tube is no longer needed
   a. Leave the chest tube connected to water seal without suction for 8 to 12 hours. Do not clamp the tube
      (1) Transilluminate to detect reaccumulation of air
      (2) Obtain radiograph or sonogram for confirmation
   b. Document absence of significant drainage of air or fluid
2. Assemble equipment
   a. Antiseptic solution
   b. Sterile gloves
   c. Scissors and forceps (if sutures applied)
   d. Petroleum gauze cut and compressed to 2-cm diameter
   e. Gauze pads, 2 × 2 in
   f. 1-in tape
3. Cleanse the skin surrounding the chest tube with antiseptic solution
4. Release tape and/or suture while holding the tube in place
5. To prevent air from entering the chest, as the tube is withdrawn and until petroleum gauze is applied, palpate the pleural entry site and hold pressure over it. After removing the tube, approximate the wound edges (a single Steri-Strip is typically sufficient for pigtail catheters) and place petroleum gauze over the site of insertion. Keep pressure on the pleural wound until the dressing is in place
6. Cover petroleum gauze with dry, sterile gauze. Limit taping to as small an area as possible so that future transillumination will be possible
7. Remove sutures, if applied, when healing is complete

D. Complications

1. Misdiagnosis with inappropriate placement (18)
2. Burn from transillumination device (19)
3. Trauma
   a. Lung laceration or perforation (**Fig. 41.15**) (20,21)
   b. Perforation of and hemorrhage from a major vessel (axillary, pulmonary, intercostal, internal mammary)
   c. Puncture of viscus within path of thoracostomy tube (22)
   d. Residual scarring

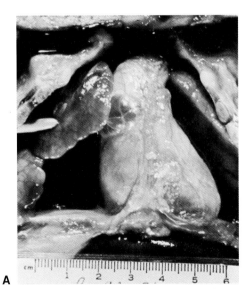 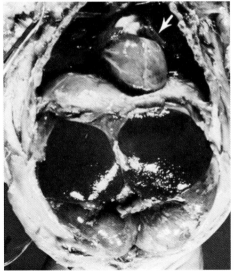

FIGURE 41.15 Postmortem examination of infants who died with uncontrolled air leaks. **A:** Perforation of the right superior lobe by a chest tube inserted without a trocar, demonstrating that virtually any tube can penetrate into the lung. **B:** Perforation of the left upper lobe by a chest tube (*arrow*).

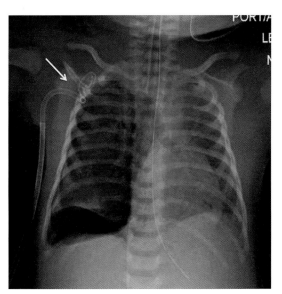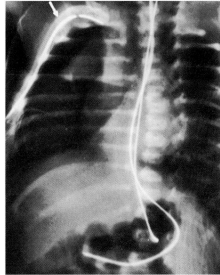

FIGURE 41.16 The thoracostomy tube is completely outside the pleural space on this slightly oblique chest film.

e. Permanent damage to breast tissue
f. Chylothorax (23)
4. Nerve damage
   a. Horner syndrome caused by pressure from the tip of a right-sided, posterior chest tube near the second thoracic ganglion at the first thoracic intervertebral space (24)
   b. Diaphragmatic paralysis or eventration from phrenic nerve injury (25)
5. Misplacement of tube
   a. Tube outside the pleural cavity in the subcutaneous tissue (**Fig. 41.16**)
   b. Side hole outside the pleural space
   c. Tip across the anterior mediastinum
6. Equipment malfunction
   a. Blockage of the tube by proteinaceous or hemorrhagic material or thrombus
   b. Leak in the evacuation system, usually at connection sites
   c. Inappropriate suction pressures (26)
      (1) Excessive pressure
         (a) Aggravation of air leak across a bronchopleural fistula
         (b) Interference with gas exchange
         (c) Suction of lung parenchyma against the holes of the chest tube
      (2) Inadequate pressure with reaccumulation of pneumothorax
7. Infection
   a. Cellulitis
   b. Inoculation of the pleura and pleural space with skin organisms, including *Candida* (27)
8. Subcutaneous emphysema secondary to leakage of tension pneumothorax through the pleural opening
9. Aortic obstruction with a posterior tube (28)

References

1. Ball CG, Lord J, Laupland KB, et al. Chest tube, complications: how well are we training our residents? *Can J Surg.* 2007;50(6):450–458.
2. Gupta AO, Ramasethu J. An innovative simulation trainer for chest tube insertion in infants. *Pediatrics.* 2014;134(3):e798–e805.
3. Kuhns LR, Bednarek FJ, Wyman ML, et al. Diagnosis of pneumothorax or pneumomediastinum in the neonate by transillumination. *Pediatrics.* 1975;56:355–360.
4. Wyman ML, Kuhns LR. Accuracy of transillumination in the recognition of pneumothorax and pneumomediastinum in the neonate. *Clin Pediatr (Phila).* 1977;16:323–324.
5. Cattarossi L, Copetti R, Brusa G, et al. Lung ultrasound diagnostic accuracy in neonatal pneumothorax. *Can Respir J.* 2016;2016:6515069.
6. Raimondi F, Rodriguez Fanjul J, Aversa S, et al. Lung ultrasound for diagnosing pneumothorax in the critically ill neonate. *J Pediatr.* 2016;175:74–78.
7. Smith J, Schumacher RE, Donn SM, et al. Clinical course of symptomatic spontaneous pneumothorax in term and late preterm newborns: report from a large cohort. *Am J Perinatol.* 2011;28(2):163–168.
8. Sathiyamurthy S, Banerjee J, Godambe SV. Antiseptic use in the neonatal intensive care unit—a dilemma in clinical practice: an evidence based review. *World J Clin Pediatr.* 2016;5(2):159–171.
9. Arda IS, Gurakan B, Aliefendioglu D, et al. Treatment of pneumothorax in newborns: use of venous catheter versus chest tube. *Pediatr Int.* 2002;44:78–82.
10. MacDonald MG. Thoracostomy in the neonate: a blunt discussion. *NeoReviews.* 2004;5:e301–e306.
11. Smith J, Schumacher RE, Donn SM, et al. Clinical course of symptomatic spontaneous pneumothorax in term and late preterm newborns: report from a large cohort. *Am J Perinatol.* 2011;28(2):163–168.

12. Kitsommart R, Martins B, Bottino MN, et al. Expectant management of pneumothorax in preterm infants receiving assisted ventilation: report of 4 cases and review of the literature. *Respir Care.* 2012;57(5):789–793.

13. Stevens TP, Harrington EW, Blennow M, et al. Early surfactant administration with brief ventilation vs. selective surfactant and continued mechanical ventilation for preterm infants with or at risk for respiratory distress syndrome. *Cochrane Database Syst Rev.* 2007;4:CD003063.

14. Bowen A, Zarabi M. Radiographic clues to chest tube perforation of neonatal lung. *Am J Perinatol.* 1985;2:43–45.

15. Mauer JR, Friedman PJ, Wing VW. Thoracostomy tube in an interlobar fissure: radiologic recognition of a potential problem. *Am J Roentgenol.* 1981;139:1155–1161.

16. Zisis C, Tsirgogianni K, Lazaridis G, et al. Chest drainage systems in use. *Ann Transl Med.* 2015;3(3):43.

17. Zidulka A. Position may reduce or stop pneumothorax formation in dogs receiving mechanical ventilation. *Clin Invest Med.* 1987;10:290–294.

18. Kesieme EB, Dongo A, Ezemba N, et al. Tube thoracostomy: complications and its management. *Pulm Med.* 2012;2012:256878.

19. Perman MJ, Kauls LS. Transilluminator burns in the neonatal intensive care unit: a mimicker of more serious disease. *Pediatr Dermatol.* 2007;24:168–171.

20. Reed RC, Waters BL, Siebert JR. Complications of percutaneous thoracostomy in neonates and infants. *J Perinatol.* 2016;36(4):296–299.

21. Brooker RW, Booth GR, DeMello DE, et al. Unsuspected transection of lung by pigtail catheter in a premature infant. *J Perinatol.* 2007;27(3):190–192.

22. Murray MJ, Brain JL, Ahluwalia JS. Neonatal pleural effusion and insertion of intercostal drain into the liver. *J R Soc Med.* 2005;98(7):319–320.

23. Kumar SP, Belik J. Chylothorax—a complication of chest tube placement in a neonate. *Crit Care Med.* 1984;12:411–412.

24. Rosegger H, Fritsch G. Horner's syndrome after treatment of tension pneumothorax with tube thoracostomy in a newborn infant. *Eur J Pediatr.* 1980;133:67–68.

25. Nahum E, Ben-Ari J, Schonfeld T, et al. Acute diaphragmatic paralysis caused by chest-tube trauma to phrenic nerve. *Pediatr Radiol.* 2001;31:444–446.

26. Grosfeld JL, Lemons JL, Ballantine TV, et al. Emergency thoracostomy for acquired bronchopleural fistula in the premature infant with respiratory distress. *J Pediatr Surg.* 1980;15:416–421.

27. Faix RG, Naglie RA, Barr M Jr. Intrapleural inoculation of candida in an infant with congenital cutaneous candidiasis. *Am J Perinatol.* 1986;3:119–122.

28. Gooding CA, Kerlan R Jr, Brasch R. Partial aortic obstruction produced by a thoracostomy tube. *J Pediatr.* 1981;98:471–473.

CHAPTER

42

Pericardiocentesis

Alan Benheim and John North

A. Definitions

1. Pericardium
   a. A double layer of mesothelial lining surrounding the heart, consisting of the visceral pericardium on the epicardial surface and the parietal pericardium as an outer layer
   b. The pericardial space, between the visceral and parietal layers, normally has a small amount of pericardial fluid (typically <5 mL for a neonate) that is thought to reduce friction
2. Pneumopericardium
   a. Collection of air in the pericardial space
3. Pericardial effusion
   a. Accumulation of excess fluid in the pericardial space
4. Pericardiocentesis
   a. A procedure to remove air or excess fluid from the pericardial space, usually through a needle, small cannula, or drainage catheter
5. Pericardial drain
   a. A catheter or other drainage device left in place to allow intermittent or continuous evacuation of air or fluid from the pericardial space
   b. Placed in select situations with recurring accumulation of air or fluid in the pericardial space

6. Tamponade
   a. Clinical condition with limited cardiac output because of external restriction of expansion of the heart, preventing normal cardiac filling, resulting in a decreased stroke volume and impaired cardiac output
   b. May be caused by:
      (1) Fluid or air in the pericardial space
      (2) Abnormalities of the pericardium (restrictive or constrictive)
      (3) Increased intrathoracic pressure associated with obstructive airway lung disease or tension pneumothorax
7. Pulsus paradoxus (**Fig. 42.1**)
   a. Respiratory variation in blood pressure, with a decrease in systolic blood pressure during spontaneous inspiration. (During positive-pressure ventilation, this is reversed, with a rise in systolic pressure during inspiration.)
   b. This finding occurs during tamponade.

B. Background

1. The heart lies within a closed space, covered by the pericardium. The pericardial space is between the two layers of the pericardium. If the pericardial space fills

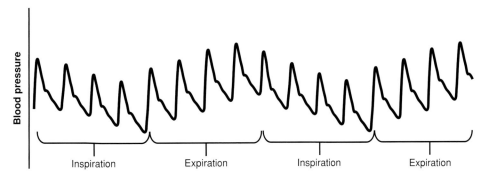

FIGURE 42.1 Pulsus paradoxus.

with excess fluid or if air accumulates, the heart has less space available, and the pressure within the pericardium increases. Increased intrapericardial pressure restricts venous return and impairs cardiac filling. The decrease in venous return and cardiac filling results in a reduced cardiac output. This clinical situation is known as cardiac tamponade (1–6).

2. Neonates are at increased risk for cardiac tamponade when there is:

a. Accumulation of air dissecting into the pericardium from the respiratory system (**Fig. 42.2**) (4,5,7,8). This risk may be higher for preterm infants whose mothers did not receive prenatal steroids (9).

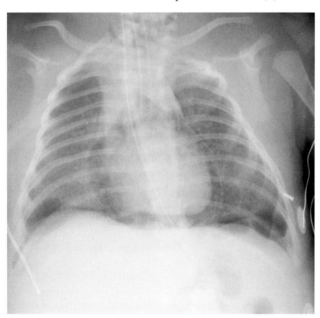

FIGURE 42.2 Chest radiograph with pneumopericardium.

b. Pericardial fluid accumulation due to perforation or transudate from umbilical or central venous catheter (Fig. 34.16, **Fig. 42.3**) (1,10–14)

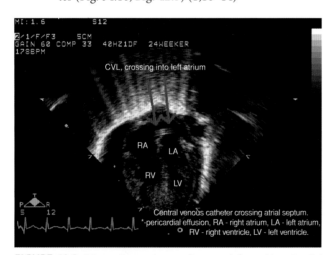

FIGURE 42.3 Echocardiogram image of preterm infant with pericardial effusion and central venous line in left atrium.

c. Hyperosmolar infusate, such as hyperalimentation (6,15)
d. Catheter tip in right atrium, especially if coiled (16,17)
e. Cannulation for extracorporeal membrane oxygenation (6,18,19)
f. Cardiac catheterization, either diagnostic or therapeutic (20)
g. Postoperative pericardial hemorrhage following cardiac surgery (2,21)
h. Postpericardiotomy syndrome, typically 1 to 3 weeks after cardiac surgery (2,21,22)
i. Pericardial effusion as part of generalized edema/hydrops (3,21)
j. Pericardial effusions due to infectious or autoimmune causes (these are less common in neonates than in older children)

3. Clinical symptoms
a. Signs of cardiac tamponade may evolve gradually or rapidly (1,3,23).
b. Symptoms may include respiratory distress, hypotension, tachycardia, and/or loss of perfusing rhythm (6,15).

4. The primary therapy for cardiac tamponade is to evacuate the pericardial space. Volume expansion and pressor agents may be of transient benefit, but they usually do not result in sustained clinical improvement (1,6,10,14,15,21,24).

5. Cardiac tamponade may require urgent treatment with pericardiocentesis in infants with severe hemodynamic compromise (1,15,21,22).

C. Indications (1,14,20–22)

1. Cardiac tamponade due to pneumopericardium
2. Cardiac tamponade due to pericardial fluid
3. Aspiration of pericardial fluid for diagnostic studies

D. Contraindications

1. There are no absolute contraindications to performing pericardiocentesis in the setting of cardiac tamponade.
2. Relative contraindications for diagnostic pericardiocentesis:
a. Coagulopathy.
b. Active infection. (However, infection may also be an indication for diagnostic pericardiocentesis in some clinical situations.)

E. Precautions

Draining a large volume from the pericardial space can alter cardiac preloading conditions significantly, and some infants may require a supplemental intravascular fluid bolus after the pericardium is drained.

F. Limitations

1. Cannot readily evacuate thrombus
2. Cannot remove mass lesions

G. Equipment

Sterile

1. Antiseptic solution
2. Aperture drape or multiple drapes to be arranged around access site
3. Swabs or gauze pads
4. Gloves
5. Local anesthetic (1% lidocaine)
6. 16- to 20-gauge IV cannula over 1- to 2-in needle; consider 22-gauge cannula over a 1-in needle for infants weighing less than 2,500 g; a 24-gauge cannula over a 0.75-in needle is appropriate for extremely low–birth-weight infants (<1,000 g)
7. Indwelling drainage catheter and 0.018-in soft-tipped guidewire (optional)
8. Three-way stopcock
9. Short IV extension tubing (optional)
10. 10- to 20-mL syringes
11. Preassembled closed drainage system as for emergency evacuation of air leaks, thoracostomy tubes described in Chapter 41 (optional)
12. Connecting tubing and underwater seal for indwelling drain (optional)
13. Specimen containers for laboratory studies, if procedure is diagnostic

Nonsterile (see also H)

1. Transillumination device (optional, for pneumopericardium)
2. Echocardiogram/sonography imaging device (optional in urgent situations)

H. Procedure (▶ Video 42.1: Pericardiocentesis)

1. If ultrasound/echocardiographic imaging is available, and if time permits, imaging can be performed to determine an optimal needle entry site and angle. In addition, the approximate distance required to reach the pericardial space can be estimated (20,25). To obtain ultrasound imaging to guide initial needle placement and course at the time of the procedure, the transducer should be placed in a sterile sheath (25). Alternatively, after a sterile field is created, ultrasound imaging can be performed from a nonsterile area of the chest to monitor the effusion during the procedure. Care should be taken to avoid moving the probe back and forth between sterile and nonsterile areas.

2. Similarly, evaluation with transillumination can be performed in cases of pneumopericardium, if time permits.

3. Cleanse skin over xiphoid, precordium, and epigastric area with antiseptic. Allow to dry.

4. Arrange sterile drapes, leaving the subxiphoid area exposed.

5. Administer local anesthesia if the patient is conscious, for example, 0.25 to 1 mL of subcutaneous 1% lidocaine instilled within 1 to 2 cm of the xiphoid process. If the baby is on a ventilator, a dose of intravenous fentanyl (1 mcg/kg) can provide sedative analgesia (see also Chapter 7).

6. Form a closed system by assembling a syringe, three-way stopcock, and extension tubing so that the stopcock is open to both the syringe and the extension tubing, but closed to the remaining side port.

7. Using the IV needle/cannula, enter the skin 0.5 to 1 cm below the tip of the xiphoid process, in the midline or slightly (0.5 cm) to the left of the midline. The needle should be at a 30- to 40-degree angle to the skin, and the tip should be directed toward the left shoulder (**Fig. 42.4A,B**). A different approach may be used in certain cases, for example, if an echocardiogram suggests that most of the fluid is right sided or apical (25).

8. Advance the needle until air or fluid is obtained.
   a. A rhythmic tug, corresponding to the heart rate, may be felt as the needle enters the pericardium.

9. If ultrasound imaging is available, needle position can be determined either by visualizing the tip of the needle within the pericardial space or by demonstrating that the amount of pericardial fluid is diminishing as fluid is aspirated (**Fig. 42.5**). Some authors have described reinfusing a small amount of the aspirated fluid while imaging to observe the location of microcavitation echoes (20,26,27). Fix the needle in position and advance the cannula over the needle into the pericardial space. Remove the needle, and connect the cannula to the closed system syringe for aspiration.

10. Aspirate as much fluid/air as possible. If the syringe fills, use the third port of the stopcock to empty the syringe, or to attach a second syringe, and then aspirate more, repeating as needed. If diagnostic studies are desired, the fluid should be transferred to appropriate specimen containers.
    a. If bloody fluid is aspirated, there could be a serosanguineous or hemorrhagic effusion, or the needle might have entered the heart (usually the right ventricle). There are a few clues that can be helpful

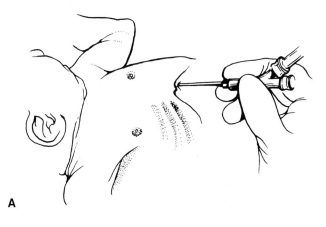

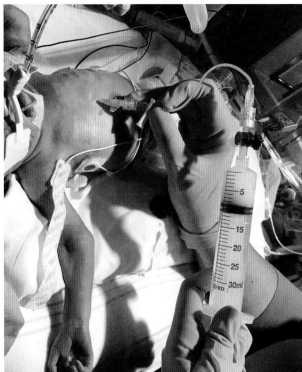

FIGURE 42.4 A: Insertion of needle/cannula attached to three-way stopcock, in the subxiphoid space, directed toward the left shoulder. **B:** Emergency pericardiocentesis in critically ill infant, showing aspiration of parenteral alimentation fluid from pericardial space.

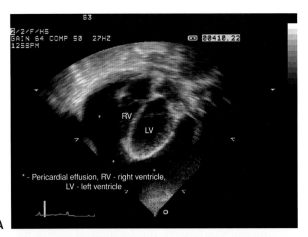

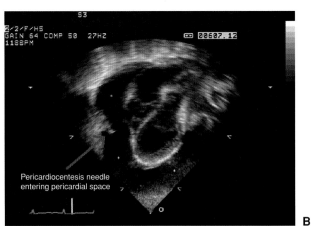

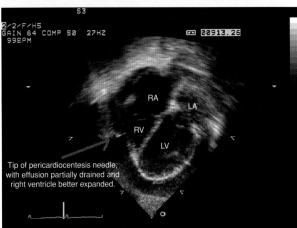

FIGURE 42.5 Echocardiogram images of pericardiocentesis. **A:** Echocardiogram image of pericardial effusion. **B:** Tip of needle in pericardial space. **C:** Pericardial effusion partially drained.

in determining whether the needle has entered the heart (see I).

b. Note that small single-lumen catheters may easily become blocked.

c. A decision will need to be made whether to leave the cannula in place for any length of time or to remove it once the pericardium has been drained. This decision will vary in individual cases, but factors to consider include the likelihood of reaccumulation and the need for repeat drainage versus the risk of infection or entry of free air with an indwelling cannula.

d. In certain cases, the operator may elect to evacuate the pericardial space directly through the needle, rather than placing a cannula.

I. Special Circumstances

1. If ultrasound imaging is available, it may be helpful in planning and guiding the needle entry site and angle, as well as anticipating the distance required to reach the pericardial space (2,20,22,25–27).

2. If transillumination is positive for free air before the procedure, it can be used to assess the adequacy of air evacuation after the procedure and to look for evidence of reaccumulation. Because pneumothorax and pneumomediastinum are potential complications, the availability of transillumination may also be helpful after the procedure. However, transillumination is not a reliable method to rule out free air or to distinguish between pericardial air and mediastinal air (5,7).

3. Initial aspiration of the pericardium may yield air, serous fluid, serosanguineous or grossly bloody fluid, or fluid resembling infusate from a central line (including parenteral nutrition fluids) (10,13). Bloody fluid raises the concern that the needle may have entered the heart. The following may be helpful in distinguishing between pericardial fluid and intracardiac blood.

a. In an infant with tamponade, aspirating 10 mL of blood from the heart will have minimal effect on the acute hemodynamics, whereas draining as little as 5 to 15 mL from the pericardial space can result in significant hemodynamic improvement within 30 seconds.

b. If ultrasound is being used, the pericardial fluid volume will appear to be decreased if the needle is correctly positioned. In some cases, one can reliably identify the needle in the pericardial space (see **Fig. 42.5**) (20).

c. Placing a few drops on a gauze swab may help distinguish the two sources, because serosanguineous fluid will separate into a central dark red zone and a more serous peripheral zone, but this can take several minutes.

d. Alternatively, a spun hematocrit can be performed rapidly if the unit has a readily available centrifuge; this also takes a few minutes.

4. Draining a large volume from the pericardial space can alter cardiac preloading conditions significantly, and some infants may benefit from intravascular fluid boluses after the pericardium is drained.

5. Pericardiocentesis is often an urgent or emergency procedure. The technique for pericardiocentesis described above applies when there is time for each step. In an infant with significant hemodynamic compromise, the operator may be forced to omit certain steps in the interest of time. This requires a judgment as to the baby's clinical status and the time delay involved for any given step, such as waiting for the ultrasound machine, preparing a larger sterile field, or assembling a three-way stopcock system. In extreme cases, this life-saving procedure might consist of pouring or swabbing Betadine over the subxiphoid area, followed by "blind" aspiration using any available needle and syringe, without anesthetic, and before any other equipment is available at the bedside (see **Fig. 42.4B**) (20).

6. To place a larger indwelling catheter that will remain in place, advance a soft-tipped 0.018-in guidewire through the cannula into the pericardial space. Leaving the guidewire in place, withdraw the cannula over the guidewire, and then advance the larger catheter over the guidewire, positioning the larger catheter so that all drainage holes are within the pericardial space. Connect to a closed tubing and drainage system. Secure in place.

J. Complications (20–22,26,27)

1. Pneumopericardium
2. Pneumomediastinum
3. Pneumothorax
4. Cardiac perforation
5. Arrhythmia
6. Hypotension (if a large effusion is drained)

References

1. Nowlen TT, Rosenthal GL, Johnson GL, et al. Pericardial effusion and tamponade in infants with central catheters. *Pediatrics*. 2002;110:137–142.
2. Tsang TS, Barnes ME, Hayes SN, et al. Clinical and echocardiographic characteristics of significant pericardial effusions following surgery and outcomes of echo-guided pericardiocentesis for management: Mayo Clinic experience. 1979–1998. *Chest*. 1999;116:322–331.
3. Tamburro RF, Ring JC, Womback K. Detection of pulsus paradoxus associated with large pericardial effusions in pediatric patients by analysis of the pulse-oximetry waveform. *Pediatrics*. 2002;109:673–677.

4. Heckmann M, Lindner W, Pohlandt F. Tension pneumopericardium in a preterm infant without mechanical ventilation: a rare cause of cardiac arrest. *Acta Paediatr*. 1998;87:346–348.

5. Hook B, Hack M, Morrison S, et al. Pneumopericardium in very low birthweight infants. *J Perinatol*. 1995;15(1):27–31.

6. Warren M, Thompson KS, Popek EJ, et al. Pericardial effusion and cardiac tamponade in neonates: sudden unexpected death associated with total parenteral nutrition via central venous catheterization. *Ann Clin Lab Sci*. 2013;43(2):163–171.

7. Cabatu EE, Brown EG. Thoracic transillumination: aid in the diagnosis and treatment of pneumopericardium. *Pediatrics*. 1979;64:958–960.

8. Bjorklund L, Lindroth M, Malmgren N, et al. Spontaneous pneumopericardium in an otherwise healthy full-term newborn. *Acta Pediatr Scand*. 1990;79:234–236.

9. Hummler HD, Parys E, Mayer B, et al. Risk indicators for air leaks in preterm infants exposed to restrictive use of endotracheal intubation. *Neonatology*. 2015;108:1–7.

10. Ramasethu J. Complications of vascular catheters in the neonatal intensive care unit. *Clin Perinatol*. 2008;35:199–222.

11. van Engelenburg KC, Festen C. Cardiac tamponade: a rare but life-threatening complication of central venous catheters in children. *J Pediatr Surg*. 1998;33:1822–1824.

12. Fioravanti J, Buzzard CJ, Harris JP. Pericardial effusion and tamponade as a result of percutaneous silastic catheter use. *Neonatal Netw*. 1998;17:39–42.

13. van Ditzhuyzen O, Ronayette D. Tamponnade cardiaque après catheterisme veineux central chez un nouveaune. *Arch Pediatr*. 1996;3:463–465.

14. Pezzati M, Filippi L, Chiti G, et al. Central venous catheters and cardiac tamponade in preterm infants. *Intensive Care Med*. 2004;30:2253–2256.

15. Weil BR, Ladd AP, Yoder K. Pericardial effusion and cardiac tamponade associated with central venous catheters in children: an uncommon but serious and treatable condition. *J Pediatr Surg*. 2010;45:1687–1692.

16. Cartwright DW. Central venous lines in neonates: a study of 2186 catheters. *Arch Dis Child Fetal Neonatal Ed*. 2004;89:F504–F508.

17. dos Santos Modelli ME, Cavalcanti FB. Fatal cardiac tamponade associated with central venous catheter a report of 2 cases diagnosed in autopsy. *Am J Forensic Med Pathol*. 2014;35(1):26–28.

18. Kurian MS, Reynolds ER, Humes RA, et al. Cardiac tamponade caused by serous pericardial effusion in patients on extracorporeal membrane oxygenation. *J Pediatr Surg*. 1999;34:1311–1314.

19. Becker JA, Short BL, Martin GR. Cardiovascular complications adversely affect survival during extracorporeal membrane oxygenation. *Crit Care Med*. 1998;26:1582–1586.

20. Tsang TS, Freeman WK, Barnes ME, et al. Rescue echocardiographically guided pericardiocentesis for cardiac perforation complicating catheter-based procedures: the Mayo Clinic experience. *J Am Coll Cardiol*. 1998;32:1345–1350.

21. Tsang TS, Oh JK, Seward JB. Diagnosis and management of cardiac tamponade in the era of echocardiography. *Clin Cardiol*. 1999;22:446–452.

22. Tsang TS, El-Najdawi EK, Seward JB, et al. Percutaneous echocardiographically guided pericardiocentesis in pediatric patients: evaluation of safety and efficacy. *J Am Soc Echocardiogr*. 1998;11:1072–1077.

23. Berg RA. Pulsus paradoxus in the diagnosis and management of pneumopericardium in an infant. *Crit Care Med*. 1990;18:340–341.

24. Traen M, Schepens E, Laroche S, et al. Cardiac tamponade and pericardial effusion due to venous umbilical catheterization. *Acta Paediatr*. 2005;94:626–628.

25. Molkara D, Tejman-Yarden S, El-Said H, et al. Pericardiocentesis of noncircumferential effusions using nonstandard catheter entry sites guided by echocardiography and fluoroscopy. *Congenit Heart Dis*. 2011;6:461–465.

26. Muhler EG, Engelhardt W, von Bernuth G. Pericardial effusions in infants and children: injection of echo contrast medium enhances the safety of echocardiographically-guided pericardiocentesis. *Cardiol Young*. 1998;8:506–508.

27. Watzinger N, Brussee H, Fruhwald FM, et al. Pericardiocentesis guided by contrast echocardiography. *Echocardiography*. 1998;15:635–640.

CHAPTER

43

Gastric and Transpyloric Tubes

Allison M. Greenleaf

A. Definitions (1)

1. Enteral feeding is defined as providing nutrients distal to the oral cavity.
2. A gastric tube is a tube inserted via the nose or mouth to the stomach.
3. A transpyloric tube is a tube passed via the nose or mouth, through the stomach and pylorus to the small intestine.

ORAL OR NASAL GASTRIC TUBES

A. Indications (2)

1. To provide a route for feeding and medication administration in the setting of neurobehavioral immaturity, physiologic instability, or respiratory compromise (3)
2. To sample gastric or intestinal contents
3. To decompress and empty the stomach

B. Types of Tubes

1. Single-lumen gastric and transpyloric tubes are made of Silastic (silicone elastomer), silicone, polyurethane, or polyvinyl chloride (PVC) and are radiopaque for location on radiography (2,4,5). They are incrementally marked in centimeters, and usually have two to four side holes at the distal end (Fig. 43.1).
   a. Available for neonates in sizes 3.5 to 8 Fr and in a variety of lengths. The smaller-diameter tubes will have slower rates of flow. Tube length will vary depending on the depth of placement and whether the tube is to be gastric or transpyloric (2,5).
   b. Single-lumen feeding tubes maybe used for occasional or intermittent decompression of the stomach (2).
2. Double-lumen (Replogle) tubes are preferable for continuous gastric decompression or for continuous suction

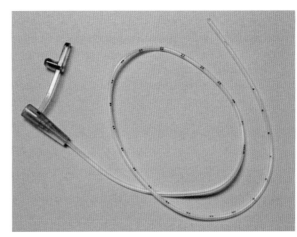

FIGURE 43.1 Silastic gastric feeding tube.

to clear secretions from the upper esophageal pouch in infants with esophageal atresia prior to surgery (6–8).
   a. The wider lumen is attached to the suction device for gastric decompression or esophageal clearing, and the second, smaller lumen is for airflow to prevent adherence of the catheter to the mucosal wall (Fig. 43.2).

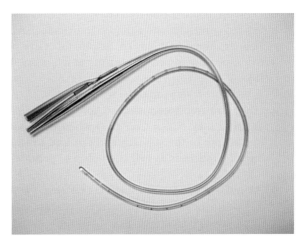

FIGURE 43.2 Double-lumen Replogle tube.

b. These catheters are also radiopaque, marked incrementally, and have multiple side holes at the distal end.

c. Available in 6, 8, and 10 Fr; vary in length. Manufacturer's recommendations should be followed for frequency of tube change.

C. Contraindications

1. Recent esophageal repair or perforation

D. Precautions

1. When determining oral or nasal placement, individual assessment must be done to weigh the risks of compromising the nasal airway as well as determine the potential impact on oral feeding.

2. Consider the size of the nares as well as the type and amount of respiratory support when determining placement.

3. Do not push against any resistance. Perforation may occur with very little force or sensation of resistance.

4. Do not instill any material before verifying tube placement.

   a. Incorrect placement of gastric and transpyloric tubes is common, with incidence ranging from 21% to 59%, and can lead to substantial morbidity and mortality (9–13).

5. Evaluate for possible esophageal perforation if any of the following occur (14):

   a. Bloody aspirate
   b. Increased oral secretion
   c. Respiratory distress
   d. Pneumothorax

6. Stop the procedure immediately if there is any respiratory compromise.

7. Silastic, silicone, and polyurethane tubes are softer and can remain in situ for up to 30 days, or per manufacturer's recommendations, although individual practice guidelines should be followed. Silastic tubes are preferred, especially in preterm infants weighing <750 g (2,15).

8. PVC tubes are stiffer and easier to insert.

   a. They are not recommended for long-term use because they stiffen over time when exposed to the acidity of the stomach and can lead to leaching of plasticizers as well as esophageal perforation (2,4,5,16).

   b. Manufacturer recommendations for frequency of tube change can vary so institutional practice guidelines should be followed.

9. Weighted, stylet-containing tubes are not recommended in the neonatal population due to the risk of perforation.

E. Equipment

1. Suction equipment
2. Cardiorespiratory monitor
3. 0.5-in hypoallergenic tape
4. Sterile water
5. 3- or 5-mL syringes
6. Stethoscope
7. Gloves
8. Infant tube of appropriate size

F. Technique

1. Wash hands and put on gloves, maintaining aseptic technique.

2. Clear infant's nose and oropharynx by gentle suctioning as necessary.

3. Monitor infant's heart rate and oxygen saturation and observe for arrhythmia or respiratory distress throughout procedure.

4. If possible, offer a pacifier and oral sucrose in accordance with unit policy to manage pain and encourage sucking and swallowing (17,18).

5. Position infant on back with head of bed elevated.

6. Measure length for insertion by measuring distance from tip of the nose to earlobe to halfway between the xiphoid and umbilicus (**Fig. 43.3**) (2,5,9,10,12,13,19).

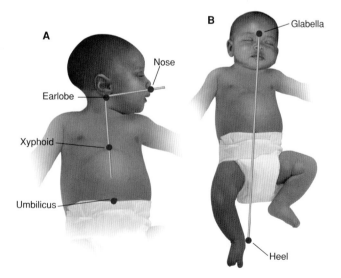

FIGURE 43.3 A: Nasogastric tube distance measurement from tip of the nose to the earlobe to halfway between the xiphoid and umbilicus. **B:** Transpyloric tube distance measurement from glabella to the heel.

7. Mark length on feeding tube with a loop of tape (**Table 43.1**).

TABLE 43.1 Guidelines for Minimum Orogastric Tube Insertion Length to Provide Adequate Intragastric Positioning in Very–Low-Birth-Weight Infants

WEIGHT (G)	INSERTION LENGTH (CM)
<750	13
750–999	15
1,000–1,249	16
1,250–1,500	17

Data from Gallaher KJ, Cashwell S, Hall V, et al. Orogastric tube insertion length in very low birth weight infants. *J Perinatol.* 1993;13:128–131.

8. Moisten end of tube with sterile water or saline.
9. Oral insertion
    a. Depress anterior portion of tongue with forefinger and stabilize head with free fingers.
    b. Insert tube along finger to oropharynx.
10. Nasal insertion (avoid this route in very–low-birth-weight infants in whom nasal tubes may be associated with increased respiratory effort and decreased ventilation) (2,3).
    a. Stabilize head. Elevate tip of nose to widen nostril.
11. Insert tip of tube, directing it toward occiput rather than toward vertex (**Fig. 43.4**).
12. Advance tube gently to oropharynx.
13. Monitor for bradycardia.
14. Tilt head forward slightly.
15. Advance tube to predetermined depth.
16. Do not push against any resistance.
17. Stop procedure if there is onset of any respiratory distress, cough, struggling, apnea, bradycardia, or cyanosis.
18. Determine location of tip using at least two measures: pH, aspirate characteristic (volume and color), external tube marking, or presence of respiratory distress. Radiograph of the abdomen to verify placement is the gold standard but is expensive and subjects neonates to additional radiation. Injecting air to verify placement is not a reliable method, as the sound of air in the respiratory tract can be transmitted to the GI tract (2,4,11–13,19,20). Measuring the pH of the aspirate as the sole method to verify tip position is not reliable, as stomach acid in infants can be weakly acidic, and the degree of acidity of the aspirate can be affected by the timing of feeding, the exact location of the tube tip in the stomach (distal vs. proximal), and timing of medication delivery (2,4,5,20).
    a. Aspirate any contents; describe and measure.
        (1) Gastric contents may be clear, milky, tan, pale green, pale yellow, or blood stained.

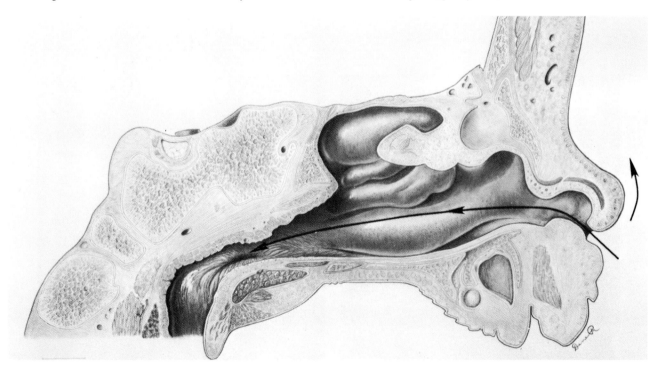

FIGURE 43.4 Anatomic view of the neonatal nasopharynx. The natural direction in tube insertion is toward the nasal turbinates, where it might stop and give an impression of obstruction. By pushing the nostril up, one can direct a tube toward the occiput with less trauma.

(2) Determine acidity by measuring pH. If the pH of the aspirate is ≤5, one can be reasonably certain the tube is in the stomach. If the pH is >5, placement should be confirmed using an additional method, such as radiography or character of secretions (4,12,19–22).

(3) Assess for any respiratory compromise or instability.

b. If there is difficulty obtaining aspirate, use a larger-sized syringe, reposition the infant, and instill a small amount of air into the tube to reposition the nasogastric tube away from the stomach wall. Avoid pushing against any resistance. If no aspirate is obtained, consider verifying placement by radiography (20).

c. Verify tube placement on all subsequent radiographs.

19. Secure indwelling tube to face with 0.5-in tape.

20. For feedings, attach to syringe.

21. For gravity drainage, attach specimen trap and position below level of stomach.

22. For decompression, a double-lumen tube, connected to low continuous suction, is preferred. Due to variations in both practice and units of pressure, specific suction pressure guidelines cannot be given, but pressure should not exceed 80 mm Hg.

23. Pinch or close gastric tube during removal to prevent emptying contents into pharynx.

24. Document patient response, observing any physiologic changes and verifying tube placement. Note the location of the tube at the nares, and document it on the chart. Check this location before each use.

G. Special Circumstances

1. Feeding with umbilical catheters in situ has been controversial; although there are insufficient data to guide practice, several NICUs feed infants with umbilical venous and/or umbilical arterial catheters in place and it is a common occurrence (23,24).

2. Tubing should be vented between feedings if continuous positive airway pressure is in place.

H. Complications

1. Apnea, bradycardia, or desaturation

2. Obstruction of obligatory nasal airway (4)

3. Irritation and necrosis of nasal mucosa (4)

4. Misplacement on insertion (**Fig. 43.5**)
   a. Coiled in oropharynx
   b. Trachea leading to aspiration (5,11,13)
   c. Esophagus
   d. Duodenum

5. Displacement after insertion because of inappropriate length or fixation
   a. Pulling back or coiling into esophagus (25)
   b. Prolapsing into duodenum (11)

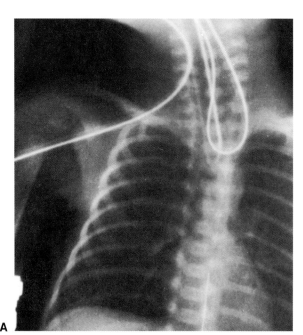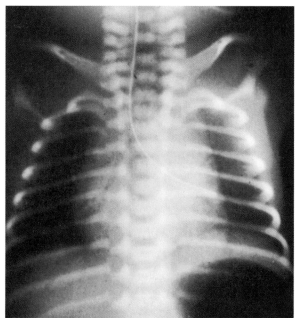

FIGURE 43.5 Radiographic examples of misplaced feeding tubes. **A:** Tube coiled in the oropharynx and upper esophagus, simulating an esophageal atresia. **B:** Tube into the left mainstem bronchus. *(continued)*

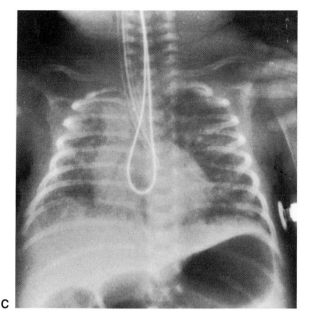

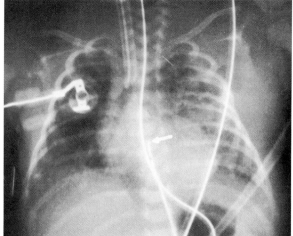

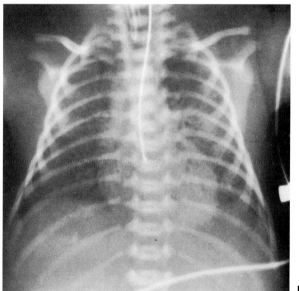

FIGURE 43.5 (*Continued*) **C:** Tube coiled in the lower esophagus. **D:** Tube doubled on itself in the stomach with its distal end in the esophagus (*arrow*). **E:** Tube in the esophagus. A rush may be heard on auscultation over the stomach when air is injected through a tube lying in this position, making an unreliable verification of gastric location.

6. Coiling and clogging of tube
7. Perforation (**Fig. 43.6**)
   a. Posterior pharynx, particularly at level of cricopharynx
   b. Esophagus
      (1) Submucosal, remaining within mediastinum
      (2) Complete into thorax
      (3) Symptoms can mimic esophageal atresia or tracheoesophageal fistula (14)
      (4) Chylothorax or pneumothorax (13)
   c. Stomach
   d. Duodenum
8. Grooved palate with long-term use of indwelling tube (13)
9. Increased gastroesophageal reflux
10. Infection (13)
11. Breakage of tube with retention of distal portion in stomach (26)

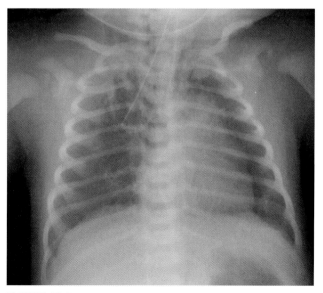

FIGURE 43.6 Chest radiograph showing esophageal perforation by an orogastric tube.

TRANSPYLORIC FEEDING TUBE

A. Indications (1,4)

1. Severe gastroesophageal reflux with risk of aspiration
2. Gastric distention with continuous positive airway pressure
3. Delayed gastric emptying
4. Gastric motility disorders
5. Sampling of duodenojejunal contents
6. Intolerance to gastric feeds

B. Contraindications

1. Clinical condition that compromises duodenojejunal integrity: necrotizing enterocolitis, fulminant sepsis, shock, recent small-bowel surgery

C. Precautions (see also Oral or Nasal Gastric Tubes, Part D)

1. Most often, if the tube does not cross the pylorus within the first 30 minutes after passage, it is unlikely to pass in the next few hours, and it may be better to restart the procedure.
2. Replace tubes per manufacturer's recommendations. If the tube is stiff on removal, replace next tube sooner.
3. If a tube has become partially dislodged, replace it rather than pushing it in farther.
4. When using feedings that tend to coagulate in tubing, it may be necessary to flush the tube periodically with air or water.
5. Use reliable infusion pumps that control rate and detect obstruction.
6. Limit infusion of hypertonic solutions and do not deliver bolus feedings beyond the pylorus.
7. Feedings must be given continuously, and not in bolus form, due to the risk of dumping syndrome and decreased ability of the small intestine to expand for larger volumes (1,4).
8. Consider the effect of continuous feedings on medication absorption.
9. Long-term use remains controversial due to concerns over short-term growth and should be used with caution (27,28).
10. There are no data to support routine use in preterm infants (27).

D. Equipment (see also Oral or Nasal Gastric Tubes, Part E)

1. Silastic tube of appropriate size. Silastic tubes are preferred over PVC tubing, as they can remain in place for a longer duration; PVC tubes are not recommended for long-term use (2,4).
2. Continuous infusion pump and connecting tubing.

E. Technique

1. Follow steps 1 through 5 above under Oral or Nasal Gastric Tubes (Part F).
2. Measure distance from glabella to heels (29). Mark point with tape on transpyloric tube (see **Fig. 43.3**).
3. Turn patient onto right side and elevate the head of the bed 30 to 45 degrees.
4. Pass transpyloric tube to predetermined depth.
5. After approximately 10 minutes with infant remaining on right side, gently aspirate through transpyloric tube. Tube may be in position within duodenum if aspirate is:
   a. Without air.
   b. Bilious (gold or yellow in color).
   c. pH >6, although this method alone is not reliable (29). (See also Oral or Nasal Gastric Tubes, Part F.)
6. Verify placement with radiograph. The tip of the tube should be just beyond the second portion of duodenum (**Fig. 43.7**) (29).
7. Avoid pushing to advance tube after initial placement. If tube is not in far enough, retape to give external slack and to allow peristalsis to carry tip to new position.
8. After verifying correct positioning, close transpyloric tube or start continuous infusion.
9. Document patient response, observing any physiologic changes and verifying tube placement.
10. Note the location of the tube at the nares and document it on the chart. Check this location before each use.

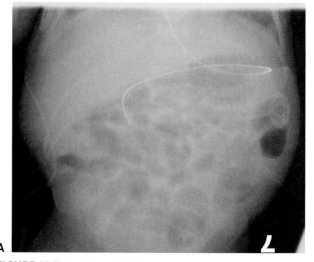

FIGURE 43.7 A: Abdominal radiograph showing appropriate position of transpyloric tube. (*continued*)

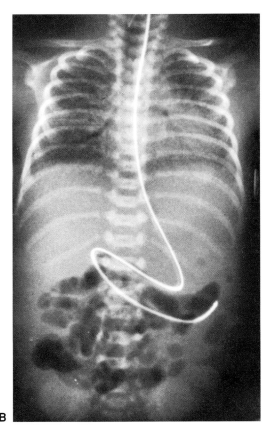

B

FIGURE 43.7 *(Continued)* **B:** Radiographic demonstration of a transpyloric feeding tube that has passed the ligament of Treitz, well below the appropriate level, increasing the risk of perforation or nutritional dumping.

11. Transpyloric tubes may also be placed with fluoroscopic guidance.

F. Special Circumstances

1. See Oral or Nasal Gastric Tubes, Part G.

G. Complications (see also Oral or Nasal Gastric Tubes, Part H)

1. The risk of aspiration with transpyloric feeding does not appear to be different from the risk with gastric feeding (27).
2. Perforation of esophagus, stomach, duodenum (30).
3. Possible interference with absorption of medications.
4. Malabsorption and GI disturbance (5,30).
   a. Risk of fat malabsorption with nasojejunal feeds.
   b. Dumping syndrome if hypertonic medications or feedings instilled too rapidly (10).
   c. GI disturbance as characterized by abdominal distention, gastric bleeding, and bilious vomiting.
5. Pyloric stenosis (31).
6. Intussusception (32).

References

1. Wessel JJ. Feeding methodologies. In: Groh-Wargo S, Thompson M, Cox JH, eds. *Nutritional Care for High-Risk Newborns*. 3rd ed. Chicago, IL: Precept Press; 2000:321–325.
2. Wallace T, Steward D. Gastric tube use and care in the NICU. *Newborn Inf Nurs Rev*. 2014;14:103–108.
3. Birnbaum R, Limperopoulos C. Nonoral feeding practices for infants in the neonatal intensive care unit. *Adv Neonatal Care*. 2009;9(4):180–184.
4. Vermilyea S, Goh VL. Enteral feedings in children: sorting out tubes, buttons and formulas. *Nutr Clin Pract*. 2016;31(1):59–67.
5. Irving SY, Lyman B, Northington L, et al. Nasogastric tube placement and verification in children: review of the current literature. *Crit Care Nurse*. 2014;34(3):67–78.
6. Replogle RL. Esophageal atresia: plastic sump catheter for drainage of the proximal pouch. *Surgery*. 1963;54:296–297.
7. Petrosyan M, Estrada J, Hunter C, et al. Esophageal atresia/tracheoesophageal fistula in very low birth weight neonates: improved outcomes with staged repair. *J Pediatr Surg*. 2009;44:2278–2281.
8. Berman L, Moss RL. Necrotizing enterocolitis: an update. *Semin Neonatal Med*. 2011;16:145–150.
9. deBoer JC, Smit BJ. Nasogastric tube position and intragastric air collection in a neonatal intensive care population. *Adv Neonatal Care*. 2009;9(6):293–298.
10. Cirgin Ellett ML, Cohen MD, Perkins SM, et al. Predicting the insertion length for gastric tube placement in neonates. *J Obstet Gynecol Neonatal Nurs*. 2011;40:412–421.
11. Quandt D, Schraner T, Bucher H, et al. Malposition of feeding tubes in neonates: Is it an issue? *J Pediatr Gastroenterol Nutr*. 2009;48:608–611.
12. Clifford P, Heimall L, Brittingham L, et al. Following the evidence: enteral tube placement and verification in neonates and young children. *J Perinat Neonatal Nurs*. 2015;29(2):149–161.
13. National Association of Children's Hospitals, ECRI Institute. *Blind Pediatric NG Tube Placements—Continue to Cause Harm*. Overland Park, KS: Child Health Patient Safety Organization Inc.; 2012.
14. Schuman TA, Jacobs B, Walsh W, et al. Iatrogenic perinatal pharyngoesophageal injury: a disease of prematurity. *Int J Pediatr Otorhinolaryngol*. 2010;74:393–397.
15. Filippi L, Pezzati M, Poggi C. Use of polyvinyl feeding tubes and iatrogenic pharyngo-oesophageal perforation in very-low-birthweight infants. *Acta Paediatr*. 2005;94(12):1825–1828.
16. Yong S, Ma JS, Chen FS, et al. Nasogastric tube placement and esophageal perforation in extremely low birth weight infants. *Pediatr Neonatol*. 2016;57:427–430.
17. Kristoffersen L, Skogvoll E, Haftsrom M. Pain reduction on insertion of a feeding tube in preterm infants: a randomized controlled trial. *Pediatrics*. 2011;127(6):e1449–e1454.
18. Chen S, Zhang Q, Xie RH. What is the best pain management during gastric tube insertion for infants aged 0–12 months: a systematic review. *J Pediatr Nurs*. 2017;34:78–83.
19. Cincinnati Children's Hospital Medical Center. Confirmation of nasogastric/orogastric tube (NGT/OGT) placement. *Best Evidence Statement (BESt)*. 2011;024:1–9.
20. Farrington M, Lang S, Cullen L, et al. Nasogastric tube placement verification in pediatric and neonatal patients. *Pediatr Nurs*. 2009;35:17–24.

21. Gilbertson HR, Rogers EJ, Ukoumunne OC. Determination of a practical pH cutoff level for reliable confirmation of nasogastric tube placement. *JPEN J Parenter Enteral Nutr.* 2011;35(4):540–544.

22. Meert KL, Caverly M, Kelm LM, et al. The pH of feeding tube aspirates from critically ill infants. *Am J Crit Care.* 2015;24(5):e72–e77.

23. Tiffany KF, Burke BL, Collins-Odoms C, et al. Current practice regarding the enteral feeding of high-risk newborns with umbilical catheters in situ. *Pediatrics.* 2003;112:20–23.

24. Hans DM, Pylipow M, Long JD, et al. Nutritional practices in the neonatal intensive care unit: analysis of a 2006 neonatal nutrition survey. *Pediatrics.* 2009;123(1):51–57.

25. Crisp CL. Esophageal nasogastric tube misplacement in an infant following laser supraglottoplasty. *J Ped Nurs.* 2006;21(6):454–455.

26. Halbertsma FJ, Andriessen P. A persistent gastric feeding tube. *Acta Paediatr.* 2010;99:162.

27. Watson J, McGuire W. Transpyloric versus gastric tube feeding for preterm infants. *Cochrane Database Syst Rev.* 2013;(2):CD003487.

28. Rosen R, Hart K, Warlaumont M. Incidence of gastroesophageal reflux during transpyloric feeds. *J Pediatr Gastroenterol Nutr.* 2011;52(5):532–535.

29. Ellett ML. Important facts about intestinal feeding tube placement. *Gastroenterol Nurs.* 2006;29:112–124.

30. Flores JC, Lopez-Herce J, Sola I, et al. Duodenal perforation caused by a transpyloric tube in a critically ill infant. *Nutrition.* 2006;22:209–212.

31. Latchaw LA, Jacir NN, Harris BH. The development of pyloric stenosis during transpyloric feedings. *J Pediatr Surg.* 1989;24:823–824.

32. Hughes U, Connolly B. Small-bowel intussusceptions occurring around nasojejunal enteral tubes—three cases occurring in children. *Pediatr Radiol.* 2001;31:456–457.

Gastrostomy

Bavana Ketha, Megan E. Beck, Kathryn M. Maselli, Thomas Sato, and A. Alfred Chahine

A. Definition

Gastrostomy is the placement of a catheter in the stomach for a variety of indications.

Although usually performed in the operating room, it is essential that the NICU staff has a good understanding of what the procedure is and the optimal care of the tube, since it has become one of the most commonly performed surgical procedures in the neonatal population (1,2). Surgical advances including endoscopy and laparoscopy have expanded the applications of gastrostomy while making placement quicker and safer (3–5).

B. Indications

1. Inability to swallow/dysphagia
    a. Neurologic impairment resulting in uncoordinated swallowing.
    b. Complex congenital malformations, e.g., esophageal atresia, Pierre Robin sequence, and chromosomal abnormalities.
2. Failure to thrive/need for supplemental feedings
    a. Anatomic intestinal anomalies, i.e., short gut syndrome.
    b. Functional intestinal dysmotility, i.e., gastrointestinal malabsorption.
    c. Malignancy/tumor.
    d. Chronic pulmonary disease, i.e., persistent pulmonary hypertension.
    e. Congenital heart disease.
    f. Glycogen storage disease (need for consistent glucose source).
    g. Chronic kidney disease.
3. Frequent aspiration
    a. Gastroesophageal reflux disease leading to pulmonary disease (in conjunction with a Nissen fundoplication).
    b. Primary hypopharyngeal aspiration.

C. Relative Contraindications

Treatable medical conditions that increase operative risks, such as active infection or coagulopathy, should be treated aggressively prior to elective gastrostomy placement.

Pure esophageal atresia often results in small stomach volumes (microgastria), thus making gastrostomy placement more difficult. Ultimately, if the patient requires gastric transposition to treat long-gap esophageal atresia, a prior gastrostomy would make the repair contraindicated.

Short-term need for enteral nutrition for a period of weeks can be met through placement of a nasogastric tube instead.

D. Preoperative Workup

Prior to operative planning, it is important to make sure that the patient meets the proper anatomical and physiologic indications for gastrostomy. An upper gastrointestinal (UGI) study would reveal any anatomic malformations like malrotation or duodenal webs, but the utility of this has been recently questioned (6–8). Identifying neonates in need of concomitant procedures such as antireflux surgeries usually requires more extensive preoperative workups such as 24-hour pH probe to quantitate the extent of the reflux and a gastric emptying study to look for impaired gastric motility (6,7,9). However, in general, the clinical picture is usually all you need to determine if the infant would benefit from only a gastrostomy or whether he/she would need a fundoplication simultaneously. If an infant is tolerating gastric feeds without any evidence of aspiration or respiratory compromise, typically that infant will do well with only a gastrostomy. If an infant is requiring transpyloric feeding because of respiratory issues, then a concomitant fundoplication may be warranted. The routine addition of a fundoplication at the time of a gastrostomy in neonates with neurologic impairment is still controversial (10,11).

E. Types of Gastrostomy

1. Open Stamm gastrostomy

    Dr. Martin Stamm described the open gastrostomy procedure in 1894, which was frequently used in premature infants and neonates. The Stamm technique, however, is now being used with less frequency secondary to its invasive approach. Current indications include altered gastric anatomy, multiple previous abdominal surgeries, concurrent laparotomy for other procedures, and unstable patients. It is performed through an upper transverse abdominal or supraumbilical midline incision. The catheter is then brought out of the skin through a separate location about halfway between the umbilicus and the costal margin on the left side **(Fig. 44.1)**. The catheters utilized in a Stamm gastrostomy include balloon, mushroom, and/or low-profile buttons.

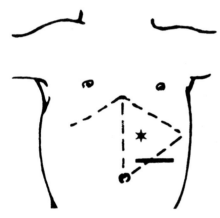

FIGURE 44.1 Anatomic landmarks for placement of a gastrostomy tube in a neonate. The tube will pass through the abdomen at a site in the center of a triangle formed by the xiphoid, umbilicus, and left costal margin.

2. Percutaneous endoscopic gastrostomy (PEG)

    Developed in 1980 by Drs. Gauderer and Ponsky, PEG has become the primary method of gastrostomy in older children and adults but is rarely used in the neonatal period for several reasons. Neonates are at higher risk of bowel injury with PEG due to lack of direct visualization. Concomitant fundoplication cannot be performed with PEG placement and patients may go on to require additional intervention. They are also at greater risk of tube dislodgement due to the inability to perform simultaneous gastropexy with PEG placement. Moreover, endoscopy is not feasible in neonates less than 3 kg due to the endoscope's size dimensions (1,4,12,13).

3. Laparoscopic gastrostomy

    Laparoscopic placement of gastrostomy tubes has become the method of choice for neonatal gastrostomy insertion (14,15). Some believe that the laparoscopic gastrostomy technique has a lower complication rate than the PEG technique in neonates and small children (14–17). It is a quick and safe technique requiring a short anesthetic and is usually very well tolerated. Most often, the tubes placed are primary button tubes that are easily maintained. They have a low profile on the outside and are held in place by a balloon inflated with a few milliliters of water **(Fig. 44.2A,B)**. The catheters vary in width (12 Fr, 14 Fr, etc.) and length of the stem from the bottom of the flange to the top of the inflated balloon (0.8 cm, 1.0 cm, 1.2 cm, etc.) **(Fig. 44.2A)**. The most commonly used size in the NICU is a 12-Fr, 0.8-cm button. A spare tube should always stay at the bedside and be given to the parents to keep at home.

4. Emergent percutaneous gastric decompression

    The ability to decompress the stomach emergently is a life-saving measure that may be required in neonates

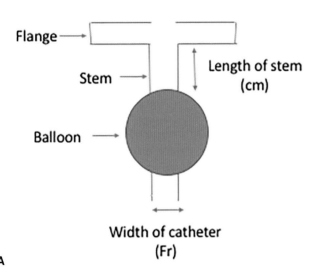

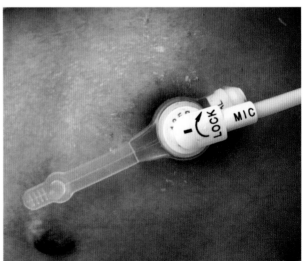

FIGURE 44.2 A: Elements of a gastrostomy button. **B:** Gastrostomy button in left upper quadrant with feeding attachment secured. (Photo courtesy of Dr. Mariana Vigiola-Cruz.)

that have severe respiratory compromise or a high probability of gastric rupture secondary to the presence of extreme gastric distention.

a. Indication
   (1) The primary indication is massive abdominal distention from preferential ventilation of the stomach rather than the stiff lungs in a premature newborn with esophageal atresia and a tracheoesophageal fistula.
b. Procedure
   (1) Prepare the abdomen with Betadine or chlorhexidine and then drape the skin in the upper left abdomen.
   (2) If possible, utilize a light to transilluminate the abdomen to locate and verify the position of the distended stomach away from liver.
   (3) Make a small wheal with 1% lidocaine to provide local anesthesia.
   (4) Using a 20- or 22-gauge catheter with needle stylet, puncture the abdominal wall at the junction of the left anterior rib cage and the lateral border of the rectus abdominis muscle **(Fig. 44.3)**.

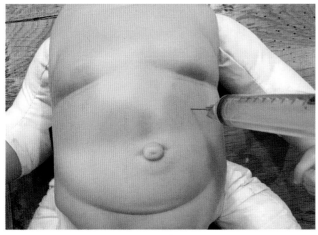

FIGURE 44.3 Simulation of emergent percutaneous gastric decompression.

   (5) Advance the needle through the wall into the stomach.
   (6) Remove the needle and advance the catheter into the stomach.
   (7) Attach a short IV extension tubing, three-way stopcock, and syringe:
      (a) Aspirate only enough air to relieve the tamponade effect and improve ventilation.
      (b) Avoid completely emptying stomach.
   (8) Secure the catheter and keep in place until surgical evaluation is possible.
   (9) Secure with tape or suture if necessary.

F. Postoperative Gastrostomy Care and Maintenance

Postoperative gastrostomy care begins immediately with meticulous attention to wound care to prevent infection and skin irritation. Initiation of feeds through the new gastrostomy tube, regardless of the method of placement, may begin within 12 to 24 hours postoperatively unless complicated by ileus, which may require further bowel rest.

Tube feeds should be started slowly and advanced to the goal rate over the next few days.

1. Maintain fixation of gastrostomy between stomach and abdomen
   a. Prevent gastric distention.
   b. Keep the gastrostomy balloon or flange pulled snugly against the stomach wall by maintaining the external bolster snug against the skin (take time to recognize and record the gastrostomy level mark at the skin if it is a tube catheter type) **(Figs. 44.4** and **44.5)**.

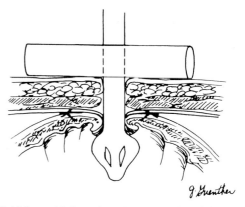

FIGURE 44.4 Good fit for a tube catheter type: A latex bolster at the gastrostomy exit stabilizes the tube perpendicular to the skin, keeping the stoma narrow to avoid leakage. Rotating the bridge around the tube allows change in contact points with the skin. Note how the flared end of the mushroom catheter is pulled to keep the stomach apposed to the stomach wall.

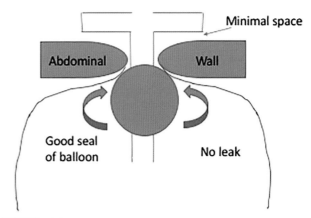

FIGURE 44.5 Good fit for a button type of gastrostomy: The distance between the external flange and the skin is minimal, allowing just enough room for a gauze. Note how the stem is long enough to allow the balloon to be apposed to the stomach to avoid leakage.

c. Avoid pressure necrosis of the abdominal wall by ensuring the external bolster is snug enough to be gently twisted around (**Fig. 44.6**).

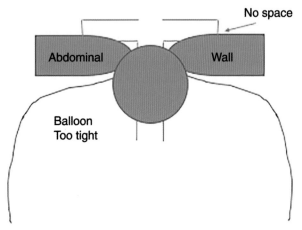

FIGURE 44.6 Gastrostomy button is too tight: The stem is too short, causing the external flange and balloon to dig into the abdominal wall. This can lead to necrosis of the abdominal wall and enlargement of the stoma.

d. Avoid inadvertent dislodgement of the gastrostomy (i.e., patient restraints, minimize tension on the gastrostomy tube by providing secondary fixation points on the skin or keeping the tube secure within the diaper).

e. Nursing staff and parents should be informed of the type of gastrostomy tube inserted, how much fluid has been placed in the retention balloon, and anticipated time of first gastrostomy tube exchange.

2. Maintain gastrostomy immobility at the insertion site to minimize the formation of granulation tissue

a. Use careful fixation to maintain the perpendicular position of the gastrostomy tube and keep some slack in the tube when it is suspended.

This prevents the amount of soft tissue stretching, tension or widening at the stoma site and thereby decreases the risk of a stoma leak.

3. Prevent migration of gastrostomy

a. Proper fixation: If not fixed on the outside with a bolster or tape, the gastrostomy tube may migrate through the pylorus or up into the esophagus. A modified nipple with a cut on the side placed around the catheter and taped to the skin and to the catheter will allow fixation of the catheter (**Fig. 44.7**).

b. Compare length of external tube with postoperative length (again checking and monitoring the level at the skin).

c. Observe for signs of obstruction

(1) Gastric distention.

(2) Feeding intolerance, nausea/vomiting.

(3) Increased drainage from oral gastric or gastrostomy tube.

(4) Bilious drainage.

(5) New-onset or increased gastroesophageal reflux.

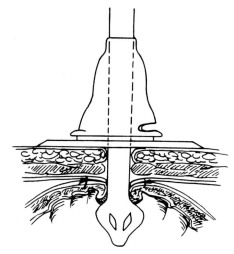

FIGURE 44.7 Fixation of a catheter type of gastrostomy without an external bolster using a modified feeding nipple: The elliptical hole at the base allows air circulation and regular cleaning of the skin as important factors in avoiding maceration of the site. (Reprinted from Kappell DA, Leape L. A method of gastrostomy fixation. *J Pediatr Surg.* 1975;10(4):523–524. Copyright © 1975 Elsevier. With permission.)

4. Minimize leak rate from the gastrostomy site

a. Maintain adequate fit of tube in stoma.

(1) If the stem of a button is too long for the abdominal wall of the baby, there will not be a good seal between the balloon and the stomach wall, leading to leaking of gastric juice, which can macerate the skin (**Fig. 44.8**).

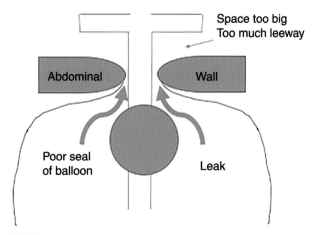

FIGURE 44.8 Leaking of gastric juice: If the stem of a button is too long for the abdominal wall of the baby, there will not be a good seal between the balloon and the stomach wall, leading to leaking of gastric juice, which can macerate the skin.

(2) Long-term gastrostomy tubes may need to be upsized if the stoma site increases in diameter.

b. Avoid local infection—continue meticulous wound care.

(1) Daily cleansing with soap and water starting 48 hours after placement.

5. Close follow-up after placement to screen for and reduce risk of catheter-related complications (see below)

G. Replacing Gastrostomy Tubes

Healing of gastrostomy sites requires at least 4 to 6 weeks for fibrosis to occur and create a well-epithelialized tract attaching the stomach to the anterior abdominal wall. This process may take several months with laparoscopic gastrostomies and PEG tubes as there are generally no sutures or fasteners deployed to form a seal between the stomach and the abdominal wall. During the initial postoperative period (2 to 4 weeks' postgastrostomy placement), loss of the tube can be treacherous in that the stomach can separate from the abdominal wall and, therefore, the surgical team should always be notified. Loss of the tube can result in an increased risk of spontaneous closure if not reintroduced promptly.

1. The steps to reintroduce a gastrostomy tube are:
   a. Replace within 4 to 6 hours to avoid stoma closure.
   b. In the initial postoperative period prior to the formation of a well-epithelialized tract, replace with a balloon-type catheter (a button or a Foley type catheter). For well-epithelialized tracts, mushroom catheter tubes or balloon-type gastrostomy tubes may be used for placement.
   c. Lubricate the catheter generously with water-soluble lubricant, and insert gently.
      (1) If resistance is felt and/or the catheter does not pass easily, stop and reassess. Attempt passing a flexible guidewire through the tract. A catheter is inserted over the wire or the stoma may be dilated by sequential dilators.
      (2) Inflate the balloon with 2 to 4 mL of water, then pull firmly against the stomach wall.
      (3) Secure with a fixation/external bolster device.
      (4) Mark outside length of catheter to help detect internal or external migration of the balloon.
2. Confirm intragastric position prior to feeding
   a. For recent gastrostomy (initial postoperative period) or if the replacement is difficult
      (1) Instill 15 to 30 mL of water-soluble contrast through the gastrostomy under fluoroscopic guidance to confirm accurate positioning.
   b. For epithelialized gastrostomy tracts
      (1) Aspirate for gastric contents and visualize the gastric contents in the tube to fluctuate with respirations and drop down with gravity.
      (2) If there is any doubt, obtain contrast study prior to initiating feeding.

H. Discontinuation of Gastrostomy (18)

1. General principles
   a. Remove gastrostomy tube and apply gauze dressing.
      (1) Spontaneous closure usually occurs in 4 to 7 days.
   b. May also approximate the skin edges with surgical tape.
2. Persistent gastrocutaneous fistula
   a. Granulation and epithelialization of gastrocutaneous tract (well-established tract).
      (1) Remove gastrostomy tube.
      (2) Cauterize the stoma granulation tissue and/or epithelium with silver nitrate.
      (3) Seal orifice with Stomahesive.
      (4) Approximate the edges with surgical tape.
   b. Persistent gastrocutaneous fistula (greater than 4 to 6 weeks).
      (1) Requires surgical closure.
      (2) If the skin is becoming macerated, replace the gastrostomy and use protective skin ointment prior to surgical closure.

I. Complications (1,18–27)

Although a commonly performed neonatal procedure, gastrostomy placement can have serious complications. Early recognition of such complications allows for prompt intervention and prevention of devastating sequelae. The complications associated with neonatal gastrostomy placement may be characterized as intraoperative, early or late.

1. Intraoperative complications
   a. Pneumoperitoneum.
      Some pneumoperitoneum is expected after the laparoscopic and open placement but is most common with PEG placement.
   b. Liver or splenic injury.
   c. Colonic placement.
   d. Hollow viscus injury.
   e. Injury to posterior wall of stomach on initial insertion or upon reinsertion (gastrostomy replacement).
   f. Bleeding.
2. Early complications (within the first 4 postoperative weeks)
   a. Most early complications are technical or mechanical in nature.
   b. Presentation may be subtle and thus requires a high index of suspicion.
   c. Symptoms range from early feeding intolerance to worsening abdominal pain/peritonitis and signs of systemic infection.
   d. Common early complications
      (1) Wound infection, dehiscence.
      (2) Prolonged ileus, gastric atony leading to feeding intolerance.
      (3) Gastric separation from anterior abdominal wall.
      (4) Intraperitoneal spillage/gastric leak leading to peritonitis.

(5) Early tube dislodgement.
(6) Early tube occlusion.
(7) Gastric outlet obstruction.
3. Late complications
   a. Prevention
      (1) Parental education is essential to long-term care and prevention of late complications (22,23).
      (2) Meticulous hygiene and appropriate perpendicular positioning are critical to avoid trauma to the skin and subcutaneous tissues.
   b. Common late complications
      (1) Dislodgement
         (a) Inadvertent removal.
         (b) Internal or external gastrostomy migration (24).
      (2) Catheter deterioration
         (a) Tube erosion/fracture.
         (b) Balloon rupture.
      (3) Tube occlusion
      (4) Granulation tissue formation
      (5) Persistent leak
4. Wound breakdown which results in the following:
   a. Granulation tissue and skin irritation.
   b. Infection.
   c. Enlargement of tract leading to loose gastrostomy with leakage.
   d. Skin ulceration.
5. Electrolyte imbalance
6. Malnutrition
   a. New-onset or worsening gastroesophageal reflux disease (25).
   b. Persistent gastrocutaneous fistula (post removal) (26).
   c. Prolapse of gastric mucosa (27).
      (1) Bleeding.
      (2) Excessive leakage.
   d. Gastric torsion around catheter.
7. Treatment of common complications
   a. Gastrostomy leak—treat early.
      (1) Remove tube for up to 24 hours to allow partial tract closure.
      (2) Replace mushroom catheter with a balloon-type catheter.
   b. Secure tube by pulling the balloon (inflated with 2 to 5 mL of water) against the abdominal wall.
      (1) Apply stomahesive around catheter.
   c. Decrease excoriation.
   d. Encourage epithelialization.
   e. Change stomadhesive every 3 to 4 days to maintain seal.
      (1) Maintain perpendicular positioning of gastrostomy tube.
      (2) Do not clamp the gastrostomy tube.
      (3) Maintain skin and stoma hygiene.
         (a) Cleanse daily with soap and water.

(4) Consider half-strength (1.5%) hydrogen peroxide for areas of fibrinous exudates.
   (a) Frequent dressing changes to maintain a dry site.
(5) Granulation tissue at gastrostomy site.
   (a) Silver nitrate
      i. Apply daily for up to 3 to 5 days.
      ii. Avoid spilling the liquefied silver nitrate onto normal adjacent skin since this would cause a chemical burn.
   (b) 0.5% Triamcinolone ointment
      i. Apply three times a day for 5 to 7 days.
   (c) Cautery
      i. May require local or general anesthesia.

References

1. Gauderer MW, Stellato TA. Gastrostomies: evolution, techniques, indications, and complications. *Curr Probl Surg.* 1986;23(9):657–719.
2. Fox D, Campagna EJ, Friedlander J, et al. National trends and outcomes of pediatric gastrostomy tube placement. *J Pediatr Gastroenterol Nutr.* 2014;59:582–588.
3. Jones VS, La Heir ER, Shun A. Laparoscopic gastrostomy: the preferred method of gastrostomy in children. *Pediatr Surg Int.* 2007;23(11):1085–1089.
4. Thatch KA, Yoo EY, Arthur LG 3rd, et al. A comparison of laparoscopic and open Nissen fundoplication and gastrostomy placement in the neonatal intensive care unit population. *J Pediatr Surg.* 2010;45(2):346–349.
5. Charlesworth P, Hallows M, Van der Avoirt A. Single-center experience of laparoscopically assisted percutaneous endoscopic gastrostomy placement. *J Laparoendosc Adv Surg Tech A.* 2010;20(1):73–75.
6. Valusek PA, St Peter SD, Keckler SJ, et al. Does an upper gastrointestinal study change operative management for gastroesophageal reflux. *J Pediatr Surg.* 2010;45:1169–1172.
7. Cuenca AG, Reddy SV, Dickie B, et al. The usefulness of the upper gastrointestinal series in the pediatric patient before anti-reflux procedure or gastrostomy tube placement. *J Surg Res.* 2011;170(2):247–252.
8. Abbas PI, Naik-Mathuria BJ, Akinkuotu AC, et al. Routine gastrostomy tube placement in children: Does preoperative screening upper gastrointestinal contrast study alter the operative plan? *J Pediatr Surg.* 2015;50(5):715–717.
9. Wheatley MJ, Wesley JR, Tkach DM, et al. Long-term follow-up of brain-damaged children requiring feeding gastrostomy: Should an anti-reflux procedure always be performed? *J Pediatr Surg.* 1991;26(3):301–305.
10. Barnhart DC, Hall M, Mahant S, et al. Effectiveness of fundoplication at the time of gastrostomy in infants with neurological impairment. *JAMA Pediatr.* 2013;167(10):911–918.
11. Puntis JW, Thwaites R, Abel G, et al. Children with neurological disorders do not always need fundoplication concomitant with percutaneous endoscopic gastrostomy. *Dev Med Child Neurol.* 2000;42:97–99.

12. Merli L, De Marco EA, Fedele C, et al. Gastrostomy placement in children: percutaneous endoscopy gastrostomy or laparoscopic gastrostomy? *Surg Laparosc Endosc Percutan Tech.* 2016;26(5):381–384.

13. Miyata S, Dong F, Lebedevskiy O, et al. Comparison of operative outcomes between surgical gastrostomy and percutaneous endoscopic gastrostomy in infants. *J Pediatr Surg.* 2017;52:1416–1420.

14. Soares RV, Forsythe A, Hogarth K, et al. Interstitial lung disease and gastroesophageal reflux disease: key role of esophageal function tests in the diagnosis and treatment. *Arq Gastroenterol.* 2001;48(2):91–97.

15. Suksamanapum N, Mauritz FA, Franken J, et al. Laparoscopic versus percutaneous endoscopic gastrostomy placement in children: results of a systematic review and meta-analysis. *J Minimal Access Surg.* 2017;13(2):81–88.

16. Liu R, Jiwane A, Varjavandi A, et al. Comparison of percutaneous endoscopic, laparoscopic and open gastrostomy insertion in children. *Pediatr Surg Int.* 2013;29(6):613–621.

17. Petrosyan M, Khalafalla AM, Franklin AL, et al. Laparoscopic gastrostomy is superior to percutaneous endoscopic gastrostomy tube placement in children less than 5 years of age. *J Laparoendosc Adv Surg Tech A.* 2016;26(7):570–573.

18. Ducharme JC, Youseff S, Tilkin R. Gastrostomy closure: a quick, easy and safe method. *J Pediatr Surg.* 1977;12:729–730.

19. Akay B, Capizzani TR, Lee AM, et al. Gastrostomy tube placement in infants and children: Is there a preferred technique? *J Pediatr Surg.* 2010;45(6):1147–1152.

20. Lantz M, Hultin Larsson H, Arnbjornsson E. Literature review comparing laparoscopic and percutaneous endoscopic gastrostomies in a pediatric population. *Int J Pediatr.* 2010;2010:507616.

21. Nah SA, Narayanaswamy B, Eaton S, et al. Gastrostomy insertion in children: percutaneous endoscopic vs. percutaneous image-guided? *J Pediatr Surg.* 2010;45(6):1153–1158.

22. Landisch RM, Colwell RC, Densmore JC. Infant gastrostomy outcomes: the cost of complications. *J Pediatr Surg.* 2016;51(12):1976–1982.

23. Correa JA, Fallon SC, Murphy KM, et al. Resource utilization after gastrostomy tube placement: defining areas of improvement for future quality improvement projects. *J Pediatr Surg.* 2014;49(11):1598–1601.

24. Fortunato JE, Cuffari C. Outcomes of percutaneous endoscopic gastrostomy in children. *Curr Gastroenterol Rep.* 2011;13:293–299.

25. Jolley SG, Tunnel WB, Hoelzer DJ, et al. Lower esophageal pressure changes with tube gastrostomy: a causative factor of gastroesophageal reflux in children? *J Pediatr Surg.* 1986;21:624–627.

26. Gordon JM, Langer JC. Gastrocutaneous fistula in children after removal of gastrostomy tube: incidence and predictive factors. *J Pediatr Surg.* 1999;34(9):1345–1346.

27. Janik TA, Hendrickson RJ, Janik JS, et al. Gastric prolapse through a gastrostomy tract. *J Pediatr Surg.* 2004;39(7):1094–1097.

Neonatal Ostomy and Gastrostomy Care

Linda C. D'Angelo, Dorothy Goodman, Kara Johnson, Laura Welch, and June Amling

Introduction

An ostomy is the construction of a permanent or temporary opening in the intestine (enterostomy) or urinary tract (urostomy) through the abdominal wall to provide fecal or urinary diversion, decompression, or evacuation (1). Gastrostomies (G-tubes) are stomas that allow direct access into the stomach and are used for feeding, medication administration, and decompression. This chapter discusses care of simple and complex enterostomies (ileostomies, colostomies), urostomies, vesicostomies, and gastrostomies (see also Chapter 44).

A. Definitions

1. **Enterostomy:** a surgical procedure in which a piece of the intestines is diverted through a stoma in the abdominal wall. The segment of the intestines diverted gives name to the subsequent ostomy: colostomy (colon) and ileostomy (ileum).
2. **Gastrostomy:** creation of an artificial external opening into the stomach for nutritional support or gastrointestinal compression. Typically, this would include an incision in the patient's epigastrium as part of a formal operation. It can be performed through surgical approach, percutaneous approach by interventional radiology, or percutaneous endoscopic gastrostomy (PEG).
3. **Ileal conduit:** a type of urinary diversion, where a small urine reservoir is created from a segment of bowel (ileum) and is brought out through an opening in the abdominal wall to drain the urine.
4. **Stoma:** surgically placed opening.
5. **Urostomy:** a urinary diversion constructed to bypass a dysfunctional portion of the urinary tract.

6. **Vesicostomy:** an opening directly from the bladder through the abdominal wall, urine flows freely through the stoma from the bladder.

ENTEROSTOMIES AND UROSTOMIES

A. Indications

Ostomies may be indicated in the neonate for a variety of congenital or acquired conditions (Table 45.1). The stoma

TABLE 45.1 Conditions Necessitating Ostomy in the Neonate

DISEASE/CONGENITAL ANOMALY	MOST COMMON LOCATION OF STOMA
Intestinal atresia	Duodenum, ileum, or jejunum
Meconium ileus	Ileum
Necrotizing enterocolitis	Ileum or jejunum
Hirschsprung disease	Sigmoid colon
Imperforate anus/anorectal malformations	Colon
Volvulus/malrotation	Ileum or jejunum
Intussusception	Ileum or jejunum
Bladder exstrophy	Bladder
Cloacal exstrophy	Bladder and colon
Epispadias	Bladder

is usually temporary, and reanastomosis of the bowel or urinary tract with closure of the stoma is performed during infancy or early childhood (2,3).

B. Types of Ostomies

1. **Enterostomies**
   a. There are several types of intestinal (enterostomy) stomas.

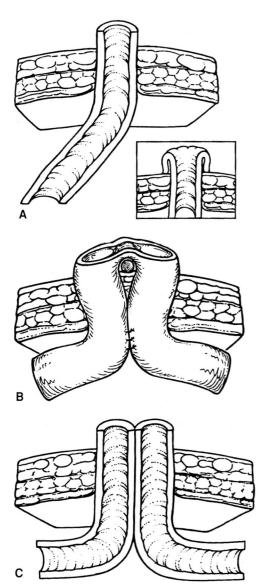

FIGURE 45.1 A: End stoma. The end of the bowel is everted at the skin surface. **B:** Loop stoma. Entire loop of bowel is brought to the skin surface and opened to create a proximal, or functioning, end and a distal, or non-functioning, end. The distal side is called a mucus fistula because of the normal mucus secretions it produces. **C:** Double-barrel stoma. Similar to a loop stoma, except the bowel is divided into two stomas, a proximal and a distal stoma. The distal stoma functions as a mucus fistula. (Reprinted from Gauderer MWL. Stomas of the small and large intestine. In: O'Neil JA, Rowe MI, Grosfeld JL, et al., eds. *Pediatric Surgery*. 5th ed. St. Louis, MO: Mosby; 1998:1349. Copyright © 1998 Elsevier. With permission.)

b. The patient's condition, the segment of bowel affected, and the size of the patient's abdomen often determine the type of stoma and its external location. **Figure 45.1** depicts the most common types of neonatal stomas and the affected section of bowel (1).

2. **Urinary diversion**
   a. Vesicostomies are the more common urinary diversion in the neonate.
   b. Ileal conduits and urostomies are more complex and are generally preformed in late infancy or early childhood.

C. Ostomy Assessment

The neonate with a stoma needs careful observation and assessment for a variety of potential complications (4). Monitoring the infant for function of the ostomy is vital in the initial postoperative period. Possible surgical complications are paralytic ileus, intestinal obstruction, anastomotic leak, and stomal necrosis. The factors to be considered during evaluation of the stoma are listed below.

1. **Stomal characteristics**
   a. **Type of stoma:** the segment of bowel from which the stoma is made.
   b. **Anatomical location**
   c. **Stomal construction:** the ostomy may be an end, loop, or double barrel (**Figs. 45.1** to **45.3**).

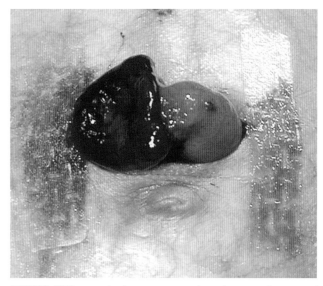

FIGURE 45.2 Immediately postoperative loop ileostomy. Segment of bowel on left is the exteriorized perforation from necrotizing enterocolitis.

d. **Size:** the stoma shape (round, oval, mushroom, or irregular) and diameter (length and width) in inches or millimeters are noted. In the early postoperative

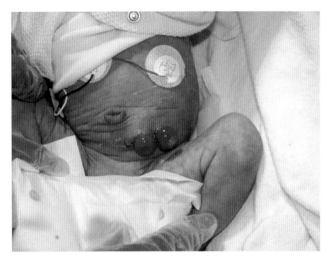

FIGURE 45.3 Premature infant with double-barrel colostomy.

period, the stoma will be edematous. After the first 48 to 72 hours, the edema should resolve and result in a reduction in size of the stoma; however, it should remain everted from the skin surface. Stomas generally continue to decrease in size over 6 to 8 weeks postoperatively. It is not uncommon for the stoma to become edematous when exposed to air while changing the pouch; this edema generally resolves quickly when the pouch is replaced.

e. **Stomal height:** the degree of protrusion of stoma from the skin. Ideally, the surgeon will evert the stoma prior to suturing it to the skin to produce an elevation, which will promote a better seal with the ostomy wafer. With the stoma elevated above the surface of the skin, the effluent will be more likely to go into the pouch instead of staying in contact with the skin (2). Eversion of the stoma, referred to as maturing the stoma, is not always possible in neonates, in whom blood supply may be tenuous, and in situations in which the bowel is markedly edematous (1,5).

2. **Viability:** a healthy stoma should be bright pink to beefy red and moist, indicating adequate perfusion and hydration (see **Fig. 45.2**). The stoma is formed from the intestine, which is very vascular and therefore may bleed slightly when touched or manipulated, but the bleeding usually resolves quickly. The stoma is not sensitive to touch because it does not have somatic afferent nerve endings (4).

a. A purple or dark brown to black stoma with loss of tissue turgor and dryness of the mucous membrane may indicate ischemia and possible stomal necrosis.

b. Distal aspect of stoma may be necrotic and later slough; the base is most indicative of a healthy stoma, and whether there is any output.

c. A pale pink stoma is indicative of anemia.

3. **Stomal complications**
a. **Bleeding**
(1) Hemorrhage during the immediate postoperative period is caused by inadequate hemostasis (4).
(2) Trauma to stoma caused by improper fitting pouch. A wafer cut too close to the stoma can injure the delicate tissue. Stomal lacerations can occur as a result of the edge of the wafer rubbing back and forth against the side of the stoma, especially as the infant's activity increases (4).

b. **Necrosis:** caused by ischemia and may be superficial or deep. Necrosis extending below the facial level may lead to perforation and peritonitis, requiring additional surgical intervention (4).

c. **Mucocutaneous separation:** caused by a breakdown of the suture line securing the stoma to the surrounding skin, leaving an open wound next to the stoma.

d. **Prolapse:** telescoping of the bowel out through the stoma. In infants, this condition is frequently related to poorly developed fascial support or excessive intra-abdominal pressure caused by crying.

e. **Retraction/recession:** the stoma is flush or recessed below the skin surface. This condition may result from insufficient mobilization of the mesentery or excessive tension on the suture line at the fascial layer, excessive scar formation, or premature removal of a support device (4).

f. **Stenosis:** the lumen of the ostomy narrows at either the cutaneous level or the fascial level. Sudden decrease in output may indicate stenosis.

4. **Peristomal skin:** peristomal skin should be intact, nonerythematous, and free from rashes. However, frequently the stoma(s) is not separate from the surgical incision (**Fig. 45.4**). There is often not enough space on the infant's abdomen for the surgeon to create separate

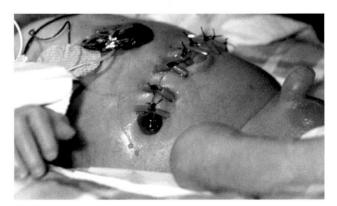

FIGURE 45.4 End ileostomy and wound closure with retention sutures posing a challenge for placing a pouch.

incisions. In addition, stomas are often in close proximity to the umbilicus, ribs, groin, and/or mucus fistula, which may interfere with pouch selection and adherence (6).

5. **Peristomal complications**
   a. **Dermatitis**
      (1) Allergic: product sensitivity.
      (2) Contact: local irritation from the procedure of cleaning and application of ostomy products.
      (3) Irritant: most common type of peristomal skin complication seen, generally are from the leakage of fecal effluent on the skin.
   b. **Infection**
      (1) Bacterial
      (2) Candidal
      (3) Fungal
      (4) Viral
   c. **Mechanical trauma:** epidermal stripping, abrasive cleansing techniques, and friction due to ill-fitting equipment are the most common causes of mechanical injury to the peristomal skin.
   d. **Hernia:** peristomal hernia appears as a bulge around the stoma that occurs when loops of the bowel protrude through a facial defect around the stoma into the subcutaneous tissue (4).

D. Enterostomy Care

1. **Immediate postoperative care**
   a. Assess stoma for adequate perfusion.
   b. Until there is output from the stoma, it is not necessary to apply an ostomy pouch.

      Keep stoma protected and moist with petrolatum gauze. When an enterostomy begins to produce, it is preferable to pouch. The pouch will protect the stoma, the peristomal skin, the suture line, and any central lines in that area. Pouching allows for qualifying and quantifying output. Before applying pouch, make sure to gently remove any residue of petrolatum gauze, which will interfere with the pouch adhesion.
   c. Cover the mucus fistula with a moisture-retentive dressing to keep it from drying out. When securing a dressing on a neonate, use low-tack adhesives. There is increased risk of skin tears in neonates, especially when they are premature with delayed epidermal barrier development. Avoid placing petrolatum gauze over the pouching surface for the stoma, as it can impede adherence.

2. **Subsequent care**
   a. Regular assessment of the stoma.
   b. Protect peristomal skin from the effects of the effluent by pouching (**Fig. 45.5**). The effluent from a small-bowel stoma contains proteolytic enzymes that can rapidly cause skin erosion. Ideally, the pouch should remain in place for at least 24 hours. In some

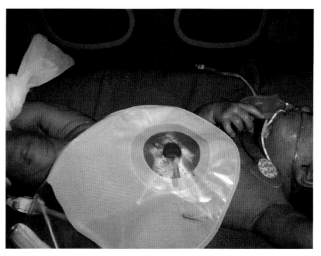

FIGURE 45.5 One-piece ostomy appliance on small newborn dwarfs this infant but provides longer wear time and holds larger volume of output than the preemie pouches previously used.

low-birth-weight neonates, the pouch may only last 12 hours. The average wear time is 1 to 3 days.
   c. The pouch *must* be changed if there is any evidence of leaking effluent under the skin barrier wafer. Frequent pouch changes, however, can result in denuded skin, especially in the premature infant (2,4,7). In situations with frequent leaking and pouch changes, expert help (certified wound ostomy continence nurse) may be required to preserve the skin and obtain acceptable wear time.
   d. In most situations powder(s) (e.g., stoma, nystatin, silver) can be used to heal the peristomal skin and provide a protective covering; then successfully pouch the stoma.
   e. In the rare instance when a pouch cannot be maintained, it may be necessary to leave the pouch off and protect the peristomal skin with a protective barrier ointment that will adhere to denuded skin, allowing the skin to heal. The barrier ointment can be covered with petrolatum-impregnated gauze; fluff gauze can then be placed on top to absorb the effluent, and changed as needed.
   f. In cases of severe skin damage, some neonatal centers stop enteral feedings briefly to limit stool production, and continue parenteral alimentation to provide adequate nutrition and allow the skin to heal (2). It is best to heal the skin, get a good seal, and then resume the feeding.
   g. Protect stoma from trauma. Measures include accurate sizing of the pouch opening to clear the stoma as the size changes. If the infant's movements cause the inner edge of the barrier to rub against the stoma, a moldable barrier between the stoma and the wafer can be used to protect the stoma.

TABLE 45.2 **Ostomy Accessory Products**

PRODUCT	INDICATIONS	PRECAUTIONS
Barrier powder	This product is used on dry, moist, and/or weepy skin. It can add extra adhesiveness to the skin. It must be sealed by patting with a moistened finger and allowed to dry. In cases of severely moist weeping skin, it may be necessary to apply powder and seal two or three times to attain a dry peristomal skin surface. It adds an additional barrier over the skin to protect from drainage. Apply in limited amounts and wipe off excess.	Protect infant from inhalation of aerosolized powder by using minimal amounts and wiping away gently; do not blow powder away.
Paste	Barrier product that is semiliquid because of addition of alcohol. Best if applied to barrier and allowed to air for 1 to 2 min to allow the alcohol to evaporate (**Fig. 45.6**).	Pastes contain alcohol and are, therefore, contraindicated for use in preemies or term neonates <2 wks old.
Skin sealants	Sealants use plasticizing agents to form a barrier on the skin that can protect from effluent and also improve adherence of some adhesives.	Most skin sealants contain alcohol and are, therefore, contraindicated for use in preemies or term neonates <2 wks old. One skin sealant that does not contain alcohol is Cavilon No Sting Barrier Film (3M, St. Paul, Minnesota) and is safe to use on neonates.
Moldable barrier	Barriers that are adhesive and can be shaped to fill in uneven spaces; generally hold up very well to corrosive effluent. Common types are Eakin Seal (ConvaTec, Princeton, New Jersey), Barrier No. 54 (Nu-Hope Laboratories, Pacoima, California), Adapt Rings (Hollister, Libertyville, Illinois), and Brava (Coloplast, Marietta, Georgia).	
Caulking strips	Similar to moldable barriers but come in narrow strips; they can be used to provide an extra barrier between the edge of the stoma and the barrier. May come in contact with stoma; soft enough that it does not injure the mucosa. Examples are Ostomy Strip Paste (Coloplast, Marietta, Georgia), Skin Barrier Caulking Strips (Nu-Hope Laboratories, Pacoima, California), and Adapt Strips (Hollister, Libertyville, Illinois).	
Belt	Elastic belt with tabs that fit to ostomy pouch of some two-piece appliances. Belt can help maintain the appliance in place by holding it firmly to abdomen. Generally used as a last resort when unable to obtain acceptable wear time.	May apply an outer covering to decrease friction to skin and aid in comfort.

E. Equipment

A variety of pouches and ostomy care supplies are available (**Table 45.2**). One-piece pouches come with a barrier and pouch attached as a single unit. Two-piece appliances have a barrier and pouch separate, with a mechanism for attaching the pouch to the wafer. The type of pouch used for a neonate is generally either an open-end pouch that allows the passage of thick or formed effluent or a urostomy pouch with a spout designed for drainage of urine or liquid effluent. The type of pouch and the need for accessory products vary depending on the anatomical location, size of the infant, the condition of the peristomal skin, abdominal size and contours, and institutional preference (**Fig. 45.6**). In general, it

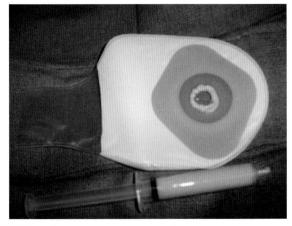

FIGURE 45.6 Barrier paste applied to wafer.

is best to keep the procedure simple and to use as few products as possible. Special consideration needs to be given to the premature infant whose skin is immature and fragile (2). Several companies manufacture pouches for neonates and premature infants (**Fig. 45.7**). Neonatal units should have several varieties to choose from in order to meet each patient's individual needs.

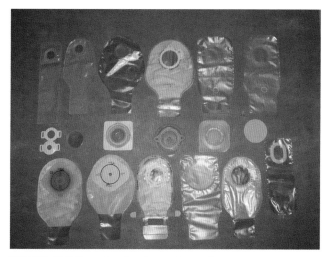

FIGURE 45.7 Examples of appliances for pouching a neonate.

Supplies

1. Clean gloves
2. Warm sterile water or normal saline
3. Clean, soft cloth
4. 2- × 2-in gauze
5. Appropriate-size pouch with closure device
6. Protective skin barrier and pouch
7. Other ostomy accessories as appropriate (see **Table 45.2**; **Fig. 45.8**)

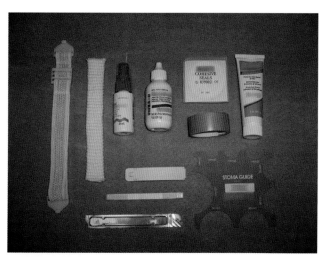

FIGURE 45.8 Examples of ostomy accessories.

8. Scissors or seam ripper
9. Stoma-measuring device

F. Applying the Pouch: Routine/ Simple Ostomies (2,6,8)

1. Remove old pouch by gently lifting up the edges and using water to loosen while pressing down gently on the skin close to the edge to reduce traction on the epidermis. Adhesive remover should not be used on a neonate <2 weeks of age. Limited use of adhesive remover, followed by thorough cleansing of the area to remove any chemical residue, is recommended only when the adhesive bond of the barrier to the skin is so strong that the skin might be injured during removal (2).

2. Use damp soft gauze or paper washcloth to gently cleanse the stoma to remove adherent stool or mucus. It is common to have a little bleeding of the stoma when it is cleansed.

3. Wash peristomal skin with water; pat dry. Soap is not recommended because it may leave a chemical residue that could cause dermatitis; furthermore, many soaps contain moisturizers that can adversely affect the adherence of the barrier to the skin. It is also not advisable to use commercial infant wipes, because most are lanolin based and contain alcohol (2).

4. Measure stoma(s) using stoma-measuring device (**Fig. 45.9**). The opening generally is cut 2 to 3 mm larger than the stoma, to limit the skin exposed to effluent. In low-birth-weight infants, in whom the mucus fistula may be immediately adjacent to the functional stoma, one pouch may be sized to fit over both the stoma and the mucus fistula. There are contraindications to pouching together in some male patients with imperforate anus, based upon the anatomy. Further discussion about pouching mucous fistula is below in F8.

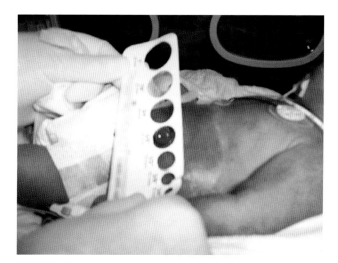

FIGURE 45.9 Measuring the stoma.

5. Trace hole size onto wafer. Cut hole(s) using small scissors or a seam ripper **(Fig. 45.10)**. After cutting and before removing the paper backing, check the fit around the stoma and trim more if needed. Run a finger along the inside of the opening to make sure there are no sharp edges; these can be cut or smoothed by rubbing with the finger. It may be necessary to trim the wafer to avoid umbilicus, groin, and other anatomical structures. Cutting small slits along the edges of the wafer may help the barrier conform to the contours of the stomach.

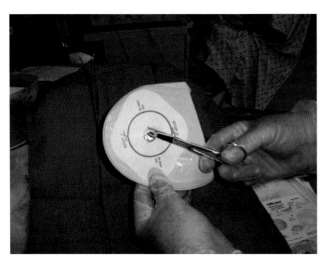

FIGURE 45.10 Cutting a hole in the wafer.

6. Warm wafer in hands to promote flexibility and enhance bonding to the skin. Avoid using a radiant heater to heat the wafer because the amount of heat absorbed cannot be controlled and may burn immature skin (2).
7. Press wafer to skin and hold for 1 to 2 minutes. Secure the edges of the wafer down to the skin to improve wear time. Avoid the use of high-tack adhesives. Pink tape is a waterproof tape that contains zinc oxide; it is very gentle and generally can be used safely. Other low-tack alternatives are silicone tape, transparent dressings, or skin barrier strips.
8. Change dressing to mucus fistula using a folded 2- × 2-in gauze piece and low-tack adhesive or secure with diaper or tubular elastic dressing. If there is an abundance of drainage from the mucus fistula and it is interfering with pouch adherence or the drainage may potentially contaminate wounds or central line sites, then the mucus fistula can be pouched. It is preferable to pouch the mucus fistula separately from the active stoma to keep the stool from contaminating the bowel anastomosis or draining into the vagina or bladder in the case of a patient with high-imperforate anus defect with fistula. It is advisable to discuss with the surgeon before placing both stomas in one pouch.

9. When an incision is within close proximity to a pouchable surface, a protective dressing (nonadherent dressing secured with a waterproof covering) should be applied to protect the incision.

G. Emptying the Pouch

1. Supplies
   a. Clean gloves
   b. Diaper or syringe for withdrawing stool/effluent
   c. 30- to 60-mL syringe for irrigating/washing the bag
   d. Tap water
   e. Cotton balls or 2 × 2 gauze
2. The pouch should be emptied when it is one-third to one-half full. Gas must also be released or vented to prevent pulling the adhesive wafer away from skin. Neonates generally produce large amounts of gas, related to increased intake with sucking and crying (2). Effluent can be drained directly into a diaper or withdrawn from the bag with a syringe. The use of two or three cotton balls or 2 × 2 gauze pad placed in an open-end pouch can improve wear time by wicking the effluent away from the barrier and also may facilitate easy drainage of the pouch. It is generally not necessary to wash the pouch, but it may be necessary to add fluid to help loosen up thick or pasty stool. For the hospitalized neonate, measurement of ostomy output is usually indicated.
3. Close the pouch with a closure device. Note: If patient will undergo magnetic resonance imaging (MRI), closure device must be approved and not contain any metal/wire.

H. Complicated Stomas and Peristomal Skin Problems (5,9–11)

Table 45.3 lists complications and interventions for treating complex stomas and common stoma problems. Note that many of items used are not generally recommended for use on premature neonates or neonates <2 weeks of age, but in situations of deterioration of the peristomal skin, they are sometimes used cautiously to prevent further deterioration and maintain an effective seal.

I. Vesicostomy Care

A vesicostomy does not require pouching; urine drains directly into the diaper. Care is similar to general perineal care of normal newborns (4). Occasionally, skin breakdown does occur; it can be treated with moisture barrier products, powders, crusting technique, open to air, and frequent diaper changes.

TABLE 45.3 **Complications and Complex Ostomies**

COMPLICATION	INTERVENTIONS
Multiple stomas	Customize pouch to fit around or accommodate stomas in bag; mucous fistulas may be in or out of pouch.
Open incision or wound	Two-piece pouches without starter hole may allow for easier customization. Keep wound as clean as possible. Use hydrocolloid wound dressing (e.g., DuoDERM, ConvaTec, Skillman, New Jersey; Replicare, Smith and Nephew, London, UK; Memphis, TN) or calcium alginate with a water-resistant cover dressing or barrier strip to protect wound from stool. Paste and powders may also be used to protect peristomal skin. In some cases it may not be possible to apply a pouch; however, the skin must be protected from caustic effluent, using a barrier such as Sensi-Care Protective Barrier (ConvaTec, Skillman, New Jersey) or Calmoseptine Ointment (Calmoseptine Inc., Huntington Beach, California).
Flush/retracted stoma	Apply paste or moldable barrier around hole in wafer. Use convex insert/convex pouch and belt to push skin back and allow stoma to protrude. May customize if commercial ones are too large.
Prolapsed stoma	Notify surgeon if evidence of compromised stoma perfusion. Protect the stoma from injury. Use caution when using a two-piece pouch with plastic flanges, the stoma could be pinched in the flanges that secure the pouch to the wafer when closed. Adjust size of hole accordingly; cover exposed skin with moldable barrier or paste. May need a larger pouch to accommodate prolapsed bowel.
Peristomal hernia	Use a flexible wafer and pouching system to adjust to contours of the skin.
Mushroom-shaped stoma	Modify opening to accommodate size of "crown"; protect skin around base with moldable barrier or paste.
Medical-associated skin damage (MASD)	Ensure that hole is cut to fit properly. Use paste/moldable barrier to protect from leakage. Apply powder to open, weepy skin. Assess for sensitivity to products. Apply topical steroids if needed to decrease inflammation, pain, and itching.
Peristomal *Candida albicans*	Appears as red, shiny, macular, papular rash that is pruritic. Apply topical antifungal powder (e.g., nystatin) to skin. The powder should be mixed with a small amount of water, painted smoothly on the skin with a cotton swab, and allowed to dry before placing the appliance. Continue to use with each pouch change until rash resolves. Dry skin completely when changing pouch. Resize pouch so that no skin is exposed.
Dehydration, metabolic acidosis, electrolyte imbalance	Monitor intake and output carefully, especially for infants with ileostomy and/or high output. Assess lab values regularly. Infants can develop electrolyte imbalance rapidly.

Data from Borkowski S. Pediatric stomas, tubes, and appliances. *Pediatr Clin North Am.* 1998;45(6):1419–1435; Craven DP, Fowler JS, Foster ME. Management of a neonate with necrotizing enterocolitis and eight prolapsed stomas in a dehisced wound. *J Wound Ostomy Continence Nurs.* 1999;26(4):214–220; Garvin G. Caring for children with ostomies and wounds. In: Wise B, McKenna C, Garvin G, et al., eds. *Nursing Care of the General Pediatric Surgical Patient.* Gaithersburg, MD: Aspen; 2000:261; Metcalfe P, Schwarz R. Bladder exstrophy: Neonatal care and surgical approaches. *J Wound Ostomy Continence Nurs.* 2004;31(5):284–292; and Wound, Ostomy and Continence Nurses Society. *Pediatric Ostomy Care: Best Practice for Clinicians.* Mount Laurel, NJ: Wound, Ostomy and Continence Nurses Society; 2011.

TABLE 45.4 **Types of Gastrostomy-Jejunostomy Tubes**

TYPE	DESCRIPTION	EXAMPLES
Temporary/ traditional	Most commonly used as initial tube following Stamm procedure; long, self-retaining catheters of latex or silicone rubber with self-retaining devices (i.e., balloon)	Malecot (Bard, Covington, Georgia) (collapsible wings), dePezzer (mushroom)
Gastrostomy feeding tubes	Silicone catheter with antimigration device and end cap	MIC (Kimberly-Clark/Ballard Medical, Draper, Utah), CORFLO (CORPAK MedSystems, Wheeling, Illinois)
Skin surface devices	Intended for use in established gastrostomy tract; have self-retaining devices, antimigration devices, and antireflux valves; two types, balloon and "Malecot type"	Bard Button (Bard, Covington, Georgia), MIC-KEY (Kimberly Clark/Ballard Medical, Draper, Utah)

Data from Borkowski S. Pediatric stomas, tubes, and appliances. *Pediatr Clin North Am.* 1998;45(6):1419–1435.

GASTROSTOMY-JEJUNOSTOMY (G-J) TUBES

A. Indications

For indications and insertion technique, see Chapter 44.

B. Types of Tubes

See **Table 45.4**.

C. Gastrostomy-Jejunostomy Tube Care (8,12)

1. **Assessment**
   a. The health care provider must know if the patient has undergone a Nissen fundoplication or other antireflux procedure together with the gastrostomy
   b. Tolerance to feedings
   c. Type and size of tube
   d. Insertion site
   e. Condition of the peristomal skin
2. **Special considerations for patients with Nissen or other antireflux procedure**
   a. Patient cannot vomit or burp.
   b. Vent tube after crying and at first sign of gagging, discomfort, or distress.
3. **G-J tube site and routine skin care** (6,8,12)
   a. Clean G-J tube site two to three times per day in the postoperative period and once per day after the site has healed. Use normal saline and sterile cotton swabs in the early postoperative period. Use mild soap and water after the site has healed. Diluted hydrogen peroxide (50% hydrogen peroxide and 50% water) is not recommended unless the site has dry, crusted blood (9).
   b. Ensure that the antimigration device is flush against skin and the G-J tube has not migrated.
   c. Position tube at 90-degree angle.
   d. A bottle nipple placed over the tube with the flanges resting on the abdominal wall may also be used to keep the tube at a 90-degree angle; secure with tape (Fig. 44.7).
   e. Stabilize gastrostomy tube to prevent excess movement of the tube. Stabilization decreases risk of stoma erosion, infection, bleeding, and development of granulation tissue.
   f. Use an anchoring/stabilizing device.
   g. Rotate device, flange of nipple, or wings of button every 4 to 8 hours to prevent pressure on skin. A silicone dressing can be used between the stoma and device in the early postoperative period to prevent shearing and absorb drainage. A one-piece shirt with snap enclosure or tubular elastic dressing can also be used to cover the tube.
   h. Assess site and peristomal skin for leaking, irritation, redness, rashes, or breakdown. Erythema and a minimal amount of clear drainage are to be expected in the 1st postoperative week.

D. Gastrostomy-Jejunostomy Tube Complications

Table 45.5 lists interventions for treating complications related to G-J tubes.

TABLE 45.5 Interventions for Gastrostomy Tube Complications

COMPLICATION	INTERVENTIONS
Leaking at insertion site	Check water volume if balloon-type catheter. Confirm that it is water not saline or air Ensure that tube is firmly secured at a 90-degree angle to prevent erosion of mucosal lining and skin. (GripLok, Hollister) Use proper feeding attachment. Ensure that tube is properly flushed and cleaned. Protect skin with skin barrier (e.g., Stomahesive wafer or powder [ConvaTec, Skillman, New Jersey], Cavilon No Sting [3M, St. Paul, Minnesota]; or hydrocolloid dressing). Use foam dressing (e.g., Hydrasorb [ConvaTec, Skillman, New Jersey], Allevyn [Smith and Nephew, London, UK; Memphis, TN], Mepilex [Mölnlycke, Gothenburg, Sweden]) or hydroconductive (e.g., Drawtex [SteadMed, Irving, Texas]) rather than gauze to "wick" moisture away from skin. If not contraindicated, consider H_2 blocker and prokinetic agent. Placing larger-size tube may temporarily control leakage but will not amend problem and is contraindicated.
Dislodgement	Institutional practices vary; in most cases do not reinsert if <2 wks postop. Contact surgeon immediately. If >2 wks postop, replace as soon as possible (see Chapter 44).
Bilious residuals	Assess for migration of tube (particularly if a Foley is being used).
Tube migration	Migration results from inadequate stabilization. Upward migration can cause vomiting and potential aspiration. Downward migration can cause gastric outlet obstruction. Migration into the small intestine can cause "dumping syndrome." When using a balloon catheter and migration is not recognized, inflation of the balloon can lead to esophageal, duodenal, or small-bowel perforation.
Pain	Assess for tube migration and secure. Vent tube. Consult surgeon if problem does not resolve.
Granulation tissue	Normal finding; caused by proliferation of granulation epithelial tissue in response to inflammation and irritation by foreign body. Prevent by stabilizing the tube. Treat by cauterizing with silver nitrate. Another treatment approach is application of triamcinolone cream 0.5%, two to three times daily until resolved.
Bleeding	Apply gentle pressure to site. Stabilize the tube. If granulation tissue is present, treat appropriately.
Irritant dermatitis	Protect skin with skin barrier (e.g., Stomahesive wafer, paste, or powder [ConvaTec, Skillman, New Jersey], Allevyn [Smith and Nephew, London, UK; Memphis, TN], iLEX paste [Medcon Biolab Technologies, Inc., Grafton, Massachusetts], or hydrocolloid dressing). Use foam dressing (e.g., Hydrasorb [ConvaTec, Skillman, New Jersey], Allevyn [Smith and Nephew, London, UK; Memphis, TN]) or hydroconductive (e.g., Drawtex [SteadMed, Irving, Texas]) rather than gauze to "wick" moisture away from skin. Assess for sensitivity to products/latex.
Peristomal (*Candida albicans*)	Apply topical antifungal to skin. Control leakage. Dry skin completely after cleaning. Patient should also be assessed for oral thrush.
Clogged tube	Flush well after medications with 5-mL lukewarm water. A small amount (3–5 mL) of carbonated soda or cranberry juice may also be poured into the tube. Allow to set for 10 min, then flush with water.
Infection	G-tube site infections are uncommon; cellulitis is treated with systemic antibiotics.

Data from Association of Women's Health, Obstetric and Neonatal Nurses, National Association of Neonatal Nurses (AWHONN). *Neonatal Skin Care: Evidence-Based Clinical Practice Guideline.* 3rd ed. Washington, DC: AWHONN; 2013; Borkowski S. Gastrostomy surgery and tubes. *Sutureline.* 2000;8:1; Borkowski S. Gastrostomy tube stabilization and security. *Sutureline.* 2005;13:8; Borkowski S. Pediatric stomas, tubes, and appliances. *Pediatr Clin North Am.* 1998;45(6):1419–1435; Crawley-Coha T. A practical guide for the management of pediatric gastrostomy tubes based on 14 years of experience. *J Wound Ostomy Continence Nurs.* 2004;31(4):193–200; Craven DP, Fowler JS, Foster ME. Management of a neonate with necrotizing enterocolitis and eight prolapsed stomas in a dehisced wound. *J Wound Ostomy Continence Nurs.* 1999;26(4):214–220; Garvin G. Caring for children with ostomies and wounds. In: Wise B, McKenna C, Garvin G, et al., eds. *Nursing Care of the General Pediatric Surgical Patient.* Gaithersburg, MD: Aspen; 2000:261; Metcalfe P, Schwarz R. Bladder exstrophy: Neonatal care and surgical approaches. *J Wound Ostomy Continence Nurs.* 2004;31(5):284–292; Rogers VE. Managing preemie stomas: More than just the pouch. *J Wound Ostomy Continence Nurs.* 2003;30(2):100–110; and Wound, Ostomy and Continence Nurses Society. *Pediatric Ostomy Care: Best Practice for Clinicians.* Mount Laurel, NJ: Wound, Ostomy and Continence Nurses Society; 2011.

References

1. Gauderer MWL. Stomas of the small and large intestine. In: O'Neil JA, Rowe MI, Grosfeld JL, et al., eds. *Pediatric Surgery*. 5th ed. St. Louis, MO: Mosby; 1998:1349.

2. Rogers VE. Managing preemie stomas: more than just the pouch. *J Wound Ostomy Continence Nurs*. 2003;30(2):100–110.

3. Metcalfe PD, Schwarz RD. Bladder exstrophy: neonatal care and surgical approaches. *J Wound Ostomy Continence Nurs*. 2004;31(5):284–292.

4. Wound, Ostomy and Continence Nurses Society. *Pediatric Ostomy Care: Best Practice for Clinicians*. Mount Laurel, NJ: Wound, Ostomy and Continence Nurses Society; 2011.

5. Craven DP, Fowler JS, Foster ME. Management of a neonate with necrotizing enterocolitis and eight prolapsed stomas in a dehisced wound. *J Wound Ostomy Continence Nurs*. 1999;26(4):214–220.

6. Borkowski S. Pediatric stomas, tubes, and appliances. *Pediatr Clin North Am*. 1998;45(6):1419–1435.

7. Garvin G. Caring for children with ostomies and wounds. In: Wise B, McKenna C, Garvin G, et al., eds. *Nursing Care of the General Pediatric Surgical Patient*. Gaithersburg, MD: Aspen; 2000:261.

8. Borkowski S. Gastrostomy tube stabilization and security. *Sutureline*. 2005;13:8. Available at https://www.aaspa.com/about/sutureline-journal.

9. Association of Women's Health, Obstetric and Neonatal Nurses, National Association of Neonatal Nurses (AWHONN). *Neonatal Skin Care: Evidence-Based Clinical Practice Guideline*. 3rd ed. Washington, DC: AWHONN; 2013.

10. Lockhat A, Kernaleguen G, Dicken BJ, et al. Factors associated with neonatal ostomy complications. *J Pediatr Surg*. 2016;51:1135–1137.

11. Brunette G. Novel pouching techniques for the neonate with fecal ostomies. *J Wound Ostomy Continence Nurs*. 2017;44(6):589–594.

12. Crawley-Coha T. A practical guide for the management of pediatric gastrostomy tubes based on 14 years of experience. *J Wound Ostomy Continence Nurs*. 2004;31(4):193–200.

CHAPTER

46

Ventriculoperitoneal Shunt Taps, Percutaneous Ventricular Taps, and External Ventricular Drains

Joshua Casaos, Rajiv R. Iyer and Edward S. Ahn

Hydrocephalus is often discovered in infancy and while not all infants with hydrocephalus require surgical intervention, this determination is based on the presence of signs and symptoms of elevated intracranial pressure (ICP). Elevation in ICP can manifest as rapidly increasing or abnormally large head circumference,j a bulging fontanelle, splayed cranial sutures, apneas and bradycardias, developmental delay, or other signs of neurologic dysfunction (1). If elevated ICP is a concern, patients with hydrocephalus are often managed by surgical implantation of a ventriculoperitoneal (VP) shunt, which allows CSF to be diverted from the ventricular system of the brain to the peritoneal cavity (2,3). VP shunts typically consist of three main components: a proximal ventricular catheter, a flow-regulating valve (programmable or nonprogrammable), and a distal peritoneal catheter (Fig. 46.1) (4).

Several types of VP shunts are available and they are implanted in the operating room by a neurosurgeon. While full-term infants with hydrocephalus can undergo VP shunting, preterm neonates are often too small to tolerate a fully functional shunt, so a temporizing device is needed. In these cases, a ventriculosubgaleal shunt (VSGS) is placed, which diverts CSF from the ventricular system into the subgaleal space of the scalp (2,5). Alternatively, a ventricular access device with a subcutaneous reservoir can be implanted and tapped periodically (see Chapter 57). Once infants reach a sufficient weight, typically 2,000 to 2,500 g, the temporizing device can be replaced with a fully functional VP shunt if CSF diversion is still required.

Certain scenarios may preclude distal shunt insertion into the peritoneum, such as abdominal infection (necrotizing enterocolitis in infants) or a history of multiple prior abdominal surgeries with poor peritoneal fluid reabsorption.

In these cases, alternative distal catheter sites can be considered, such as the right atrium of the heart, pleural cavity, and others.

SHUNT TAP

VP shunt dysfunction can occur due to abnormalities in any component of the system (proximal catheter, valve, distal catheter). Patients with dysfunctional shunts demonstrate signs and symptoms of elevated ICP, as well as diagnostic imaging that is often concerning for enlarged ventricles. Concern for obstruction or infection may be an indication for investigation of the functionality of a shunt with a *shunt tap*. This procedure can be performed relatively quickly at

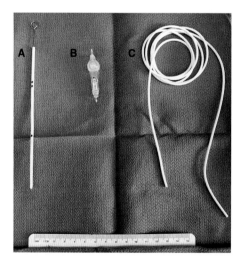

FIGURE 46.1 VP shunt components consisting of a proximal catheter and stylet (**A**), a flow-regulating valve (**B**), and a distal peritoneal catheter (**C**).

353

the bedside and can serve both diagnostic and therapeutic purposes.

A. Indications

1. Interrogation of shunt functionality when malfunction is suspected
2. CSF withdrawal for temporary ICP relief in a distally occluded shunt (valve or distal catheter malfunction)
3. Other possible indications depending on clinical scenario:
   a. To obtain CSF
      (1) For evaluation of shunt infection: cell count, Gram stain, culture, glucose, protein
      (2) For cytology: assessment of malignant cells in CSF
      (3) Note: VP shunts are typically not used as CSF access devices, as shunt taps carry a procedural risk of infection and shunt dysfunction. Therefore, when infants with a VP shunt present to the ER with fever of unknown origin and meningitis is suspected, a lumbar puncture is often the preferred route of CSF acquisition in patients with communicating hydrocephalus

   b. The injection of agents for shunt patency/function studies, such as radionuclide shuntograms
   c. Administration of medications:
      (1) Antibiotics, chemotherapeutic agents (this is often accomplished with a permanent Ommaya reservoir rather than a VP shunt)

B. Relative Contraindications

1. Infection over the entry site
2. Lack of appropriate diagnostic imaging such as a CT scan or MRI to ensure safety of the shunt tap (e.g., shunt tip within a body of CSF to be withdrawn)

C. Equipment (Fig. 46.2)

1. Sterile gown, gloves, drapes, mask
2. Hair clippers (if necessary)
3. Antiseptic (Betadine, chlorhexidine, DuraPrep, etc.)
4. 25-gauge butterfly needle with associated tubing
5. 3-, 5-, 10-, or 20-mL syringes depending on ventricular size, ICP
6. CSF collection tubes

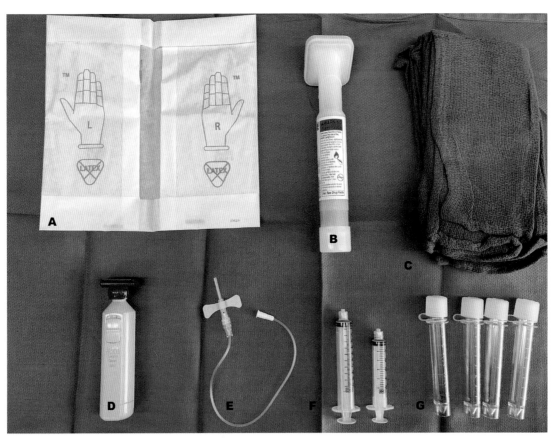

FIGURE 46.2 Necessary equipment for a shunt tap including: mask and hairnet (not pictured), sterile gloves (**A**), antiseptic (**B**), sterile towels (**C**), hair clippers (**D**), butterfly needle (**E**), 5- or 10-mL syringe (**F**), CSF collection tubes (**G**).

7. Optional: manometer: a physical manometer, often used for lumbar punctures, can be attached to butterfly tubing to directly measure ICP in cm H_2O. This can also be approximated with the shunt tubing length held vertically after the tap.

D. Preprocedure Care

1. Obtain informed consent (risk of hemorrhage, infection, shunt malfunction)
2. Check labs for hematologic abnormalities that can alter clotting function (i.e., coagulation factors, platelets, etc.)
3. Position infant such that shunt valve is easy to access (**Fig. 46.3**)

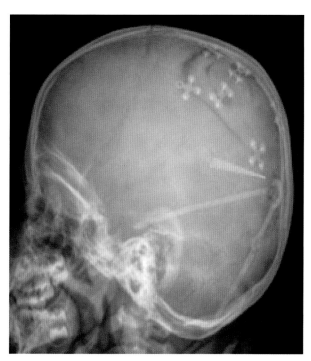

FIGURE 46.3 Radiograph demonstrating location of proximal catheter and shunt reservoir (*yellow arrowhead*).

   a. Ancillary staff and parents may assist with infant positioning
4. Check insertion site for infection

E. Procedure

1. Shave hair over shunt if necessary
2. Prep area with antiseptic and create a working sterile field with all necessary equipment
3. Drape out a small sterile field over the shunt valve
4. Locate shunt reservoir and enter the center of the reservoir with butterfly needle (**Fig. 46.4**). Be careful not to pierce the bottom of the reservoir as plastic can occlude the needle and give a false result.

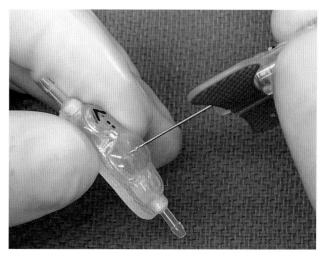

FIGURE 46.4 Photograph of needle entering the shunt reservoir in correct fashion for a shunt tap. Scalp is not depicted.

5. Observe for spontaneous CSF flow into butterfly tubing. If there is spontaneous flow, the proximal end is likely not completely obstructed.
   a. Opening pressure can be measured with manometer (normal ventricular pressure is <15 cm of H_2O in a recumbent patient)

     Alternatively, the butterfly tubing may be placed upright and straightened to act grossly as a manometer to estimate ventricular pressure. CSF overflowing from the end of the tubing suggests abnormally elevated ventricular pressure, which is suggestive of **partial proximal, valve, or distal catheter malfunction** (1). CSF of varying amounts can be aspirated until the closing pressure returns to a normal range.
   b. Placing the butterfly tubing below the level of the shunt valve and observing the drip interval has been shown to be effective in assessing proximal shunt functionality.
6. If there is no spontaneous flow, connect a 3- or 5-mL syringe to the tubing and attempt to gently aspirate CSF. No flow may indicate proximal occlusion, a neurosurgical emergency, and preparation should be made to take the patient to the operating room for shunt revision. Easily obtaining fluid with gentle aspiration may indicate low ICP.
7. Collect all CSF and send for studies: Gram stain, cell count, cultures, glucose, and protein.

F. Complications

Risks associated with a shunt tap are relatively low but must be considered and families must be informed of them (6).

1. **Infection**
   a. Any exposure of the shunt system to foreign material carries a risk of infection

2. **Shunt malfunction**
   a. Aggressive (or any) aspiration within the shunt reservoir could result in shunt malfunction
3. **Hemorrhage**
   a. Although uncommon, scalp bleeding associated with a shunt tap can result in blood entry into the shunt system and could affect shunt functionality

FONTANELLE TAP/PERCUTANEOUS VENTRICULAR PUNCTURE

A fontanelle tap or percutaneous ventricular puncture can also be performed in infants who require urgent ventricular decompression, and have an open anterior fontanelle, but no VP shunt. The procedure is performed by the neurosurgeon at the bedside, using a technique similar to the shunt tap. Fontanelle taps are similar to shunt taps, except that in this situation, the procedure makes use of the infants' open fontanelle to directly puncture the lateral ventricle with a butterfly needle.

A. Indication

Urgently required ventricular decompression in the setting of infantile hydrocephalus (7–9).

B. Preprocedure

Careful analysis of diagnostic imaging, such as ultrasound or MRI, can help determine the length of needle entry required to reach the lateral ventricle.

C. Procedure

1. **Prepare as for sterile procedure:** wear hat and mask, wash hands, wear sterile gown and gloves.
2. Prepare infant's scalp with antiseptic and cover with sterile drapes, leaving anterior fontanelle accessible.
3. Insert 25-gauge butterfly needle through the anterolateral aspect of the anterior fontanelle (away from midline, avoiding the superior sagittal sinus). Prior to needle insertion, the skin can be pulled taut such that the point of entry over the skin and fontanelle is interrupted, thus avoiding a direct tract from skin surface to ventricle and reducing the risk of postprocedure CSF leak.
4. Once the ventricular system is entered, determine pressure; CSF can be aspirated and sent for laboratory studies. Typically no more than 10 mL/kg/tap of CSF is drained, with the goal of restoring a soft fontanelle (10).

EXTERNAL VENTRICULAR DRAIN

An external ventricular drain (EVD) is a temporary intraventricular catheter connected to an external drainage system as well as a pressure transducer capable of providing ICP measurement (**Figs. 46.5** and **46.6**) (11–13).

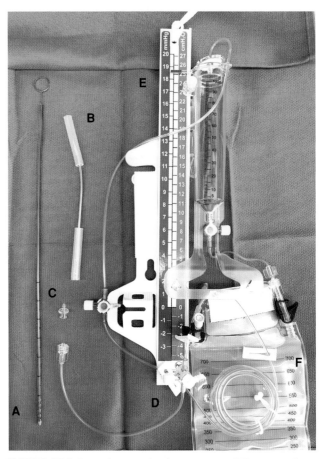

FIGURE 46.5 External ventricular drainage system/ICP monitor. Setup includes: ventricular catheter and stylet (**A**), tunneling trocar (**B**), connector (**C**), drainage system tubing and three-way stopcock (**D**), CSF drainage system (**E**), CSF collection bag (**F**).

A. Indications

1. Acute hydrocephalus
2. ICP monitoring
3. Shunt infection
4. Postoperative diversion of CSF

B. Relative Contraindications

1. Mass lesion in catheter pathway
2. Coagulopathy/thrombocytopenia (14)
3. Slit ventricles (if EVD required in this scenario, surgeons may elect to place an EVD with neuronavigation in the operating room)

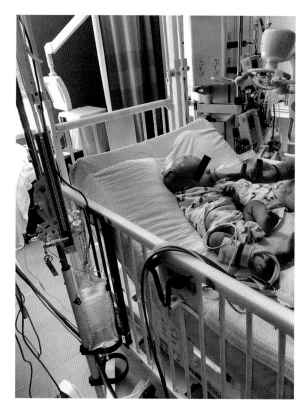

FIGURE 46.6 Photograph of EVD setup at the patient bedside, demonstrating CSF drainage system/ICP monitor, CSF collection bag, and associated tubing and connections.

C. Equipment

1. Sterile gown, gloves, drapes, mask
2. Antiseptic
3. 1% lidocaine
4. Cranial access kit (including clippers, gauze, sterile saline, scalpel, cranial twist drill, needle driver, forceps, scissors, suture)
5. Ventricular catheter
6. External drainage collection system

D. Preprocedure Care

1. Obtain informed consent.
2. Review the imaging, carefully noting the ventricular size and distance of the ventricle from skull or skin surface, as well as the skull thickness, if possible.
3. Review laboratory results, assessing for coagulopathy or thrombocytopenia.
4. Generally, placement of an EVD on the right side (nondominant hemisphere) is preferred, although there are exceptions to this rule. The preferred site of entry is at Kocher point, which in adults, is a point on the skull 2 to 3 cm from midline and 10 to 11 cm posterior to the nasion. Alternatively, external landmarks

of the midpupillary line and anterior to the coronal suture can be used (15). Because of smaller and more variable head sizes in infants, rigid measurements can be suboptimal and instead, these external landmarks are preferable in determining the insertion site. Other insertion sites have also been described, but are rarely used at the bedside.

E. Procedure

1. Position patient supine with head at the edge of the bed with easy access for the surgeon.
2. Mark, prep, and sterilely drape the planned incision according to the points described above.
3. After injecting local anesthetic, make a skin incision (usually vertical, can be horizontal) approximately 2 cm in length, and place a self-retaining retractor.
4. Use a twist drill with the appropriate length to create a fenestration in the skull, being careful not to plunge the drill once the inner table of the skull is reached.
5. Pierce the dura with a needle and place the intraventricular catheter in the lateral ventricle by directing the catheter perpendicular to surface of brain, and aligning the catheter with the medial canthus of the ipsilateral eye and a point immediately anterior to the external auditory meatus (EAM)/tragus (16,17). This trajectory allows the catheter tip to end in the frontal horn of the lateral ventricle near the foramen of Monro at about 6-cm depth into the skull. After placement, ensure CSF return from the catheter.
6. Tunnel the distal end of the catheter away from insertion site under the skin and secure the catheter at the exit site.
7. Close the incision and connect the EVD catheter to external drainage system. The drain should be leveled to the EAM.
   a. Height of the drainage bag in relation to the EAM regulates flow. Depending on the indication for the EVD, different drainage methods are possible. For example, a "pop-off" pressure can be set on the EVD drainage system such that drainage will occur once a certain ICP threshold is met, which is often used in the trauma setting to help control ICP through CSF drainage. Hourly drainage goals, such as a 5- to 10-cc/hr goal, may be useful in conditions such as intraventricular hemorrhage, infection, or postoperative settings, in which debris or blood clearance is the goal.
8. Place sterile, occlusive dressings. It is helpful to place translucent dressings to visualize the totality of the catheter system in the event that interrogation is necessary.
9. Imaging may or may not be necessary to confirm catheter location. A well-defined ICP waveform is also

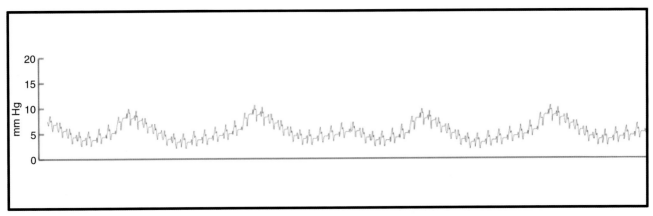

FIGURE 46.7 Depiction of a normal ICP waveform with associated cardiorespiratory variations.

helpful in determining EVD functionality and adequacy of placement.

F. Management

EVD malfunction can include obstruction and infection (18). If problems arise with the EVD, malfunction can be observed as change or loss of ICP waveform (**Fig. 46.7**), or a lack of CSF drainage from adequately sized ventricles.

1. **Possible causes**
   a. Improper connections
   b. Wet-air filter on drip chamber, which can affect flow and pressure readings
   c. Occlusion of the proximal catheter by debris (blood, cells, protein, choroid plexus)
      (1) Test and assess as below
   d. Dislodgement or migration of proximal catheter from ventricle
      (1) Test and assess as below
   e. Air in the system (air lock)
      (1) This can be resolved by allowing a specific amount of CSF to drain and therefore expelling the air from the system.
2. To test for proximal obstruction, the drainage bag/collection system can be lowered, and the system can be assessed for increased CSF flow. Adequate flow suggests that there is no proximal catheter obstruction.
3. A distal or proximal catheter flush can be performed under sterile conditions if debris is thought to be causing catheter or tube obstruction.
   a. A small volume of saline (about 1 cc of preservative-free saline, if proximal) is gently flushed using a three-way stopcock. The distal system is usually tested first. CSF flow is checked after flushing by lowering the collection system after opening the stopcock. If no flow can be obtained after this maneuver, and the clinical scenario warrants, the EVD may require replacement.

G. Monitoring

1. The EVD should be checked every hour for functionality as well as ICP measurement. Gradual or abrupt changes in ICP, neurologic examination, or CSF output may warrant further investigation, including diagnostic imaging when appropriate.
2. Assess for normal ICP waveform cardiorespiratory variation (**Fig. 46.7**).

H. Complications

1. Hemorrhage (subdural hematoma, epidural hematoma, tract hemorrhage)
2. Infection (warrants treatment with IV or intrathecal antibiotics, catheter replacement)
3. Malposition (may warrant repositioning/replacement)

References

1. Kahle KT, Kulkarni AV, Limbrick DD Jr, et al. Hydrocephalus in children. *Lancet.* 2016;387(10020):788–799.
2. Kumar N, Al-Faiadh W, Tailor J, et al. Neonatal post-haemorrhagic hydrocephalus in the UK: a survey of current practice. *Br J Neurosurg.* 2017;31(3):307–311.
3. Kulkarni AV, Drake JM, Kestle JR, et al. Predicting who will benefit from endoscopic third ventriculostomy compared with shunt insertion in childhood hydrocephalus using the ETV success score. *J Neurosurg Pediatr.* 2010;6(4):310–315.
4. Chari A, Czosnyka M, Richards HK, et al. Hydrocephalus shunt technology: 20 years of experience from the Cambridge Shunt Evaluation Laboratory. *J Neurosurg.* 2014;120(3):697–707.
5. Koksal V, Oktem S. Ventriculosubgaleal shunt procedure and its long-term outcomes in premature infants with post-hemorrhagic hydrocephalus. *Childs Nerv Syst.* 2010;26(11):1505–1515.
6. Miller JP, Fulop SC, Dashti SR, et al. Rethinking the indications for the ventriculoperitoneal shunt tap. *J Neurosurg Pediatr.* 2008;1(6):435–438.

7. Kreusser KL, Tarby TJ, Kovnar E, et al. Serial lumbar punctures for at least temporary amelioration of neonatal posthemorrhagic hydrocephalus. *Pediatrics.* 1985;75(4):719–724.

8. Levene MI. Ventricular tap under direct ultrasound control. *Arch Dis Child.* 1982;57(11):873–875.

9. Whitelaw A, Lee-Kelland R. Repeated lumbar or ventricular punctures in newborns with intraventricular haemorrhage. *Cochrane Database Syst Rev.* 2017;4:CD000216.

10. Garton HJ, Piatt JH Jr. Hydrocephalus. *Pediatr Clin North Am.* 2004;51(2):305–325.

11. Ngo QN, Ranger A, Singh RN, et al. External ventricular drains in pediatric patients. *Pediatr Crit Care Med.* 2009;10(3):346–351.

12. Walker CT, Stone JJ, Jacobson M, et al. Indications for pediatric external ventricular drain placement and risk factors for conversion to a ventriculoperitoneal shunt. *Pediatr Neurosurg.* 2012;48(6):342–347.

13. Bratton S, Chestnut R, Ghajar J, et al. Guidelines for the management of severe traumatic brain injury. VII. Intracranial pressure monitoring technology. *J Neurotrauma.* 2007;24:S45–S54.

14. Davis JW, Davis IC, Bennink LD, et al. Placement of intracranial pressure monitors: Are "normal" coagulation parameters necessary? *J Trauma.* 2004;57(6):1173–1177.

15. Tillmanns H. Something about puncture of the brain. *Br Med J.* 1908;2:983–984.

16. O'Neill BR, Velez DA, Braxton EE, et al. A survey of ventriculostomy and intracranial pressure monitor placement practices. *Surg Neurol.* 2008;70(3):268–273.

17. Becker DP, Nulsen FE. Control of hydrocephalus by valve-regulated venous shunt: avoidance of complications in prolonged shunt maintenance. *J Neurosurg.* 1968;28(3):215–226.

18. Muralidharan R. External ventricular drains: Management and complications. *Surg Neurol Int.* 2015;6(Suppl 6): S271–S274.

Transfusions

47

Delayed Cord Clamping and Cord Milking

Anup C. Katheria, Debra A. Erickson-Owens, and Judith S. Mercer

A. Definitions

1. **Placental transfusion:** Placental transfusion is the transfer of residual placental blood to the baby during the first few minutes of life. A placental transfusion will supply the infant with whole blood, red blood cells, and stem cells. This occurs in both term and preterm infants.
2. **Delayed umbilical cord clamping (DCC):** The practice of DCC is waiting to clamp the umbilical cord for a specific time period.
3. **Umbilical cord milking (UCM)**
    a. Intact umbilical cord milking (I-UCM): The practice of I-UCM is when the umbilical cord is grasped between the thumb and forefinger and firmly milked (or stripped) pushing blood from the placental end toward the infant several times before clamping the umbilical cord.
    b. Cut umbilical cord milking (C-UCM): The practice of C-UCM is when a long segment (typically 30 to 40 cm) of umbilical cord is immediately clamped and cut (near the introitus or at the cord insertion site on the placenta), untwisted and slowly milked toward the infant before clamping at the base of the cord.
4. **Immediate cord clamping (ICC):** The practice of immediately clamping the umbilical cord after birth. ICC does not support placental transfusion and leaves a large amount of the infant's blood volume behind in the placenta.

B. Background

1. The decision of when to clamp and cut the umbilical cord may have both short- and long-term effects on the newborn. In the first few minutes after birth, a delay in clamping the umbilical cord or milking the cord can result in a significant return of blood volume from the placenta to the infant. This blood, the infant's own blood, can serve as a major source of warm, oxygenated blood volume, iron-rich red blood cells, and millions of stem cells (1).
2. Placental transfusion via DCC or UCM provides a number of short- and long-term benefits.
    a. Early hematologic advantages (2–5).
    b. Additional iron which can boost infant iron stores out to 4 to 6 months of age (6,7). This may prevent iron deficiency anemia and has been shown to increase white matter growth in the infant's developing brain (8).
    c. Both UCM and DCC also have hemodynamic benefits in term and preterm infants including improved blood pressure and less inotropic use (5).
    d. Improved systemic and cerebral blood flow as measured by heart ultrasound and cerebral oximetry (9,10).
    e. Improved neurodevelopmental outcomes in term infants at 4 years of age and in preterm infants at 18, 24, and 42 months of age (11–13).
    f. A recent meta-analysis suggests that DCC results in a 30% reduction in all-cause mortality for preterm infants (14).

C. Factors That Can Either Support or Hinder Placental Transfusion

1. Timing of cord clamping: Infants who receive ICC can leave up to 30% (term infants) or 50% (preterm infants <30 weeks) of their blood volume behind in the placenta (1).

2. Gravity: While recent studies suggest that placing the infant on the abdomen does not affect the amount of a placental transfusion, holding the infant above the level of the placenta slows placental transfusion while holding an infant below accelerates it (15).

3. Maternal uterine contractions and use of uterotonic medications (1). Frequent uterine contractions (spontaneous or stimulated by uterotonic medications) can accelerate a transfusion to the infant (16).

4. International and national health care organizations have published opinion papers supporting DCC.
    a. Various institutions across the world (American College of Obstetricians and Gynecologists [ACOG], Royal College of Obstetricians and Gynaecologists [RCOG], International Liaison Committee on Resuscitation [ILCOR], American Academy of Pediatrics [AAP], European Association of Perinatal Medicine [EAPM], World Health Organization [WHO], American College of Nurse-Midwives [ACNM]) have developed and implemented DCC guidelines (6,17–23).
    b. UCM has only been recommended by the European Task Force on Resuscitation (21).

D. Indications

1. Delayed cord clamping (DCC)
    a. To facilitate placental transfusion for infants of all gestational ages.
    b. Supports transfer of whole blood, red cells, and stem cells from placenta to the newborn in the first few minutes of life.
        (1) Can be used at all modes of delivery. DCC may be less effective with a cesarean section. A cut uterus may not effectively contract around the placenta to keep the placental pressure high. Some obstetrical providers may be uncomfortable waiting several minutes because of concerns with uterine bleeding.
        (2) There also may be clinical situations where waiting 30 to 60 seconds may be unacceptable. In all of these situations, UCM may be a preferred option.

2. UCM
    a. To accelerate placental transfusion when the clinical situation does not allow a delay in cord clamping.
    b. Preferred in "cut and run" clinical situations such as cesarean section.

E. Concerns and Widely Held Beliefs

1. Overtransfusion
    a. Yao et al. demonstrated that overtransfusion does not occur (16).

b. The residual blood is the infant's own blood volume that has been circulating continuously throughout pregnancy.
    c. There is a finite blood volume available.

2. Symptomatic polycythemia
    a. DCC is associated with asymptomatic (benign) polycythemia requiring no treatment (24).
    b. In examining the evidence over the past 30 years, there has been no association between DCC (and milking) and symptomatic polycythemia (2,14).

3. Jaundice
    a. The concern is that the infants will receive too many red blood cells leading to jaundice and hyperbilirubinemia requiring treatment.
    b. The most recent Cochrane review on term infants reports no increase in clinical jaundice although a 2% increase of infants needing phototherapy was noted (1–3).
    c. In the last 15 published randomized controlled trials, hyperbilirubinemia requiring treatment was not any greater in the DCC or milked groups compared to ICC (1,3,14).

4. Hypothermia
    a. Hypothermia from DCC has not been reported in any studies.
    b. Mercer et al. demonstrated no significant difference in temperatures of term infants at 15 minutes after birth or preterm infants on admission to the NICU (3,25).

5. Delay in neonatal resuscitation
    a. Clinicians must understand that gas exchange is occurring at the placental level, so the nonbreathing infant is not becoming more hypoxic after birth.
    b. Breathing in preterm infants only occurs in 40% of infants at 20 seconds, 70% at 40 seconds, and 90% at 60 seconds (20).
    c. If urgent resuscitation is needed (hypotonic, pale, and apneic infants), milking the cord (I-UCM or C-UCM) can be performed in a timely fashion and will not interfere with resuscitation (26).
    d. Assisted ventilation during DCC has not shown any clinical benefits over DCC alone in preterm infants with 60 seconds of DCC (27).

6. Viral infections (hepatitis B, C, and HIV)
    While no subset studies exist, numerous trials have included these groups of mothers with no reported increases in transmission. The blood obtained by DCC or UCM is the same blood that was circulating in the fetus in utero. The WHO recommendations on umbilical cord clamping do not consider HIV infection in the mother or unknown HIV status to be a contraindication for DCC (22).

F. Contraindications

1. Monochorionic placentation

---

[1]Theoretical and not substantiated by evidence.

[2]Conditions where the evidence is not available.

a. There is a theoretical concern of an acute twin-twin transfusion occurring after delivery of one twin into the other twin. Based on this theory, almost all trials have excluded this population.

b. However, there are no published trials demonstrating this occurrence. Compared to dichorionic placentation, monochorionic twins are at a higher risk of intraventricular hemorrhage and may benefit from a placental transfusion.

2. Complete placental abruption
   a. With a complete abruption, there is concern about newborn blood loss.
   b. However, there are case reports of keeping the cord intact and holding the placenta above the infant so whatever remaining blood in the placenta is transfused to the infant (28).

3. Umbilical cord prolapse and bleeding placenta accreta
   a. In both clinical situations, the infant is at risk for extreme hypovolemia and hypoxia due to compression of the umbilical vein but not the firmer umbilical arteries.
   b. While such infants would benefit from restoration of blood volume, these infants are often too depressed to receive DCC.
   c. Cord milking may be useful in this circumstance, but there are no studies to date in this subgroup.

G. Equipment

1. No special equipment is required.
2. Some hospital facilities have begun to use a special resuscitation trolley or cart in the labor room or operating room. This trolley is placed next to the delivery bed or operating room table and resuscitation efforts can be conducted while maintaining an intact umbilical cord during the first few minutes of life (29).

H. Special Circumstances

The goal in special clinical circumstances is to support an intact cord to facilitate placental transfusion. The following special circumstances are part of everyday clinical practice and strategies are offered for the clinician to consider.

1. Shoulder dystocia
   a. Shoulder dystocia is an obstetrical emergency and often infants are hypovolemic following delivery.
   b. Immediately after birth, hold the infant at or below the perineum. Dry, and then stimulate the infant per Neonatal Resuscitation Program (NRP) recommendations.
   c. If there is a "need for resuscitation," one can milk the cord several times before clamping to provide a placental transfusion.

2. Nuchal cord
   a. Most nuchal cords are benign. However, when the cord is very tight around the neck, body, or limbs of the fetus, hypovolemia can result.
   b. When the cord cannot be reduced, use of the somersault maneuver (**Fig. 47.1**) can support an intact cord and allow restoration of blood volume by placental transfusion (1).
   c. Cutting of the cord prior to delivery of the shoulders is strongly discouraged.
   d. If the baby has poor tone or is very pale, the infant should be placed on the bed or held in a "football hold" on the OB provider's nondominant forearm and hand.
   e. The infant can be dried and stimulated while he or she receives a placental transfusion until tone returns and the infant is breathing.
   f. Most resuscitations can be done at the perineum.
   g. Once the infant has good tone and color, the infant can be placed on the maternal abdomen without cutting the cord (30).

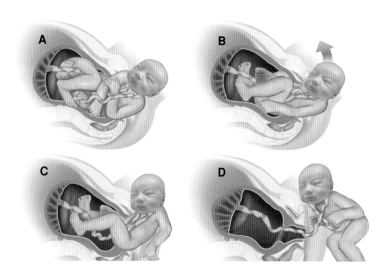

FIGURE 47.1 The somersault maneuver is all about keeping the cord intact. **A:** A nuchal cord is noted after the head delivers. It is not easily reducible over the head and is too tight to push down over the shoulders. **B:** As the infant is born, the head is kept as close to the perineum (or thigh) as possible. **C:** "Folding" the baby up toward the symphysis as it is born. **D:** The cord is gently unwound from around the neck and the infant can be resuscitated as needed with an intact cord.

3. Cord blood collection
   a. ACOG suggests that cord blood collection should not alter the timing of cord clamping (31).
   b. Considering the emerging evidence supporting DCC and UCM, parents should receive "balanced and accurate" information regarding the advantages and disadvantages of cord blood banking.
4. Cord gas collection
   Milking the cord prior to cord gas collection is recommended. The cord can then be clamped and cut and the usual technique for cord gas (arterial and/or venous) collection can be followed.

I. Technique

1. DCC (see ▶ **Video 47.1**):
   DCC is a technique that supports placental transfusion. Cord clamping time is delayed allowing a return of the residual placental blood volume to the infant. Recommendations for the duration of delaying/deferring cord clamping following birth vary. The WHO recommends "at least 1 to 3 minutes" (14); ACOG and AAP recommend at least 30 to 60 seconds (6,18), the ACNM recommends 5 minutes if baby is being held skin-to-skin with mother and 2 minutes if baby is held below the level of the introitus (23). In the United Kingdom, the NICU guidelines suggest cord clamping "not before 5 minutes" (17). Some midwifery groups advocate "Wait for White," or waiting until cord pulsations cease or the cord is flat and white.
   a. *Vaginal delivery*
      (1) Hold infant at or below the level of the placenta or skin-to-skin on the maternal abdomen.
      (2) Wrap in warmed blanket or place skin-to-skin and cover with blanket.
      (3) Evaluate the infant following NRP recommendations. If there is no need for resuscitative measures, then consider the following:
         (a) Preterm infants (<37 weeks' gestation)
            i. Leave cord intact for 45 to 120 seconds before clamping
         (b) Term infants
            i. Leave the cord intact at least 2 to 3 minutes if infant is held at perineum.
            ii. Leave cord intact at least 5 minutes if the infant is held skin-to-skin.
            iii. If cord is too short to facilitate a delay, then consider cord milking.
   b. *Cesarean section*
      (1) Dry and then wrap infant in warmed sterile blanket
      (2) Preterm infants (<37 weeks)
         (a) Hold infant below level of placenta

         (b) Leave cord intact for 45 to 120 seconds before clamping
         (c) Pass infant to pediatric provider and usual care at the radiant warmer
      (3) Term infants
         (a) Place infant on sterile drapes, between mother's thighs.
         (b) To reduce maternal blood loss put Greene-Armytage uterine clamps over each uterine incision angle and on any myometrial bleeding vessels (A. Weeks, personal communication January 31, 2018); if the OB provider is concerned about bleeding, UCM may be preferred.
         (c) Leave cord intact for at least 2 to 3 minutes.
         (d) Pass infant to pediatric provider and usual care at the radiant warmer.
      (4) Milking (see ▶ **Videos 47.2** and **47.3**)
         (a) Milking is a technique used to accelerate placental transfusion when time and the clinical situation prevent delay.
   c. *Two milking techniques*: I-UCM and C-UCM (can be used at vaginal delivery or cesarean section)
      (1) I-UCM
         (a) Hold infant at or below the level of the placenta.
         (b) Grasp the umbilical cord between the thumb and fore finger of dominant hand.
         (c) Firmly milk the cord toward infant three to five times.
         (d) Clamp and cut cord after completion of milkings.
      (2) C-UCM (32)
         (a) Clamp and cut the umbilical cord approximately 30 to 40 cm away from the infant's umbilicus and within 30 seconds. Performed by the OB provider.
         (b) Bring the infant and attached cord segment to the radiant warmer.
         (c) Untwist the cord. Performed by the pediatric provider.
         (d) Firmly milk the entire length of the cord once toward the infant. Performed by the pediatric provider.
   d. *Vaginal delivery (using the I-UCM technique)*
      (1) Preterm (<37 weeks)
         (a) Wrap infant in a prewarmed blanket or towel.
         (b) Place infant on a clean pad between the mother's legs or in a "football hold" using your nondominant forearm and hand.
         (c) Firmly milk the cord (over 2 seconds allowing the cord to refill) from the perineum to the infant's umbilicus three to four times.
         (d) Pass to the pediatric staff for further evaluation.

(2) Term

   (a) Place infant on clean pad between mother's legs or in a "football hold" using your non-dominant hand and forearm.

   (b) Firmly milk the cord (over 2 seconds allowing the cord to refill) from the perineum to the infant's umbilicus five times.

   (c) Pass the stable infant to the mother for skin-to-skin placement. If the infant is unstable, pass to pediatric staff for further evaluation.

e. *Cesarean section (using the I-UCM technique)*

   (1) Preterm (<37 weeks)

   (a) Wrap infant in a prewarmed sterile blanket or towel.

   (b) Place infant on the sterile field or in a "football hold" using your nondominant hand and forearm.

   (c) Firmly milk the cord (over 2 seconds allowing the cord to refill) close to the cord insertion site on the placenta to the infant's umbilicus three to four times.

   (d) Pass to the pediatric staff for further evaluation.

   (2) Term

   (a) Place infant on sterile drapes between mother's legs.

   (b) Firmly milk the cord (over 2 seconds allowing the cord to refill) close to the cord insertion site on the placenta to the infant's umbilicus five times. Usually completed in 10 to 15 seconds.

   (c) Continue usual infant care.

J. Complications

1. There have been no adverse effects reported with either DCC or UCM in term infants. DCC is associated with a decrease in hospital mortality in preterm infants (14).

2. While higher bilirubin levels have been reported with both methods, with a slight increase in requirement for phototherapy, there has not been any increase in need for exchange transfusion or in long-term morbidity.

3. During UCM or DCC, if the cord should tear, immediately clamp both ends of the torn portions of the cord.

References

1. Mercer JS, Erickson-Owens DA. Rethinking placental transfusion and cord clamping issues. *J Perinat Neonatal Nurs.* 2012;26(3):202–217.

2. McDonald SJ, Middleton P, Dowswell T, et al. Effect of timing of umbilical cord clamping of term infants on maternal and neonatal outcomes. *Cochrane Database Syst Rev.* 2013;7:CD004074.

3. Mercer JS, Erickson-Owens DA, Collins J, et al. Effects of delayed cord clamping on residual blood volume, hemoglobin, bilirubin levels in term infants: a randomized controlled trial. *J Perinatol.* 2017;37(3):260–264.

4. Erickson-Owens DA, Mercer JS, Oh W. Umbilical cord milking in term infants delivered by cesarean section: a randomized controlled trial. *J Perinatol.* 2012;32(8):580–584.

5. Rabe H, Diaz-Rossello JL, Duley L, et al. Effect of timing of umbilical cord clamping and other strategies to influence placental transfusion at preterm birth on maternal and infant outcomes. *Cochrane Database Syst Rev.* 2012;(8):CD003248. doi:10.1002/14651858.CD003248.pub3.

6. American College of Obstetricians and Gynecologists (ACOG). Committee opinion no.684: delayed umbilical cord clamping after birth. *Obstet Gynecol.* 2017;129(1):e5–e10.

7. Andersson O, Hellstrom-Westas L, Andersson D, et al. Effect of delayed versus early umbilical cord clamping on neonatal outcomes and iron status at 4 months: a randomized controlled trial. *BMJ.* 2011;343:d7157.

8. Erickson-Owens D, Mercer J, Deoni S, et al. The effects of delayed cord clamping on 12-month brain myelin content: a randomized controlled trial. *2nd Congress of joint European Neonatal Societies (jENS) Conference.* 2017; Abstract 534.

9. Sommer R, Stonestreet B, William Oh, et al. Hemodynamics effecting delayed cord clamping in premature infants. *Pediatrics.* 2012;129(3):e667.

10. Katheria AC, Leone TA, Woelkers D, et al. The effects of umbilical cord milking on hemodynamics and neonatal outcomes in premature neonates. *J Pediatr.* 2014;164(5):1045–1050.

11. Andersson O, Lindquist B, Lindgren M, et al. Effect of delayed cord clamping on neurodevelopment at 4 years of age: a randomized controlled trial. *JAMA Pediatr.* 2015;169(7):631–638.

12. Mercer JS, Erickson-Owens DA, Vohr BR, et al. Effects of placental transfusion on neonatal and 18-month outcomes in preterm infants: a randomized controlled trial. *J Pediatr.* 2016;168:50–55.

13. Rabe H, Sawyer A, Amess P, et al. Neurodevelopmental outcomes at 2 and 3.5 years for very preterm babies enrolled in a randomized trial of milking the umbilical cord versus delayed cord clamping. *Neonatology.* 2016;109(2):113–119.

14. Fogarty M, Osborn DA, Askie L, et al. Delayed versus early umbilical cord clamping for preterm infants: a systematic review and meta-analysis. *Am J Obstet Gynecol.* 2018;218(1):1–18.

15. Yao AC, Lind J. Effect of gravity on placental transfusion. *Lancet.* 1969;2(7619):505–508.

16. Yao AC, Moinian M, Lind J. Distribution of blood between infant and placenta after birth. *Lancet.* 1969;2(7626):871–873.

17. Royal College of Obstetricians and Gynaecologists (RCOG). Guidelines. Clamping of the umbilical cord and placental transfusion (Scientific Impact Paper #14). 2015. *www.rcog.org.uk.*

18. American Academy of Pediatrics (AAP). Delayed umbilical cord clamping after birth. *Pediatrics.* 2017;139(6). doi:10.1542/peds.2017-0957.

19. Wyllie J, Perlman JM, Kattwinkel J, et al. Part 7: Neonatal resuscitation: 2015 International consensus on cardiopulmonary resuscitation and emergency cardiovascular care science with treatment recommendations. *Resuscitation.* 2015;95:e169–e201.

20. Perlman JM, Wyllie J, Kattwinkel J, et al. Part 7: Neonatal resuscitation: 2015 International consensus on cardiopulmonary resuscitation and emergency cardiovascular care science with treatment recommendations. *Circulation*. 2015;132(16 suppl 1):S204–S241.

21. Sweet DG, Carnielli V, Greisen G, et al. European consensus guidelines on the management of respiratory distress syndrome—2016 Update. *Neonatology*. 2017;111(2): 107–125.

22. World Health Organization (WHO). *Guideline: Delayed Umbilical Cord Clamping for Improved Maternal and Infant Health and Nutrition Outcomes*. Geneva: World Health Organization; 2014. http://www.who.int/nutrition/publications/guidelines/cord_clamping/en/.

23. American College of Nurse-Midwives (ACNM). Position statement: delayed umbilical cord clamping. 2014. *www.midwife.org.*

24. Hutton EK, Hassan ES. Late vs. early clamping of the umbilical cord in full-term neonates: systematic review and meta analysis of controlled trials. *JAMA*. 2007;297(11):1241–1252.

25. Mercer JS, Vohr BR, McGrath MM, et al. Delayed cord clamping in very preterm infants reduces the incidence of intraventricular hemorrhage and late-onset sepsis: a randomized controlled trial. *Pediatrics*. 2006;117(4):1235–1242.

26. Katheria AC, Truong G, Cousins L, et al. Umbilical cord milking versus delayed cord clamping in preterm infants. *Pediatrics*. 2015;136:61–69.

27. Katheria AC, Brown MK, Rich W, et al. Placental transfusion in newborns who need resuscitation. *Front Pediatr*. 2017;5(1):1.

28. Cook LMS. Placental transfusion for neonatal resuscitation after a complete abruption. *AWHONN Connections*. 2015. https://awhonnconnections.org/2015/06/09/placental-transfusion-for-neonatal-resuscitation-after-a-complete-abruption/.

29. Thomas MR, Yoxall CW, Weeks AD, et al. Providing newborn resuscitation at the mother's bedside: assessing the safety, usability and acceptability of a mobile trolley. *BMC Pediatr*. 2014;14:135.

30. Mercer JS, Skovgaard RL, Peareara-Eaves J, et al. Nuchal cord management and nurse-midwifery practice. *J Midwifery Women Health*. 2005;50(5):373–379.

31. American College of Obstetricians and Gynecologists (ACOG). Committee opinion no 648: umbilical cord blood banking. *Obstet Gynecol*. 2015;126(6):e127–e129.

32. Hosono S, Mugishima H, Takahashi S, et al. One-time umbilical cord milking after cord cutting has same effectiveness as multiple-time umbilical cord milking in infants born at 29 weeks of gestation: a retrospective study. *J Perinatol*. 2015;35(8):590–594.

Transfusion of Blood and Blood Products

Jennifer L. Webb, Yunchuan Delores Mo, Cyril Jacquot, and Naomi L. C. Luban

OVERVIEW

Blood Products Utilized in Neonates

1. Red blood cells (RBCs)
2. Fresh or reconstituted whole blood (WB)
3. Platelet concentrates derived from WB or plateletpheresis
4. Fresh-frozen plasma (FFP), plasma frozen within 24 hours (FP24), or thawed plasma
5. Cryoprecipitate
6. Granulocyte concentrates derived from granulocytapheresis

Sources of Blood Products

1. Banked donor blood and blood products
2. Directed donor transfusions
3. Autologous fetal blood transfusions (delayed cord clamping)

Indications, requirements, and transfusion techniques differ for each procedure and component. Simple transfusions are discussed in this chapter. Exchange transfusions are discussed in Chapter 49. Complications common to all blood products are listed later in this chapter.

A. Precautions (1)

1. Whenever possible, obtain informed consent prior to transfusions, delineating risks, benefits, and alternatives to transfusion.
2. Limit use of transfusions to justified indications.
3. Select the blood product appropriate for infant's condition.

4. Confirm with proper identifiers at bedside that blood product is for correct patient. Maintain all records relevant to collection, preparation, transfusion, and clinical outcome.
5. Avoid excessive transfusion volume or rate for current patient size unless acute blood loss or shock dictates rapid transfusion.
6. Store blood and blood products appropriately. Freezing and lysis may occur if RBCs are stored in unmonitored refrigerators.
   a. Use blood bank refrigerator which is continuously monitored and maintained within a specific temperature storage of RBCs, WB, thawed plasma, and thawed cryoprecipitate until the time of transfusion.
   b. Temperature should be controlled at 1° to 6°C with constant temperature monitors and alarm systems.
   c. Refrigerator should be quality controlled at least daily.
   d. Refrigerator should be designated for blood products only.
   e. Store platelets at 20° to 24°C with continuous agitation until the time of transfusion.
   f. Store frozen plasma at ≤−18°C.
7. RBCs and WB should be out of refrigeration for <4 hours to minimize risk of bacterial contamination and RBC hemolysis.
8. Use approved blood-warming devices for RBCs and WB. Syringes for aliquots must not be warmed in water baths because of the risk of contamination.
9. Stop transfusion if transfusion reaction is suspected. Symptoms may include:
   a. Tachycardia, bradycardia, or arrhythmia
   b. Tachypnea
   c. Systolic blood pressure increases of >15 mm Hg, unless this is the desired effect

d. Temperature above 38°C and/or increase in temperature of ≥1°C
e. Hyperglycemia or hypoglycemia
f. Cyanosis
g. Skin rash, hives, or flushing
h. Hematuria/hemoglobinuria
i. Hyperkalemia

10. Transfuse RBCs cautiously in infants with incipient or existing cardiac failure (2).
    a. Monitor heart rate, blood pressure, and peripheral perfusion.
    b. Consider partial exchange transfusion if the patient cannot tolerate the increase in blood volume from simple transfusion
       (1) With hemoglobin level <5 to 7 g/dL
       (2) With cord hemoglobin <10 g/dL

11. Prevent fluctuations in glucose during or after RBC transfusion (3).
    a. In infants weighing <1,200 g or in other unstable infants, to prevent hypoglycemia
       (1) Do not discontinue parenteral glucose administration
       (2) Establish separate IV line for blood administration
    b. As transfused blood may have elevated glucose concentration, expect rebound hypoglycemia in infants with hyperinsulinism or after large glucose load from exchange transfusion.

B. Pretransfusion Testing and Processing (1)

1. Blood group and Rh type
   a. Maternal ABO blood group and Rh type: Screen maternal serum for unexpected antibodies.
   b. Infant's ABO blood group and Rh type: Screen infant's serum for unexpected antibodies if maternal blood is unavailable.
   c. Cord blood may be used for initial testing.
   d. Infant's blood group is determined from the red cells alone, because the corresponding anti-A and anti-B isoagglutinins are usually weak or absent in neonatal serum.

2. Cross-matching
   a. Compatible blood may be low–anti-A, anti-B titer group O Rh-negative blood, or blood of the infant's ABO group and Rh type (except in alloimmune hemolytic disease of the newborn).
   b. Conventional cross-match is not required if the infant is <4 months old and no unexpected antibodies are detected with the initial sample.
   c. Compatibility testing for repeated small-volume transfusions is usually unnecessary because formation of alloantibodies is extremely rare in the first 4 months of life.
   d. If antibody screen (indirect antiglobulin test [IAT]) is positive in mother or infant:

(1) Serologic investigation to identify antibody(ies) is necessary.
(2) Full compatibility testing is required.
(3) If anti-A or anti-B detected in the infant's sample, infant should receive RBCs lacking A or B antigen until antibody screen is negative.

e. If infant has received large volumes of plasma or platelets, passive acquisition of antibodies may occur; cross-matching of RBCs is recommended.
f. If directed donor blood from a parent is used, cross-matching is required.

3. Specifically processed products (4)
   a. CMV safe products
      (1) Cytomegalovirus (CMV) seronegative or leukodepleted (LD) blood is recommended for infants with birth weight ≤1,200 g born to seronegative mothers or those with unknown serostatus (5) (see "Complications" Section).
      (2) Use of universal LD and/or CMV seronegative products is institution specific (6).
   b. Irradiation to prevent transfusion-associated graft-versus-host disease (TA-GVHD) (7)
      (1) WB, PRBCs, previously frozen RBCs, granulocyte and platelet concentrates, and fresh plasma have been implicated in TA-GVHD; LD products have also been implicated.
      (2) Clinical indications for irradiated blood components are listed in **Table 48.1**.

TABLE 48.1 **Clinical Indications for Irradiated Blood Components (2,46)**

1. Intrauterine transfusion (IUT) or postnatal transfusion in neonate who had received IUT
2. Premature infants, variably defined by weight and postgestational age
3. Congenital immunodeficiency suspected or confirmed
4. Neonatal exchange transfusion recipients
5. Hematologic/solid organ malignancy
6. Significant immunosuppression related to chemotherapy, radiation, or hematopoietic stem cell transplant
7. Recipient of familial blood donation
8. Recipient of HLA-matched or cross-match–compatible platelets or granulocytes

From Wong EC, Punzalan RC. Neonatal and pediatric transfusion practice. In: Fung MK, ed. *Technical Manual of the American Association of Blood Banks*. 19th ed. Bethesda, MD: AABB Press; 2017:613; From Overview of Special Products. In: Wong EC, Rosef SD, King K, et al., eds. *Pediatric Transfusion: A Physician's Handbook*. 4th ed. Bethesda, MD: AABB Press; 2015:185.

(3) Some institutions provide irradiated blood products to all neonates to avoid TA-GVHD in patients with undiagnosed immunodeficiency.

C. Equipment

1. Blood product (see Appendix E)
2. Cardiorespiratory monitor
3. Blood and blood administration set: All blood and blood components must be filtered immediately prior to transfusion to remove blood clots and particles that are potentially harmful to the recipient
   a. Transfusion services may supply RBCs and occasionally platelets and cryoprecipitate, prefiltered to the neonatal intensive care unit (NICU).
   b. If not prefiltered, administration sets with inline filter of 120- to 260-μm pore size may be used for all products (standard size is 170 to 260 μm).
   c. Microaggregate filters, 20- to 40-μm pore size are infrequently used in the NICU.
      (1) Usefulness questionable and unnecessary if LD and/or additive solution RBCs used
      (2) Must follow manufacturer's instructions
      (3) Some only function if product is dripped
      (4) Not advisable for syringe administration as they may cause hemolysis
   d. Leukodepletion (2,4,6)
      (1) Removes 99.9% of white blood cells (WBCs)
      (2) Must follow manufacturers instruction if performing at bedside
      (3) Prestorage LD (performed by collecting facility) preferred to poststorage (bedside) LD
      (4) Attenuation/abrogation of CMV and other viruses such as Epstein–Barr virus (EBV) and human T-lymphotrophic virus (HTLV) I/II harbored in WBCs
4. Sterile syringe (if blood is not already aliquoted into a syringe)
5. Blood warmer not needed for small-volume transfusions
6. Automated syringe pump with appropriate tubing and needle (8–14)
   a. Least hemolysis occurs with peristaltic pumps, but syringe pumps may be used for precise, small volume administration.
   b. Vascular access: RBCs may be transfused through 24-, 25-, or 27-gauge needles and short catheters, and there is growing evidence supporting the safety of intermittent transfusions through 24- or 27-gauge PICC lines; however, historically, those have not been the preferred access for transfusion.
   c. The amount of hemolysis that results from infusion of RBCs is directly proportionate to the age of the blood and the rate of transfusion, and inversely proportional to needle size.
   d. Hyperkalemia, hemoglobinuria, and renal dysfunction may result if hemolyzed blood is transfused.
7. Normal saline flush (1 mL or more) to clear IV solution from line.

RED BLOOD CELL TRANSFUSIONS

A. Indications

1. Guidelines and justifications for transfusions are controversial because there are few studies that address the appropriateness of various transfusion triggers in neonates. Therefore, indications for RBC transfusion vary among different institutions.
2. Current guidelines for neonatal RBC transfusion therapy are given in **Table 48.2** (15,16). In general:

TABLE 48.2 Guidelines for Transfusion of RBCs in Patients <4 Months of Age (15,29)

CLINICAL STATUS	TARGET HEMATOCRIT (%)
For severe cardiopulmonary disease (requiring mechanical ventilation with FiO$_2$ >0.35)	>40–45
For moderate cardiopulmonary disease	>30–40
For major surgery	>30–35
For infants with stable anemia with unexplained apnea/bradycardia, tachycardia, or poor growth	>20–25

Definitions for level of severity of cardiopulmonary disease may be defined individually by institution.
Modified from Fasano RM, Paul W, Luban NL. Blood component therapy for the neonate. In: Martin R, Fanaroff A, eds. *Fanaroff & Martin's Neonatal-Perinatal Medicine*. 10th ed. St. Louis, MO: Elsevier; 2014:1344–1361; Strauss RG. How I transfuse red blood cells and platelets to infants with the anemia and thrombocytopenia of prematurity. *Transfusion*. 2008;48:209–217.

   a. Infants with significant cardiopulmonary disease require more RBC transfusion support.
   b. Infants receiving minimal cardiopulmonary support, with acceptable weight gain, and with minimal episodes of apnea and bradycardia, require less RBC support.
3. Liberal versus conservative RBC transfusion
   a. Studies on liberal versus conservative RBC transfusion practices have demonstrated mixed results in terms of clinical benefit of liberal transfusion practices toward preventing apneic episodes and immediate neurologic sequelae (17,18).
   b. Long-term neurodevelopmental benefit has not been ascertained for either transfusion practice and evidence is conflicting (19–21).
   c. Observational studies have documented a temporal relationship between RBC transfusions with the occurrence of necrotizing enterocolitis (NEC)

in premature infants; however, prospective studies and meta-analyses have shown a protective effect of transfusions (22–28).

d. The relationship between RBC transfusions and NEC in premature infants is being evaluated further.

B. Contraindications

1. None absolute
2. Exert caution in patient with:
   a. Volume overload
   b. Congestive heart failure
   c. T-activation (see Section "Complications of Blood Transfusions") (3,29)

C. Technique

1. Determine total amount of blood needed.
   a. Calculate volume of blood for transfusion. Most infants are transfused 10 to 15 mL/kg of RBCs, which will increase the hemoglobin by 2 to 3 g/dL.
   b. RBC volume required = (EBV × [Hct desired − Hct observed])/Hct of RBC unit
      (1) Hct is hematocrit
      (2) EBV is the estimated patient's blood volume 80 to 85 mL/kg in full-term infants and approximately 100 to 120 mL/kg in preterm infants
      (3) RBC units collected in citrate-phosphate-dextrose-adenine (CPDA-1) have an Hct of approximately 70%, RBCs in extended-storage additive solutions (AS) have an Hct ≤60%
2. Include volume of blood needed for dead space of tubing, filter, pump mechanism (varies from system to system; may be as much as 30 mL).
3. Obtain blood product (see Appendix E).
   a. Several studies have documented the safety of using PRBCs stored in extended-storage AS for small-volume, intermittent transfusions (30–32).
   b. Transfusions of ≤15 mL/kg of CPDA-1 or AS RBCs stored to maximum outdate (35 or 42 days) deliver approximately 0.3 mEq/kg of K^+ which does not pose a significant risk to most neonates when transfused slowly over 2 to 4 hours (2,3).
   c. A randomized controlled trial showed no benefit to using ≤7-day-old blood as compared to standard-of-care transfusion practice for intermittent transfusions in premature infants (33).
   d. Use of split RBC packs effectively limits donor exposures, and these are safe for use in neonatal small-volume transfusions up to the outdate (2,34,35). This practice requires sterile connecting devices, and either transfer packs or syringe sets that permit multiple aliquots to be removed (**Figs. 48.1** and **48.2**).

e. Avoid use of old RBCs for large-volume transfusions (including massive and exchange transfusions as well as extracorporeal membrane oxygenation [ECMO] circuit priming), unless the additive is removed by inverted storage or centrifugation; risks of hyperosmolality, hyperglycemia, hypernatremia, hyperkalemia, hyperphosphatemia are postulated (3,31,36).
   f. Despite concerns about AS, infants on ECMO have tolerated RBCs stored in AS well (37).
4. Verify whether cross-matched product is necessary or un–cross-matched product is adequate.
5. Verify appropriateness of blood selected for infant by comparing blood product and unit tag (integral to blood unit) information, patient identification, and orders. Barcode reading devices are advisable.
   a. Confirm informed consent has been obtained (if possible)—Note: Should obtain informed consent even if two physicians sign for initial transfusion (emergency situation). Refer to institutional policy.
   b. Confirm recipient identity using two identifiers.
   c. Verify information on blood unit tag and blood bag/syringe.

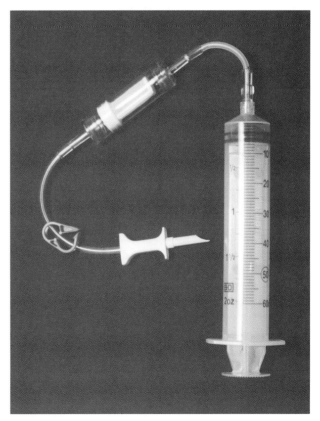

FIGURE 48.1 Neonatal syringe set with filter. (Courtesy of Charter Medical Ltd., Winston-Salem, North Carolina.) This system, when used with sterile connection technology, provides a closed delivery system that maintains primary unit outdate. Syringe blood aliquots (PRCBs, plasma) must be administered to the patient within 24 hours and syringe platelet aliquots within 4 hours.

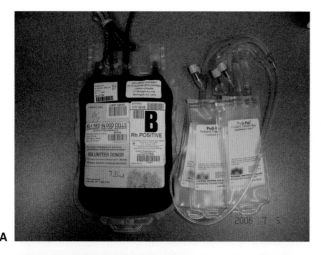

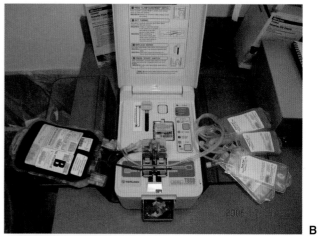

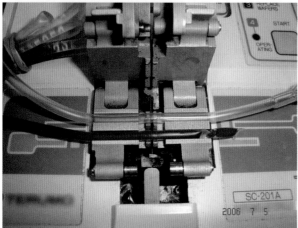

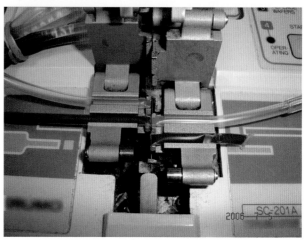

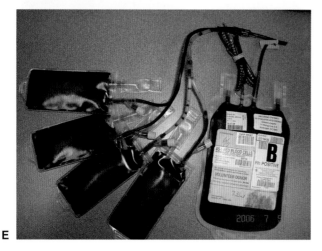

FIGURE 48.2 Use of a sterile connecting device. **A:** An adult RBC unit is shown along with a set of pediatric transfer bags. The transfer bags can be attached by spiking the unit, causing it to expire in 24 hours; alternatively, the transfer bags can be connected using a sterile connection device. **B, C:** The separate tubings are loaded into the tubing holders of the device. The covers are closed. **D:** A welding wafer heated to about 500°F melts through the tubing. The tubing holders realign and the welding wafer retracts allowing the tubing ends to fuse together. **E:** The unit can now be aliquoted as needed. Because a functionally closed system has been maintained, the expiration date of the blood has not changed.

d. Blood group and type of both donor and recipient
e. Expiration date and time of product
f. Product meets restrictions as ordered by physician or by institutional guidelines
6. Restrictions that may be evident on the blood product and transfusion tag include:
a. CMV: Tested/untested
b. Irradiated: Yes/no

c. Directed (familial) donation: Yes/no
d. RBC antigen-negative: Yes/no
e. Sickle tested-negative: Yes/no
f. Other restrictions specified: Yes/no
7. Warming RBCs.
a. There is no need to warm small-volume RBC aliquots, particularly if the transfusion is given over 2 to 3 hours.

b. RBCs may be warmed by placing the syringe beside the infant in the warm-air incubator for 30 minutes prior to transfusion.

c. Inappropriate warming by exposure of blood to heat lamps or phototherapy lights may produce hemolysis. Shielding the RBC component and tubing from UV light (used for phototherapy) are recommended (38,39).

8. Adhere to aseptic technique throughout procedure.

9. If prefiltered RBCs are provided by the blood bank in a syringe, attach tubing directly to syringe.

10. If RBCs are provided in a bag, use large-bore needle (18 gauge or larger) to withdraw volume into syringe. Filter should be placed between bag and syringe (**Fig. 48.1**).

11. Prime tubing with blood. Clear syringe and tubing of bubbles, and mount into infusion device.

12. Verify patency of vascular access.

13. Clear line into patient with normal saline.

14. Record and monitor vital signs.

15. Determine spot glucose test. Repeat hourly as needed.

16. Begin transfusion at controlled rate: 3 to 5 mL/kg/hr.

17. Gently invert container of blood every 15 to 30 minutes to minimize sedimentation if RBCs are provided in a bag. This step is not required for syringes since they contain prefiltered RBCs.

18. Stop transfusion if any adverse change in condition occurs.

19. At end of infusion, clear blood from line with saline.

20. Check recipient hemoglobin and hematocrit, if necessary, at least 2 hours after transfusion.

21. If posttransfusion hematocrit/hemoglobin is not up to expected level, consider:
   a. Low hematocrit of RBC unit (extended-storage AS vs. CPDA-1 units)
   b. Inappropriate calculation of transfusion requirement
   c. Ongoing blood loss or hemolysis in the recipient (hemolytic disease of the newborn, G6PD deficiency, hereditary membranopathy, etc.)
   d. Transfusion reaction
   e. Hemolysis from T-activation
   f. Hemolysis from extrinsic damage (mechanical) to RBCs
   g. Hemolysis due to ABO or other RBC incompatibility. Testing may show:
      (1) Infant has circulating anti-A, anti-B, or anti-AB, which is bound to A or B antigens on transfused RBCs.
      (2) Direct anti-globulin (DAT) test negative initially but now positive.
      (3) Unexpected increase in bilirubin or LDH.
      (4) Infant has RBC antibody other than ABO on repeat type and screen (IAT).

FRESH OR RECONSTITUTED WHOLE BLOOD TRANSFUSIONS

A WB unit contains approximately 450 to 500 mL of blood and 63 to 70 mL of anticoagulant-preservative solution. Fresh WB is defined as WB refrigerated for up to 48 hours from the time of collection. WB stored longer than 48 hours has decreasing levels of coagulation factors V and VIII, does not contain functional platelets or granulocytes, and has a progressively higher concentration of K^+. Reconstituted WB is prepared by adding a unit of RBCs to a compatible unit of FFP and may be preferable to the use of stored WB (29,40).

A. Indications

1. Massive transfusion for acute blood loss in excess of 25% of total blood volume (TBV) when restoration of blood volume and oxygen-carrying capacity are needed simultaneously

2. Exchange transfusions

3. Cardiopulmonary bypass (CPB)

4. ECMO

5. Continuous hemofiltration

6. There currently exists no consensus within the United States on the use of fresh WB, reconstituted WB, or reconstituted *fresh* WB (RFWB) for CPB pump priming or postoperative transfusion support in neonates with congenital heart disease
   a. Randomized controlled trials have questioned the use of WB (41) and have suggested an advantage in clinical outcomes in infants with congenital heart disease receiving RFWB during CPB surgery (42). However, observational data suggest fresh WB in patients <2-year old undergoing complex cardiac surgery may limit subsequent donor exposures (43).
   b. Additional prospective studies are warranted to determine optimal age and type of WB units for neonates undergoing CPB surgery.
   c. Units or components <7 to 14 days are generally acceptable for large volume priming of extracorporeal/CPB circuits, with fresher units being preferable (2).
   d. Fresh WB is not universally available.

B. Precautions (3,4,31)

1. Not suitable for simple transfusion for anemia.

2. Not suitable for correction of coagulation factor deficiencies.

3. Hyperkalemia may result from rapid transfusion of large volumes.

4. Anticoagulant (citrate) effects must be considered for large volume and consideration given to calcium repletion (44).

5. Platelet count needs to be monitored closely following large-volume exchange transfusion due to lack of platelets in reconstituted WB.
6. Reconstitution of WB to desired hematocrit may take time, so early notification to the blood bank is critical.
7. Warming of product(s) may be necessary due to large volume administered, but should not delay transfusion.

C. Equipment and Technique

1. Same as for RBCs.
2. The rate of transfusion may be increased to 10 to 20 mL/kg/hr to replace acute blood loss.
3. Inline filters often used for complex mechanical procedures (CPB, ECMO).

PLATELET TRANSFUSIONS

A. Indications

1. The platelet count at which transfusion is recommended must be individualized since hemostatic competence is determined not only by the quantity of platelets but also by platelet function, vascular integrity, coagulation factor levels, and underlying clinical conditions (**Table 48.3**).
2. A recent controlled trial reported that infants randomized to higher platelet transfusion threshold (50,000/μL) had higher occurrence of a new major bleeding episode or death than infants randomized to the lower threshold (25,000/μL) (46).

B. Contraindications (47)

1. Autoimmune thrombocytopenic purpura (neonatal ITP)
2. Heparin-induced thrombocytopenia (HIT)
3. Bleeding due to coagulopathy only (i.e., vitamin K deficiency)
4. Bleeding due to anatomic defect or controllable with direct pressure/local measures (i.e., surgical bleeding)

C. Precautions

1. Use type-specific (e.g., Rh-negative) platelets when the potential for sensitization is present (i.e., in Rh-negative female). Although platelets do not have Rh antigens, products may be contaminated by small numbers of RBCs (significantly fewer in apheresis vs. WB-derived units which may cause Rh sensitization) (48).
2. Use platelets from donor with ABO-compatible plasma whenever possible. Isohemagglutinins in ABO-incompatible plasma may result in hemolysis, a positive direct antiglobulin test (DAT), and shorter in vivo platelet survival than anticipated.

TABLE 48.3 Guidelines for Platelet Transfusion in Neonates (2,5,45)

With Thrombocytopenia
1. Platelet count $<25 \times 10^9$/L in neonate with failure of platelet production in the absence of bleeding
2. Platelet count $<50 \times 10^9$/L in stable premature infant:
   - With active bleeding
   - Invasive procedure with failure of platelet production
   - Extremely low–birth-weight (<1,000 g) infants within the first week of life
3. Platelet count $<50 \times 10^9$/L in neonates with (or presumed) NAIT[a]
4. Platelet count $<100 \times 10^9$/L in sick premature infant:
   - With active bleeding
   - Invasive procedure in patient with disseminated intravascular coagulation

Without Thrombocytopenia
1. Active bleeding in association with qualitative platelet defect
2. Unexplained, excessive bleeding in a patient undergoing cardiopulmonary bypass
3. Patient undergoing extracorporeal membrane oxygenation:
   - With a platelet count of $<100 \times 10^9$/L
   - With higher platelet counts and bleeding

[a]NAIT, neonatal alloimmune thrombocytopenia.
Adapted from Wong EC, Punzalan RC. Neonatal and pediatric transfusion practice. In: Fung MK, ed. *Technical Manual of the American Association of Blood Banks*. 19th ed. Bethesda, MD: AABB Press; 2017:613; Wong EC, Paul WM. Intrauterine, neonatal, and pediatric transfusion therapy. In: Mintz PD, eds. *Transfusion Therapy: Clinical Principles and Practice*. Bethesda, MD: AABB Press; 2011:209; New EV, Berryman J, Bolton-Maggs PH, et al. Guidelines on transfusion for fetuses, neonates, and older children. *Br J Haematol*. 2016;175:784–828.

---

3. Certain diseases (e.g., neonatal alloimmune thrombocytopenia [NAIT]) require antigen-negative platelet products to achieve optimal platelet count increments. However, random donor platelets may be used in the interim to sustain platelet counts and minimize bleeding complications such as intraventricular hemorrhages.
4. Transfuse platelets as soon after preparation as possible. Platelets should never be refrigerated or warmed.
5. Platelets should not be infused through arterial lines.

D. Equipment and Technique

1. Platelets
   a. WB-derived platelet concentrate (5.5×10^{10} platelets in 40 to 70 mL of plasma)
      (1) Separated from WB by centrifugation within 8 hours of blood draw and resuspended in plasma
      (2) Shelf life of 5 days
   b. Volume-reduced platelets
      (1) Standard platelet concentrate further concentrated to a volume of 15 to 20 mL by centrifugation

(2) Associated with loss of platelets and possible decrease in platelet function

(3) Shelf life reduced to 4 hours

(4) Use only if the infant has oliguria or severe volume load sensitivity, or if the unit contains ABO-incompatible plasma

c. Apheresis platelets (3×10^{11} platelets in volume of 250 mL of plasma)

(1) Automated collection instrument removes only platelets and returns RBCs and plasma to donor

(2) Usually LD before storage

(3) Repeat donations from same donor every 48 hours permissible under select circumstances

(4) High yield of platelets

(5) More expensive product

(6) Useful when multiple platelet transfusions of a particular phenotype are required, as in NAIT or for patients on ECMO

(7) May be typed for HLA or HPA antigens in case of NAIT

(8) Maternal or antigen-negative platelets from another donor may be transfused for NAIT. All maternal plateletpheresis products should be washed, irradiated, and resuspended in ABO group-compatible plasma or saline prior to transfusion

2. Calculate volume to transfuse based on type of platelet product

a. 10 to 15 mL/kg of a WB-derived platelet concentrate provides 10×10^9 platelets/kg and should increase platelet count by approximately 50×10^9/L in the absence of ongoing consumption. Similar calculations may be used for apheresis platelets, but studies do not confirm posttransfusion increments.

b. Equivalent unit (EU) calculations are preferred over mL/kg dosing for apheresis platelets.

c. 1 EU is the volume of a platelet aliquot that has a minimum platelet content of 5.5×10^{10} platelets (approximately one WB-derived platelet concentrate).

d. The standard dose based on this method is 1 EU per 5 to 10 kg, with a minimum dose of 1 EU. Volume reduction may be necessary for some extremely low–birth-weight infants.

e. Other products (cross-matched or HLA-matched platelets) may be indicated for platelet refractoriness. Irradiation is indicated when familial and/or HLA-matched units are used.

3. Required equipment

a. Blood administration set with a 120- to 260-μm inline filter, unless platelets have been prefiltered while drawing into a syringe. Specific sets designed for plasma/platelets have inline filters with reduced surface area to increase platelet transfusion efficacy

b. Sterile syringe for automated pump infusion. Use of a syringe technique will increase damage to platelets. Administer by drip if clinically feasible

c. Automated syringe pump

d. Connecting IV tubing

e. IV access, preferably through 23-gauge or larger needle or through umbilical venous catheter (due to risk of catheter-associated thrombosis, institutional policies may prohibit platelet transfusion through umbilical venous catheters) (49)

f. Normal saline flush solution

E. Technique for Platelet Administration by Automated Syringe

1. Estimate the volume of platelets in a single bag by weight to determine fluid load to patient.

2. Confirm correct platelet product.
   a. Patient and unit identification
   b. Patient and donor ABO blood group and Rh type
   c. Other modifications: irradiation, volume reduction, etc.

3. Aseptically attach the following components in sequence
   a. Platelet concentrate or aliquot bag
   b. Platelet administration set, including filter
   c. Three-way stopcock
   d. Transfusion syringe

4. Draw sufficient volume of platelets for transfusion and tubing dead space into syringe. Clear air bubbles.

5. Remove syringe from three-way stopcock and attach to connecting tubing.

6. Establish IV access. If infant is at risk for hypoglycemia with interruption of continuous glucose source, start new IV or monitor closely throughout infusion.

7. Clear IV of glucose solution with a minimum of 1 mL of normal saline.

8. Attach connecting tubing and syringe to IV line.

9. Monitor patient's vital signs.

10. Infuse platelets over 1- to 2-hour period or over shorter duration if tolerated by infant.

11. After infusion is complete, flush IV line with 1 mL of normal saline before restarting glucose solution.

12. Determine survival time of transfused platelets by obtaining platelet counts within 15 to 60 minutes and/or 24 hours posttransfusion if concern for platelet refractoriness.

F. Complications

1. Hemolysis in sensitized patients with antibodies not detected by IAT

2. Rh sensitization in Rh-negative recipient (50)

3. Volume overload

4. Allergic reactions, including hypotension

5. Transfusion-related acute lung injury (TRALI) (51)

6. Possible increased morbidity in NEC (52)

Complications discussed in more detail in "Complications of Blood Products" Section.

GRANULOCYTE TRANSFUSIONS

A. Indications

1. Granulocyte transfusions are infrequently administered because of improvements in antimicrobial medications and supportive care as well as increasing use of recombinant granulocyte- and granulocyte/macrophage-stimulating factors.
2. Granulocyte transfusion may be considered in the following conditions; however, reduction in morbidity or mortality has not been confirmed in randomized trials (53).
    a. Neonates <14 days old with bacterial sepsis and absolute neutrophil count (ANC) (+ band count) <1,700/uL, and older neonates with bacterial sepsis and ANC (+ band count) <500/uL.
    b. Neutropenic neonates with fungal disease not responsive to standard antifungal therapy.

B. Equipment and Technique

1. Granulocyte concentrates for neonatal use are prepared by automated granulocytapheresis, and should contain 1 to 2×10^9 neutrophils/kg in a volume of 10 to 15 mL/kg. Steroid- and G-CSF-mobilized donors are preferred.
2. Daily transfusions are indicated until there is clinical improvement and evidence of recovery of neutrophil counts.
3. Components must be ABO/Rh and cross-match–compatible with the recipient due to significant RBC contamination.
4. Products should be irradiated and preferably CMV negative if the recipient is also seronegative.
5. The product should not be refrigerated or warmed above room temperature.
6. Infusions should be given as soon as possible after collection. For patients with small blood volumes, products may be split into two or more doses depending on total yield for multiple infusions as long as sufficient time remains in the shelf life (see Precautions below).
7. Standard 120- to 260-µm filters should be used for infusion; microaggregate and LD filters must be avoided to prevent inadvertent removal of leukocytes.

C. Precautions

1. Storage of product for >8 hours is associated with a rapid decrease in WBC function, resulting in decreased efficacy of the product. The product expires 24 hours from the time of collection.
2. Fever, alloimmunization, TRALI, and CMV infection have all been reported complications (53).

PLASMA PRODUCTS AND CRYOPRECIPITATE

A. Indications (2,54)

1. Plasma (including FFP, FP24, and thawed plasma)
    Clinically significant bleeding or for correction of hemostatic defects prior to invasive procedures in the presence of the following:
    a. Complex factor deficiency unresponsive to vitamin K replacement
    b. Isolated congenital factor deficiency for which virus-inactivated plasma-derived or recombinant factor concentrates are unavailable
    c. Similarly, for acquired single or combined factor deficiencies, FFP or FP24 may be used when virus-inactivated plasma-derived or recombinant factor concentrates are unavailable
    d. Support during the management of disseminated intravascular coagulation
2. Cryoprecipitate
    a. Congenital or acquired dys- or hypofibrinogenemia[1]
    b. Congenital FXIII deficiency in the absence of FXIII concentrate[1]
    c. Bleeding associated with von Willebrand disease and hemophilia A when virally inactivated plasma-derived or recombinant factor products are unavailable.

B. Contraindications

1. No absolute contraindications
2. Exert caution when the possibility of volume overload exists.
3. Use with caution in the setting of NEC and/or T-activation as transfusion may aggravate hemolysis (55).
4. Not indicated for hypovolemic shock in the absence of bleeding, nutritional support, treatment of immunodeficiency, or prevention of intraventricular hemorrhage.

C. Equipment and Technique

See Platelet Transfusions.

1. Cross-matching is not required because type-specific or universally compatible AB-negative product is usually issued.
2. Plasma dosing is 10 to 20 mL/kg; multiple transfusions may be required until the underlying condition resolves.
3. Once thawed, FFP or FP24 should be transfused within 6 hours for labile factor replacement.

---

[1]In the presence of active bleeding or planned invasive procedures.

4. In cases for which repeated plasma transfusions are required, a thawed unit from a single donor may be divided into smaller aliquots and used within 24 hours if stored between 1°C and 6°C.

5. A dose of 1 unit of cryoprecipitate per 5 kg patient weight will increase the total fibrinogen by approximately 100 mg/dL in the absence of ongoing consumption.

6. 1 unit of cryoprecipitate contains approximately 12 to 20 mL.

DIRECTED DONOR TRANSFUSIONS

A. Potential Problems

Directed donations provide no known benefit in terms of increased safety and may pose unique immunologic and serologic risks to the neonate (29,47).

1. Possible increased risk of transmitting infectious disease because directed donors are often first-time or infrequent donors with no track record of safety, unlike established volunteer donors, whose screening tests are negative repeatedly.

2. Possibility of serologic incompatibility between the recipient baby and the family donors.
   a. Maternal plasma may contain alloantibodies directed against paternal RBC, leukocyte, platelet, and HLA antigens, which may result in significant hemolytic, thrombocytopenic, or pulmonary reactions (56).
   b. Paternal blood cells may express antigens to which the neonate may have been passively immunized by transplacental transfer of maternal antibodies.
   c. Routine pretransfusion testing may not detect these serologic incompatibilities (private epitopes).

3. Although biologic parents may be interested in donating for their infants, many are likely to be ineligible for medical or serologic reasons (57).

B. Precautions

1. Directed donors must be screened as stringently as volunteer donors (e.g., hemoglobin criteria, travel history, medications, etc.).

2. If maternal RBCs or platelets are transfused, they should be irradiated and undergo plasma reduction or washing.

3. Fathers and paternal blood relatives should preferably not serve as donors for blood components containing cellular elements (RBCs, platelets, or granulocytes); if their use is unavoidable, a full antiglobulin cross-match should be performed to detect incompatibilities.

4. All blood components obtained from first- or second-degree relatives should be irradiated prior to transfusion to prevent TA-GVHD.

AUTOLOGOUS FETAL BLOOD TRANSFUSIONS

The placenta contains 75 to 125 mL of blood at birth depending on the gestational age of the infant. Autologous transfusion in an infant can occur by collection, storage, and reinfusion of autologous cord blood, or by delaying cord clamping, a successful variation of autologous transfusion. Both maneuvers potentially provide a substantial volume of fetal blood for the neonate, eliminating the potential risks of anemia, transfusion-transmitted diseases, and TA-GVHD (58). The American College of Obstetricians and Gynecologists currently recommends a delay in umbilical cord clamping in vigorous term and preterm infants for at least 30 to 60 seconds after birth (59) (Chapter 47).

Autologous stored cord blood has been used for open heart surgery and cardiopulmonary circuit priming (60). However, other reports have shown that only a minority of allogeneic RBC transfusions to the infant are spared and that collection/storage costs may not justify the benefits. Additional large, randomized, controlled clinical trials are needed to validate the safety and efficacy of this process before it can become routine practice (61).

A. Indications

1. Delivery room resuscitation of infants with shock and profound anemia, when O Rh-negative RBCs are not immediately available. Delaying cord clamping has been shown to instantly increase RBC mass and circulating blood volume, while decreasing the immediate need of RBC transfusions and possibly the incidence of intraventricular hemorrhage and NEC in the preterm infant (58,62,63).

2. Source of cord blood for freezing for hematopoietic reconstitution.

B. Contraindications

Cord blood collection and storage should not be performed if there is concern for maternal bacteremia as this increases the risk of contaminated products (64). Such scenarios include:

1. Maternal infection
2. Chorioamnionitis
3. Sepsis
4. Hepatitis, HIV
5. Prolonged rupture of membranes >24 hours

C. Complications

1. Bacterial sepsis from contaminated collection (65).
2. Insufficient collection volumes from infants weighing <1,000 g.

3. Over-/undercollection for volume of anticoagulant used (clotting and/or hemolysis can occur in the stored unit).
4. Concern for volume overload to the neonate if cord clamping is delayed; however, no evidence of this in controlled trials.

COMPLICATIONS OF BLOOD TRANSFUSIONS

Transfusions are safer now than ever before, but they are not risk-free.

1. Transmission of infectious diseases: The potential risk of transfusion-transmitted infections in the United States has been dramatically reduced by extensive donor screening and laboratory testing. Current transfusion-transmitted disease testing for allogeneic blood donation includes: Hepatitis B surface antigen (HBsAg) and core antibody (anti-HBc); anti–hepatitis C (anti-HCV), HIV-1/HIV-2 antibodies (anti–HIV-1/2), HTLV-I/HTLV-II antibodies, syphilis (FTA-Abs) and *Trypanosoma cruzi* antibodies; and nucleic acid testing (NAT) for HIV-1/2, hepatitis B virus, HCV, West Nile virus (WNV), and most recently Zika virus (66).
   a. Viruses: Risk varies geographically (66,67)
      (1) HIV: Estimated potential risk in the United States from a blood donor with negative serologic tests is 1 in 2.1 million (67).
      (2) HTLV I and II: Risk estimated at 1 in 2.99 million units transfused (68).
      (3) Hepatitis B virus: Risk 1 in 750,000 to 1 million units transfused (67).
      (4) Hepatitis C virus: Risk 1 in 1.9 million units transfused (67).
      (5) Hepatitis A virus: Risk <1 in 1 million (likely underreported), asymptomatic in newborn, but may cause symptomatic infection in adults who are in contact with infected neonates (69).
      (6) Zika virus: Associated with microcephaly and other fetal abnormalities when placental transmission occurs in acutely infected pregnant women (70). Blood donations in the United States have been screened with an unlicensed nucleic acid test starting in fall 2016 (71). In a preliminary analysis of 466,834 donations, five donors tested positive. The FDA cleared the first approved Zika virus detection test based on viral RNA in the plasma of blood donors in October 2017.
      (7) CMV: Transmitted by cellular blood products (not FFP, FP24, or cryoprecipitate). Risk factors for neonatal transfusion-acquired CMV (TA-CMV) include birth weight <1,200 g, exposure to ≥50 mL of blood, and maternal CMV seronegativity. Risk of TA-CMV from CMV-seronegative or effectively leukoreduced components ("CMV-safe") is <1% to 4% (72,73).
      (8) WNV: Very low risk (1 case in over 35 million units screened during periods of WNV activity [April to December]) (74).
      (9) Hepatitis G, parvovirus B-19, EBV.
   b. Bacteria
      (1) Platelet concentrates and RBCs are most often implicated
      (2) Frequency:
      Approximately 1 per 38,500 U transfused with low prevalence of septic reactions (1 in 250,000) for RBCs (75).
      Approximately 1 per 5,000 U transfused with septic reactions in 1 in 116,000 for platelets, when pretransfusion bacterial screening (i.e., BacT/ALERT system) is employed. Other safety improvements include more thorough donor-skin scrubbing prior to venipuncture and implementation of diversion pouch for first 50 mL of blood (more likely to contain skin plug and bacterial flora) (76). Lower bacterial contamination rates and septic reactions exist for apheresis platelets compared to WB-derived platelets (77).
      (3) Some sites perform point of issue testing on platelets with assays detecting bacterial cell wall components (78,79).
      (4) Organisms:
      Common RBC contaminants include *Yersinia enterocolitica, Serratia* spp., and *Pseudomonas* spp., *Enterobacter* spp., *Campylobacter* spp., and *Escherichia coli*. All have the potential to cause endotoxin-mediated shock in recipients.
      Common platelet contaminants include *Staphylococcus aureus, Staphylococcus epidermidis, Bacillus* spp., *Diphtheroid bacilli*, and *Streptococci*. Most fatal cases of bacterial contaminated platelets involve gram-negative organisms.
      (5) Often a result of contamination by skin flora at time of venipuncture. However, some cases may be due to asymptomatic transiently bacteremic donors (e.g., recent dental procedure).
      (6) *Treponema pallidum*: No new transfusion-transmitted cases reported in >50 years (66).
   c. Protozoa
      (1) Malaria: Rare in the United States but reported even in nonendemic areas (66).
      (2) Babesiosis (donations collected in regions with high prevalence undergo testing for Babesia microti) (80).
      (3) Chagas disease (*Trypanosoma cruzi*).

d. Prions: Creutzfeldt–Jakob
   (1) Few proven cases of transfusion-transmitted new-variant Creutzfeldt–Jakob disease at present. Those described have been in the United Kingdom (81).
   (2) Most blood collection centers attempt to minimize the risk by excluding donors considered to be at higher risk for possibly harboring the infection, by family and travel/residence history, and specific medical history.

e. Pathogen reduction
   (1) All-encompassing term for several techniques (e.g., photochemical activation, solvent/detergent treatment) that broadly inactivate or destroy pathogens by targeting cellular membranes or nucleic acid replication (82).
   (2) Proactive approach to ensuring blood supply safety against emerging infectious organisms.
   (3) Technologies at various stages of development: solvent/detergent treatment currently in use for plasma product derivatives, INTERCEPT (photochemical activation) recently FDA-approved for use in processing platelets/plasma.
   (4) Limited data on use in pediatric/neonatal patients. Concerns exist about photochemical activation's potentially detrimental effects on coagulation factors in plasma and, on platelet function (83). Other unanticipated adverse effects may not have been characterized yet.

2. Hemolytic reactions
   a. **Acute hemolytic immunologic reactions:** Rare, because of absence in infant of naturally occurring anti-A or anti-B antibodies, and infrequent post-transfusion red cell alloimmunization despite multiple transfusions (84).
   b. **T-activation:** A form of immune-mediated hemolysis associated with the transfusion of adult blood containing naturally occurring anti-T antibodies, into neonates with exposure of a normally masked Thomsen–Friedenreich (T) cryptantigen on their RBC surface. T-activation can present with evidence of intravascular hemolysis following transfusion of blood products, or unexplained failure to achieve the expected posttransfusion hemoglobin increment (3,29).
      (1) Commonly observed in premature infants with NEC and/or sepsis (55).
      (2) Suspect T-activation in neonates at risk with intravascular hemolysis, hemoglobinuria, hemoglobinemia following transfusion of blood products, or unexpected failure to achieve post-transfusion hemoglobin increment.
      (3) Routine cross-matching techniques will not detect T-activation when monoclonal ABO antiserum is used.
      (4) Diagnosis: Minor cross-match of neonatal T-activated red cells with donor anti–T-containing serum, discrepancies in forward and reverse blood grouping, confirmed by specific agglutination tests using peanut lectins *Arachis hypogea* and *Glycine soja.*
      (5) Use washed red cells and platelets, and low-titer anti-T plasma (if available) only when hemolysis is confirmed.

3. Nonimmunologic causes of hemolysis
   a. Mechanical, through excessive infusion pressure through small needles or 20- to 40-µm filters
   b. Accidental overheating or freezing of blood
   c. Simultaneous administration of incompatible drugs and fluids (hyperosmolar or hypoosmolar effect)
   d. Transfusion of abnormal donor cells (glucose 6-phosphate dehydrogenase deficiency, hereditary spherocytosis)

4. Other immunologic/nonimmunologic reactions
   a. TA-GVHD (See processing with irradiation for risk factors and prevention page 369)
      (1) Seen 3 to 30 days following transfusion of a cellular component. Symptoms include fever; generalized, erythematous rash with/without progression to desquamation; diarrhea; hepatitis (mild to fulminant liver failure); respiratory distress; and severe pancytopenia
      (2) High mortality rate (80% to 100%)
   b. TRALI:
      (1) Secondary to transfusion of donor blood containing anti-HLA or anti-neutrophil antibodies directed against recipient leukocytes, causing complement activation with microvascular lung injury and capillary leak.
      (2) Presents within 4 hours of transfusion with respiratory distress due to noncardiogenic pulmonary edema, hypotension, fever, and severe hypoxemia.
      (3) Reported only rarely in neonates due to the difficulty in distinguishing TRALI from other causes of respiratory deterioration in sick infants; however, it is documented in the setting of a directed blood transfusion between mother and infant (85).
      (4) Mitigation strategies: plasma and platelets currently only collected from male donors, women who have never been pregnant, or women who test negative on HLA antibody screening test (86).
   c. Transfusion-associated circulatory overload (TACO)
      (1) Nonimmune alteration in pulmonary compliance and blood pressure due to volume overload
      (2) Presents with respiratory distress, cardiogenic pulmonary edema, and hypertension
      (3) Diuresis may be helpful

5. Adverse metabolic effects
   a. Hyperkalemia
      (1) Blood that is irradiated and then refrigerator-stored may have K⁺ levels of 30 to 50 mEq/L or higher in the supernatant plasma.
      (2) Small-volume transfusions of stored red cells do not cause clinically significant elevations in serum K⁺ levels.
      (3) Life-threatening hyperkalemia has been described in sick infants and in those receiving rapid infusions of large volumes of stored red cells (3).
      (4) Washed or fresh (<14 days) red cells are recommended for infants with profound hyperkalemia, renal failure, or when large volumes are transfused rapidly.
      (5) For ECMO, prebypass filtration during circuit prime helps normalize electrolytes (87).
      (6) Other measures to reduce risk of hyperkalemia: anticipating and replacing blood loss before significant hemodynamic compromise occurs and using larger-bore (>23 gauge) peripheral intravenous catheters rather than central venous access (88).
   b. Hypoglycemia or hyperglycemia
   c. Hypocalcemia
   d. Alterations in acid–base balance with large-volume transfusions

References

1. AABB. *Standards for Blood Banks and Transfusion Services.* 31st ed. Bethesda, MD: AABB Press; 2018.
2. Wong EC, Punzalan RC. Neonatal and pediatric transfusion practice. In: Fung MK, ed. *Technical Manual of the American Association of Blood Banks.* 19th ed. Bethesda, MD: AABB Press; 2017:613–640.
3. Fasano RM, Paul WM, Pisciotto PT. Complications of neonatal transfusion. In: Popovsky MA, ed. *Transfusion Reactions.* 4th ed. Bethesda, MD: AABB Press; 2012:471–518.
4. Girelli G, Antoncecchi S, Casadei AM, et al. Recommendations for transfusion therapy in neonatology. *Blood Transfus.* 2015;13(3):484–497.
5. Wong EC, Paul WM. Intrauterine, neonatal, and pediatric transfusion therapy. In: Mintz PD, ed. *Transfusion Therapy: Clinical Principles and Practice.* Bethesda, MD: AABB Press; 2011:209.
6. Fergusson D, Hébert PC, Lee SK, et al. Clinical outcomes following institution of universal leukoreduction of blood transfusions for premature infants. *JAMA.* 2003;289(15): 1950–1956.
7. Kopolovic I, Ostro J, Tsubota H, et al. A systematic review of transfusion-associated graft-versus-host disease. *Blood.* 2015;126(3):406–414.
8. Wong EC, Schreiber S, Criss VR, et al. Feasibility of red blood cell transfusion through small bore central venous catheters used in neonates. *Pediatr Crit Care Med.* 2004;5(1):69–74.
9. Nakamura KT, Sato Y, Erenberg A. Evaluation of a percutaneously placed 27-gauge central venous catheter in neonates weighing less than 1200 grams. *JPEN J Parenter Enteral Nutr.* 1990;14(3):295–299.
10. Oloya RO, Feick HJ, Bozynski ME. Impact of venous catheters on packed red blood cells. *Am J Perinatol.* 1991;8(4):280–283.
11. Frey B, Eber S, Weiss M. Changes in red blood cell integrity related to infusion pumps: a comparison of three different pump mechanisms. *Pediatr Crit Care Med.* 2003;4(4):465–470.
12. Frelich R, Ellis MH. The effect of external pressure, catheter gauge, and storage time on hemolysis in RBC transfusion. *Transfusion.* 2001;41(6):799–802.
13. Repa A, Mayerhofer M, Cardona F, et al. Safety of blood transfusions using 27 gauge neonatal PICC lines: an in vitro study on hemolysis. *Klin Padiatr.* 2013;225(7):379–382.
14. Repa A, Mayerhofer M, Worel N, et al. Blood transfusions using 27 gauge PICC lines: a retrospective clinical study on safety and feasibility. *Klin Padiatr.* 2014;226(1):3–7.
15. Strauss RG. How I transfuse red blood cells and platelets to infants with the anemia and thrombocytopenia of prematurity. *Transfusion.* 2008;48(2):209–217.
16. Widness JA. Treatment and prevention of neonatal anemia. *Neoreviews.* 2008;9(11):526–533.
17. Kirpalani H, Whyte RK, Andersen C, et al. The premature infants in need of transfusion (PINT) study: a randomized, controlled trial of a restrictive (low) versus liberal (high) transfusion threshold for extremely low birth weight infants. *J Pediatr.* 2006;149(3):301–307.
18. Bell EF, Strauss RG, Widness JA, et al. Randomized trial of liberal versus restrictive guidelines for red blood cell transfusion in preterm infants. *Pediatrics.* 2005;115(6):1685–1691.
19. Whyte RK, Kirpalani H, Asztalos EV, et al. Neurodevelopmental outcome of extremely low birth weight infants randomly assigned to restrictive or liberal hemoglobin thresholds for blood transfusion. *Pediatrics.* 2009;123(1):207–213.
20. McCoy TE, Conrad AL, Richman LC, et al. Neurocognitive profiles of preterm infants randomly assigned to lower or higher hematocrit thresholds for transfusion. *Child Neuropsychol.* 2011;17(4):347–367.
21. Keir A, Pal S, Trivella M, et al. Adverse effects of red blood cell transfusions in neonates: a systematic review and meta-analysis. *Transfusion.* 2016;56(11):2773–2780.
22. El-Dib M, Narang S, Lee E, et al. Red blood cell transfusion, feeding and necrotizing enterocolitis in preterm infants. *J Perinatol.* 2011;31(3):183–187.
23. Paul DA, Mackley A, Novitsky A, et al. Increased odds of necrotizing enterocolitis after transfusion of red blood cells in premature infants. *Pediatrics.* 2011;127(4):635–641.
24. Singh R, Visintainer PF, Frantz ID 3rd, et al. Association of necrotizing enterocolitis with anemia and packed red blood cell transfusions in preterm infants. *J Perinatol.* 2011;31(3):176–182.
25. Hay S, Zupancic JA, Flannery DD, et al. Should we believe in transfusion-associated enterocolitis? Applying a GRADE to the literature. *Semin Perinatol.* 2017;41(1):80–91.
26. Rai SE, Sidhu AK, Krishnan RJ. Transfusion-associated necrotizing enterocolitis re-evaluated: a systematic review and meta-analysis. *J Perinat Med.* 2018;46(6):665–676.
27. Wallenstein MB, Arain YH, Birnie KL, et al. Red blood cell transfusion is not associated with necrotizing enterocolitis: a

review of consecutive transfusions in a tertiary neonatal intensive care unit. *J Pediatr*. 2014;165(4):678–682.

28. Patel RM, Knezevic A, Shenvi N, et al. Association of red blood cell transfusion, anemia, and necrotizing enterocolitis in very low-birth-weight Infants. *JAMA*. 2016;315(9):889–897.

29. Fasano RM, Said M, Luban NL. Blood component therapy for the neonate. In: Martin R, Fanaroff A, eds. *Neonatal-Perinatal Medicine*. 10th ed. St. Louis, MO: Elsevier; 2014:1344–1361.

30. Jain R, Jarosz C. Safety and efficacy of AS-1 red blood cell use in neonates. *Transfus Apher Sci*. 2001;24(2):111–115.

31. Luban NL, Strauss RG, Hume HA. Commentary on the safety of red cells preserved in extended-storage media for neonatal transfusions. *Transfusion*. 1991;31(3):229–235.

32. Strauss RG, Burmeister LF, Johnson K, et al. Feasibility and safety of AS-3 red blood cells for neonatal transfusions. *J Pediatr*. 2000;136(2):215–219.

33. Fergusson DA, Hébert P, Hogan DL, et al. Effect of fresh red blood cell transfusions on clinical outcomes in premature, very low-birth-weight infants: The ARIPI randomized trial. *JAMA*. 2012;308(14):1443–1451.

34. Luban NL. Neonatal red blood cell transfusions. *Vox Sang*. 2004;87(Suppl 2):184–188.

35. Mangel J, Goldman M, Garcia C, et al. Reduction of donor exposures in premature infants by the use of designated adenine-saline preserved split red blood cell packs. *J Perinatol*. 2001;21(6):363–367.

36. Luban NL. Massive transfusion in the neonate. *Transfus Med Rev*. 1995;9(3):200–214.

37. Yuan S, Tsukahara E, De La Cruz K, et al. How we provide transfusion support for neonatal and pediatric patients on extracorporeal membrane oxygenation. *Transfusion*. 2013;53(6):1157–1165.

38. Luban NL, Mikesell G, Sacher RA. Techniques for warming red blood cells packaged in different containers for neonatal use. *Clin Pediatr (Phila)*. 1985;24(11):642–644.

39. Strauss RG, Bell EF, Snyder EL, et al. Effects of environmental warming on blood components dispensed in syringes for neonatal transfusions. *J Pediatr*. 1986;109(1):109–113.

40. Bandarenko N, King KE, et al. Blood components. In: *Blood Transfusion Therapy: A Physician's Handbook*. 12th ed. Bethesda, MD: AABB Press; 2017.

41. Mou SS, Giroir BP, Molitor-Kirsch EA, et al. Fresh whole blood versus reconstituted blood for pump priming in heart surgery in infants. *N Engl J Med*. 2004;351(16):1635–1644.

42. Gruenwald CE, McCrindle BW, Crawford-Lean L, et al. Reconstituted fresh whole blood improves clinical outcomes compared with stored component blood therapy for neonates undergoing cardiopulmonary bypass for cardiac surgery: A randomized controlled trial. *J Thorac Cardiovasc Surg*. 2008;136(6):1442–1449.

43. Jobes DR, Sesok-Pizzini D, Friedman D. Reduced transfusion requirement with use of fresh whole blood in pediatric cardiac surgical procedures. *Ann Thorac Surg*. 2015;99(5):1706–1711.

44. Ogunlesi TA, Lesi FE, Oduwole O. Prophylactic intravenous calcium therapy for exchange blood transfusion in the newborn. *Cochrane Database Syst Rev*. 2017;10:CD011048.

45. New HV, Berryman J, Bolton-Maggs PH, et al. Guidelines on transfusion for fetuses, neonates and older children. *Br J Haematol*. 2016;175(5):784–828.

46. Curley A, Stanworth SJ, Willoughby K, et al. Randomized Trial of Platelet-Transfusion Thresholds in Neonates. *N Engl J Med*. 2019;380(3):242–251.

47. Wong EC, Roseff SD, King KE. Blood components. In: *Pediatric Transfusion: A Physician's Handbook*. 4th ed. Bethesda, MD: AABB Press; 2014:1.

48. Cid J, Lozano M, Ziman A, et al. Low frequency of anti-D alloimmunization following D+ platelet transfusion: The anti-D alloimmunization after D-incompatible platelet transfusions (ADAPT) study. *Br J Haematol*. 2015;168(4):598–603.

49. Narang S, Roy J, Stevens TP, et al. Risk factors for umbilical venous catheter-associated thrombosis in very low birth weight infants. *Pediatr Blood Cancer*. 2009;52(1):75–79.

50. Cid J, Lozano M. Risk of Rh(D) alloimmunization after transfusion of platelets from D+ donors to D- recipients. *Transfusion*. 2005;45(3):453.

51. Sanchez R, Toy P. Transfusion related acute lung injury: a pediatric perspective. *Pediatr Blood Cancer*. 2005;45(3):248–255.

52. Kenton AB, Hegemier S, Smith EOB, et al. Platelet transfusions in infants with necrotizing enterocolitis do not lower mortality but may increase morbidity. *J Perinatol*. 2005;25(3):173–177.

53. Pammi M, Brocklehurst P. Granulocyte transfusions for neonates with confirmed or suspected sepsis and neutropenia. *Cochrane Database Syst Rev*. 2011(10):CD003956.

54. Poterjoy BS, Josephson CD. Platelets, frozen plasma, and cryoprecipitate: What is the clinical evidence for their use in the neonatal intensive care unit? *Semin Perinatol*. 2009;33(1):66–74.

55. Moh-Klaren J, Bodivit G, Jugie M, et al. Severe hemolysis after plasma transfusion in a neonate with necrotizing enterocolitis, Clostridium perfringens infection, and red blood cell T-polyagglutination. *Transfusion*. 2017;57(11):2571–2577.

56. Elbert C, Strauss RG, Barrett F, et al. Biological mothers may be dangerous blood donors for their neonates. *Acta Haematol*. 1991;85(4):189–191.

57. Jacquot C, Seo A, Miller PM, et al. Parental versus non-parental-directed donation: an 11-year experience of infectious disease testing at a pediatric tertiary care blood donor center. *Transfusion*. 2017;57(11):2799–2803.

58. Kc A, Rana N, Målqvist M, et al. Effects of delayed umbilical cord clamping vs early clamping on anemia in infants at 8 and 12 months: a randomized clinical trial. *JAMA Pediatr*. 2017;171(3):264–270.

59. ACOG, Committee on Obstetric Practice. Committee opinion No. 684: Delayed umbilical cord clamping after birth. *Obstet Gynecol*. 2017;129(1):e5–e10.

60. Choi ES, Cho S, Jang WS, et al. Cardiopulmonary bypass priming using autologous cord blood in neonatal congenital cardiac surgery. *Korean Circ J*. 2016;46(5):714–718.

61. Cure P, Bembea M, Chou S, et al. 2016 proceedings of the National Heart, Lung, and Blood Institute's scientific priorities in pediatric transfusion medicine. *Transfusion*. 2017;57(6):1568–1581.

62. Rabe H, Reynolds G, Diaz-Rossello J. A systematic review and meta-analysis of a brief delay in clamping the umbilical cord of preterm infants. *Neonatology*. 2008;93(2):138–144.

63. Christensen RD, Carroll PD, Josephson CD. Evidence-based advances in transfusion practice in neonatal intensive care units. *Neonatology*. 2014;106(3):245–253.

64. Clark P, Trickett A, Stark D, et al. Factors affecting microbial contamination rate of cord blood collected for transplantation. *Transfusion.* 2012;52(8):1770–1777.

65. Eichler H, Schaible T, Richter E, et al. Cord blood as a source of autologous RBCs for transfusion to preterm infants. *Transfusion.* 2000;40(9):1111–1117.

66. Stramer SL, Galel SA. Infectious disease screening. In: Fung MK, ed. *Technical Manual of the American Association of Blood Banks.* 18th ed. Bethesda, MD: AABB Press; 2017:161–205.

67. Zou S, Stramer SL, Dodd RY. Donor testing and risk: current prevalence, incidence, and residual risk of transfusion-transmissible agents in US allogeneic donations. *Transfus Med Rev.* 2012;26(2):119–128.

68. Bihl F, Castelli D, Marincola F, et al. Transfusion-transmitted infections. *J Transl Med.* 2007;5:25.

69. Hughes JA, Fontaine MJ, Gonzalez CL, et al. Case report of a transfusion-associated hepatitis A infection. *Transfusion.* 2014;54(9):2202–2206.

70. Shirley DT, Nataro JP. Zika virus infection. *Pediatr Clin North Am.* 2017;64(4):937–951.

71. Williamson PC, Linnen JM, Kessler DA, et al. First cases of Zika virus-infected US blood donors outside states with areas of active transmission. *Transfusion.* 2017;57(3pt2):770–778.

72. Nichols WG, Price TH, Gooley T, et al. Transfusion-transmitted cytomegalovirus infection after receipt of leukoreduced blood products. *Blood.* 2003;101(10):4195–4200.

73. Strauss RG. Optimal prevention of transfusion-transmitted cytomegalovirus (TTCMV) infection by modern leukocyte reduction alone: CMV sero/antibody-negative donors needed only for leukocyte products. *Transfusion.* 2016;56(8):1921–1924.

74. Groves JA, Shafi H, Nomura JH, et al. A probable case of West Nile virus transfusion transmission. *Transfusion.* 2017;57(3pt2):850–856.

75. Hong H, Xiao W, Lazarus HM, et al. Detection of septic transfusion reactions to platelet transfusions by active and passive surveillance. *Blood.* 2016;127(4):496–502.

76. Eder AF, Kennedy JM, Dy BA, et al. Bacterial screening of apheresis platelets and the residual risk of septic transfusion reactions: The American Red Cross experience (2004–2006). *Transfusion.* 2007;47(7):1134–1142.

77. Fang CT, Chambers LA, Kennedy J, et al. Detection of bacterial contamination in apheresis platelet products: American Red Cross experience, 2004. *Transfusion.* 2005;45(12): 1845–1852.

78. Jacobs MR, Smith D, Heaton WA, et al. Detection of bacterial contamination in prestorage culture-negative apheresis platelets on day of issue with the Pan Genera Detection test. *Transfusion.* 2011;51(12):2573–2582.

79. Heaton WA, Good CE, Galloway-Haskins R, et al. Evaluation of a rapid colorimetric assay for detection of bacterial contamination in apheresis and pooled random-donor platelet units. *Transfusion.* 2014;54(6):1634–1641.

80. Moritz ED, Winton CS, Tonnetti L, et al. Screening for Babesia microti in the U.S. Blood Supply. *N Engl J Med.* 2016;375(23):2236–2245.

81. Ludlam CA, Turner ML. Managing the risk of transmission of variant Creutzfeldt Jakob disease by blood products. *Br J Haematol.* 2006;132(1):13–24.

82. Prowse CV. Component pathogen inactivation: a critical review. *Vox Sang.* 2013;104(3):183–199.

83. Hess JR, Pagano MB, Barbeau JD, et al. Will pathogen reduction of blood components harm more people than it helps in developed countries? *Transfusion.* 2016;56(5):1236–1241.

84. Turkmen T, Qiu D, Cooper N, et al. Red blood cell alloimmunization in neonates and children up to 3 years of age. *Transfusion.* 2017;57(11):2720–2726.

85. Yang X, Ahmed S, Chandrasekaran V. Transfusion-related acute lung injury resulting from designated blood transfusion between mother and child: a report of two cases. *Am J Clin Pathol.* 2004;121(4):590–592.

86. Otrock ZK, Liu C, Grossman BJ. Transfusion-related acute lung injury risk mitigation: an update. *Vox Sang.* 2017;112(8):694–703.

87. Delaney M, Axdorff-Dickey RL, Crockett GI, et al. Risk of extracorporeal life support circuit-related hyperkalemia is reduced by prebypass ultrafiltration. *Pediatr Crit Care Med.* 2013;14(6):e263–e267.

88. Lee AC, Reduque LL, Luban NL, et al. Transfusion-associated hyperkalemic cardiac arrest in pediatric patients receiving massive transfusion. *Transfusion.* 2014;54(1):244–254.

CHAPTER

49

Exchange Transfusions

Jayashree Ramasethu

Advances in pre- and postnatal care have led a marked decline in the frequency of exchange transfusions (ET) in the United States and other developed countries (1–4). ET remains a vital therapeutic procedure primarily for the prevention of devastating neurodevelopmental complications from bilirubin encephalopathy and is also useful for a number of other indications. In developing countries, the burden of severe neonatal jaundice is high and ET rates remain elevated (5).

A. Definitions

1. ET: replacing the infant's blood with donor blood by repeatedly exchanging small aliquots of blood over a short time period.

B. Indications

1. Significant unconjugated hyperbilirubinemia in the newborn due to any cause, when intensive phototherapy fails or there is risk of acute bilirubin encephalopathy (6).

   a. Immediate ET may avert brain injury even when there are intermediate or advanced signs of acute bilirubin encephalopathy (7).

   b. **Figure 49.1** indicates the total serum bilirubin levels at which ET is recommended for infants of 35 or more weeks' gestation.

   c. In resource-limited settings where laboratory testing may not be easily available, a combination of bilirubin levels and clinical criteria has been proposed to determine the threshold for ET (8).

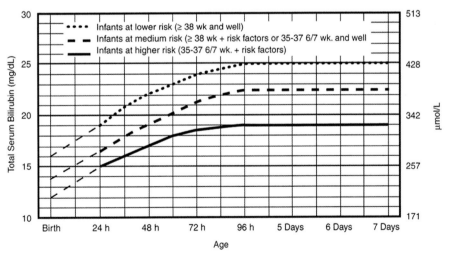

FIGURE **49.1** Guidelines for exchange transfusion in infants 35 or more weeks' gestation. (Reprinted with permission from American Academy of Pediatrics Subcommittee on Hyperbilirubinemia. Management of hyperbilirubinemia in the newborn infant 35 or more weeks of gestation. *Pediatrics.* 2004;114(1):297–316. Erratum: *Pediatrics.* 2004; 114(4):1138. Copyright © 2004 by the AAP.)

- The dashed lines for the first 24 hours indicate uncertainty due to a wide range of clinical circumstances and a range of responses to phototherapy.
- Immediate exchange transfusion is recommended if infant shows signs of acute bilirubin encephalopathy (hypertonia, arching, retrocollis, opisthotonos, fever, high pitched cry) or if TSB is ≥5 mg/dL (85 µmol/L) above these lines.
- Risk factors - isoimmune hemolytic disease, G6PD deficiency, asphyxia, significant lethargy, temperature instability, sepsis, acidosis.
- Measure serum albumin and calculate B/A ratio (See legend)
- Use total bilirubin. Do not subtract direct reacting or conjugated bilirubin
- If infant is well and 35-37 6/7 wk (median risk) can individualize TSB levels for exchange based on actual gestational age.

d. Indications for ET in more immature infants are variable and highly individualized, although some countries have attempted to establish uniform guidelines (9–11) (see **Table 49.1**).

TABLE 49.1 Suggested Use of Phototherapy and Exchange Transfusion in Preterm Infants <35 Weeks' Gestation

	INITIATE PHOTOTHERAPY	EXCHANGE TRANSFUSION
Gestational Age (Wk)	Total Serum Bilirubin (mg/dL)	Total Serum Bilirubin (mg/dL)
<28 0/7	5–6	11–14
28 0/7–29 6/7	6–8	12–14
30 0/7–31 6/7	8–10	13–16
32 0/7–33 6/7	10–12	15–18
34 0/7–34 6/7	12–14	17–19

Use postmenstrual age for phototherapy; e.g., when a 29 0/7-wk infant is 7 days old, use the TSB for 30 0/7 wks.

Use total bilirubin—do not subtract direct or conjugated bilirubin from the total.

Use the lower range of listed TSB levels for infants at greater risk of bilirubin toxicity (lower gestational age, serum albumin level <2.5 g/dL, rapidly rising TSB level, suggesting hemolytic disease, or those who are clinically unstable).

Infants considered to be clinically unstable may have one or more of the following: blood pH <7.15, blood culture positive sepsis during the previous 24 hrs, apnea and bradycardia requiring bagging or intubation during the previous 24 hrs, hypotension requiring pressor support in the previous 24 hrs, or mechanical ventilation at the time of blood sampling.

The wider ranges and overlapping of values in the ET column reflect the degree of uncertainty in making these recommendations.

Recommendations for ET apply to infants who are receiving intensive phototherapy to the maximal surface area but whose TSB levels continue to increase to the levels indicated.

For all infants, ET is recommended if the infant shows signs of acute bilirubin encephalopathy (i.e., hypertonia, arching, retrocollis, opisthotonus, high-pitched cry) although it is recognized that these signs rarely occur in very low–birthweight infants.

Reprinted by permission from Nature: Maisels MJ, Watchko JF, Bhutani VK, et al. An approach to the management of hyperbilirubinemia in the preterm infant less than 35 weeks of gestation. *J Perinatol.* 2012; 32(9):660–664. Copyright © 2012 Springer Nature.

2. Alloimmune hemolytic disease of the newborn (HDN) (12)
   a. For correction of severe anemia and hyperbilirubinemia
   b. In addition, in infants with alloimmune HDN, ET replaces antibody-coated neonatal red cells with antigen-negative red cells that should have normal in vivo survival and removes free maternal antibody in plasma
3. Severe anemia with congestive cardiac failure or hypervolemia (13)
4. Polycythemia (14,15)
   Although partial exchange transfusion reduces the packed cell volume and hyperviscosity in neonates with polycythemia, there is little evidence of long-term benefit from the procedure
5. Uncommon indications where ET has been used for therapy
   a. Congenital leukemia/hyperleukocytosis (16,17)
   b. Extreme thrombocytosis (18)
   c. Neonatal hemochromatosis/gestational alloimmune liver disease (19)
   d. Severe hypertriglyceridemia or hyperlipidemia (20)
   e. Hyperammonemia (hemodialysis is more effective) (21)
   f. Lead poisoning (22)
   g. Drug overdose or toxicity (23)
   h. Removal of antibodies and abnormal proteins (24)
   i. Neonatal sepsis (25,26)
   j. Malaria and babesiosis (27)

C. Contraindications

1. When alternatives such as simple transfusion or phototherapy would be just as effective with less risk.
2. When patient is unstable and the risk of the procedure outweighs the possible benefit.
   Partial ET, particularly to correct severe anemia associated with cardiac failure or hypervolemia, can be used to stabilize the patient's condition before a complete or double-volume ET is performed.
3. When a contraindication to placement of necessary lines outweighs indication for ET. Alternative access should be sought if ET is imperative.

D. Equipment

1. Infant care center (see Chapter 4, Maintenance of Thermal Homeostasis)
   a. Automatic and manually controlled heat source
   b. Temperature monitor
   c. Cardiorespiratory monitor
   d. Pulse oximeter for oxygen saturation monitoring
2. Resuscitation equipment and medication (immediately available)
3. Infant restraints
4. Orogastric tube
5. Suctioning equipment
6. Equipment for central and peripheral vascular access
7. Blood warmer and appropriate cartridge

8. Sterile exchange transfusion equipment
   a. Disposable set with special four-way stopcock *or*
   b. Assemble the following equipment
      (1) Two three-way stopcocks with locking connections
      (2) 5-, 10- or 20-mL syringes
      (3) Waste receptacle (empty IV bottle or bag)
      (4) IV connecting tubing to attach stopcocks to blood warmer and to waste receptacle
9. Appropriate blood product (see Section F)
10. Syringes and tubes for pre- and post-exchange blood tests
11. Heparinized saline 1 unit heparin/mL to flush syringes used for the exchange

E. Precautions

1. Stabilize infant before initiating exchange procedure.
2. Do not start ET until personnel are available for monitoring and as backup for other emergencies.
3. Monitor infant closely during and after procedure.
4. Do not rush procedure—stop or slow if patient becomes unstable.
5. Use blood product appropriate to clinical indication. Use freshest blood available, preferably less than 5 to 7 days.
6. Check potassium level of donor blood if patient has hyperkalemia or renal compromise.
7. Use only thermostatically controlled blood-warming device that has passed quality control for temperature and alarms. Be sure to review operating and safety procedures for specific blood warmer.
8. Do not apply excessive suction if it becomes difficult to draw blood from catheter. Reposition catheter or replace syringes, stopcocks, and any adapters connected to line.
9. Leave anticoagulated, banked blood in catheter or clear line with heparinized saline if the procedure is interrupted.
10. Clear catheter with heparinized saline if administering calcium.

F. Preparation for Total or Partial Exchange Transfusion

Blood Product and Volume

Blood Product

1. Communicate with blood bank or transfusion medicine specialist to determine most appropriate blood product for transfusion.
   a. Plasma-reduced whole blood or packed red cells reconstituted with plasma are usually used (28).
   b. Blood may be anticoagulated with citrate phosphate dextrose (CPD or CPDA1) or heparin (heparinized blood is not licensed for use in the United States). Additive anticoagulant solutions are generally avoided; if there is no other option, packed red cells stored in additive solutions may be washed or hard-packed prior to reconstitution for ET (see Chapter 48).
   c. Hematocrit (Hct) may be adjusted within the range of 45% to 60%, depending on desired end result. Hct between 40% and 45% is preferred when the indication for the ET is hyperbilirubinemia. Higher Hct levels may be requested when correcting anemia.
   d. Blood should be as fresh as possible (<7 days).
   e. Irradiated blood is recommended for all ET to prevent graft-versus-host disease. There is a significant increase in potassium concentration in stored irradiated units, so irradiation should be performed as close to the transfusion as possible (<24 hours).
   f. Standard blood-bank screening is particularly important, including sickle cell preparation, HIV, Hepatitis B, and CMV.
   g. Donor blood should be screened for glucose-6-phosphate dehydrogenase (G-6-PD) deficiency and sickle hemoglobin (HbS) in population endemic for these conditions (29).
2. In presence of alloimmunization, for example, Rh, ABO, special attention to compatibility testing is necessary (12,28).
   a. If delivery of an infant with severe HDN is anticipated, O Rh-negative blood cross-matched against the mother may be prepared before the baby is born.
   b. Donor blood prepared after the infant's birth should be negative for the antigen responsible for the hemolytic disease, and should be cross-matched against the infant.
   c. In ABO HDN, the blood must be type O and either Rh negative or Rh compatible with the mother and the infant. The blood should be washed free of plasma or have a low titer of anti-A or anti-B antibodies. Type O cells may be used with AB plasma, but this results in two donor exposures per ET.
   d. In Rh HDN, the blood should be Rh negative, and may be O group or the same group as the infant.
   e. In cases of rare blood group incompatibilities when the specific antigen negative blood is unavailable, the least incompatible blood may be used for the ET (30).
   f. Uncross-matched packed red blood cells have been suggested for emergency ET infants with intermediate/advanced bilirubin encephalopathy to reduce bilirubin levels quickly, but this may not be efficacious. The efficacy of ET in clearing bilirubin from plasma and the extravascular space is a direct function of the mass of albumin exchanged, and the low albumin content of packed red blood

cells may fail to prevent ongoing bilirubin neuro-toxicity (31).

3. In infants with polycythemia, the optimal dilutional fluid is isotonic saline rather than plasma or albumin (32).

Volume of Donor Blood Required

1. Whenever possible, use no more than the equivalent of one whole unit of blood for each procedure, to decrease donor exposure

2. Quantity needed for total procedure = Volume for the actual ET + volume for tubing dead space and blood warmer (usually an additional 25 to 30 mL)

3. Double volume ET for removal of bilirubin, antibodies, etc.

$$2 \times \text{infant's blood volume} = 2 \times 80 - 120 \text{ mL/kg}$$

(Infant's blood volume in preterm infant $\cong$ 100 to 120 mL/kg, in term infant $\cong$ 80 to 85 mL/kg)
Exchanges approximately 85% of infant's blood volume **(Fig. 49.2)**

4. Single-volume ET: Exchanges approximately 60% of infant's blood volume **(Fig. 49.2)**

5. Partial ET for correction of severe anemia

$$\text{Volume (mL)} = \frac{\text{Infants blood volume} \times (\text{Hb desired} - \text{Hb initial})}{\text{Hb of PRBC} - \text{Hb initial}}$$

6. Single volume or partial ET for correction of polycythemia

$$\text{Volume (mL)} = \frac{\text{Infants blood volume} \times \text{desired HCT change}}{\text{Initial HCT}}$$

Preparation of Infant

1. Place infant on warmer with total accessibility and controlled environment. ET may be performed on small preterm infants in warm incubators, provided a sterile field can be maintained and catheters are easily accessible.

2. Restrain infant suitably. Sedation and pain relief are not usually required. Conscious infants may suck on a pacifier during the procedure.

3. Connect physiologic monitors, and establish baseline values (temperature, respiratory and heart rates, oxygen saturation by pulse oximetry).

4. Empty infant's stomach.
   a. Do not feed for 4 hours prior to procedure, if possible.
   b. Place orogastric tube, and remove gastric contents, and leave on open drainage.

5. Start peripheral IV line for glucose and medication infusion.
   a. Extra IV line may be necessary for emergency medications.
   b. Exchange procedure may interrupt previous essential infusion rate through umbilical venous catheter (UVC); run parenteral fluids through peripheral IV line.
   c. If prolonged, lack of enteral feeds or parenteral glucose will lead to hypoglycemia.

6. Stabilize infant prior to starting exchange procedure, for example, give packed-cell transfusion when severe hypovolemia and anemia are present, or modify ventilator or ambient oxygen as required.

7. The use of albumin infusions prior to ET to improve bilirubin binding remains controversial (33).

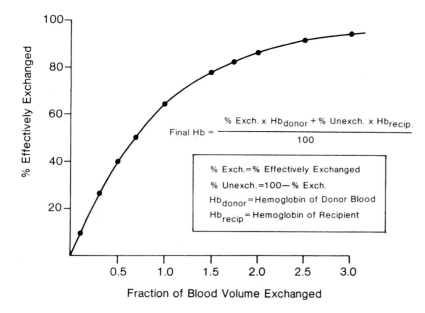

$$\text{Final Hb} = \frac{\% \text{ Exch.} \times \text{Hb}_{donor} + \% \text{ Unexch.} \times \text{Hb}_{recip.}}{100}$$

% Exch. = % Effectively Exchanged
% Unexch. = 100 − % Exch.
Hb_{donor} = Hemoglobin of Donor Blood
Hb_{recip} = Hemoglobin of Recipient

FIGURE 49.2 Graph depicting the effectiveness of exchange transfusion against the fraction of blood volume exchanged. The formula permits the calculation of the final hemoglobin.

Establish Access for ET

1. Push–Pull technique: central access—usually through UVC. Note: A single-lumen UVC is preferred; increased resistance is noted when using a double-lumen UVC.
2. Isovolumetric exchange: Simultaneous infusion of donor blood through venous line and removal of baby's blood through arterial line. This technique may be better tolerated in sick or unstable neonates because there is less fluctuation of blood pressure and cerebral hemodynamics (34). The technique is also favored when only peripheral vascular access is available or preferred for various reasons. The femoral vein and external jugular vein have been used as alternative access sites when the UVC is not accessible (35,36).
   a. Infusion of donor blood may be through UVC or peripheral intravenous catheter.
   b. Removal of baby's blood may be from umbilical arterial or venous catheter, or peripheral arterial catheter, usually a radial arterial line.

Pre-Exchange Laboratory Tests on Infant's Blood

Tests are based on clinical indications

1. Note that diagnostic serologic tests on the infant, such as studies to evaluate unexplained hemolysis, antiviral antibody titers, neonatal metabolic screening, or genetic tests should be drawn prior to the ET.
2. Hemoglobin, Hct, platelets
3. Electrolytes, calcium, blood gas
4. Glucose
5. Bilirubin total and direct
6. Coagulation profile

Prepare Blood

1. Verify identification of blood product (see Chapter 48)
   a. Type and cross-match data
   b. Expiration date
   c. Donor and recipient identities
2. Attach blood administration set to blood-warmer tubing and to blood bag
3. Place cartridge into blood warmer
4. Allow blood to run through blood warmer

G. Technique (▶ Video 49.1: Exchange Transfusion)

Exchange Transfusion by Push–Pull Technique Through Special Stopcock With Preassembled Tray

1. Read instructions provided by manufacturer carefully.

2. Wear head cover and mask. Scrub as for major procedure. Wear sterile gown and gloves.
3. Open preassembled equipment tray, using aseptic technique.
4. Identify positions on special stopcock in clockwise rotation (**Figs. 49.3** and **49.4**). The direction that the handle is pointing indicates the port that is open to syringe. The special stopcock allows clockwise rotation in the order used: (1) withdraw from patient, (2) clear to waste bag, (3) draw new blood, (4) inject into patient. Always rotate in clockwise direction to follow proper sequence, and keep connections tight.

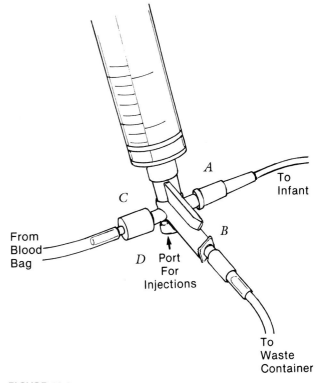

FIGURE 49.3 Special four-way stopcock. **A:** Male adapter to infant line. **B:** Female adapter to waste container. **C:** Attachment to blood tubing. **D:** "Off" position (180 degrees from adapter to waste container), allowing injection through rubber-stoppered port "*below*" syringe. The stopcock is used in clockwise rotation when correctly assembled.

   a. Male adapter to umbilical or peripheral catheter
   b. Female adapter to the extension tubing to which waste bag will be attached
   c. Connection to tubing for attachment to blood-warmer cartridge
   d. Neutral "off" position in which additives may be administered through rubber stopper (180 degrees from waste receptacle port)
5. Follow steps as illustrated by manufacturer to make all connections to blood and waste bags.
6. With stopcock open to blood source, clear all air into syringe. Turn in clockwise direction 270 degrees and evacuate into waste.
7. Turn stopcock to "off," and replace onto sterile field.

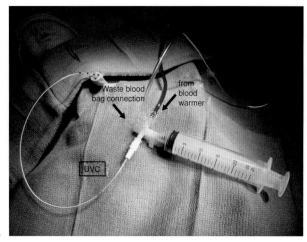 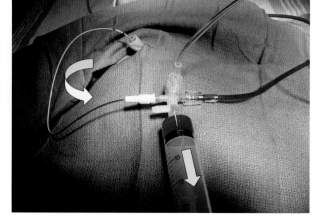

FIGURE 49.4 A, B: ET using special four-way stopcock.

8. Use pre-existing UVC or insert UVC, as described in Chapter 32, Umbilical Vein Catheterization.
   a. Place a single-lumen UVC whenever possible. The internal lumen of a double-lumen UVC is smaller and makes it more difficult to perform the ET.
   b. Consider central venous pressure (CVP) measurement, using pressure transducer, in unstable baby.
   c. Place catheter in inferior vena cava (IVC) and verify position by radiograph.
   d. If catheter cannot be positioned in IVC, it may still be used cautiously in an emergency, when placed in the umbilical vein, if adequate blood return is obtained.
9. Have an assistant document all vital signs, volumes, and other data, on the exchange record.
10. Draw blood for diagnostic studies and pre-exchange laboratory studies.
11. Check peripheral glucose levels every 60 minutes. Monitor cardiorespiratory status, continuous pulse oximetry. Determine blood gases as often as indicated by preexisting clinical condition and stability.
12. Usual rate of removal and replacement of blood during the ET is 5 mL/kg over a 2- to 4-minute cycle.
13. If infant is hypovolemic or has low CVP, start exchange with transfusion of aliquot into catheter. If infant is hypervolemic or has high CVP, start by withdrawing precalculated aliquot.
14. Remeasure CVP if indicated. Expect rise as plasma oncotic pressure increases, if CVP low at start.
15. Ensure that the stages of drawing and infusing blood from and into the infant are done slowly, taking at least a minute each to avoid fluctuations in blood pressure. Rapid fluctuations in arterial pressure in the push–pull technique may be accompanied by changes in intracranial pressure (34). Rapid withdrawal from the umbilical vein induces a negative pressure that may be transmitted to the mesenteric veins and contribute to the high incidence of ischemic bowel complications.

16. Gently agitate the blood bag every 10 to 15 minutes to prevent red cell sedimentation, which may lead to exchange with relatively anemic blood toward the end of the exchange.
17. The use of calcium supplementation during ET is common, but may not be necessary or advantageous (37). Consider giving calcium supplement:
    a. When hypocalcemia is documented.
    b. With symptoms or signs of hypocalcemia.
       (1) Change in Q-Tc interval.
       (2) Agitation and tachycardia: These symptoms are not reliably correlated with ionized calcium levels.

       The effect of intravenous calcium may last only a few minutes. Intravenous calcium may also cause bradycardia or cardiac arrest. Calcium will reverse the effect of the anticoagulant in the donor blood and may cause clotting of the catheter, so administration through a peripheral IV catheter is preferred. If calcium is given through the UVC, prior to administration, clear the line of donor blood with 0.9% NaCl. Give 1 mL of 10% calcium gluconate per kg body weight. Administer slowly, with careful observation of heart rate and rhythm. Clear catheter again with 0.9% NaCl.
18. Perform calculated number of passes, until desired volume has been exchanged.
19. Be sure there is adequate volume of donor blood remaining to infuse after last withdrawal, if a positive intravascular balance is desired.
20. Clear umbilical catheter of banked blood and withdraw amount of infant's blood needed for laboratory testing, including re-crossmatching.
21. Infuse IV fluids with 0.5 to 1 unit heparin/mL of fluid through UVC if further ET is anticipated.
22. Total duration for double-volume ET: 90 to 120 minutes.
23. Document procedure in patient's hospital record.

Exchange Transfusion Using a Single Umbilical Line and Two Three-Way Stopcocks in Tandem

The principles and techniques for using either the special stopcock or two three-way stopcocks in tandem are the same. It is important to ensure that all junctions are tight to produce a closed, sterile system. It is also essential to understand the working positions of the stopcocks before starting the exchange.

1. Scrub as for major procedure. Wear sterile gown and gloves.
2. Attach stopcock and tubing in sequence (**Fig. 49.5**).
   a. Proximal stopcock
      (1) Umbilical catheter
      (2) IV extension tubing to sterile waste container
   b. Distal stopcock
      (1) Tubing from blood-warming cartridge
      (2) 10- or 20-mL syringe
3. Clear lines of air bubbles.
4. Start exchange record.
5. Follow steps of push–pull technique until exchange is completed.

Exchange Transfusion by Isovolumetric Technique (Central or Peripheral Lines)

1. Scrub as for major procedure.
2. Select two sites for line placement, and insert as per Section 5, Vascular Access.

a. Venous for infusion
   (1) UVC or
   (2) Peripheral IV that is at least 23 gauge
b. Arterial for removal
   (1) Umbilical artery catheter
   (2) Peripheral, usually radial if infant's size permits
3. Connect arterial line to three-way stopcock.
   a. Use short, connecting IV tubing to extend peripheral line.
   b. Attach additional connecting tubing to stopcock and place into sterile waste container.
   c. Attach empty 3- to 10-mL syringe to stopcock, for withdrawal of blood.
      An additional stopcock may also be placed on this port so that a syringe of heparinized saline (5 units/mL) may be attached for use as needed. Be cautious about total volume infused.
4. Connect venous catheter to single, three-way stopcock, which in turn connects to empty 5- to 10-mL syringe and to blood-warming cartridge.
5. Start exchange-transfusion record.
6. Withdraw and discard blood from arterial side at rate of 2 to 3 mL/kg/min, and infuse at same rate into venous side. The blood from the warmer cartridge may be run through an infusion pump which will measure the volume infused per hour and the cumulative volume delivered. Keep flow as steady as possible, and volumetrically equal for infusion and removal.

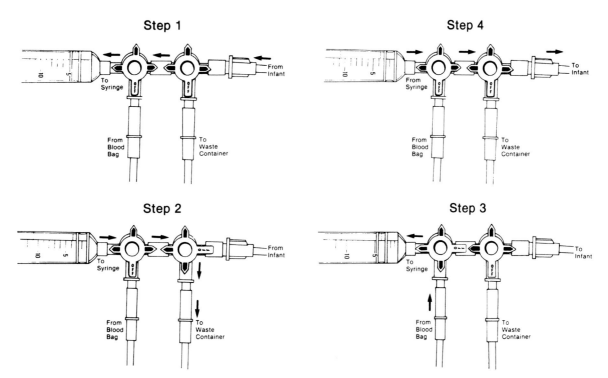

FIGURE 49.5 Three-way stopcocks in tandem. *Step 1:* Stopcocks positioned for withdrawing blood from infant. *Step 2:* Stopcocks positioned for emptying withdrawn blood to waste container. *Step 3:* Stopcocks positioned for filling syringe from blood bag. *Step 4:* Stopcocks positioned for injecting blood into infant line.

7. Intermittently, flush arterial line with heparinized saline to clear.

   The heparin solution remaining in tubing will be removed with next withdrawal, thus reducing significantly the total heparin dose actually received by the patient.

8. Follow steps as for push–pull technique until exchange is complete.

9. Fully automated simultaneous umbilical arteriovenous ET has been performed in term and late preterm infants (38).

10. Total duration for isovolumetric ET: 45 to 60 minutes, may be longer in sick, unstable infant.

H. Postexchange for All Techniques

1. Continue to monitor vital signs closely for at least 6 to 12 hours.

2. Rewrite orders: Adjust any drug dosages as needed to compensate for removal by exchange.

3. Keep infant NPO for at least 4 hours. Restart feeds if clinically stable. Monitor abdominal girth and bowel sounds every 3 to 4 hours for next 24 hours if exchange has been performed using umbilical vascular lines. Observe for signs of feeding intolerance.

4. Monitor serum glucose levels every 2 to 4 hours for 24 hours.

5. Repeat blood gases as often as clinically indicated.

6. Measure serum ionized calcium levels and platelet counts in sick or preterm infants immediately after the ET and then as indicated.

7. Repeat hemoglobin, Hct, and bilirubin measurements approximately 4 hours after exchange, and further as clinically indicated. A double-volume ET replaces 85% of the infants' blood volume, but eliminates only about 50% of the intravascular bilirubin. Equilibration of intra- and extravascular bilirubin, and continued breakdown of sensitized and newly formed red cells by persisting maternal antibody results in a rebound of bilirubin levels following initial ET, and may necessitate repeated ET in severe HDN.

I. Complications

1. Risk of death or permanent serious sequelae is estimated to be less than 1% in healthy infants, but as high as 12% in sick infants. There may be some uncertainty in ascribing adverse events to the ET in infants who are already critically ill (2–4,39).

2. Many of the adverse events are hematologic or biochemical laboratory abnormalities which may be asymptomatic. The most common adverse effects noted during or soon after the ET, usually in infants who are preterm and/or sick:

   a. Apnea and/or bradycardia
   b. Hypocalcemia
   c. Thrombocytopenia (<50, 000 in 10% of healthy infants, up to 67% in infants <32 weeks gestational age)
   d. Metabolic acidosis
   e. Vascular spasm

3. Complications reported from ET are related to the blood transfusion and to complications of vascular access (Chapters 31–33, 36, 48).

4. Potential complications include:

   a. Metabolic: hypocalcemia, hypo- or hyperglycemia, hyperkalemia.
   b. Cardiorespiratory: apnea, bradycardia, hypotension, hypertension.
   c. Hematologic: thrombocytopenia, dilutional coagulopathy, neutropenia, disseminated intravascular coagulation.
   d. Vascular catheter related: vasospasm, thrombosis, embolization.
   e. Gastrointestinal: feeding intolerance, ischemic injury, necrotizing enterocolitis
   f. Infection: omphalitis, septicemia

References

1. Bhutani VK, Meng NF, Knauer Y, et al. Extreme hyperbilirubinemia and rescue exchange transfusion in California from 2007 to 2012. *J Perinatol.* 2016;36:853–857.

2. Steiner LA, Bizzarro MJ, Ehrenkrantz RA, et al. A decline in the frequency of neonatal exchange transfusions and its effect on exchange transfusion related morbidity and mortality. *Pediatrics.* 2007;120:27–32.

3. Chessman JC, Bowen JR, Ford JB. Neonatal exchange transfusions in tertiary and non-tertiary hospital settings, New South Wales, 2001–2012. *J Paediatr Child Health.* 2017;53:447–450.

4. Chitty HE, Ziegler N, Savoia H, et al. Neonatal exchange transfusions in the 21st century: a single hospital study. *J Paediatr Child Health.* 2013;49:825–832.

5. Slusher TM, Zamora TG, Appiah D, et al. Burden of severe neonatal jaundice: a systematic review and meta-analysis. *BMJ Paediatr Open.* 2017;25;1(1):e000105.

6. American Academy of Pediatrics. Subcommittee on hyperbilirubinemia. Clinical practice guideline. Management of hyperbilirubinemia in the newborn infant 35 or more weeks gestation. *Pediatrics.* 2004;114:297–316.

7. Hansen TW, Nietsch L, Norman E, et al. Reversibility of acute intermediate phase bilirubin encephalopathy. *Acta Paediatr.* 2009;98:1689–1694.

8. Olusanya BO, Iskander IF, Slusher TM, et al. A decision-making tool for exchange transfusions in infants with severe hyperbilirubinemia in resource-limited settings. *J Perinatol.* 2016;36:338–341.

9. Maisels MJ, Watchko JF, Bhutani VK, et al. An approach to the management of hyperbilirubinemia in the preterm infant less than 35 weeks of gestation. *J Perinatol.* 2012;32:660–664.

10. Van Imhoff DE, Dijk PH, Hulzebos CV; BARTrial study group, Netherlands Neonatal research Network. Uniform treatment thresholds for hyperbilirubinemia in preterm infants: background and synopsis of a national guideline. *Early Hum Dev.* 2011;87:521–525.

11. Morioka I. Hyperbilirubinemia in preterm infants in Japan: new treatment criteria. *Pediatr Int.* 2018;60:684–690.

12. Ree IMC, Smits-Wintjens VEHJ, van der Bom JG, et al. Neonatal management and outcome in alloimmune hemolytic disease. *Expert Rev Hematol.* 2017;10:607–616.

13. Naulaers G, Barten S, Vanhole C, et al. Management of severe neonatal anemia due to fetomaternal transfusion. *Am J Perinatol.* 1999;16:193–196.

14. Ozek E, Soll R, Schimmel MS. Partial exchange transfusion to prevent neurodevelopmental disability in infants with polycythemia. *Cochrane Database Syst Rev.* 2010;20:CD 005089.

15. Hopewell B, Steiner LA, Ehrenkranz RA, et al. Partial exchange transfusion for polycythemia hyperviscosity syndrome. *Am J Perinatol.* 2011;28:557–564.

16. Hayasaka I, Cho K, Morioka K, et al. Exchange transfusion in patients with down syndrome and severe transient leukemia. *Pediatr Int.* 2015;57:620–625.

17. Kuperman A, Hoffmann Y, Glikman D, et al. Severe pertussis and hyperleukocytosis: Is it time to change for exchange? *Transfusion.* 2014;54:1630–1633.

18. Park ES, Kim SY, Yeom JS, et al. Extreme thrombocytosis associated with transient myeloproliferative disorder with Down Syndrome with t(11;17)(q13;q21). *Pediatr Blood Cancer.* 2008;50:643–644.

19. Okada N, Sanada Y, Urahashi T, et al. Rescue case of low birth weight infant with acute hepatic failure. *World J Gastroenterol.* 2017;23:7337–7342.

20. Rodríguez-Castaño MJ, Iglesias B, Arruza L. Successful exchange transfusion in extremely preterm infant after symptomatic lipid overdose. *J Neonatal Perinatal Med.* 2018;11:199–202.

21. Chen CY, Chen YC, Fang JT, et al. Continuous arteriovenous hemodiafiltration in the acute treatment of hyperammonaemia due to ornithine transcarbamylase deficiency. *Ren Fail.* 2000;22:823–836.

22. Chinnakaruppan NR, Marcus SM. Asymptomatic congenital lead poisoning- case report. *Clin Toxicol (Phila).* 2010;48:563–565.

23. Sancak R, Kucukoduk S, Tasdemir HA, et al. Exchange transfusion treatment in a newborn with phenobarbital intoxication. *Pediatr Emerg Care.* 1999;15:268–270.

24. Dolfin T, Pomerance A, Korzets Z, et al. Acute renal failure in a neonate caused by the transplacental transfer of a nephrotoxic paraprotein: successful resolution by exchange transfusion. *Am J Kidney Dis.* 1999;34:1129–1131.

25. Pugni L, Ronchi A, Bizzarri B, et al. Exchange transfusion in the treatment of neonatal septic shock: a ten-year experience in a neonatal intensive care unit. *Int J Mol Sci.* 2016;17(5):pii: E695.

26. Aradhya AS, Sundaram V, Kumar P, et al. Double volume exchange transfusion in severe neonatal sepsis. *Indian J Pediatr.* 2016;83:107–113.

27. Virdi VS, Goraya JS, Khadwal A, et al. Neonatal transfusion malaria requiring exchange transfusion. *Ann Trop Pediatr.* 2003;23:205–207.

28. American Association of Blood Banks. *Standards for Blood Banks and Transfusion Services.* 31st ed. Bethesda, MD: AABB; 2018.

29. Samanta S, Kumar P, Kishore SS, et al. Donor blood glucose 6-phosphate dehydrogenase deficiency reduces the efficacy of exchange transfusion in neonatal hyperbilirubinemia. *Pediatrics.* 2009;123:e96–e100.

30. Li BJ, Jiang YJ, Yuan F, et al. Exchange transfusion of least incompatible blood for severe hemolytic disease of the newborn due to anti-Rh17. *Transfus Med.* 2010;20:66–69.

31. Watchko JF. Emergency release uncross-matched packed red blood cells for immediate double volume exchange transfusion in neonates with intermediate to advanced acute bilirubin encephalopathy: Timely but insufficient? *J Perinatol.* 2018;38:947–953.

32. De Waal KA, Baerts W, Offringa M. Systematic review of the optimal fluid for dilutional exchange transfusion in neonatal polycythemia. *Arch Dis Child Fetal Neonatal Ed.* 2006;91: F7–F10.

33. Ahlfors CE. Pre exchange transfusion administration of albumin: an overlooked adjunct in the treatment of severe neonatal jaundice? *Indian Pediatr.* 2010;47:231–232.

34. van de Bor M, Benders MJ, Dorrepaal CA, et al. Cerebral blood volume changes during exchange transfusions in infants born at or near term. *J Pediatr.* 1994;125:617–621.

35. Weng YH, Chiu YW. Comparison of efficacy and safety of exchange transfusion through different catheterizations: femoral vein versus umbilical vein versus umbilical artery/vein. *Pediatr Crit Care Med.* 2011;12:61–64.

36. Chen HN, Lee ML, Tsao LY. Exchange transfusion using peripheral vessels is safe and effective in newborn infants. *Pediatrics.* 2008;122:e905–e910.

37. Ogunlesi TA, Lesi FE, Oduwole O. Prophylactic intravenous calcium therapy for exchange blood transfusion in the newborn. *Cochrane Database Syst Rev.* 2017;10:CD011048.

38. Altunhan H, Annagür A, Tarakçi N, et al. Fully automated simultaneous umbilical arteriovenous exchange transfusion in term and late preterm infants with neonatal hyperbilirubinemia. *J Matern Fetal Neonatal Med.* 2016;29:1274–1278.

39. Patra K, Storfer-Isser A, Siner B, et al. Adverse events associated with neonatal exchange transfusion in the 1990s. *J Pediatr.* 2004;144:626–631.

Miscellaneous Procedures

CHAPTER

50

Whole-Body Cooling

Ela Chakkarapani and Marianne Thoresen

Moderate therapeutic hypothermia (HT; rectal or esophageal temperature 33.5°C) initiated within 6 hours of birth and continued for 72 hours reduces death or disability in neonates with moderate or severe hypoxic ischemic encephalopathy (HIE) with a number needed to treat (NNT) of 7 (95% CI 5 to 10); and NNT for an additional beneficial outcome in reducing neurodevelopmental disability in survivors of 8 (95% CI 5 to 14) (1–5). Benefits of HT persist into early childhood with increased proportion of cooled children having IQ >85 (6,7), and less severe cerebral palsy (8).

HT is typically administered in newborn infants as whole-body cooling (WBC) using different types of mattresses or wraps around the body (3,4), or as selective head cooling (SHC) using a "coolcap" around the head (2) with water circulating within the "coolcap." Selective head cooling (SHC) is an excellent technique and Cool-Cap was the first to show neuroprotection by cooling term newborns after moderate or severe perinatal asphyxia. Trends in Protective Hypothermia have moved quickly towards Total Body Hypothermia, and servo controlled units, which is not the case with Cool-Cap which is a non-servo controlled device. The Cool-Cap SHC equipment is currently not supported commercially.

A. Indications (2,4) (see Fig. 50.1)

1. To decrease death or disability in the following group of infants
   a. ≥35 weeks' gestation newborn infants <6 hours of age (5)
   b. Evidence of asphyxia (at least one of the four criteria below must be met)
      (1) Apgar score at 10 minutes of age ≤5
      (2) Worst arterial or capillary or venous pH within 60 minutes of life ≤7.0
      (3) Arterial or capillary or venous base deficit within 60 minutes of life ≥16 mmol/L
      (4) Ventilated or resuscitated for at least the first 10 minutes after birth
          AND c OR d AND e

   c. Moderate or severe encephalopathy characterized by:
      (1) Abnormal consciousness—lethargy or stupor or coma *and*
      (2) Hypotonia or abnormal reflexes (including oculomotor or pupillary abnormalities), or decreased/absent spontaneous activity, or abnormal (distal flexion/complete extension/decerebrate) posture, or absent/weak suck, or incomplete/absent Moro *or*
   d. Clinical seizures *and*
   e. A 30 minutes abnormal background activity or electrical seizures in amplitude-integrated electroencephalogram (aEEG) within the first 6 hours of life
2. If pH is between 7.01 and 7.15 or base deficit between 10 and 15.9 mmol/L or blood gas unavailable and/or aEEG is unavailable or not used as entry criteria, the following criteria can be used (3):
   a. ≥35 weeks' gestation within <6 hours of age *and*
   b. any <u>one</u> of the following
      (1) Acute perinatal event such as cord prolapse, uterine rupture, late or variable decelerations
      (2) Apgar scores ≤5 at 10 minutes
      (3) Prolonged resuscitation: chest compressions and/or intubation and/or mask ventilation at 10 minutes
          and
   c. Any one of the following
      (1) Clinical seizures
      (2) Encephalopathy defined as one or more signs in at least three of the following six categories: Level of consciousness, spontaneous activity, posture, tone, primitive reflexes, autonomic system (**Fig. 50.1**)

B. Special Circumstances

1. *Cooling beyond 6 hours of age*: In a recent trial (9), 21 centers randomized 168 term infants, who failed the 6-hour time-window, to HT (*n* = 83) and normothermia (*n* = 85) over 8 years. Participants had a median (range) postnatal

Clinical Pathway for Commencing Therapeutic Hypothermia

Inclusion criteria*: gestation ≥ 35 weeks, birth weight ≥1,800 g
Exclude: severe chromosomal /congenital anomalies

Cord or 1st blood gas within 1 hour:
pH ≤7.0 or base deficit ≥16 mEq/L

Blood gas not available **or**
Cord or 1st blood gas within 1 hour:
pH 7.01–7.15 or base deficit 10–15.9 mEq/L
And
Acute perinatal event (e.g., placenta abruption, cord prolapse or severe FHR abnormality)
And
Apgar Score ≤5 at 10 minutes **or**
Continued need for ventilation initiated at birth and continued for at least 10 minutes

Neurologic Evidence of Moderate / Severe Encephalopathy
Seizures or Presence of one or more signs in 3 of 6 categories

Category	Moderate Encephalopathy	Severe Encephalopathy
Level of consciousness	Lethargic	Stupor/coma
Spontaneous activity	Decreased activity	No activity
Posture	Distal flexion, full extension	Decerebrate
Tone	Hypotonia (focal, general)	Flaccid
Primitive reflexes		
Suck	Weak	Absent
Moro	Incomplete	Absent
Autonomic system		
Pupils	Constricted	Dilated/nonreactive
Heart rate	Bradycardia	Variable
Respirations	Periodic breathing	Apnea

*Note: Therapeutic hypothermia should be started as quickly as possible within 6 hours of birth. Hypothermia initiated 6–24 hours after birth may have benefit but there is uncertainty about its effectiveness.

FHR = Fetal heart rate

FIGURE 50.1 Clinical pathway for commencing therapeutic hypothermia. (Derived from Shankaran S, Laptook AR, Ehrenkranz RA, et al. Whole-body hypothermia for neonates with hypoxic-ischemic encephalopathy. *N Engl J Med*. 2005;353:1574–1584; Jacobs SE, Morley CJ, Inder TE, et al. Whole-body hypothermia for term and near-term newborns with hypoxic- ischemic encephalopathy: a randomised controlled trial. *Arch Pediatr Adolesc. Med.* 2011;165(8):692–700; Laptook AR, Shankaran S, Tyson JE, et al. Effect of therapeutic hypothermia initiated after 6 hours of age on death or disability among newborns with hypoxic-ischemic encephalopathy: a randomized clinical trial. *JAMA.* 2017;318(16):1550–1560.; and MedStar Georgetown University Hospital Neonatal Intensive Care Unit.)

age of 16 hours (6–24) at the commencement of intervention. Death or disability was comparable between the HT (24.4%) and normothermic group (27.9%) (N-1 Chi squared = 0.25). Experimental studies demonstrate that the therapeutic effect of hypothermia declines linearly up to 9 hours following hypoxic insult and is negligible beyond 9 hours (10,11). These results indicate that cooling should be commenced before 6 hours of age.

2. *Cooling mild HIE:* There is currently no published evidence to support using HT for infants with mild HIE (12).

3. *Cooling longer (5 days) or deeper (32°C):* A four group randomized study found that neither cooling for 5 days or cooling down to 32°C had better outcome than the current protocol of 33.5°C for 3 days. This study was stopped early due to futility (13). Outcome of the 50% who underwent the treatment was recently published confirming the above (14).

C. Contraindications

1. Preterm infants born less than 35 weeks' gestation due to lack of data regarding the safety and benefit of TH.

Hypothermia may be associated with coagulopathy, hypo- or hyperglycemia in preterm infants between 34 and 35 weeks' gestation with HIE (15).

2. Major congenital anomalies. However, local guidelines might differ. Some centers offer HT to term infants with surgical, cardiac, chromosomal, or sudden unexpected postnatal collapse, who have suffered significant perinatal asphyxial encephalopathy and whose intensive care will be continued (e.g., infant with surgical conditions including ventilated asphyxiated infant with tracheoesophageal fistula requiring imminent surgery) (16,17), have a cardiac condition (e.g., infant with transposition of great arteries with tight atrial septum leading to HIE), have a chromosomal condition (e.g., infant with trisomy 21 with perinatal asphyxia), and infants suffering postnatal collapse (e.g., sudden unexpected neonatal cardiorespiratory arrest leading to HIE) (17) unless low body temperature might adversely influence the effect(s) of other required treatments (18).

3. Syndromes involving brain dysgenesis, when known.

4. Infants in moribund state.

5. Birth weight below second percentile.

D. Cooling at Birth

1. If the infant fulfills criteria (b) in A by 10 minutes of age, initiate passive HT and core temperature monitoring.
   a. Switch off heater in the open warmer/transport incubator.
   b. Do not wrap or cover the head with hat (19).
   c. Insert rectal or esophageal temperature probe as early as possible.

E. Securing Rectal or Esophageal Temperature Sensor

Rectal Temperature Sensor

1. Measure and mark the rectal temperature sensor (tape bridge) (**Fig. 50.2A**).
2. Lubricate the first 5 cm before insertion (**Fig. 50.2B**).

3. Insert to 6 cm into the infant's rectum. Clean the peri-anal region followed by smearing the under surface of the thigh with a no-sting barrier film (Sorbaderm/Cavilon) (**Fig. 50.2C**).
4. Stick a hydrocolloid dressing (7 × 3 cm) (duoDERM) on the under surface of both thighs (**Fig. 50.2D**).
5. Fix the temperature sensor over the hydrocolloid dressing with another (5 × 5 cm) hydrocolloid dressing (**Fig. 50.2E**).
6. Insert a second rectal probe to 6 cm (**Fig. 50.2 E**), to be connected to the patient monitor to double check the readings from the rectal probe connected to the cooling machine.

Esophageal Temperature Sensor

1. Insert esophageal probe, preferably via the nostril. If not possible, insert orally. Measure from tip of the nose to ear lobe and to xiphoid then subtract 2 cm

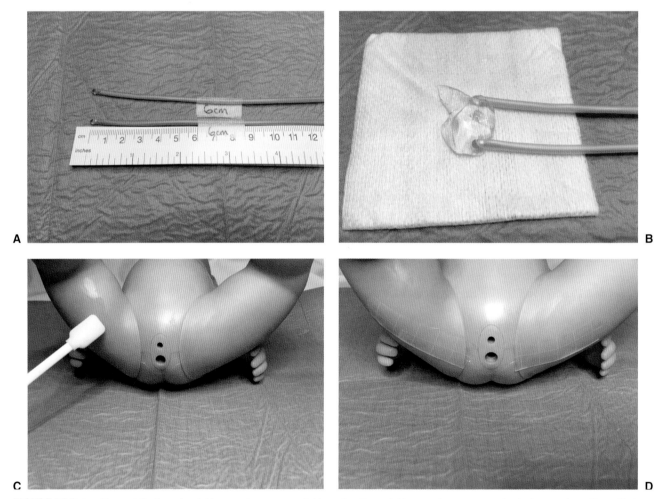

FIGURE 50.2 Insertion and fixation of rectal temperature sensors. **A:** Measuring the rectal temperature sensor probe to 6 cm and marking with tape. **B:** Lubrication of the tip of the temperature sensor. **C:** Smearing the under surface of the thigh with no-sting barrier film after cleaning the perianal region. **D:** Sticking a hydrocolloid dressing on the surface of the thigh. (*continued*)

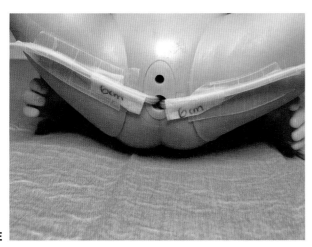

E

FIGURE 50.2 (*Continued*) **E:** Securing two rectal temperature sensors on the side of the thigh.

to calculate the length of insertion. This length will position the tip of the sensor 2 cm above the diaphragm.

2. Obtain a CXR to confirm the position of the tip of the esophageal probe. Attach the esophageal probe to the extension that connects to the cooling machine.

F. Supportive Intensive Care With HT

1. Provide airway support and monitoring: Appropriate respiratory support with ventilator or continuous positive airway pressure, and monitoring of pulse oximetry, pulmonary function, end-tidal CO_2, and arterial blood gases.

2. Maintain PCO_2 corrected for temperature >35 mm Hg (20) (PCO_2 at 33.5°C is approximately PCO_2 at 37°C × 0.83). Keep CO_2 at normal range of 35 to 50 mm Hg when analyzed at 33.5°C. If analyzed at 37°C, use a range of 42 to 60 mm Hg. Avoid unnecessary exposure to high oxygen concentration (21).

3. Provide cardiac monitoring and support: Arterial blood pressure, cardiac output, and function monitoring (if available). Support cardiac function and perfusion with inotropes and volume as necessary. Heart rate is normally reduced by approximately 10 beats/1°C during HT; however, inotropic support will increase the heart rate (22). Expected heart rate for infants cooled to 33.5°C will be 80 to 100 beats per minute (22).

4. Provide aEEG and EEG monitoring: Use single- or two-channel aEEG recording to assess the background activity, pattern, and monitor the time to normalization of background pattern (23–25); identify seizures preferably using continuous EEG/aEEG to diagnose subclinical seizures (26), and monitor the effect of anticonvulsants. Some units use multichannel EEG.

5. Actively monitor and treat clinical and electrical seizures, because seizures worsen neurodevelopmental outcome independent of the severity of hypoxic-ischemic brain injury (27). The serum drug levels of anticonvulsants should be monitored closely because of liver impairment in infants with neonatal encephalopathy and potential HT-induced reduction in metabolism (28).

6. Monitor blood glucose from birth and treat hypoglycemia. Hypoglycemia is common in severely asphyxiated infants, particularly within the first 24 hours (29) and is associated with adverse long-term neurodevelopment (30).

7. Monitor serum electrolytes and maintain serum magnesium ≥1 mmol/L, as this may improve the neuroprotection (31).

8. Treat coagulopathy.

9. Sedate the cooled infants with appropriate sedatives to avoid cold stress. Experimental evidence shows that lack of sedation during HT may abolish the neuroprotective effect (32).

10. Monitor urine output. Catheterization may be necessary to maintain accurate fluid balance in sedated cooled infants.

11. Monitor core, surface, and scalp temperature (if on head cooling) every 15 minutes of maintaining HT during rewarming in manual modes. In servo modes, core, surface, and scalp temperatures can be monitored every 30 minutes during maintenance phase of HT.

12. Monitor skin for changes, and change the position of the infant (right lateral, left lateral, supine, and slight tilt of upper body) every 6 hours to avoid pressure sores or fat necrosis from poorly perfused tissue (3) and improve perfusion/ventilation within different areas of the lung.

G. Selective Head Cooling

SHC with mild systemic hypothermia (rectal temperature 34° to 35°C) was the first FDA approved cooling method in clinical use (34) and aims to selectively reduce the temperature of the brain more than the rest of the body, seeking to minimize potential systemic adverse effects of HT (35,36). It is currently not feasible to accurately measure temperature in different parts of the brain, and the large size of the infant's head can preclude achieving significant cooling in the deep brain using a cooling cap without reducing core temperature (37). There is no evidence to suggest that either of the cooling methods (SHC or WBC) is superior to the other; however, servo-controlled WBC is easier than SHC and is most commonly used.

In the SHC with mild systemic hypothermia, while the head is cooled using a cooling cap, the body is warmed using an overhead radiant warmer. Advantages of SHC includes achieving a lower temperature in the cortex and as the body is warm, babies are more comfortable. Disadvantages include lack of servo-control in maintaining the core temperature, which makes the technique labor intensive. SHC with normothermia might be useful to investigate in preterm infants with hypoxic ischemic encephalopathy.

H. Whole-Body Cooling

WBC can be achieved by:

1. Passive cooling.
2. Cooling with simple adjuncts such as water bottles, gloves filled with water, gels, or fan.
   These methods are effective, but they are more difficult to use and are labor intensive. It is difficult to achieve stable temperature over a long period.
3. Manually controlled cooling machine and mattress.
4. Servo-controlled cooling machines with body wrap or mattress.
   a. Temperature, blood pressure, and heart rate variation during cooling with manual and servo-controlled WBC and manual SHC are shown in **Figure 50.3**.

Passive Cooling

After perinatal asphyxia, the metabolism of infants is naturally low, and the core temperature will fall unless active warming is commenced (38). When perinatal asphyxia is likely in an infant at birth, passive cooling should be initiated as soon as ventilation is established (39). This method of cooling can be effective for days, depending on the environmental temperature and frequent control of cooling sources. Passive cooling is usually only used until active cooling equipment is available (40). Passive cooling is used in peripheral centres who do not have servo-controlled cooling machine to commence cooling on babies who fulfil cooling criteria or on asphyxiated babies who have inconclusive neurological examination or mild encephalopathy until the babies could either be assigned to full therapeutic hypothermia protocol or rewarmed.

Technique

1. No radiant warmer or other methods of warming should be initiated.
2. Keep the infant uncovered (small diaper may remain in place).

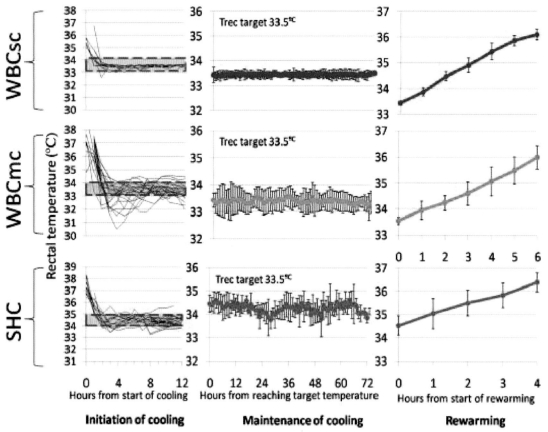

FIGURE 50.3 Variability in the rectal temperature during initiation, maintenance, and rewarming phase of HT. SHC, selective head cooling manual (CoolCap *n* = 21); WBCmc, whole-body cooling manual control (Tecotherm *n* = 25); WBCsc, whole-body cooling servo-controlled (CritiCool *nv* = 28).

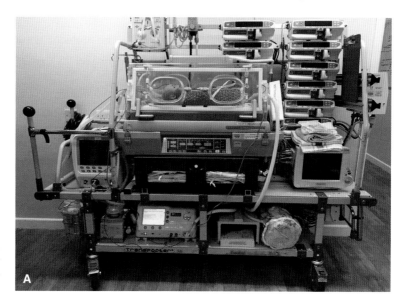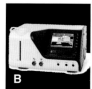

FIGURE 50.4 Cooling during transport using Tecotherm (**A**) or CritiCool mini (**B**). CritiCool can operate using battery for 1 hour.

3. Monitor core temperature with rectal or esophageal probe. If overcooling occurs, infant can be rewarmed slowly with a heat source (e.g., warm water bottles, overhead heating [with heat shield to the head]) (see **Fig. 50.17**).
4. Maintain ambient temperature below 26°C.

Pitfalls

1. Continuous core temperature monitoring is required to avoid excessive cooling (40,41).
2. Variability of core temperature during passive HT is high (40).

I. Cooling During Transport

1. Refer the infant to a center offering therapeutic HT as soon as possible.
2. Provide the required cardiorespiratory support, and use passive or other (*see G, I*) cooling method to achieve the target temperature early (44) and maintain target temperature using servo control during transport by ambulance (45) or aircraft (**Fig. 50.4**) (46).

Cooling With Adjuncts

1. *Gloves/bottles filled with tap water* (**Fig. 50.5**)

Technique

a. Expose the infant fully and place in an open crib.
b. Remove all heat sources.
c. Maintain ambient temperature between 25°C and 26°C.
d. Use three rubber water bottles, filled with cold tap water, to form a mattress *and/or*
e. Place rubber gloves filled with water at approximately 10°C next to the groins, axillae, and neck (35).

f. Monitor core temperature (rectal or esophageal) for 72 hours duration of HT.
g. Apply blankets and change gloves and/or water bottles as frequently as necessary to maintain core temperature at 33.5 ± 0.5°C.
h. Rewarming can be achieved passively by discontinuing active cooling and monitoring the rise in core temperature.
i. Gradual rewarming using external heat source, as for passive cooling, can be used with appropriate shield to protect the head (**Figs. 50.17**).

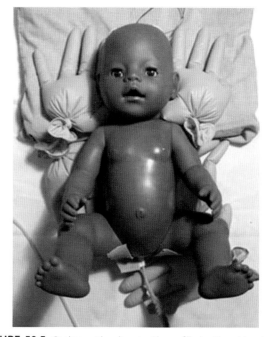

FIGURE 50.5 Cooling with adjuncts. Gloves filled with cold water are placed around the head, trunk, and legs to cool the infant, along with rectal temperature monitoring.

Pitfalls

a. Maintain minimal variation in ambient temperature.
b. Some, but relatively less, variability in core temperature compared with passive cooling.
c. Frequent monitoring is required to determine when the gloves/water bottles need replacing.

2. *Gels (5)* (**Fig. 50.6**)

Technique

a. Expose the infant to the ambient temperature in an open crib with an overhead warmer turned off.
b. Apply two refrigerated gel packs (12 cm × 12 cm, at 7° to 10°C) across the chest and/or under the head and shoulders.
c. Remove one gel pack when the core temperature falls below 35°C.
d. Remove the next gel pack when the core temperature falls below 34.5°C.
e. Turn on the radiant warmer and manually adjust the heater output every 15 to 30 minutes if the core temperature falls below 33.5°C and use appropriate shield to protect the head (see **Fig. 50.17**).
f. Reapply gel packs if core temperature rises above 34°C.
g. After 72 hours, increase the radiant warmer heater output to achieve rewarming by 0.5°C every 1 hour.

Phase Changing Material (42)

a. Phase change material based on Glauber salt can maintain a steady temperature by storing or releasing thermal energy providing a natural feedback.
b. Hypothermia can be induced and maintained with phase change material achieving a set temperature of 32°C.

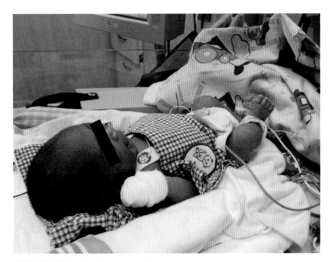

FIGURE 50.6 Cooling with refrigerated gel packs placed under the head and across the chest and trunk.

c. Phase change material is likely to be effective when the ambient temperature is <28°C and requires nursing input (43).

Pitfalls

a. High variability of core temperature.
b. Intensive monitoring and support required to maintain the desired core temperature.

Cooling Using a Servo-Controlled Cooling Machine

The servo-controlled cooling systems cool and maintain the core temperature by altering the temperature of the cooling fluid automatically, based on the core and surface temperature feedback to the system. The infant can be placed inside an incubator or preferably in an open bed.

1. The CritiCool (MTRE Advanced Technologies Ltd, Yavne, Israel) Temperature management unit (**Fig. 50.7**)
   a. *Other equipment*
      (1) Power cable
      (2) Connecting tubes
      (3) Cure wrap (MTRE Advanced Technologies Ltd, Yavne, Israel)
      (4) Sterile or 0.22 micron filtered water
      (5) Rectal temperature probe × 2 (reusable) or adapter with single-use rectal probes or esophageal temperature probe (E)
      (6) Skin temperature probe (reusable) or adapter with single-use probes
      (7) Layered bubble wrap pillow.
   b. *Modes available*
      (1) Cooling
      (2) Controlled rewarming (for slow rewarming)
      (3) Normothermia (for fast rewarming)
      (4) Empty (to empty the system)
   c. *Mode selection*
      (1) Press the MENU key
      (2) Select the MODE SELECT option to display the MODE SELECT panel
      (3) Use up/down arrows to select the required mode
      (4) Click OK to activate the mode
   d. *Technique using cooling mode*
      (1) Position CritiCool unit and lock front wheels.
      (2) Fill tank of the temperature management unit with sterile or 0.22 micron filtered water to between the two red lines (**Fig. 50.7A,B**).
      (3) Select the size of the CureWrap ("cooling jacket") appropriate to the size of the infant (<3.5 kg and >3.5 kg) (**Fig. 50.7C**).
      (4) Connect the connecting tubes to the temperature management unit and the CureWrap (**Fig. 50.7A**).

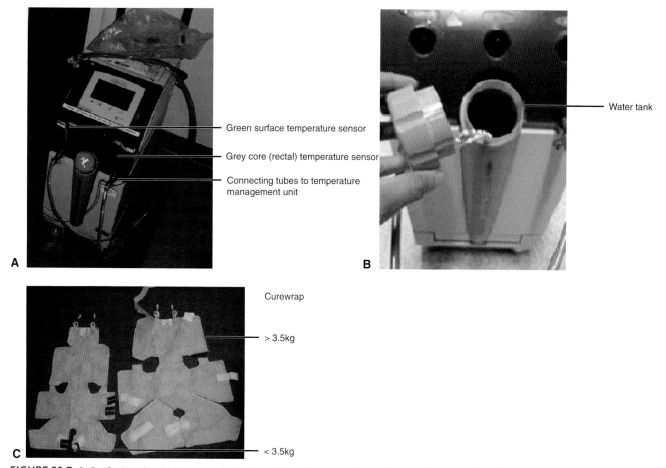

Green surface temperature sensor

Grey core (rectal) temperature sensor

Connecting tubes to temperature management unit

Water tank

Curewrap

> 3.5kg

< 3.5kg

FIGURE 50.7 A: CritiCool machine. **B:** Water tank to be filled with sterile water to the area between the two red lines. **C:** CureWrap with the Velcro fasteners for infants <3.5 kg and >3.5 kg.

(5) Pull the collar off the female end of the connecting tube and insert over the male connector to the CureWrap.

(6) Connect the connecting tubes to the metallic sockets in front of the temperature management unit.

(7) Switch on the temperature management unit after connecting the power cable. A prompt to confirm mode will appear with an audio alarm.

(8) CureWrap will fill with water; ensure the CureWrap is filled with water prior to wrapping and securing on infant.

(9) Confirm neonatal cooling mode (**Fig. 50.8A**).

(a) The default set core temperature in the management unit is 33.5°C.

(b) Water will not flow in the wrap without a valid core temperature reading.

(10) Connect grey temperature sensor into Core socket and green temperature sensor into surface socket (**Fig. 50.7A**).

(11) Circulation is confirmed when the "flow icon" (top right of display) is rotating (**Fig. 50.8B**).

(12) Place the infant in the supine position on the CureWrap (which is shaped to fit the infant) in an open crib/bed.

(13) Undress the infant down to a small diaper.

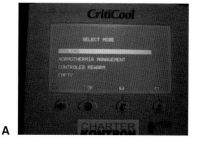

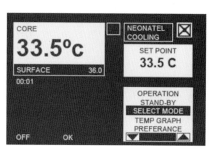

FIGURE 50.8 Setting up CritiCool for neonatal cooling and automatic rewarming mode. **A,B:** LCD display on the CritiCool.

(14) Insert the rectal or esophageal temperature probe (grey sensor) supplied with the equipment (see *E* and **Fig. 50.2A**).

(15) Insert a second calibrated rectal probe to 6 cm, alongside the previous probe. The second probe is connected to a separate patient monitor to serve as a means to double check the rectal temperature.

(16) Secure both the rectal temperature sensors (see *E*).

(17) Cover the infant's legs and the trunk with the CureWrap, and secure with the Velcro straps (see **Fig. 50.9C**).

(18) Expose the umbilicus to allow insertion of umbilical lines and monitoring for bleeding (**Fig. 50.9C**).

(19) Place six layers of bubble wrap between the head and the head portion of the wrap (**Fig. 50.9A–C**).

    (a) This insulates the head from the cycling temperature in the CureWrap (19).

    (b) Keeping the head exposed in an open bed maintains the superficial brain colder (19).

    (c) The experimental evidence indicates that the fluctuation in the mattress temperature every 12 minutes induces similar fluctuations in the superficial brain temperature.

(20) Secure the surface temperature probe to the forehead with tape (**Fig. 50.9C**).

(21) Monitor core and surface temperature every 15 minutes during induction of HT and rewarming, and every 30 to 60 minutes during maintenance phase of HT.

(22) After 72 hours of HT, rewarm using either the *manual* or *controlled* mode.

e. *Technique using manual mode*

During the *manual mode*, the user increases the set core temperature in the CritiCool by 0.2° to 0.3°C per 30 minutes to increase the core temperature by 0.4° to 0.5°C per hour. Rewarming degree and duration can be individualized to infant's clinical condition in this mode.

(1) To select *controlled rewarm mode*, press *menu*, select *mode*, press ▲ to move up or to move down, and highlight the controlled rewarm option. Press *OK* (**Fig. 50.10A**).

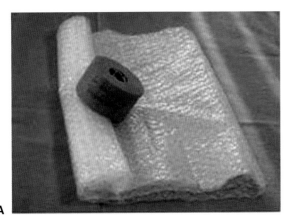

A

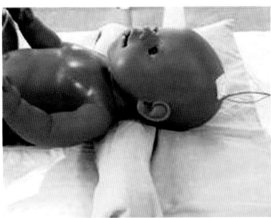

B

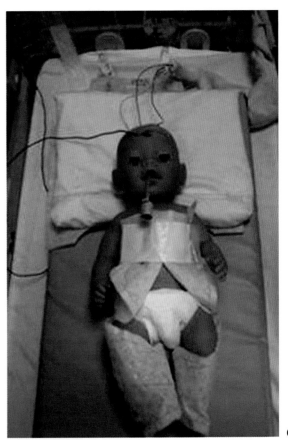

C

FIGURE 50.9 Insulating the head with bubble wrap. **A:** Pillow is prepared with six layers of bubble wrap. **B:** The layers of bubble wrap are rolled at one end to form a neck roll. **C:** CureWrap placed around the doll; bubble wrap pillow is covered with sheet; the neck rests on the neck roll; aEEG electrode is fixed in the parietal (P3) position.

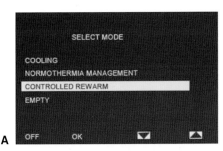

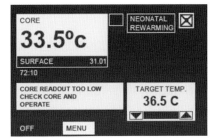

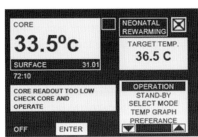

FIGURE 50.10 LCD display on the Critical for rewarming modes (**A–C**).

(a) The message "CORE readout too low check core and operate" will appear (**Fig. 50.10B**).
(b) Core, skin, and target temperatures are shown on the monitor of the temperature management unit (**Fig. 50.10B**). The water will no longer be circulating in the wrap.
(c) The default target temperature is 36.5°C; however, the set target temperature can be varied between 36°C and 38°C, using the ▲ or ▼ arrows below the target temperature read out (**Fig. 50.10B**).
(2) To start controlled rewarming, press *menu* and use the ▲ or ▼ arrows to select *Operation* (**Fig. 50.10C**).
(3) Once *Operation* is highlighted, press the *Enter* button to confirm (**Fig. 50.10C**).
(4) Once normothermia achieved, leave the infant on the wrap for 12 hours.
(5) If the infant is in a crib in which the temperature of the mattress can be increased, increase the temperature of the mattress to 1°C above the infant core temperature at the end of the 12-hour period and remove the wrap.
(6) Keep the infant's head uncovered and placed on the bubble wrap pillow to insulate the head from the heated mattress.
(7) Infant may be dressed in one layer of clothing.
(8) Monitor the rectal temperature for 24 hours after achieving normothermia (approximately 36.5°C rectal) to avoid hypo- or hyperthermia.
f. Precautions
(1) The CureWrap must be applied loosely (allow a space of a finger width between the skin and the wrap) around the trunk to avoid impeding ventilation and pressure on the skin from the monitoring leads between the wrap and skin (**Fig. 50.11**).

(2) Skin care must be performed a minimum of every 8 hours.
(3) An alarm will alert the user if the rectal or surface probes become dislodged.
(4) An alarm will sound if there is insufficient water in the temperature management unit.
g. Advantages
(1) Rapid initiation of HT.
(2) No overshoot of core temperature during induction.
(3) Variability of core temperature during maintenance and rewarming phase is minimal (47).
(4) Better hemodynamic stability in terms of blood pressure and heart rate than manual cooling (see **Fig. 50.3**, upper panel).
(5) Easy downloading of all temperature data.

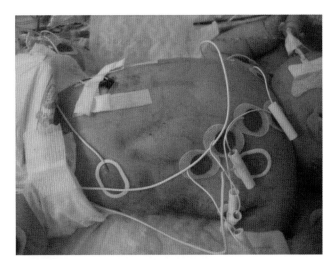

FIGURE 50.11 Impressions on the skin produced by ECG lead under the wrap, which are the result of applying the CureWrap too tightly.

2. *Tecotherm Neo (Fig. 50.12) (TECCOM GmbH, Halle/Salle, Germany)*
   a. Equipment
      (1) Mains cable
      (2) Tecotherm Neo cooling unit
      (3) Cooling mattress
      (4) Mattress connecting hoses
      (5) Rectal temperature probe × 2
      (6) Lubricating jelly
      (7) Skin temperature probe × 1
      (8) Coolant fluid
      (9) Coolant fill-up set
      (10) Pillow of six-layered bubble wrap
   b. *Modes Available*
      (1) *Servo-control complete treatment mode:* Duration of treatment, rate of cooling/warming as well as the target temperature can be set by the user. Whole cycle of treatment will be completed and the final temperature is reached.
      (2) *Servo-control mode (constant rectal temperature):* Target temperature, time to get to the target temperature, and the duration to maintain the target temperature can be set. Rate of change to allow even cooling/warming can be set.
      (3) *Constant mattress temperature mode:* Temperature of the mattress can be maintained at a set temperature. No servo-control.
   c. Technique
      (1) Connect the mains cable to the power and switch on.
      (2) Connect the fill-up set to the cooling unit (**Fig. 50.12B**).

(3) Keep the fill-up set above the cooling unit so that the coolant fills up the cooling unit.
(4) Connect the mattress to the cooling unit with the connecting hose (**Fig. 50.12A,C**).
(5) Connect the rectal temperature probe and the skin temperature probe to the cooling unit (**Fig. 50.12C**).
(6) Set the Tecotherm Neo to programmable servo-controlled mode (this completes the induction and maintains the temperature at the target of 33.5°C for 72 hours, followed by servo-controlled rewarming to 37°C over 7 hours).
(7) Undress the infant down to small diaper.
(8) Secure two rectal temperature probes to 6 cm (see **Fig. 50.2**), and tape to the side of the thigh as previously described in E.
(9) Secure the skin temperature probe on the forehead.
(10) Place the infant supine on the mattress and encircle the baby with the mattress, in a closed unheated incubator or an open crib/bed (**Figs. 50.12 and 50.13**).
(11) Secure the mattress at the front of the infant with the supplied ties (**Figs. 50.12C and 50.13**).
(12) Place the pillow between the head and the mattress (**Fig. 50.13**) (19). Alarms are activated if there is no power, low fluid, no flow of fluid, rectal temperature is out of range by 0.5°C, and for system failure.

Tecotherm Neo

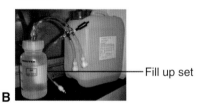

— Cooling unit
— Rectal temperature sensor
— Skin temperature sensor
— Coolant fill up set connector

Coolant

— Fill up set

Tecotherm Neo set up for cooling

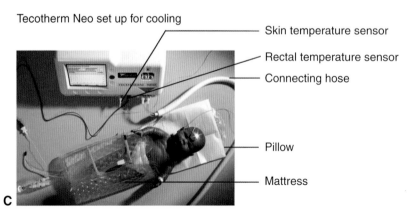

— Skin temperature sensor
— Rectal temperature sensor
— Connecting hose
— Pillow
— Mattress

FIGURE 50.12 Tecotherm Neo–servo-controlled. **A:** Cooling unit. **B:** Coolant. **C:** Tecotherm Neo setup for cooling.

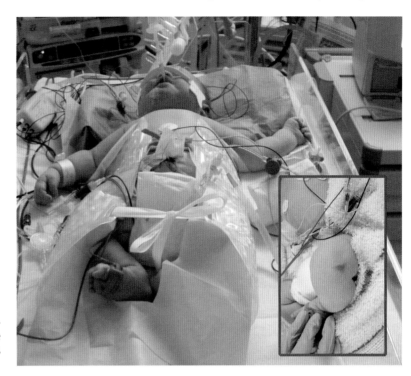

FIGURE 50.13 Tecotherm Neo–servo-controlled cooling. Reusable cooling mattress was wrapped around the lower body. *Insert* shows red pressure area on the knee, where the mattress was wrapped too tight.

d. Precautions

Avoid tight wrapping of mattress. This can lead to excessive pressure on the skin (**Fig. 50.13**).

e. Advantages

(1) Rapid initiation of HT.

(2) No overshoot of core temperature during induction (47).

(3) Variability of core temperature during maintenance and rewarming phase is minimal.

(4) Easy downloading of all temperature data with USB memory stick.

3. *Blanketrol III* (Cincinnati Sub-Zero Products, Inc., Cincinnati, Ohio) (**Fig. 50.14**)

a. Equipment

(1) Blanketrol III unit

(2) Hyper/hypothermia blanket

(3) Dry sheet, bath blanket or Disposal-Cover

(4) Connecting hose

(5) 400-series probe

(6) Lubricating jelly

(7) Connector cable for the disposable probes

(8) Distilled water (do not use tap water or deionized water)

b. *Cooling modes available.*

(1) Manual mode (**Fig. 50.15B**): Operation based on temperature of circulating water relative to the set blanket/water temperature.

(2) Auto control (**Fig. 50.15F**): Monitors patient temperature and delivers maximum heating or cooling therapy to bring patient's temperature to the set point.

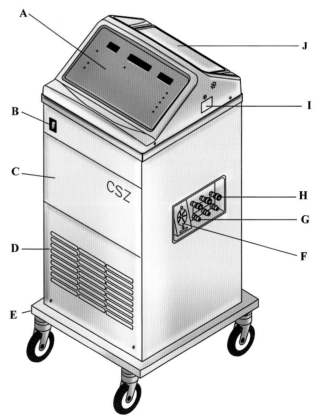

FIGURE 50.14 Blanketrol III. **A:** Control panel. **B:** Power switch (I–on; O–off). **C:** Storage drawer. **D:** Grill. **E:** Protective bumper. **F:** Water flow indicator. **G:** Male outlet coupling. **H:** Female return coupling. **I:** Patient probe jack. **J:** Water fill tank.

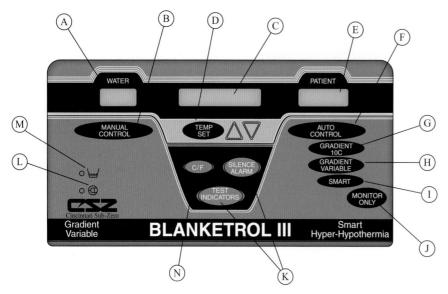

FIGURE 50.15 Blanketrol III membrane control panel (115-volt unit). A, Water temperature; B, Manual control of circulating water temperature; C, LCD status display; D, Temperature set button; E, Patient temperature; F, Auto control mode; G, Gradient 10c mode; H, Gradient variable mode; I, Smart function; J, Monitor patient temperature; K, Test indicator (confirm all the indicators are working) and silence alarm; L, Power failure (LED on the side flashes with audible alarm when power has been interrupted); M, Low water symbol; N, Celsius or Fahrenheit.

(3) Gradient 10C (**Fig. 50.15G**): Heats or cools the patient with water 10°C above or below the patient's temperature, until the patient reaches the desired set temperature.

(4) Gradient 10C smart (**Fig. 50.15G,I**): Heats or cools the patient with water 10°C above or below the patient's temperature and increases the gradient 5°C until set temperature is reached. When the patient's temperature deviates from set point after having reached the target temperature, the gradient returns to 10°C.

(5) Gradient variable (**Fig. 50.15H**): Same as Gradient 10C mode, except that the gradient can be determined by user. Smart mode can be added to Gradient.

(6) Variable: The gradient increases by 5°C beyond the specified gradient until the set temperature is reached. When the infant's temperature deviates from set point after having reached the target temperature, the gradient returns to the specified gradient.

(7) Monitor only (**Fig. 50.15J**): Displays the patient temperature without heating or cooling or circulating the water.

(8) The cooling system is activated by pressing *Temp Set* and setting the target temperature, followed by pressing the mode selector. To change to *Monitor Only*, press the appropriately labeled button (**Fig. 50.15J**).

c. WBC gradient variable mode technique

(1) Place the Blanketrol III unit in the patient area, accessible to the correct power source.

(2) Check the level of the distilled water in the reservoir. Lift the cover of the water fill opening and check that the water is visibly touching the strainer (**Fig. 50.14J**).

(3) Check that the power switch is in the *off* position (**Fig. 50.14B**).

(4) Insert the plug into a properly grounded receptacle.

(5) Lay the hyper/hypothermia blanket flat (**Fig. 50.16**) with the hose routed, without kinks, toward the unit.

(6) Cover the blanket with a dry sheet or disposable cover (**Fig. 50.16**), if single patient use blanket such as MAXI-THERM (Cincinnati Sub-Zero Products, Inc., Cincinnati, Ohio).

(7) Connect the blanket to the Blanketrol III unit: Attach the quick-disconnect female coupling of the connecting hose to the male outlet coupling on the cooling unit (**Fig. 50.14G**) and the male coupling to the female return coupling (**Fig. 50.14H**) by pushing back the collar of the female coupling while connecting to the male coupling, followed by releasing the collar.

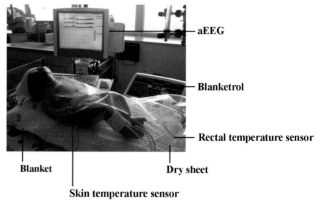

FIGURE 50.16 Blanketrol III setup for cooling.

(8) Gently pull the connecting hose to ensure a positive connection, that there are no twists in the connecting hose, and that the blanket is flat.

(9) Initiate **precooling:** Precooling may not be necessary if the infant's temperature has already been lowered (e.g., by passive hypothermia during transport).

    (a) Switch on the cooling machine (**Fig. 50.14B**).

    (b) Press *Temp Set* (**Fig. 50.15D**).

    (c) Use the up (Δ) or down (∇) arrows by the side of *Set Temp* (**Fig. 50.15**) and set the temperature to 33.5°C.

    (d) Press *Manual Control* (**Fig. 50.15B**).

    (e) Listen for the compressor to activate.

    (f) Check the water flow indicator (**Fig. 50.14F**) to confirm that water is circulating.

    (g) Place the infant on the blanket (**Fig. 50.16**).

    (h) Place patient temperature monitoring probes.

d. Rectal temperature sensor

    (1) Mark a 400-series probe at 6 cm from the tip with tape/indelible pen (see **Fig. 50.2**).

    (2) Insert rectal probe 6 cm into the rectum, and secure to leg using DuoDERM/Tegaderm and tape, as described in E (see **Fig. 50.2**).

e. Esophageal temperature

    (1) Measure a 400-series probe from nose/midline of the mouth to ear and then to an imaginary line between the nipples.

    (2) Mark this position on the probe with tape/indelible pen.

    (3) Insert the probe via mouth or nose up to the mark.

    (4) Secure the probe to the upper lip.

        (a) Connect the rectal or esophageal probe to black cable jack.

        (b) Connect black cable to probe outlet in Blanketrol (**Fig. 50.14I**).

        (c) Initiate **induction** of HT (*Gradient Variable* mode)

    (5) After 1 minute, press *Temp Set* (**Fig. 50.14D**).

    (6) Press the Δ/∇ (**Fig. 50.14**) button to set the temperature to **33.5°C.**
        The status display (**Fig. 50.15C**) will read **33.5°C.**

    (7) Press *Gradient Variable* (**Fig. 50.15H**).

    (8) Press Δ/∇ (Fig. 45.20) to **20°C.**

    (9) Press the *Gradient Variable* (Fig. 50.22H) again.

    (10) Listen for the activation of the pump.

    (11) Check that the water flow indicator (**Fig. 50.14F**) is rotating.

    (12) Place the dry sheet or disposable cover over the infant, to decrease convection losses and fluctuations in water temperature in blanket (**Fig. 50.16**).

(13) Monitor temperature displays. The *Patient* display (**Fig. 50.15E**) will show the infant's actual temperature.

    (a) The *Water* display (**Fig. 50.15A**) will show the actual temperature of the circulating water.

    (b) The *Status* display (**Fig. 50.15C**) will show the mode of operation and set temperature.

    (c) Monitor core temperature every 15 minutes to determine when the target temperature is reached.

f. Maintain HT (gradient variable mode)

    (1) Press *Temp Set* (**Fig. 50.15D**).

    (2) Press the Δ/∇ (**Fig. 50.15**) button to maintain core temperature at **33.5°C.**

    (3) Press *Gradient Variable* (**Fig. 50.15H**).

    (4) Press the Δ/∇ (**Fig. 50.15**) button to **5°C** to minimize the temperature fluctuations between the patient and the water in the cooling blanket.

    (5) Press the *Gradient Variable* (**Fig. 50.15H**) again.

    (6) Listen for the activation of the pump.

    (7) Check that the water flow indicator (**Fig. 50.14F**) is rotating.

g. *Initiate manual* **rewarming** *after 72 hours of HT*

    (1) Press *Temp Set* (**Fig. 50.15D**).

    (2) Press Δ button to **0.5°C.**

    (3) Increase 0.5°C every hour until the core temperature is 36.5°C.

    (4) Press *Gradient Variable* (**Fig. 50.15H**).

    (5) Press Δ to 5°C to minimize the temperature fluctuations between the patient and the water in the cooling blanket.

    (6) Press *Gradient Variable* (**Fig. 50.15H**).

    (7) Listen for the activation of the pump.

    (8) Check that the water flow indicator (**Fig. 50.14F**) is rotating.

h. Initiate post-rewarming care

    When the rectal temperature has been 36.5°C for 60 minutes, the Blanketrol can be set to *Monitor Only* and the infant can be kept normothermic (36.5 ± 0.2°C) with a servo-controlled overhead radiant warmer and overhead reflective shield (**Fig. 50.17**).

    (1) Press *Monitor Only* (**Fig. 50.15J**).

    (2) Keep core temperature probe in place for 24 hours after completion of cooling.

    (3) For radiant warmer, use servo control.
        Place the skin probe over the liver, right upper quadrant, below ribs.
        Set servo to achieve axillary temperature of 36.5 ± 0.2°C.

    (4) Cover the face and head with a reflective shield to prevent elevation of the superficial brain temperature (**Fig. 50.16**).
        Alternatively, the infant can be warmed in a Babytherm infant warmer (Dräger Medical

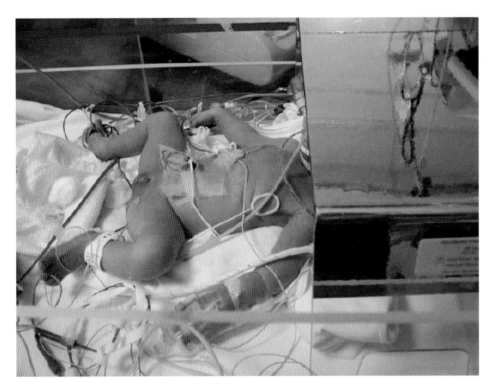

FIGURE 50.17 Baby with head under heat shield to protect the head from direct overhead heating.

Inc., Telford, Pennsylvania) or any "hot cot," which has the option of increasing the temperature of the mattress, by setting the temperature of the cot at the same temperature that the water in the Blanketrol was set at to maintain the infant normothermic.

(5) Place a six-layered bubble wrap "pillow" between the infant's head and the hot cot, to prevent elevation of the superficial brain temperature (**Fig. 50.9B,C**).

(6) Discontinue hourly core temperature monitoring after 24 hours, and resume routine 4 hourly temperature monitoring.

i. Precautions

(1) Do not use deionized water. The majority of deionizers do not maintain a neutral pH of 7. This results in acidification of water, which can deteriorate the battery and the copper refrigeration line, ultimately leading to a leak in the refrigeration system.

(2) Do not use alcohol, as it may cause blanket deterioration.

(3) Do not overfill the reservoir in Blanketrol.

(4) Check for leaks in the blanket and hose. Water leaks can be a risk for infection.

(5) If the *Check Probe* alarm activates, confirm that the core temperature probe has not fallen out.

If the core temperature probe is in place, consider changing the temperature cable rather than the temperature probe.

(a) Connect new temperature cable to Blanketrol (**Fig. 50.14I**) and to the temperature probe.

(b) Turn the machine off and back on.

(c) Press the *Temp Set* switch (**Fig. 50.15D**).

(d) Press $\Delta\nabla$ until most recent set point is reached.

(e) Press *Auto Control* (**Fig. 50.15F**).

4. ArcticSun 5000 Temperature Management System ArcticSun is able to precisely control temperature by monitoring the patient's core temperature every second and adjusting the water temperature every 2 minutes automatically without intervention

Cooling is achieved using a neonatal pad which is light weight with optional and adjustable abdominal foam straps. This is claimed to support the baby.

J. Rewarming

1. Rewarming is carried out after 72 hours of hypothermia.

2. Rewarming is generally achieved at a rate of 0.5°C/hr, when it is carried out with a cooling unit.

3. Rewarming without cooling equipment (covering with blanket or warm gloves, etc.) should be undertaken with continuous monitoring of rectal temperature to ensure it does not occur faster than 0.5°C/hr.

4. If seizures occur during rewarming (48), temporarily suspend rewarming until seizures cease with anticonvulsants; if the seizures are refractory to anticonvulsants, cooling again by 0.5 to 1°C may be necessary

(this may decrease the mismatch between cerebral oxygen delivery and consumption (49) and prevent further seizures). The rewarming can be continued at a rate of 0.2°C/hr after a seizure-free period (39).

K. Postrewarming Care

1. Monitor core temperature for 24 hours to avoid hyper- or hypothermia.
2. Protect the infant's head from heat source with a bubble-wrap pillow (in case of a heated crib or mattress) and a head shield (if a radiant warmer is used) (see **Figs. 50.9B** and **Fig. 50.17**).
3. Avoid placing the infant in an incubator, as this may cause an increase in superficial brain temperature.

L. Complications of Hypothermia

1. Increased levels of sedatives, anticonvulsants, and neuromuscular blocking agents due to individually decreased clearance of drugs metabolized in the liver (39,50,51).
2. Infants who are not well sedated will be uncomfortable due to the cold stress, and cooling may be painful. Therefore, cooled babies should be kept comfortable. Stress may reduce the effectiveness of cooling (32).
3. Thrombocytopenia (1)
4. Subcutaneous fat necrosis (52). This complication is rare (0.9% to 2.8%) and should be avoidable (33). This occurs in infants with macrosomia, hemodynamic instability (52), thrombocytopenia, and altered calcium levels. Subcutaneous fat necrosis is usually self-limiting.
5. Most predictors of outcome (except MRI, neurologic examination on/after day 12) after perinatal asphyxia that are validated for normothermic infants are less predictive for cooled infants; hence, cutoff values and interpretations are different (53).

Acknowledgments

Dr. Sonia Bonifacio, University of California, San Francisco, who kindly shared experience with Blanketrol cooling equipment and provided **Figures 50.14,** to **50.16,** and Dr. Terrie Inder, Washington University, St. Louis, MO, who provided **Figure 50.6.**

References

1. Jacobs SE, Berg M, Hunt R, et al. Cooling for newborns with hypoxic ischaemic encephalopathy. *Cochrane Database Syst Rev (Online)*. 2013;1:CD003311.
2. Gluckman PD, Wyatt JS, Azzopardi D, et al. Selective head cooling with mild systemic hypothermia after neonatal encephalopathy: multicentre randomised trial. *Lancet*. 2005;365(9460):663–670.
3. Shankaran S, Laptook AR, Ehrenkranz RA, et al. Whole-body hypothermia for neonates with hypoxic-ischemic encephalopathy. *N Engl J Med*. 2005;353(15):1574–1584.
4. Azzopardi DV, Strohm B, Edwards AD, et al. Moderate hypothermia to treat perinatal asphyxial encephalopathy. *N Engl J Med*. 2009;361(14):1349–1358.
5. Jacobs SE, Morley CJ, Inder TE, et al. Whole-body hypothermia for term and near-term newborns with hypoxic-ischemic encephalopathy: a randomized controlled trial. *Arch Pediatr Adolesc Med*. 2011;165(8):692–700.
6. Shankaran S, Pappas A, McDonald SA, et al. Childhood outcomes after hypothermia for neonatal encephalopathy. *N Engl J Med*. 2012;366(22):2085–2092.
7. Azzopardi D, Strohm B, Marlow N, et al. Effects of hypothermia for perinatal asphyxia on childhood outcomes. *N Engl J Med*. 2014;371(2):140–149.
8. Jary S, Smit E, Liu X, et al. Less severe cerebral palsy outcomes in infants treated with therapeutic hypothermia. *Acta Paediatr*. 2015;104(12):1241–1247.
9. Laptook AR, Shankaran S, Tyson JE, et al. Effect of therapeutic hypothermia initiated after 6 hours of age on death or disability among newborns with hypoxic-ischemic encephalopathy: a randomized clinical trial. *JAMA*. 2017;318(16):1550–1560.
10. Sabir H, Scull-Brown E, Liu X, et al. Immediate hypothermia is not neuroprotective after severe hypoxia-ischemia and is deleterious when delayed by 12 hours in neonatal rats. *Stroke*. 2012;43(12):3364–3370.
11. Gunn AJ, Bennet L, Gunning MI, et al. Cerebral hypothermia is not neuroprotective when started after postischemic seizures in fetal sheep. *Pediatr Res*. 1999;46(3):274–280.
12. El-Dib M, Inder TE, Chalak LF, et al. Should therapeutic hypothermia be offered to babies with mild neonatal encephalopathy in the first 6 h after birth? *Pediatr Res*. 2019;85(4):442–448.
13. Shankaran S, Laptook AR, Pappas A, et al. Effect of depth and duration of cooling on deaths in the NICU among neonates with hypoxic ischemic encephalopathy: a randomized clinical trial. *JAMA*. 2014;312(24):2629–2639.
14. Shankaran S, Laptook AR, Pappas A, et al. Effect of depth and duration of cooling on death or disability at age 18 months among neonates with hypoxic-ischemic encephalopathy: a randomized clinical trial. *JAMA*. 2017;318(1):57–67.
15. Rao R, Trivedi S, Vesoulis Z, et al. Safety and short-term outcomes of therapeutic hypothermia in preterm neonates 34–35 weeks gestational age with hypoxic-ischemic encephalopathy. *J Pediatr*. 2017;183:37–42.
16. Chakkarapani E, Harding D, Stoddart P, et al. Therapeutic hypothermia: surgical infant with neonatal encephalopathy. *Acta Paediatr*. 2009;98(11):1844–1846.
17. Smit E, Liu X, Jary S, et al. Cooling neonates who do not fulfil the standard cooling criteria—short- and long-term outcomes. *Acta Paediatr*. 2015;104(2):138–145.
18. Thoresen M. Hypothermia after perinatal asphyxia: selection for treatment and cooling protocol. *J Pediatr*. 2011;158 (2 Suppl):e45–e49.
19. Liu X, Chakkarapani E, Hoque N, et al. Environmental cooling of the newborn pig brain during whole-body cooling. *Acta Paediatr*. 2011;100(1):29–35.

20. Pappas A, Shankaran S, Laptook AR, et al. Hypocarbia and adverse outcome in neonatal hypoxic-ischemic encephalopathy. *J Pediatr.* 2011;158(5):752–758.

21. Sabir H, Jary S, Tooley J, et al. Increased inspired oxygen in the first hours of life is associated with adverse outcome in newborns treated for perinatal asphyxia with therapeutic hypothermia. *J Pediatr.* 2012;161(3):409–416.

22. Chakkarapani E, Thoresen M, Liu X, et al. Xenon offers stable haemodynamics independent of induced hypothermia after hypoxia-ischaemia in newborn pigs. *Intensive Care Med.* 2012;38(2):316–323.

23. Thoresen M, Hellstrom-Westas L, Liu X, et al. Effect of hypothermia on amplitude-integrated electroencephalogram in infants with asphyxia. *Pediatrics.* 2010;126(1):e131–e139.

24. Skranes JH, Lohaugen G, Schumacher EM, et al. Amplitude-integrated electroencephalography improves the identification of infants with encephalopathy for therapeutic hypothermia and predicts neurodevelopmental outcomes at 2 years of age. *J Pediatr.* 2017;187:34–42.

25. Liu X, Jary S, Cowan F, et al. Reduced infancy and childhood epilepsy following hypothermia-treated neonatal encephalopathy. *Epilepsia.* 2017;58(11):1902–1911.

26. Boylan GB, Kharoshankaya L, Wusthoff CJ. Seizures and hypothermia: importance of electroencephalographic monitoring and considerations for treatment. *Semin Fetal Neonatal Med.* 2015;20(2):103–108.

27. Glass HC, Glidden D, Jeremy RJ, et al. Clinical neonatal seizures are independently associated with outcome in infants at risk for hypoxic-ischemic brain injury. *J Pediatr.* 2009;155(3):318–323.

28. Wood T, Thoresen M. Physiological responses to hypothermia. *Semin Fetal Neonatal Med.* 2015;20(2):87–96.

29. Nadeem M, Murray DM, Boylan GB, et al. Early blood glucose profile and neurodevelopmental outcome at two years in neonatal hypoxic-ischaemic encephalopathy. *BMC Pediatr.* 2011;11:10.

30. Basu SK, Kaiser JR, Guffey D, et al. Hypoglycaemia and hyperglycaemia are associated with unfavourable outcome in infants with hypoxic ischaemic encephalopathy: a post hoc analysis of the CoolCap Study. *Arch Dis Child Fetal Neonatal Ed.* 2016;101(2):F149–F155.

31. Bhat MA, Charoo BA, Bhat JI, et al. Magnesium sulfate in severe perinatal asphyxia: a randomized, placebo-controlled trial. *Pediatrics.* 2009;123(5):e764–e769.

32. Thoresen M, Satas S, Loberg EM, et al. Twenty-four hours of mild hypothermia in unsedated newborn pigs starting after a severe global hypoxic-ischemic insult is not neuroprotective. *Pediatr Res.* 2001;50(3):405–411.

33. Chakkarapani E. Cooled infants with encephalopathy: Are heavier infants with weaker heart at a cutaneous disadvantage? *Acta Paediatr* 2016;105(9):996–998.

34. Gunn AJ, Gluckman P, Wyatt JS, et al. Selective head cooling after neonatal encephalopathy—author's reply. *The Lancet.* 2005;365(9471):1619–1620.

35. Thoresen M, Whitelaw A. Cardiovascular changes during mild therapeutic hypothermia and rewarming in infants with hypoxic-ischemic encephalopathy. *Pediatrics.* 2000;106(1 Pt 1):92–99.

36. Thoresen M, Simmonds M, Satas S, et al. Effective selective head cooling during posthypoxic hypothermia in newborn piglets. *Pediatr Res.* 2001;49(4):594–599.

37. Van Leeuwen GM, Hand JW, Lagendijk JJ, et al. Numerical modeling of temperature distributions within the neonatal head. *Pediatr Res.* 2000;48(3):351–356.

38. Burnard ED, Cross KW. Rectal temperature in the newborn after birth asphyxia. *Br Med J.* 1958;2(5106):1197–1199.

39. Thoresen M. Supportive care during neuroprotective hypothermia in the term newborn: adverse effects and their prevention. *Clin Perinatol.* 2008;35(4):749–763.

40. Hallberg B, Olson L, Bartocci M, et al. Passive induction of hypothermia during transport of asphyxiated infants: a risk of excessive cooling. *Acta Paediatr.* 2009;98(6):942–946.

41. Kendall GS, Kapetanakis A, Ratnavel N, et al. Passive cooling for initiation of therapeutic hypothermia in neonatal encephalopathy. *Arch Dis Child Fetal Neonatal Ed.* 2010;95(6):F408–F412.

42. Thomas N, Chakrapani Y, Rebekah G, et al. Phase changing material: an alternative method for cooling babies with hypoxic ischaemic encephalopathy. *Neonatology.* 2015;107(4):266–270.

43. Montaldo P, Pauliah SS, Lally PJ, et al. Cooling in a low-resource environment: lost in translation. *Semin Fetal Neonatal Med.* 2015;20(2):72–79.

44. Thoresen M, Tooley J, Liu X, et al. Time is brain: starting therapeutic hypothermia within three hours after birth improves motor outcome in asphyxiated newborns. *Neonatology.* 2013;104(3):228–233.

45. O'Reilly KM, Tooley J, Winterbottom S. Therapeutic hypothermia during neonatal transport. *Acta Paediatr.* 2011;100(8):1084–1086; discussion e1049.

46. Weiss MD, Tang A, Young L, et al. Transporting neonates with hypoxic-ischemic encephalopathy utilizing active hypothermia. *J Neonatal Perinatal Med.* 2014;7(3):173–178.

47. Hoque N, Chakkarapani E, Liu X, et al. A comparison of cooling methods used in therapeutic hypothermia for perinatal asphyxia. *Pediatrics.* 2010;126(1):e124–e130.

48. Battin M, Bennet L, Gunn AJ. Rebound seizures during rewarming. *Pediatrics.* 2004;114(5):1369.

49. van der Linden J, Ekroth R, Lincoln C, et al. Is cerebral blood flow/metabolic mismatch during rewarming a risk factor after profound hypothermic procedures in small children? *Eur J Cardiothorac Surg.* 1989;3(3):209–215.

50. Sunjic KM, Webb AC, Sunjic I, et al. Pharmacokinetic and other considerations for drug therapy during targeted temperature management. *Crit Care Med.* 2015;43(10):2228–2238.

51. Roka A, Melinda KT, Vasarhelyi B, et al. Elevated morphine concentrations in neonates treated with morphine and prolonged hypothermia for hypoxic ischemic encephalopathy. *Pediatrics.* 2008;121(4):e844–e849.

52. Courteau C, Samman K, Ali N, et al. Macrosomia and hemodynamic instability may represent risk factors for subcutaneous fat necrosis in asphyxiated newborns treated with hypothermia. *Acta Paediatr.* 2016;105(9):e396–e405.

53. Sabir H, Cowan FM. Prediction of outcome methods assessing short- and long-term outcome after therapeutic hypothermia. *Semin Fetal Neonatal Med.* 2015;20(2):115–121.

Removal of Extra Digits and Skin Tags

Jessica S. Wang and Stephen B. Baker

A. Definitions

1. **Polydactyly:** A condition characterized by more than five digits in one hand, usually due to a mutation in the HOX gene or disruption in the upper limb developmental pathway (1).
   a. **Postaxial (ulnar sided):** Accessory digit on the ulnar aspect of the hand **(Fig. 51.1A)**. More common in those of African descent (1:143) and may present as a well-developed (type A) or rudimentary/pedunculated (type B) digit (2,3).

b. **Preaxial (radial):** Duplication of the thumb **(Fig. 51.1B)**. This condition is more common in Asians (2.2:1,000) and usually presents in a unilateral fashion (2,4). Most cases are sporadic (2,4).

2. **Preauricular tag/accessory tragus:** A rare (1.7:1,000) congenital defect characterized by malformation of the cartilaginous projection anterior to the opening of the ear (5). Clinical presentation includes a 3- to 10-mm skin-colored papule located in the preauricular region. The lesion may be unilateral or bilateral and appear pedunculated or sessile (5).

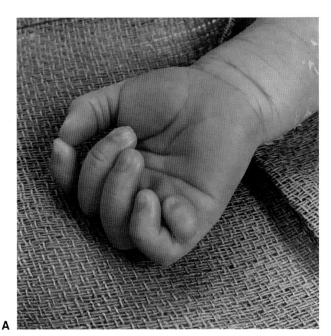
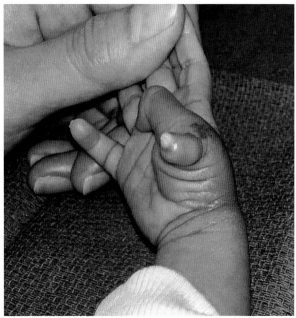

A   B

FIGURE 51.1 A: Postaxial polydactyly (type B) with stalk. **B:** Preaxial polydactyly with rudimentary nail.

B. Indications

1. **Polydactyly**
   a. All require surgical intervention to improve aesthetic and functional outcomes (2,4).
   b. Surgical excision is the preferred treatment modality.
      (1) In-office surgical excision is an excellent option for the rudimentary/pedunculated accessory digit, allowing the patient to forgo general anesthesia and undergo treatment at as early as 2 weeks of age (6).
      (2) Although suture ligation can be used to treat pedunculated digits with a thin stalk, this method suffers from high rates of amputation neuromas, residual rudimentary supernumerary digits, secondary bacterial infections, and need for revision procedures (7,8).
2. **Preauricular tag**
   Surgical excision is the most common treatment to optimize aesthetic outcomes (5).

C. Precautions

1. For well-developed accessory digits, referral to a hand surgeon is needed to determine the anatomic level of duplication and ensure proper musculotendinous reconstruction (4).
2. In preaxial polydactyly, the radial thumb is resected and ulnar thumb kept in order to preserve the ulnar collateral ligament, which plays an important role during pinch (4).
3. Preauricular tags may be associated with congenital syndromes (i.e., Goldenhar, Treacher Collins, VACTERL, etc.) and permanent hearing loss (5,9). As a result, a thorough family history and newborn hearing screen should be obtained, with a low threshold for genetic testing.

D. Equipment (Fig. 51.2)

1. Povidone-iodine skin cleanser
2. Sterile towels/drapes, gauze, and gloves

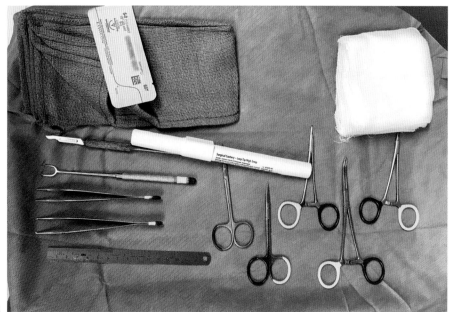

FIGURE 51.2 Equipment for office-based excision of duplicated digit. Set includes (**A**) sterile towels, Adson forceps, double-prong skin hooks, ruler, no. 15 blade scalpel, Iris scissors, suture scissors, needle driver, 5-0 chromic gut suture, and (**B**) loop tip cautery.

3. Sterile instruments
   a. Adson forceps
   b. Double-prong skin hook
   c. Ruler
   d. Scalpel with no. 15 blade
   e. Curved Iris scissors
   f. Suture scissors
   g. Needle driver
   h. 5-0 chromic gut suture
   i. Loop tip/high temperature surgical cautery
4. Local anesthetic
   a. 1% lidocaine with epinephrine (no more than 10 mL)
5. 3M Steri-Strips

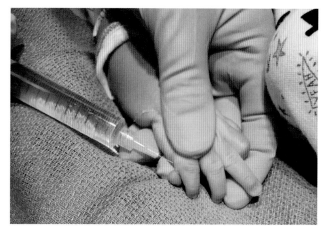

FIGURE 51.3 Injection of lidocaine with epinephrine into base of duplicated digit.

E. Procedure or Technique

Polydactyly

1. Prepare the surgical area with an alcohol swab, and inject the base of the accessory digit with 0.5 mL of 1% lidocaine with 1:100,000 epinephrine (**Fig. 51.3**). Allow 10 minutes for the local anesthetic to take effect.
2. Prepare the hand with povidone-iodine solution, then drape the surgical field with sterile towels.
3. Perform the procedure under 2.5 to 3.5× loupe magnification for best results. Place the accessory digit on gentle extension, and excise the base of the digit using curved Iris scissors or a no. 15 scalpel.
4. If a vessel is encountered in the stalk and bleeding occurs, use electrocautery for hemostasis.

5. If a digital nerve is encountered in the stalk, trim the nerve back sharply and bury within deeper tissues.
6. Close the skin with 5-0 chromic sutures and dress with Steri-Strips (**Fig. 51.4**).

Preauricular Tag

1. Prepare the surgical area with an alcohol swab, and perform a ring block around the ear with 1 mL of 1% lidocaine with 1:100,000 epinephrine. Allow 10 minutes for the local anesthetic to take effect.
2. Prepare the entire auricular area with povidone-iodine solution, then drape the surgical field with sterile towels.

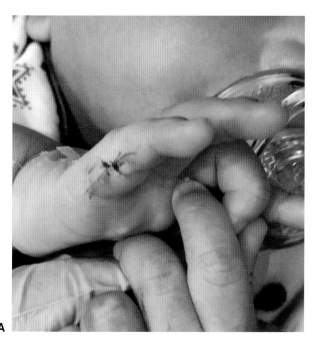 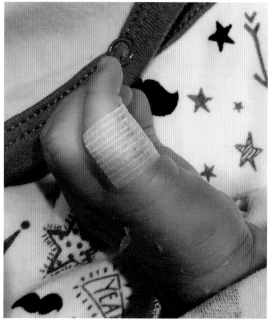

A   B

FIGURE 51.4 A: Status post excision of duplicated digit. Incision closed with 5-0 chromic gut suture. **B:** Post excision of duplicated digit. Incision closed with Steri-Strip.

3. Perform the procedure under 2.5 to 3.5× loupe magnification for best results. Grasp the accessory tragus with forceps, and make an elliptical incision around the lesion using a no. 15 scalpel.
4. Dissect down to subcutaneous tissue with Iris scissors, and remove the lesion with the subcutaneous tissue.
5. Identify and remove the protruding accessory cartilage deep to the subcutaneous tissue using Iris scissors or a scalpel.
6. Obtain hemostasis with electrocautery.
7. Close the skin with 5-0 chromic sutures.

F. Complications

1. Wound dehiscence
2. Wound infection
3. Residual aesthetic deformity
4. Postsurgical neuroma

References

1. Janis J. *Essentials of Plastic Surgery*. 2nd ed. Thieme Medical Publishers; 2014:1367. Rerrieved from https://www.thieme.com/books-main/plastic-surgery/product/3714-essentials-of-plastic-surgery-second-edition.

2. Brown DL, Borschel GH, Levi B. *Michigan Manual of Plastic Surgery*. Lippincott Williams & Wilkins; 2014:624. Retrieved from https://shop.lww.com/Michigan-Manual-of-Plastic-Surgery/p/9781451183672.
3. Kozin SH, Zlotolow DA. Common pediatric congenital conditions of the hand. *Plast Reconstr Surg*. 2015;136(2):241e–257e.
4. Oda T, Pushman AG, Chung KC. Treatment of common congenital hand conditions. *Plast Reconstr Surg*. 2010;126(3):121e–133e.
5. Bahrani B, Khachemoune A. Review of accessory tragus with highlights of its associated syndromes. *Int J Dermatol*. 2014;53(12):1442–1446.
6. Carpenter CL, Cuellar TA, Friel MT. Office-based post–axial polydactyly excision in neonates, infants, and children. *Plast Reconstr Surg*. 2016;137(2):564–568.
7. Leber GE, Gosain AK. Surgical excision of pedunculated supernumerary digits prevents traumatic amputation neuromas. *Pediatr Dermatol*. 2003;20(2):108–112.
8. Mullick S, Borschel GH. A selective approach to treatment of ulnar polydactyly: preventing painful neuroma and incomplete excision. *Pediatr Dermatol*. 2010;27(1):39–42.
9. Roth DA, Hildesheimer M, Bardenstein S, et al. Preauricular skin tags and ear pits are associated with permanent hearing impairment in newborns. *Pediatrics*. 2008;122(4):e884–e890.

Neonatal Circumcision

Sarah A. Holzman, Aaron Krill, and Louis Marmon

A. Indications

Newborn male circumcision is one of the oldest formally recorded surgical procedures as well as among the most controversial (1–4). Many physicians and lay people consider neonatal circumcision to be routine, but rare severe complications have been reported. Despite the perceived simplicity of the procedure, meticulous attention to anatomic landmarks, wound care, and follow-up is necessary.

B. Contraindications (4,5)

1. Age <1 day (i.e., before complete physical adaptation to extrauterine life has occurred).
2. Any current illness.
3. Temperature instability.
4. Prematurity (<37 weeks' gestation).
5. Bleeding diathesis or family history of bleeding disorder.
6. Abnormality of urethra or penile shaft since the foreskin may be essential for later reconstruction (e.g., hypospadias, chordee, very small penis). *Note: The identification of a megameatus or hypospadias after retraction of an intact-appearing foreskin is not a contraindication to neonatal circumcision (6).*
7. Local infection.
8. Lack of truly "informed" parental consent (see Chapter 3).
9. Prior to infant receiving vitamin K.

Disclaimer: The following discussions of the equipment, analgesia, and procedures are guidelines and are not intended to replace supervised instruction of the various circumcision techniques. Newborn circumcisions should only be performed by experienced personnel.

C. Equipment (7–9)

1. Most frequently required
   a. *Sterile*

   (1) Gloves
   (2) Cup with antiseptic
   (3) 4 × 4-inch gauze pads
   (4) Small, flexible, blunt probe
   (5) Two curved mosquito hemostats
   (6) Large, straight hemostat
   (7) Tissue scissors
   (8) Scalpel
   b. *Nonsterile*
   (1) Infant restraint to immobilize lower extremities is usually required. Can use commercially available equipment (Circumstraint Newborn Immobilizer, Olympic Medical) (see Chapter 5).
   (2) An acceptable alternative is swaddling that provides adequate genitalia exposure.
2. Analgesia

   The current recommendation is that neonatal circumcisions be performed under local anesthesia (4). In the past, neonatal circumcision had been performed without anesthesia, but this is no longer recommended. Kirya and Werthmann initially reported the efficacy and safety of dorsal penile blocks in 1978 (10). A randomized controlled trial showed that anesthesia with ring block, dorsal nerve block, or EMLA cream was superior to placebo. A ring block was found to be more effective than dorsal nerve block alone or EMLA cream during foreskin separation and incision (11).
   a. Equipment for injected analgesia
   (1) Local anesthetic: 1 mL of 1% lidocaine hydrochloride without epinephrine in a tuberculin syringe with a 1.2-cm × 27-gauge needle.
   (2) Alcohol or iodine-based skin prep.
   (3) Sterile gauze.
   b. Topical analgesia
   (1) Topical anesthesia options include eutectic mixture of lidocaine-prilocaine local anesthetic (EMLA) and topical lidocaine 4% (LMX4) cream. Topical anesthesia has been shown to reduce neonatal stress indicators during circumcision and reduces crying time (12,13).

LMX4 cream should be placed 20 minutes (14) and EMLA cream 60 minutes prior to circumcision (15). LMX4 may have some advantage over EMLA cream with faster onset of action and no risk of methemoglobinemia (14).

(2) Oral sucrose and oral analgesics (acetaminophen) may be similar to placebo and are not sufficient alone for procedural pain control. However, positioning and a sucrose pacifier should be used as adjuncts for pain control (4).

3. Optional circumcision equipment
   a. Sterile fine-tipped marking pen.
   b. Sterile gauze impregnated with petroleum jelly (e.g., Vaseline).
4. Additional sterile equipment for use with Gomco clamp
   a. Gomco circumcision clamp (Gomco Surgical Manufacturing Corp., Buffalo, New York) (5), size 1 to 2 cm for average newborn glans. 1.3 cm is the most commonly used size (sizes range from 1 to 3.5 cm). Must use a size that is large enough to protect the glans (16).
   b. No. 11 scalpel blade and holder.
   c. A small safety pin (optional but helpful).
5. Additional sterile equipment for use with Plastibell
   a. Plastibell plastic cone (Hollister, Libertyville, Illinois). Available in presterilized packs. Size range based on size of glans penis: 1.1, 1.3, and 1.5 cm. A linen suture is included in the pack **(Fig. 52.1)**. Must assure that the size of the bell is not too large to prevent proximal migration of the bell with excessive loss of penile skin, nor so small that it could impair penile circulation.

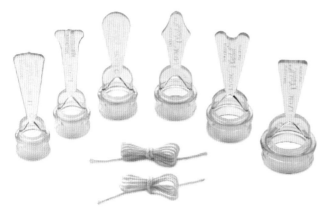

FIGURE 52.1 Plastibell with linen suture.

   b. Scissors capable of cutting through plastic.

D. Precautions

1. Obtain fully informed consent (see Chapter 3). This includes a discussion of the expected postoperative appearance, required postoperative care, potential complications, and indications to contact their health care provider.
2. Mandatory "time-out" to confirm correct patient and procedure.
3. Never circumcise at time of delivery. The timing of neonatal circumcision is dependent upon the patient's total gestational age, weight, and size.
4. Be sure to allow adequate time for wound observation prior to discharge.
5. Do not use local anesthetic containing epinephrine.
6. Identify the coronal sulcus and urethral meatus during the procedure.
7. Ensure that inner epithelium is completely separated from glans penis and that the prepuce can be retracted to visualize entire circumference of coronal sulcus.
8. **Never use electrocautery**! (17)
9. Do not use a tight circumferential dressing.
10. Recheck wound prior to discharging patient and within 1 to 2 weeks after circumcision. Residual skin should retract completely and the entire coronal sulcus must be visible to avoid postcircumcision adhesions.
11. When Plastibell is used, parents should be told to contact their health care provider if ring has not fallen off within 10 days.
12. Infants do not have to be NPO for a prolonged period prior to circumcision; however, the procedure should not be performed immediately after a feeding.

E. Techniques

A complete description of formal surgical foreskin excision has been excluded from this discussion because of the requirement to use sutures and the associated increased risk of bleeding compared with methods that involve crushing of tissue.

Ritual circumcisions are often performed using a Mogen clamp, Gomco clamp, or some type of "shield" that protects the glans. The Mogen technique usually does not require a dorsal incision or sutures (18).

1. Immobilize the patient and prepare region under aseptic procedures (see Chapters 5 and 6).
2. Perform penile dorsal nerve block.
   a. Familiarity with the anatomy of dorsal nerves of penis is required **(Fig. 52.2)** (9). Although only the two dorsal penile nerves are targeted by the injection of lidocaine, the ventral penile nerve is also blocked by infiltration through the subcutaneous tissue. Additional anesthesia ventrally is recommended to block the perineal nerves (a branch of the pudendal nerve).
   b. Identify dorsal nerve roots at 10 and 2 o'clock positions.

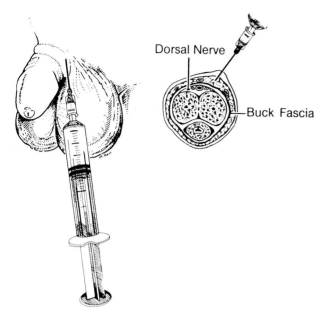

FIGURE 52.2 Penis is stabilized at angle of 20 to 25 degrees from midline. The formation of a lidocaine ring is shown (see text).

c. Identify by palpation the symphysis pubis and corpora cavernosa at the penile base.

d. Estimate depth of pubic bone from penile base to indicate necessary depth of injection (should not exceed 0.5 cm). Although the ideal area for infiltration corresponds to the 2 and 10 o'clock positions, 1 cm distal to the penile base, if the base is buried in pubic fat, the injection must be done at the junction of pubic and pelvic skin.

e. Stabilize organ with gentle traction, at an angle of 20 to 25 degrees from midline.

f. Pierce skin over one of dorsal nerves at penile root, and advance carefully posteromedially (0.25 to 0.5 cm) (see **Fig. 52.2**) into subcutaneous tissue to avoid lodging in the erectile tissue. After entering skin, needle should not meet resistance and tip should remain freely movable. If the tip of the needle is not freely mobile, it is probably embedded in the corpora cavernosum beneath the dorsal nerve and should be withdrawn slightly.

g. Aspirate to rule out intravascular position.

h. Slowly infiltrate area with 0.2 to 0.4 mL of lidocaine (never infiltrate as needle is advanced or withdrawn).

i. Repeat procedure at other dorsolateral position. After infiltration, a small lidocaine ring forms (see **Fig. 52.2**). The swelling is minimal and does not interfere with the circumcision procedure.

j. Wait 3 to 5 minutes for optimal analgesia. Analgesia is usually obtained after 3 minutes and typically disappears within 20 to 30 minutes. However, there is individual variation, and testing of the prepuce with a hemostat is suggested prior to dissection.

3. Locate coronal sulcus (**Fig. 52.3A**). Marking the position of the sulcus with ink on the outer prepuce of the penile shaft prior to the procedure can be helpful in demarcating this vital landmark but is not always necessary.

4. Use mosquito hemostat to dilate preputial ring (**Fig. 52.3B**).

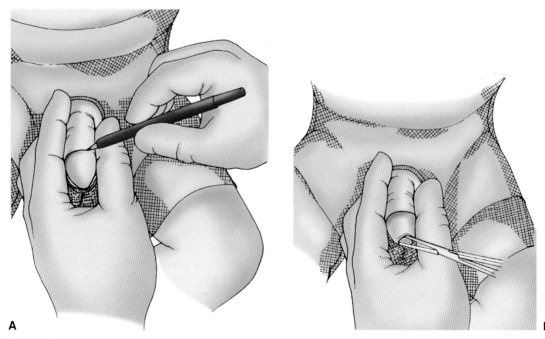

A **B**

FIGURE 52.3 Circumcision. **A:** Marking the position of the coronal sulcus. **B:** Dilating the preputial ring. (*continued*)

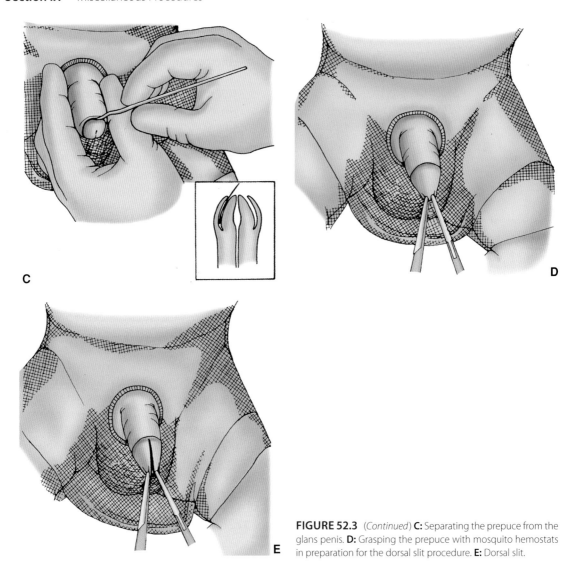

FIGURE 52.3 (*Continued*) **C:** Separating the prepuce from the glans penis. **D:** Grasping the prepuce with mosquito hemostats in preparation for the dorsal slit procedure. **E:** Dorsal slit.

5. Use blunt probe or the tip of the hemostat to separate inner epithelium of prepuce from glans penis (**Fig. 52.3C**). Failure to do this completely may result in a concealed penis.
6. Perform dorsal slit if desired.

    This step is not mandatory if there is adequate separation of the glans from the prepuce and the bell can be easily passed through the preputial ring and applied onto the glans.

    a. Grasp rim of prepuce on lateral aspects at 2 and 10 o'clock positions with mosquito hemostats, approximately 2 to 4 mm apart (**Fig. 52.3D**).
    b. Visualize urethral meatus.
    c. Place lower blade of large, straight hemostat between prepuce and glans in the dorsal midline with the tip 3 to 4 mm distal (not proximal) to corona, making sure to avoid urethra.
    d. Close hemostat for 5 to 10 seconds to crush foreskin in dorsal midline.
    e. Use tissue scissors to cut prepuce along crush line (**Fig. 52.3E**).
    f. Check that prepuce is completely freed from entire surface of glans and that the coronal sulcus is completely visualized.
7. Complete circumcision using either the Gomco or bell device.

Circumcision With Gomco Circumcision Clamp

1. Check clamp to ensure that all parts are present, fit well, and are in good working order.
2. Assemble clamp, ensuring that yoke (arm) articulates correctly with baseplate.
3. Draw prepuce backward gently to expose entire glans penis.
4. Break down all residual adhesions and observe position of meatus. If meatus is abnormal, cease at this point.

5. Sponge glans dry with gauze swabs.
6. Select stud (bell) of adequate size (see C), and place over glans (**Fig. 52.4A**).
7. Pull prepuce over stud.
8. Approximate edges of foreskin if dorsal slit is performed (sterile safety pin may be used).
9. Observe amount of skin remaining under baseplate for accuracy.

   Proper placement of prepuce over stud is essential. Pulling too taut may lead to removal of excessive penile skin. Insufficient tension may lead to incomplete circumcision.

10. Place baseplate of clamp over stud (with pin perpendicular to shaft of penis) so that prepuce is sandwiched between them (**Fig. 52.4B**).

11. Continue to pull upward on stud until entire prepuce is drawn through baseplate and stud engages with baseplate.
12. Hook yoke (arm) of clamp under side arms on shaft of stud and bolt firmly to baseplate after checking position of prepuce between stud and baseplate (**Fig. 52.4C**).
13. Remove safety pin.
14. Wait 10 minutes for hemostasis.
15. Hemostasis is produced by pressure between baseplate and rim of stud. If the clamp is removed before 10 minutes has elapsed, wound edge hemostasis may be inadequate. If significant bleeding occurs during the procedure, remove the device and search for bleeding vessel to control—avoid blindly placing sutures.
16. Remove prepuce with scalpel held parallel to and flush with upper surface of baseplate. Never use electrocautery;

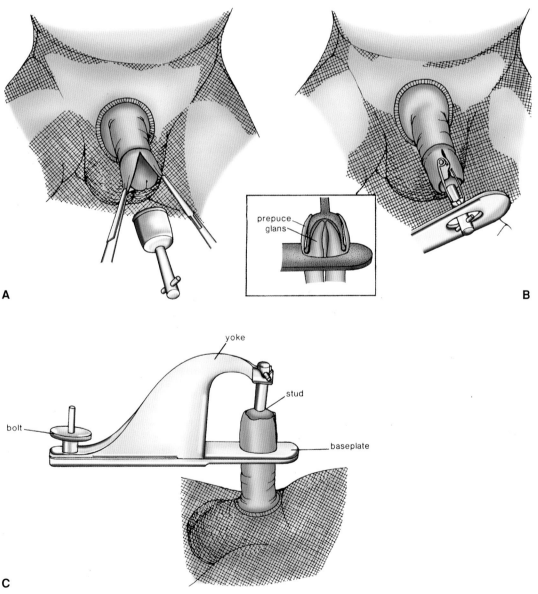

FIGURE 52.4 Circumcision with a Gomco clamp. **A:** Placing the stud over the glans. **B:** Placing the baseplate of the clamp over the stud until the stud engages with the baseplate (*inset*). **C:** Gomco clamp in position for circumcision.

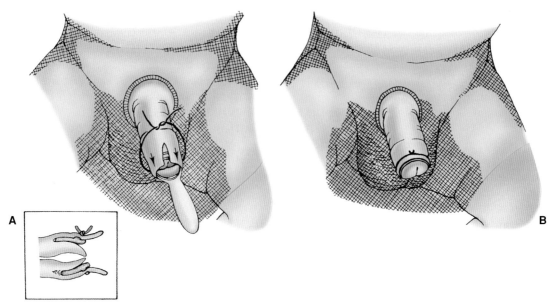

FIGURE 52.5 Circumcision with a Plastibell. **A:** The prepuce is pulled forward onto the bell. *Inset:* The prepuce is compressed into the groove by the circumferential suture. **B:** Appearance of the completed circumcision.

however, use of an ultrasound dissection scalpel has been described as a safe alternative to electrocautery (8).

17. Loosen bolt on clamp and remove.

Circumcision With Plastibell

1. Select bell of correct size.
2. Cone should fit snugly without pressure on glans.
3. Grooved rim of bell should be just distal to apex of dorsal slit.
4. If necessary, cut small segment out of cone so that it clears frenulum.
5. Hold prepuce firmly in place over cone (**Fig. 52.5A**).
6. Tie suture tightly around rim of bell so that prepuce is firmly compressed into groove.
7. Trim prepuce distal to ligature with tissue scissors. Use outer rim of cone as guide.
8. Break off cone handle. Tissue beneath ligature will undergo necrosis and separate from bell in 5 to 8 days (maximum 10 to 12 days) (**Fig. 52.5B**).

Circumcision With Mogen (Crushing) Clamp (Fig. 52.6)

1. Assure the device is in good working order. The screw must be tight and the lever arm must fit and lock securely within the groove on the opposite side to provide adequate approximation of the two halves of the device in the midline.
2. Dilate the opening of the prepuce to allow retraction of the foreskin and complete exposure of the glans.
3. Completely separate the foreskin from the glans and coronal sulcus with a blunt probe or the tip of a hemostat.

4. Return the foreskin to the original position.
5. Attach the tip of one small straight hemostat to the 6 o'clock position of the foreskin distal to the frenulum.
6. Slide a second open small straight hemostat along the dorsal midline foreskin (12 o'clock position). The lower jaw of the hemostat is positioned superior to the glans with the inner serrated surface touching the overlying foreskin assuring that the hemostat has not entered the meatus and urethra.
7. The tip of this dorsal hemostat is positioned approximately 3 to 4 mm distal (not proximal) to the corona and then the hemostat is closed.
8. The Mogen clamp is opened and oriented along the patient's midline. The grooved undersurface is toward the penis with the smooth upper surface visible superiorly.
9. Place the hemostats holding the foreskin within the "V" created by the open arms of the Mogen clamp. The tips of the hemostats should be almost touching the upper smooth aspect of the Mogen clamp.
10. Slide the hemostats and foreskin as far as possible toward the apex of the "V" maintaining the hemostats in line. The clamp will be oriented at a slight angle created by the different positions of the tips of the two hemostats.
11. Pulling the foreskin too taut may lead to removal of excessive penile skin. Insufficient tension may lead to incomplete circumcision.
12. It is important to confirm that the tips of the glans and meatus are separated from the undersurface of the Mogen.
13. Close and lock the Mogen clamp; and again assure that the glans and meatus are not within the clamp.
14. Cut the foreskin along the upper smooth surface of the Mogen clamp with a scalpel blade. Never cut below the Mogen clamp.

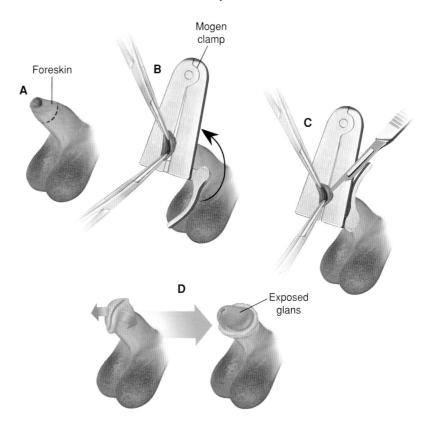

FIGURE 52.6 Circumcision using Mogen clamp.

15. Keep the Mogen clamp closed for at least 30 seconds for adequate hemostasis.
16. Unlock and remove the Mogen clamp. Then gently separate and retract the crushed skin and mucosa to completely expose the glans and sulcus.
17. Apply ointment to the site and tightly close the diaper.
18. Reexamine the circumcision site within 10 minutes to assure adequate hemostasis and positioning.

F. Postcircumcision Care

1. The typical postoperative appearance includes:
   a. Ecchymosis at the base of the penis (especially if injected local anesthetic is utilized) that resolves within weeks.
   b. Asymmetric circumferential edema of the mucosa that may take months to resolve.
   c. Dried blood at the junction of the mucosa and penile skin.
   d. Yellow/white crust or mucus-appearing discharge at the circumcision site, the mucosa, and the glans. This should not be confused with an infectious process (edema, erythema, and induration of the shaft and base of penis extending onto the suprapubic region). It will resolve within weeks and does not require treatment other than routine postcircumcision care.
2. Routine care
   a. *Optional:* Dress with loose, noncircumferential sterile gauze impregnated with Vaseline.

(1) Gough and Lawton (9) have shown that the addition of tincture of benzoin to the dressing adversely affected wound healing and the addition of topical antibiotic did not produce better results than those achieved with ordinary paraffin gauze.
   b. *Postprocedure:* Apply tight diaper for 1 hour. Check for bleeding every 30 minutes for 2 hours.
   c. For 24 hours after circumcision, check (or instruct parents to check) for bleeding, excessive swelling, and difficulty voiding.
   d. Diapers may be changed as per parent's regular routine.
   e. Apply a lubricant such as petroleum jelly to the circumcision site with each diaper change until the edema and discharge have resolved.
   f. Wash infant with cloth for 3 days postcircumcision. Subsequent immersion into water is permitted if no other issues.
   g. Acetaminophen may be administered for mild pain. Some pediatricians do not recommend the use of this medication in this age group.
   h. Infants with a prominent suprapubic fat pad may develop a "buried penis" appearance following the circumcision. This predisposes the development of adhesions secondary to drying of the mucous between the glans and mucosa. These adhesions are prevented by retraction of the fat pad to expose the glans and the application of a lubricant to the area with each diaper change until the fat pad resolves.

G. Complications

The overall incidence of complications associated with circumcision ranges from approximately 0.2% to 7%. Complication rates for neonatal circumcisions are lower than for older children (18–41).

1. Postoperative bleeding

    Postoperative bleeding is usually the result of inadequate local hemostasis. Other less common causes include underlying coagulopathies (e.g., unrecognized neonatal hepatitis (20) or hereditary clotting disorders.

    a. Continuous ooze

    (1) Apply manual pressure for 5 to 10 minutes. Check that the string on the Plastibell is in place and is sufficiently tight.

    (2) If continued oozing:

    (a) Apply topical thrombin (Thrombostat) on absorbable gelatin sponge (Gelfoam) or oxidized cellulose (Oxycel, Surgicel). Do not use a tight circumferential dressing.

    (b) Silver nitrate and epinephrine have also been used topically to control bleeding. To avoid local ischemia or systemic effects, do not exceed a 1:100,000 concentration of epinephrine.

    b. Active hemorrhage or uncontrolled ooze

(1) Surgical assessment and ligation of bleeding vessel if present.

(2) Consider underlying coagulopathy.

H. Other Complications (Fig. 52.7)

1. **Traumatic complications that require urologic consultation**

    a. Urethral laceration during dorsal slit procedure (avoided by keeping urethra in view at all times during the procedure).

    b. Injury to meatus and glans.

    c. Amputation: Requires immediate urologic care. Amputated tissues are placed in moist sterile saline-soaked gauze and transported with patient to the emergency room.

    d. Loss of penis (most commonly due to injuries related to cautery or amputation of glans (19,21,22)).

    e. Cyanosis/necrosis of glans penis caused by overly tight Plastibell, misplaced sutures, or overly tight circumferential bandage (8,23).

    f. Urethrocutaneous fistula associated with use of Gomco clamp or Plastibell (most commonly caused by using a Plastibell or clamp of incorrect size or failure to recognize congenital megalo-ureter) (24).

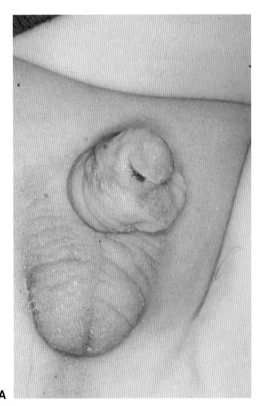 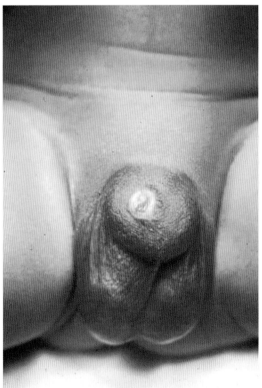

A   B

FIGURE 52.7 Complication of circumcision. **A:** Glans injury 6 months after circumcision. **B:** Trapped penis following contraction of wound after circumcision. (*continued*)

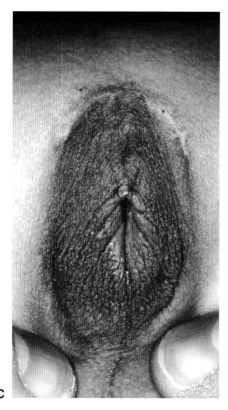

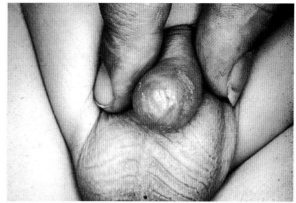

FIGURE 52.7 (*Continued*) **C:** Penile amputation following cautery injury during circumcision. **D:** Cicatrix following circumcision.

g. Rare reports of death exist secondary to anesthetic (1), infection, and hemorrhage (20).

2. **Early complications**
   a. Infection (25–27).
      More common with the Plastibell. Most are mild and respond to wet to dry dressings and Sitz baths, but fatalities have been reported.
   b. Lymphedema and venous stasis.
   c. Urinary retention (28).
   d. Tight (or occlusive) dressing or glanular prolapse through ring of Plastibell (29).
   e. Adhesions: Often associated with prominent suprapubic fat pad (see F).

3. **Late complications that require urologic consultation**
   a. Incomplete circumcision (most common complication).
   b. Recurrent phimosis.
   c. Skin bridge between penile shaft and glans.
   d. Concealed penis. Usually associated with prominent suprapubic fat pad and cicatrix at circumcision site (30).
   e. Meatal complications (e.g., meatal stenosis and meatitis (31)).
   f. Poor patient selection. Circumcision of hypospadias or micropenis.
   g. Chordee, most commonly is the result of dense ventral scarring from inflammation. Less commonly due to removal of excess skin from shaft or secondary to a skin bridge.

h. Inclusion cyst of prepuce.
i. Lymphedema (32).
j. Venous stasis (33).
k. Wound dehiscence (see **Fig. 52.6**) (34).
   (1) Treated with local care including the application of antiseptic (iodophor, or antibiotic ointment) and not with grafting or burying the penis in scrotum. The site will gradually heal by secondary intention.

I. Mechanical Device Failures

1. Mechanical problems with Gomco clamp (35) include loss of a part, warping of the plate with multiple use, the arm breaking during tightening, and grooves and nicks at junction of bell and plate.
2. Displacement with lodging of Plastibell around penile shaft or glans penis (10).
3. Inadequate closure and locking of the Mogen clamp due to a loose screw or worn lever arm.

J. Anesthetic Complications

1. Reports of methemoglobinemia following exposure to prilocaine, procaine, benzocaine, and lidocaine (36).
2. Hematoma from anesthetic injection. Reported cases have resolved spontaneously.
3. Seizures (37).

References

1. Gairdner D. The fate of the foreskin—a study of circumcision. *Br Med J.* 1949;2:1433–1437.
2. Foddy B. Medical, religious and social reasons for and against an ancient rite. *J Med Ethics.* 2013;39(7):415.
3. Sorokan ST, Finlay JC, Jefferies AL. Newborn male circumcision. *Paediatr Child Health.* 2015;20(6):311–320.
4. American Academy of Pediatrics Task Force on Circumcision. Circumcision policy statement. *Pediatrics.* 2012;130:585–586.
5. Concodora CW, Maizels M, Dean GE, et al. Checklist assessment tool to evaluate suitability and success of neonatal clamp circumcision: a prospective study. *J Pediatr Urol.* 2016;12(4):235.e1–e5.
6. Chalmers D, Wiedel CA, Siparsky GL, et al. Discovery of hypospadias during newborn circumcision should not preclude completion of the procedure. *J Pediatr.* 2014;164(5):1171–1174.
7. Sinkey RG, Eschenbacher MA, Walsh PM, et al. The GoMo study: a randomized clinical trial assessing neonatal pain with Gomco vs Mogen clamp circumcision. *Am J Obstet Gynecol.* 2015;212(5):664.e1–e8.
8. Fette A, Schleef J, Haberlik A, et al. Circumcision in pediatric surgery using an ultrasound dissection scalpel. *Technol Health Care.* 2000;8:75–80.
9. Gough DCS, Lawton N. Circumcision—which dressing? *Br J Urol.* 1990;65:418–419.
10. Kirya C, Werthmann MW Jr. Neonatal circumcision and penile dorsal nerve block—a painless procedure. *J Pediatr.* 1978;92:998–1000.
11. Lander J, Brady-Fryer B, Metcalfe JB, et al. Comparison of ring block, dorsal nerve block, and topical anesthesia for neonatal circumcision: a randomized controlled trial. *JAMA.* 1997;278:2157–2162.
12. Woodman PJ. Topical lidocaine-prilocaine versus lidocaine for neonatal circumcision: a randomized controlled trial. *Obstet Gynecol.* 1999;93(5 pt 1):775–779.
13. Taddio A, Ohlsson K, Ohlsson A. Lidocaine-prilocaine cream for analgesia during circumcision in newborn boys. *Cochrane Database Syst Rev.* 1999;(2):CD000496.
14. Lehr VT, Cepeda E, Frattarelli DA, et al. Lidocaine 4% cream compared with lidocaine 2.5% and prilocaine 2.5% or dorsal penile block for circumcision. *Am J Perinatol.* 2005;22(5):231–237.
15. Sharara-Cami R, Lakissian Z, Charafeddine L, et al. Combination analgesia for neonatal circumcision: a randomized controlled trial. *Pediatrics.* 2017;140(6):pii: e20171935. doi:10.1542/peds.2017-1935.
16. Seleim HM, Elbarbary MM. Major penile injuries as a result of cautery during newborn circumcision. *J Pediatr Surg.* 2016;51(9):1532–1537.
17. Reynolds RD. Use of the Mogen clamp for neonatal circumcision. *Am Fam Physician.* 1996;54(1):177–182.
18. El Bcheraoui C, Zhang X, Cooper CS, et al. Rates of adverse events associated with male circumcision in U.S. medical settings, 2001 to 2010. *JAMA Pediatr.* 2014;168(7):625–634.
19. Essid A, Hamazaoui M, Sahli S, et al. Glans reimplantation after circumcision accident. *Prog Urol.* 2005;15:745–747.
20. Hiss J, Horowitz A, Kahana T. Fatal haemorrhage following male ritual circumcision. *J Clin Forensic Med.* 2000;7:32–34.
21. Cook A, Khoury AE, Bagli DJ, et al. Use of buccal mucosa to simulate the coronal sulcus after traumatic penile amputation. *Urology.* 2005;66:1109.
22. Barnes S, Ben Chaim J, Kessler A. Postcircumcision necrosis of the glans penis: Gray scale and color Doppler sonographic findings. *J Clin Ultrasound.* 2007;35(2):105–107.
23. Bode CO, Ikhisemojie S, Ademuyiwa AO. Penile injuries from proximal migration of the Plastibell circumcision ring. *J Pediatr Urol.* 2010;6(1):23–27.
24. Limaye RD, Hancock RA. Penile urethral fistula as a complication of circumcision. *J Pediatr.* 1968;72:105–106.
25. Gesundheit B, Grisaru-Soen G, Greenberg D, et al. Neonatal genital herpes simplex type 1 infection after Jewish ritual circumcision: modern medicine and religious tradition. *Pediatrics.* 2004;114:e259–e263.
26. Kirkpatrick BV, Eitzman DV. Neonatal septicemia after circumcision. *Clin Pediatr (Phila).* 1974;13:767–768.
27. Woodside JR. Necrotizing fasciitis after neonatal circumcision. *Am J Dis Child.* 1980;134:301–302.
28. Pearce I. Retention of urine: an unusual complication of the Plastibell device. *Br J Urol Int.* 2000;85:560–561.
29. Horowitz J, Sussheim A, Scalettar HE. Abdominal distention following ritual circumcision. *Pediatrics.* 1976;57:579.
30. Trier WC, Drach GW. Concealed penis—another complication of circumcision. *Am J Dis Child.* 1973;125:276–277.
31. Mackenzie AR. Meatal ulceration following neonatal circumcision. *Obstet Gynecol.* 1966;28:221–223.
32. Yildirim S, Taylan G, Akoz T. Circumcision as an unusual cause of penile lymphedema. *Ann Plast Surg.* 2003;50:665–666.
33. Ly L, Sankaran K. Acute venous stasis and swelling of the lower abdomen and extremities in an infant after circumcision. *Can Med Assoc J.* 2003;169:216–217.
34. Van Duyn J, Warr WS. Excessive penile skin loss from circumcision. *J Med Assoc Ga.* 1962;51:394–396.
35. Feinberg AN, Blazek MA. Mechanical complications of circumcision with a Gomco clamp. *Am J Dis Child.* 1988;142:813–814.
36. Peker E, Cagan E, Dogan M, et al. Methemoglobinemia due to local anesthesia with prilocaine for circumcision. *J Pediatr Child Health.* 2010;46(6):362–363.
37. Moran LR, Hossain T, Insoft RM. Neonatal seizures following lidocaine administration for elective circumcision. *J Perinatol.* 2004;24:395–396.
38. Mano R, Nevo A, Sivan B, et al. Post-ritual circumcision bleeding—characteristics and treatment outcome. *Urology.* 2017;105:157–162.
39. Srinivasan M, Hamvas C, Coplen D. Rates of complications after newborn circumcision in a well-baby nursery, special care nursery, and neonatal intensive care unit. *Clin Pediatr (Phila).* 2015;54(12):1185–1191.
40. Pippi Salle JL, Jesus LE, Lorenzo AJ, et al. Glans amputation during routine neonatal circumcision: mechanism of injury and strategy for prevention. *J Pediatr Urol.* 2013;9(6 Pt A):763–768.
41. Brook I. Infectious complications of circumcision and their prevention. *Eur Urol Focus.* 2016;2(4):453–459.

53

Drainage of Superficial Abscesses

Maame Efua S. Sampah and Manuel B. Torres

A. Indications

1. Therapeutic

Definitive treatment for soft tissue abscess is surgical incision and drainage, which allows free flow of purulent material from the abscess cavity (1). Needle aspiration alone is significantly less likely to resolve an abscess (2).

2. Diagnostic

For neonates, drainage also provides specimen for Gram stain and culture, which allows identification of microbes and susceptibility testing to guide antibiotic therapy.

B. Contraindications

1. Patients with inflammatory skin changes and areas of swelling or induration without an abscess collection should not undergo incision and drainage (**Fig. 53.1**)

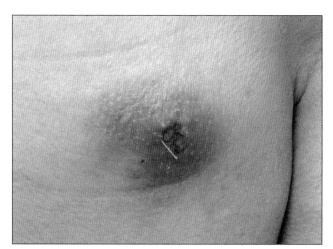

FIGURE 53.1 Superficial abscess over left gluteal region.

(3). Fluctuance on physical examination, may be absent in up to 50% of patients (4). Ultrasound and needle aspiration are useful adjuncts to determine if a pus pocket is present (5).

2. It is important to differentiate abscesses from vascular and lymphatic malformations such as hemangiomas and cystic hygromas as incision of such lesions may lead to grave complications. Ultrasound and careful physical examination are helpful to make the correct diagnosis in this instance (6).

3. Defer drainage of abscesses located on the face, breast, genital, and perirectal areas, complicated hand abscesses as well as those in close proximity to large vessels and nerves, to a surgeon.

4. Neonates with bleeding disorder must undergo correction of coagulopathy prior to drainage.

C. Principles

1. While specimen for cultures may generally be obtained by swabbing purulent material, isolation of anaerobic organisms specifically is better achieved by needle aspiration following skin prep prior to incision and drainage.

2. For better cosmetic outcome, make use of natural skin creases in planning the incision. Abscesses may however be much larger than they appear on the surface and may require longer incisions than expected.

3. The abscess should be left open to heal by secondary intention. Avoid primary closure.

4. While drainage is the mainstay of treatment for superficial abscesses in neonates, antibiotics are associated with clinical improvement and prevent recurrence, subsequent drainage, and secondary spread (7,8).

5. Blood cultures should be obtained prior to initiation of antibiotics.

D. Equipment

Sterile

1. Gloves
2. Drapes
3. Gauze squares
4. No. 11 blade and scalpel holder
5. Curved hemostats
6. Forceps
7. Saline solution
8. Antiseptic solution or prep pads (povidone-iodine or chlorhexidine)
9. 3- to 10-mL syringe, 25- or 27-gauge needle
10. Culture swab/specimen tube with occluding cap
11. Needleless 30- to 60-mL syringe with 19-gauge intravenous (IV) catheter or needleless irrigation device with splash protection
12. Packing material (e.g., iodoform or plain gauze packing tape)
13. Local anesthetic (e.g., 1% lidocaine) for large abscesses
14. Dressing of choice

Nonsterile

1. Eye protection/face mask

E. Technique

1. Obtain informed consent.
2. Ensure appropriate hand hygiene. Don protective eyewear and nonsterile gloves.
3. Prepare the skin with disinfecting agent of choice and allow it to dry (see Chapter 6).
4. Put on sterile gloves and apply sterile drapes at the site.
5. Local anesthetic may now be injected at the site, if indicated, using the 27-gauge needle.
6. Take the 25-gauge (or 23-gauge) sterile needle, attach the syringe, and introduce the tip through the skin into the area of maximal edema or fluctuance, while pulling back on the syringe. Purulent material aspirated should be sent for cultures. Ultrasound guidance may be used during this step.
7. Make a stab incision at the point of needle entry and extend the incision over the entire length of the abscess cavity, conforming to the natural folds of the skin.
8. Evacuate all material from the abscess cavity by applying gentle compression.
9. Dissect bluntly within the abscess cavity using curved hemostats to break up loculations, identify foreign bodies, and ensure proper drainage **(Fig. 53.2A)**. Do **not** probe with a gloved finger, which may be injured by a sharp foreign body. Dissecting with a sharp instrument

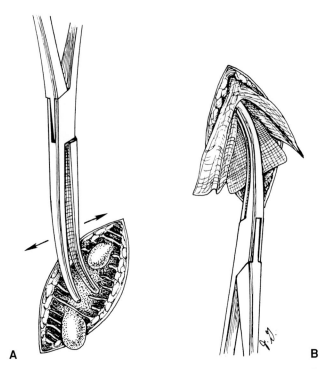

FIGURE 53.2 Drainage of a superficial abscess. **A:** Breaking the septa with a clamp. **B:** Packing the wound.

such as a scalpel may cause tissue damage or create a false passage or fistula. Dissection of the wound is painful and may require additional analgesia.
10. Using a needleless 30- to 60-mL syringe with 19-gauge IV catheter, irrigate the abscess cavity with copious saline solution until all visible pus is removed.
11. For abscess cavities greater than or equal to 5 cm, insert packing material to prevent closure of wound margins **(Fig. 53.2B)**. Tight packing will cause tissue necrosis and should be avoided. Generally, packing for small wounds does not appear to prevent the need for further drainage procedures (9).
12. Apply sterile dressing.

F. Complications

1. Bleeding: Bleeding from subcutaneous tissues is usually self-limited. Wound packing provides some tamponade effect.
2. Recurrence: Look for local predisposing factors such as foreign material in cases of recurrence following initial drainage. Radiographs should be obtained. Recurrence should be treated in the same way as the initial episode.

References

1. Liu C, Bayer A, Cosgrove SE, et al. Clinical practice guidelines by the Infectious Diseases Society of America for the

treatment of methicillin-resistant *Staphylococcus aureus* infections in adults and children. *Clin Infect Dis.* 2011;52:e18–e55.

2. Ramakrishnan K, Salinas R, Higuita N. (2015, September 15). Superficial abscess over left gluteal region [Digital image]. https://www.aafp.org/afp/2015/0915/p474.html. Accessed January 16, 2019.

3. Gaspari RJ, Resop D, Mendoza M, et al. A randomized controlled trial of incision and drainage versus ultrasonographically guided needle aspiration for skin abscesses and the effect of methicillin-resistant Staphylococcus aureus. *Ann Emerg Med.* 2011;57(5):483.e1–491.e1.

4. Iverson K, Haritos D, Thomas R, et al. The effect of bedside ultrasound on diagnosis and management of soft tissue infections in a pediatric ED. *Am J Emerg Med.* 2012;30(8):1347–1351.

5. Stevens DL, Bisno AL, Chambers HF, et al; Infectious Diseases Society of America. Practice guidelines for the diagnosis and management of skin and soft tissue infections: 2014 update by the Infectious Diseases Society of America. *Clin Infect Dis.* 2014;59(2):e10–e52.

6. Blaivas M, Adhikari S. Unexpected findings on point-of-care superficial ultrasound imaging before incision and drainage. *J Ultrasound Med.* 2011;30:1425–1430.

7. Daum RS, Miller LG, Immergluck L, et al. A placebo-controlled trial of antibiotics for smaller skin abscesses. *N Engl J Med.* 2017;376:2545–2555.

8. Hogan PG, Rodriguez M, Spenner AM, et al. Impact of systemic antibiotics on staphylococcus aureus colonization and recurrent skin infection. *Clin Infect Dis.* 2018;66: 191–197.

9. Leinwand M, Downing M, Slater D, et al. Incision and drainage of subcutaneous abscesses without the use of packing. *J Pediatr Surg.* 2013;48:1962–1965.

CHAPTER

54

Wound Care

Kara Johnson, Laura Welch, and June Amling

Neonates in the intensive care unit are susceptible to alterations in the integumentary system as a result of medical/surgical procedures, application of medical devices, and congenital defects (1–3). The skin is an organ that acts as the first line of defense against the invasion of bacteria and toxins, absorption of chemicals from topical products, and plays a vital role in water and electrolyte excretion, insulation, thermoregulation, and tactile sensations. Neonatal skin is fragile and can be easily damaged, particularly in extremely preterm infants (4).

A. Definitions

1. **Wound:** an injury to living tissue caused by a cut, blow, or other impact; typically one in which the skin is cut or broken, where damage is caused to underlying tissue(s).
2. **Periwound:** tissue surrounding the wound edge.
3. **Partial thickness skin injury:** superficial; epidermis and possibly partial loss of dermis.
4. **Full thickness skin injury:** total loss of epidermis and dermis. Extends into subcutaneous tissue; may extend to muscle, fascia, bone, or cartilage.
5. **Pressure injury:** localized damage to the skin and underlying soft tissue over a bony prominence or related to a medical device. The injury occurs as a result of intense and or prolonged pressure or pressure in combination with shear.
6. **Shear:** force exerted parallel to the tissue. One layer of tissue slides over another, deforming adipose and muscle tissue and disrupting blood flow.
7. **Friction:** resistance to motion in a parallel direction resulting in a mechanical disruption of the epidermal skin layer.
8. **Tear:** separation of the epidermis from the dermis or separation of both the epidermis and dermis from underlying tissue.

9. **Aseptic technique:** free from pathogenic microorganisms, purposeful prevention of the transfer of organisms. Use sterile gloves and sterile instruments.
10. **Clean technique:** reduction in number of overall microorganisms, purposeful prevention of direct contamination of materials/supplies. Use clean gloves and sterile instruments.

B. Integumentary Assessment Scales

Careful assessment of the skin is an important element of the neonatal physical examination. Nutritional status, organ function, and disease processes are also important to note in the head to toe assessment. It is imperative for clinicians to be familiar with normal variances in the skin of the newborn infant.

1. **Neonatal skin risk assessment scale (NSRAS):** is a risk assessment tool that evaluates neonates' risk for skin breakdown. The scale is based on the Braden scale (adult) for predicting pressure injuries (5)
   a. Subscales
      (1) Six subscales: general physical condition, mental status, mobility, activity, nutrition, and moisture
   b. Scoring
      (1) Subscales are scored from 1 to 4 points
      (2) Total scores range 6 to 24 points
      (3) Higher scores indicate better skin function, and are therefore indicative of lower risk for pressure injury development
2. **Neonatal skin condition score (NSCS):** evaluates the neonate's (preterm to full term) overall skin condition, and is used as a skin care guideline (6)
   a. Subscales
      (1) Three subscales: dryness, erythema, and skin breakdown/excoriation

b. Scoring
   (1) Subscales are scored from 1 to 3 points
   (2) Total scores range from 3 to 9 points
   (3) Higher scores indicate impaired integumentary function

C. Types of Wounds

Common wound etiologies for the hospitalized neonate are categorized in **Table 54.1**.

TABLE 54.1 Neonatal Wound Types

CATEGORY	TYPES OF WOUNDS
Traumatic	■ Epidermal striping ■ Tearing from adhesives/friction ■ Forceps injury ■ Shearing injuries ■ Abrasions
Surgical	■ Primary incisions ■ Dehisced surgical sites
Contact excoriation	■ Diaper dermatitis (DD) ■ Ostomy or fistula effluent ■ Medical adhesive –related skin injury (MARSI) ■ Moisture associated skin damage (MASD) ■ Irritant contact dermatitis
Extravasation injury	■ Refer to Chapter **30**
Burn/thermal injury	■ Chemical burns ■ Heat probes ■ Laryngoscope bulbs
Pressure injuries	■ Breakdown over bony prominences ■ Medical device–related pressure injuries
Ischemic injuries	■ Amniotic banding in utero ■ Arterial lines ■ Extracorporeal membrane oxygenation ■ Coagulopathy injuries
Congenital conditions	■ Aplasia cutis congenita ■ Epidermolysis bullosa ■ Gastroschisis/omphalocele ■ Spina bifida ■ Vesicular bullous lesions

Adapted with permission from Thames Valley Neonatal ODN Quality Care Group. Guideline framework for neonatal wound care. Thames Valley & Wessex Neonatal Operational Delivery Network. 2012. https://www.networks.nhs.uk/nhs-networks/thames-valley-wessex-neonatalnetwork/documents/guidelines/Wound%20Guideline.pdf.

D. Wound Assessment

A systematic wound assessment is essential, providing information and evaluation of healing and the efficacy of prescribed treatment. At a minimum, wound assessments should include the following (7–11).

1. Wound type (**Table 54.1**)
2. Anatomical location
3. Wound measurements
   a. General measuring techniques
      (1) Clock method is frequently used, where the patient's head is referenced as 12:00 and the feet are 6:00
      (2) Patient position
         (a) Place the patient in the same anatomical position for each measurement
         (b) Do not stretch or pull wound edges for measurement
      (3) Documentation format: length × width × depth in centimeters (**Fig. 54.1**)

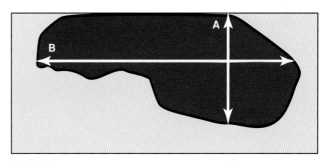

FIGURE 54.1 Measuring length and width. Measuring length from head to toe (*A*), and width from left to right (*B*) of a wound. (Reprinted with permission from Primaris Business Solutions.)

   (a) Length: measure the longest point from head (12:00) to toe (6:00)
   (b) Width: measure from left (9:00) to right (3:00) at the greatest width
   (c) Depth is the measurement of the deepest part of the visible wound bed (**Fig. 54.2**)

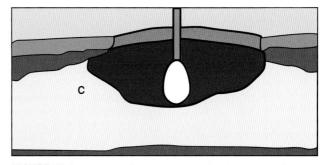

FIGURE 54.2 Measuring depth (*c*). (Reprinted with permission from Primaris Business Solutions.)

4. Tunneling and undermining
   a. Tunneling (sinus tract): a channel of tissue loss that can extend in any direction away from the wound through soft tissue, muscle, and to bone. The tunnel or tract may result in dead space, delaying wound healing (**Fig. 54.3**)

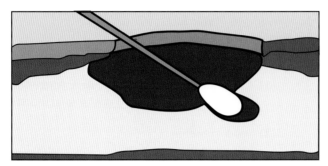

FIGURE 54.3 Measuring tunneling. (Reprinted with permission from Primaris Business Solutions.)

   b. Undermining: tissue destruction underneath intact skin at the wound edge. Wound edges are not attached to the wound base, rather, overhang the periphery of the tissue (**Fig. 54.4**)

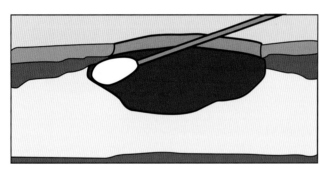

FIGURE 54.4 Measuring undermining. (Reprinted with permission from Primaris Business Solutions.)

5. How to measure depth/tunneling and undermining
   a. Supplies
      (1) Clean gloves
      (2) Sterile water or normal saline
      (3) Sterile, cotton-tipped applicator
      (4) Measuring tape in centimeters
   b. Procedure
      (1) Technique: Clean
      (2) Wash hands, don clean gloves
      (3) Moisten sterile cotton-tipped applicator with sterile water or normal saline
      (4) Place applicator to measure depth or into the tunnel(s) or undermined areas
      (5) Grasp applicator with thumb and index finger at point where it meets skin level
      (6) Place next to centimeter ruler to determine measurement
      (7) Repeat for each tunnel

   c. Documentation
      (1) Use the clock method (12:00/head)
      (2) Indicate at which hour on the clock there is a tunnel/undermining
      (3) Document length of tunnel(s) in centimeters
      (4) Document area(s) of undermining in centimeters and how far back the undermining goes
6. Wound bed description
   After cleaning the wound, describe wound bed appearance. As wound bed tissue is identified, identify each type that is present as a percentage (e.g., 60% granulation, 25% slough, 15% eschar)
   a. Pale pink/dusky (poor perfusion): investigate perfusion and if hemoglobin/hematocrit are low
   b. Pink/pearly pink (epithelial tissue): new skin growth
   c. Red (granulation tissue): vascular connective tissue
      (1) Hypergranulation: when granulation tissue proliferates and overlaps, occurs as a result of extended inflammatory response, excessive moisture, or moisture combined with friction
      (2) Friable tissue: tissue that bleeds easily with minimal stimulation
   d. Green or green/yellow (infected): potential infection
   e. Yellow (slough): accumulation of nonviable (dead) debris
      (1) Adherent to loosely adherent: soft, thick, or stringy debris; attached to wound base
      (2) Nonadherent: thick, mucinous substance, scattered clumps of debris throughout the wound bed; easily separated from wound base
   f. Black (necrotic): avascular, nonviable tissue
      (1) Adherent, soft: soggy tissue, strongly attached to wound base
      (2) Adherent, hard: firm, strongly attached to wound base and edges
      (3) Stable eschar: leathery, dry and hard; adhered to underlying subcutaneous tissue, no exudate, fluctuance, or surrounding cellulitis
      (4) Unstable eschar: softening, spongy, slimy, nonadherent to underlying wound bed; boggy feel, underlying exudate, and/or surrounding cellulitis
   g. Exudate
      (1) Quantity
         (a) None: no exudate, dry wound
         (b) Scant/minimal: wound bed is moist no drainage from wound bed
         (c) Moderate: periwound tissue and wound bed are wet
         (d) Heavy: periwound tissue and wound bed are saturated
      (2) Type
         (a) Serous: thin, light colored, clear wound fluid with no visible pus, blood, or debris

(b) Serosanguineous: thin, pale red to pink

(c) Sanguineous (bloody): thin, bright red, appearing to be entirely blood

(d) Purulent: thin or thick, opaque/tan/yellow, pus-like appearance. May be malodorous

(3) Odor

(a) None

(b) Smell is noticeable with removal of dressing

(c) At all times

h. Periwound: issues involving the periwound can delay wound healing and increase pain

(1) Condition of the skin

(a) Intact versus nonintact

(b) Indurated: abnormal firmness

(c) Crepitus: air or gas accumulation

(d) Rash: eczema, infection, candida

(e) Hyperkeratosis: callus-like tissue formation at wound edge

(f) Epibole: thickened and rolled wound edges

(2) Hydration

(a) Maceration: overhydrated, reduces barrier function

(b) Dry/flaking/cracked

(3) Color

(a) Erythema

(b) Pigmentation

    i. Hypopigmentation

    ii. Hyperpigmentation

(c) Dusky

(4) Edema

(a) Pitting

(b) Nonpitting

i. Pain

(1) None

(2) Intermittent

(3) Constant

(4) Only with dressing changes

(5) Worse with dressing changes

E. Wound Cultures

Diagnosis of an infected wound should be done in conjunction with observable signs of local and systemic infection. Careful consideration should be given to differentiate between signs of infection, which are not to be confused with the inflammatory stage of healing. Treatment is not required for wounds that are contaminated or colonized, but is needed for wounds that are critically colonized or infected (11). The gold standard for wound cultures is a quantitative biopsy; however, the swab technique is most commonly utilized in clinical practice because it is a noninvasive and cost-effective way to identify wound organisms and tailor antimicrobial therapy.

1. Wound bacteria classification

a. Contamination: the presence of nonreplicating bacteria in an open wound that does not interfere with wound healing

b. Colonization: the presence of replicating bacteria within the wound bed that do not interfere with wound healing and do not cause injury to the host

c. Critical colonization: the presence of replicating bacteria within/on the wound bed surface that interfere with wound healing and cause injury to the host

(1) The acronym "NERDS" indicates superficial wound surface involvement, topical antimicrobial treatment is indicated (12)

(a) Nonhealing wound

(b) Exudative wound

(c) Red and bleeding wound

(d) Debris

(e) Smell

d. Infected: bacteria levels are high on the wound surface and also invade viable tissues, eliciting a host response

(1) The acronym "STONES" indicates deep periwound and systemic infection, systemic antibiotics are indicated (12)

(a) Size is bigger

(b) Temperature increased

(c) Osteomyelitis suspicion (probes to or has exposed bone)

(d) New areas of breakdown

(e) Erythema/exudate

(f) Smell

2. Swab wound culture

a. Indications

(1) Local signs/symptoms of infection: pus, malodorous, increased exudate, redness, induration, pain

(2) Systemic signs/symptoms of infection: fever, leukocytosis, sudden elevation in serum glucose

(3) Lack of wound healing after 2 weeks in a clean wound, despite optimal treatment

b. Contraindications

(1) Do not culture: avascular tissue, necrotic debris, or hard eschar

c. How to: swab wound culture, Levine method (13,14)

(1) Supplies:

(a) Clean gloves

(b) Swab culturette(s): bacterial, fungal, viral, Gram stain

(c) Sterile water or normal saline

(d) Absorbent pad for excess cleaning solution, wound debris, and exudate

(e) Sterile gauze

(2) Procedure:

(a) Technique: clean

(b) Wash hands, don clean gloves

(c) Remove old dressing

(d) Remove gloves, wash hands, don clean gloves

(e) Cleanse the wound with sterile water or normal saline

    i. Moisten sterile gauze pad

    ii. Wipe wound surface to remove surface debris

(f) Gently pat wound bed dry with new sterile gauze

(g) Remove gloves, wash hands, don clean gloves

(h) Using culturette, swab 1 cm² of viable tissue for 5 seconds with enough force to produce exudate and elicit minimal bleeding

    i. For dry wound beds, moisten swab with culture medium, sterile water, or normal saline prior to obtaining culture

F. Wound Healing

There are two ways for soft tissue in the body to heal: by regeneration or by scar tissue formation (connective tissue repair). The depth of the wound and tissue layers lost dictate whether the wound will heal by regeneration (partial thickness skin injuries) or by scar formation (full thickness skin injuries) (11).

1. Wounds heal by one of the following intentions

  a. Primary intention: surgical closure, all skin layers are approximated by staples, sutures, or skin adhesives. There is minimal risk of infection or delayed healing because the wound is closed (intact bacterial barrier)

  b. Secondary intention: wounds that are left open to heal through the process of granulation, contraction, and epithelialization. Wound contraction is necessary in order to decrease the size of the defect, resulting in greater scar formation. These wounds are at a greater risk for infection and delayed healing

  c. Tertiary (delayed primary) intention: there is a delay between injury and surgical closure (usually when there is suspected infection or gross edema present). These wounds frequently begin healing by secondary intention, but then are surgically closed so that a limited amount of granulation tissue is required

2. Moist wound healing is essential, mimicking the function of the epidermis

  a. Advantages

    (1) Faster rates of healing

    (2) Decreased pain

    (3) Diminished scaring

    (4) Cost effective

  b. Contraindications

    (1) Dry gangrene

    (2) Palliative care, when healing is not realistic

    (3) When necrotic tissue provides protection of deeper structures

G. Wound Cleansing

Limited research exists about the safety and efficiency of wound products in the neonatal population (7,15–17). Careful consideration of local skin irritation and absorption related systemic effects are critical with product selection in the neonate. Wounds should be cleansed, not rubbed, as rubbing damages fragile epithelializing and granulating tissue.

1. Cleaning solutions: before using any cleaning solution, it should be warmed to body temperature or at least be room temperature

  a. Sterile saline: sterile saline is preferred; it can be used on all wound types

  b. Wound cleanser: there are several antiseptic formulations that are noncytotoxic, nonirritating, fragrance free, and no-rinse. These pH balanced cleansers are designed to not only cleanse and remove debris from the wound bed, but to optimally prepare the wound bed for healing

    (1) Infants ≤32 weeks: cleanse only with sterile saline/water during the first week of life (9)

    (2) Infants >32 weeks: nonirritating, pH neutral to mildly acidic formulations (e.g., normal saline, formulated antimicrobial wound cleanser) (9)

  c. Avoid the use of cytotoxic antiseptics (e.g., hydrogen peroxide, acetic acid, sodium hypochlorite) to irrigate neonatal wounds; there is potential for tissue damage and systemic absorption

2. Wound cleaning

  a. Supplies:

    (1) Clean gloves

    (2) Cleaning solution

    (3) Absorbent pad for excess cleaning solution and debris

    (4) Sterile gauze

    (5) 50 to 60 mL sterile syringe, if irrigating

  b. Procedure: wound cleansing

    (1) Technique: clean

    (2) Wash hands, don clean gloves

    (3) Remove old dressing

    (4) Remove gloves, wash hands, don clean gloves

    (5) Cleanse the wound with sterile water or normal saline

      (a) Moisten sterile gauze pad

      (b) Gently wipe wound surface to remove surface debris

(6) Gently pat wound bed and periwound dry with new sterile gauze

(7) Proceed to prescribed wound treatment plan

c. Procedure: wound irrigation

(1) Technique: Clean

(2) Follow Procedure: wound cleansing, steps 1 to 3

(3) Fill sterile syringe with cleaning solution

(4) Trickle cleaning solution into wound bed

   (a) Do not apply pressure when pushing solution through syringe

(5) Gently pat wound bed and periwound dry with new sterile gauze

(6) Proceed to prescribed wound treatment plan

H. Wound Dressing Selection

There are several factors that can impact dressing selection. It is important to select the most appropriate wound dressing to achieve optimal wound healing.

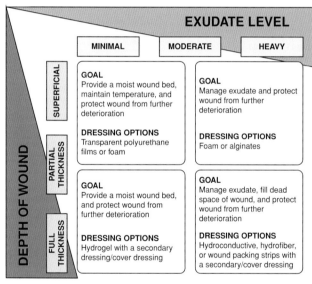

FIGURE 54.5 Wound dressing treatment objectives. (Adapted from Emory Nursing WOCNEC Faculty. *Skin and Wound Core Content Manual*. Atlanta, GA: Emory University; 2017. Copyright © 2018 Children's National Medical Center.)

1. General dressing principles **(Fig. 54.5)**
   a. If it is too wet, absorb it
   b. If it is too dry, hydrate it
   c. If there is a hole, fill it
   d. If there is necrotic tissue, remove it
   e. If there is healthy tissue, protect it

2. Considerations for dressing selection **(Table 54.2)**
   Wound dressings should provide a moist wound environment while managing exudate, remove barriers to wound healing (e.g., nonviable tissue), eliminate dead space, and may provide antimicrobial coverage. As the wound heals, dressing characteristics should be reevaluated to ensure the dressing type is still appropriate for the wound. Additionally, clinicians must understand compatibility with wound products and dressings to optimize healing outcomes

3. Periwound protection
   a. Moisture associated skin damage (MASD): skin injury resulting from prolonged exposure to urine/stool, perspiration, mucous, or exudate
      (1) Protection: use of a liquid skin barrier or hydrocolloid dressing (18)
   b. Medical adhesive–related skin injury (MARSI): injury from medical adhesives when the skin to adhesive attachment is stronger than the skin to skin attachment
      (1) Protection: for dressings with adhesive properties, use a liquid skin barrier or hydrocolloid dressing. Use an adhesive remover when applicable. Refer to **Table 54.3** for frequently used skin barriers, adhesives, and adhesive removers

4. Primary dressing: comes into direct contact with the wound

5. Secondary dressing: used to secure the primary dressing, when necessary

I. Negative Pressure Wound Therapy

Negative Pressure Wound Therapy (NPWT) systems are utilized to create an environment that promotes wound healing by secondary or tertiary intention, to prepare the wound bed for closure, promote granulation tissue formation and perfusion, and remove exudate and infectious materials. At this time, the U.S. Food and Drug Administration (FDA) (19) has not cleared the use of this system for the neonate, infant, or pediatric population. There are no established guidelines on the safety and efficacy of NPWT within these age groups, but there is growing expert opinion/case reports/panel expert opinions supporting use of NPWT in neonates (20–22).

1. NPWT in the neonate
   a. Wound etiologies: treatment of surgical site dehiscence, pressure injuries (PIs), and extremity wounds (20–22)
   b. Foam selection: refer to **Table 54.4**
   c. Pressure settings: pressure setting guidelines within the neonatal and pediatric population are based upon literature and panel expert opinion
      (1) Pressure settings can range from 25 to 125 mm Hg
      (2) NPWT pressure settings can be titrated up/down by 25 mm Hg increments

TABLE 54.2 Wound Dressings

DRESSING CLASS	EXAMPLE(S)	INDICATION	FEATURES	PRECAUTION
Alginate	Algisite M Medihoney	**Wound Type:** PI*, surgical dehiscence, tunnels/undermining **Thickness:** partial, full **Exudate:** moderate, heavy	Promotes autolytic debridement Highly absorptive Atraumatic removal Cut to fit Hemostatic (minimal) properties Safe for infected wounds Requires secondary dressing	Not intended for wounds that are dry, necrotic Alginates containing calcium use cautiously, secondary to systemic absorption
Contact layer	Mepitel	**Wound Type:** PI, surgical dehiscence, skin tears **Thickness:** superficial, partial, full **Exudate:** none, minimal, moderate	Protects epithelial tissue Exudate transfer Wound dressing interface Conformable to wound bed May use with topical treatment Safe for infected wounds Requires secondary dressing	Not intended for wounds that are clean, dry, covered in eschar, or have viscous exudate Do not use when debriding Not intended to be changed daily
Foam (polyurethane foam and composite)	Mepilex Allevyn Thin	**Wound Type:** PI, surgical incisions **Thickness:** partial, full **Exudate:** moderate, heavy	Atraumatic removal Pressure redistribution Provides thermal insulation Safe for infected wounds Requires secondary dressing, unless a composite	Not intended for wounds that are dry, covered in eschar (unless using for protection), have sinus tracks/tunneling
Hydrocolloid (gelatin, pectin, and/or carboxymethyl cellulose)	Duoderm Medihoney	**Wound Type:** PI, skin tears **Thickness:** superficial, partial **Exudate:** minimal, moderate	Promotes autolytic debridement Water resistant Impermeable Moldable Gels on contact with exudate Cut to fit Periwound protection Pressure redistribution (minimal)	Not intended for wounds that are infected, have tunnels/undermining, heavy exudate May cause maceration and epidermal stripping, use skin barrier film prior Use with caution in infected wounds
Hydroconductive	Drawtex	**Wound Type:** PI, surgical dehiscence, tunnels/undermining **Thickness:** partial, full **Exudate:** moderate, heavy	Highly absorbent Cut to fit Safe for infected wounds Requires secondary dressing	Not intended for wounds that are dry-minimal exudate, eschar
Hydrofiber/gelling fiber (sodium carboxymethyl cellulose)	Aquacel	**Wound Type:** PI, surgical dehiscence, tunnels/undermining **Thickness:** partial, full **Exudate:** moderate, heavy	Promotes autolytic debridement Flexible Gel on contact with exudate Aids in granulation tissue formation Safe for infected wounds Requires secondary dressing	Not intended for wounds that are dry-minimal exudate, eschar Hypergranulation risk

TABLE 54.2 Wound Dressings (*Continued*)

DRESSING CLASS	EXAMPLE(S)	INDICATION	FEATURES	PRECAUTION
Hydrogel	Solosite Medihoney	**Wound Types:** PI, surgical dehiscence, tunnels/undermining **Thickness:** partial, full **Exudate:** none, minimal	Promotes autolytic debridement Atraumatic Insoluble in water Provides moisture Promotes granulation and epithelialization Fills dead space Requires secondary dressing	Not intended for wounds that are viral lesions, heavy exudate May overhydrate/macerate wound/periwound (apply skin barrier film first)
Nonadherent	Telfa Primapore	**Wound Types:** PI, surgical dehiscence, skin tears, fragile skin **Thickness:** partial, full **Exudate:** none, minimal	Atraumatic removal Cut to fit Provides cover for topical therapy Safe for infected wounds Requires secondary dressing	Not intended for wounds that are heavily exudating
Transparent polyurethane film	Tegaderm Opsite	**Wound Types:** skin tears **Thickness:** superficial, partial, full **Exudate:** none, minimal	Promotes autolytic debridement Conformable Waterproof Impermeable to bacteria/contaminants Moisture vapor/oxygen transmission	Not intended for wounds that are infected, moderately to heavily exudating Risk of epidermal stripping (apply skin barrier film first)

*Pressure injuries.

This table does not endorse any product. It is intended to provide an at a glance reference for products (product list is not all inclusive). Always refer to manufacture information for Warnings and Precautions for specific products. Specific products may have different indications, contraindications, or warnings. Silver (Ag) products are contraindicated for patients with silver or iodine sensitivity. Silver products should be removed prior to magnetic resonance imaging (MRI) scans. Certain silver dressing cannot be used with collagenase ointments because they deactivate the collagenase.

Source: Copyright © 2018 Children's National Medical Center.

TABLE 54.3 Skin Barrier Films, Creams, Adhesives and Adhesive Removers

CATEGORY	EXAMPLE(S)	FUNCTION	PRECAUTIONS
Skin barrier film (nonalcohol based, plastic polymer)	No Sting Skin Prep	Provides a protective layer between the epidermis and adhesive Reduces the risk of MASD*, epidermal stripping, irritation from adhesives	Use with caution in neonates <30 days of life
Skin barrier cream (petrolatum, silicone, zinc based)	Vaseline Aquaphor Desitin	Protects against MASD, epidermal stripping, irritation/friction	Residual cream/ointment should not be removed prior to reapplication
Adhesives/bonding agents (silicone based)	Adapt Medical Adhesive Spray	Increase the stickiness of adhesives, also known as tackifiers Limit use to protecting skin under tape for critical tubes (e.g., endotracheal tubes)	The use of these products for routine adhesive application is not recommended Not approved in neonates ≤30 days of age Can cause contact irritant dermatitis
Adhesive remover (silicone based)	Adapt Medical Adhesive Remover	Prevent discomfort and skin disruption when adhesives are removed from the skin	Avoid alcohol-based remover, case reports of toxicity and skin injury

*Moisture associated skin damage.

This table does not endorse any product. It is intended to provide an at a glance reference for products (product list is not all inclusive). Always refer to manufacture information for Warnings and Precautions for specific products. Specific products may have different indications, contraindications, or warnings.

Source: Copyright © 2018 Children's National Medical Center.

TABLE 54.4 V.A.C. Foam Selection

WOUND CATEGORY	BLACK (POLYURETHANE) HYDROPHOBIC	WHITE (POLYVINYL ALCOHOL) HYDROPHILIC	SILVER (POLYURETHANE) MICROBONDED SILVER
Sternal	X	X	X
Omphalocele/gastroschisis	X	X	
Enterocutaneous fistula	X	X	
Abdominal compartment syndrome	X		
Spinal incision	X	X	X
Pressure injury	X		X
Extremity wounds	X		X
Fasciotomy wounds	X		X

Keswani SG. Managing neonatal and pediatric wounds and infections (power point slides). Retrieved from WOCN Annual Conference: Montreal, Canada, June 4–8, 2016.

2. Contraindications
   a. Wounds with exposed vessels, organs, tendons, and nerves
   b. Untreated osteomyelitis
   c. Nonenteric and unexplored fistulas
   d. Necrotic tissue with eschar present
   e. Sensitivity to silver (Ag⁺), do not use the V.A.C. GranuFoam Silver Dressing
   f. Malignancy in the wound

J. Diaper Dermatitis

Diaper dermatitis (DD) is a frequent and significant problem among neonates that results in pain, increased risk of infection, and additional hospital costs. DD develops as a result of overhydration, leading to disruption of the acid mantel and creation of an alkaline environment. Additional factors that cause breakdown are bacterial content and enzyme activity from urine and stool, with friction from the diaper rubbing against the overhydrated skin (23,24).

1. Prevention strategies
2. General management principles (**Fig. 54.6**)
3. Crusting technique
   a. Supplies
      (1) Clean gloves
      (2) Cleaning solution
      (3) Clean soft cloth
      (4) Skin barrier powder
      (5) Skin barrier wipe
      (6) Barrier cream
      (7) Nonadherent dressing
   b. Procedure
      (1) Technique: clean
      (2) Wash hands, don clean gloves
      (3) Clean the affected area with cleaning solution
      (4) Gently pat area until completely dry with a clean soft cloth
      (5) Apply a thin sprinkling of selected skin barrier powder to the raw/excoriated areas
      (6) Using a blotting/dabbing technique, blot powder with the skin barrier wipe
         (a) Initially powder may appear to be dissolving
      (7) Repeat steps 4, 5, two to four times, until you achieve a "crust"
         (a) A whitish crust will appear
      (8) Allow the area to dry for a few seconds
         (a) Test for dryness by gently brushing your finger over the area; it will feel rough but dry
      (9) Apply a thick layer of barrier cream over crusting
      (10) Apply nonadherent dressing over barrier cream
      (11) Secure new diaper

PICTURE EXAMPLE	DESCRIPTION OF SKIN	GOALS OF TREATMENT	PRODUCTS USED	TREATMENT PLAN (GIVE EACH THERAPY 48 hrs AND REASSESS TREATMENT PLAN)
	No Evidence of Diaper Dermatitis – Intact skin, no erythema	– Prevent skin breakdown – Provide skin barrier for "at-risk" patients – Educate caregivers	– Clean, soft cloth – Cleaning solution – Skin barrier cream	– Cleanse skin with each diaper change – For "at-risk" patients, apply barrier cream with each diaper change – Patients "at-risk" for skin breakdown: sensitive skin, immunosuppression, withdrawal symptoms, frequent stooling, infectious or caustic stools (antibiotic therapy, chemotherapy, and surgical interruption of the gastrointestinal system)
	Candida Diaper Dermatitis – With or w/out erythema – Yeast present (red, raised, scattered dotty/oval lesions)	– Prevent skin breakdown – Treat candida – Provide skin barrier – Educate caregivers	– Clean, soft cloth – Cleaning solution – Antifungal skin barrier cream or ointment	– Cleanse affected area with cleaning solution and pat dry with soft cloth (no commercial diaper wipes) – Apply a thick layer of antifungal barrier cream/ointment, and cover with nonadherent dressing – If no improvement after 48 hrs, change antifungal ointment or use the crusting technique with an antifungal powder and liquid skin barrier. May cover with skin barrier cream and nonadherent dressing
	Mild Diaper Dermatitis – Erythema present – Intact skin – No yeast present	– Prevent skin breakdown – Provide skin barrier – Reduce existing erythema – Educate caregivers	– Clean, soft cloth – Cleaning solution – Skin barrier cream containing zinc oxide	– Cleanse affected area with cleaning solution and pat dry with soft cloth (no commercial diaper wipes) – Apply a thick layer of skin barrier cream and cover with nonadherent dressing – If no improvement after 48 hrs, initiate treatment for moderate diaper dermatitis
	Moderate Diaper Dermatitis – Nonintact skin – Top layer of epidermis loss – Small/moderate surface area involvement	– Prevent further skin breakdown – Provide skin barrier – Enhance epithelization – Educate caregivers	– Clean, soft cloth – Cleaning solution – Skin barrier cream containing zinc oxide – Crusting supplies: liquid skin barrier, stoma, or silver, powder	– Cleanse affected area with cleaning solution and pat dry with soft cloth (no commercial diaper wipes) – Implement the crusting technique with stoma powder and a liquid skin barrier to the affected areas. Apply a thick layer of skin barrier cream over the crusting, and cover with a nonadherent dressing – If no improvement after 48 hrs, initiate treatment for severe diaper dermatitis
	Severe Diaper Dermatitis – Nonintact skin – Denuded areas, weepy raw skin, may contain ulcerations – Large surface area involvement – Persistent DD unresolved with other treatment methods	– Prevent further skin breakdown – Provide skin barrier – Enhance epithelization – Educate caregivers	– Clean, soft cloth – Cleaning solution – Cholestyramine powder – Skin barrier cream containing zinc oxide – Antifungal powder Treatment Options: – Cyanoacrylate-based liquid skin barrier (e.g., Marathon) – Petroleum-based skin barrier (e.g., Ilex) and petroleum jelly – Crusting supplies: liquid skin barrier, stoma, or silver powder	– Cleanse affected area with cleaning solution and pat dry with soft cloth (no commercial diaper wipes) – Options for treatment strategies based on severity of DD (therapies may be combined in some situations) – Initial treatment plan: mix equal parts of cholestyramine, zinc oxide, and antifungal powder. Apply a thick layer of the mixture to affected areas and cover with nonadherent dressing Treatment options if no improvement after 48 hrs: • Apply a thin layer of the liquid skin barrier to affected areas and allow to dry completely. Apply a thick layer of barrier cream over liquid skin protectant and cover with a nonadherent dressing. Reapply liquid skin barrier as needed • Apply petroleum based skin barrier (e.g., Ilex) and cover with a thin layer of petroleum jelly. Cover with nonadherent dressing • Crust with silver powder and liquid skin barrier. Apply a thick layer of skin barrier cream over the crusting, and cover with a nonadherent dressing

FIGURE 54.6 Diaper dermatitis. (Copyright © 2018 Children's National Medical Center.)

K. Pressure Injuries

The National Pressure Ulcer Advisory Panel (NPUAP) defines PIs as localized damage to the skin and underlying soft tissue over a bony prominence or related to a medical device (25). The injury occurs as a result of intense and/or prolonged pressure, or pressure in combination with shear.

1. Staging: PIs require staging in accordance with "NPUAP Pressure Injury Stages" definitions **(Fig. 54.7)**
   a. Numeric stages (1–3,26): when the deepest visible or palpable level of tissue injury or damage can be observed
   b. Unstageable (UTS): used when the deepest anatomic structures of the injury cannot be identified.
   c. Deep tissue pressure injury (DTPI): injuries that result from intense and/or prolonged pressure and shear forces at the bone–muscle interface
   d. Mucosal membrane pressure injuries (MMPIs): observed on mucous membranes with history of a medical device in use at the location of the injury. MMPIs cannot be staged due to the anatomy of mucosal tissue
2. Neonates at-risk for pressure injuries (PIs)
   a. Pressure-related PIs
      (1) Frequently locations: occiput, ears, heels
      (2) General prevention
         (a) Frequent inspection of bony prominences, heels, and occiput
            i. Conduct inspections more frequently in neonates who have signs of edema or are vulnerable to fluid shifts
         (b) Frequent repositioning
            i. Utilize repositions and repositioning aids
         (c) Pressure redistribution
            i. Prophylactic dressings: foam or hydrocolloid over high-risk locations
   b. Medical device–related PIs (MDRPIs): describes an etiology; appropriate staging is still required
      (1) >90% of MDRPIs are documented in premature infants (27)
      (2) High-risk medical devices: oxygen delivery devices, extracorporeal membrane oxygenation (ECMO) cannulas, pulse oximetry probes, near-infrared spectroscopy (NIRS) leads, feeding tubes, and vascular access devices
   c. General prevention
      (1) Remove device as soon as medically able
         (a) Frequent inspection of skin around and under medical devices
         (b) Ensure tubing or monitoring lead lines are not under the neonates' occiput, ears, or back
      (2) Device rotation/repositioning
      (3) Prophylactic dressings
         (a) Hydrocolloid dressing
            i. Secure device tubing/line to hydrocolloid with a cloth tape
         (b) Thin foam dressing
            i. Thicker foam is recommended when a medical device cannot be rotated or offloaded
   d. Oxygen delivery device PI prevention
      (1) Continuous positive airway pressure (CPAP): gold-standard noninvasive ventilation in the preterm infant (1,3,28)
         (a) Equipment: bi-nasal prong, nasal face mask
         (b) Prevention: silicone-based skin adhesive followed by a hydrocolloid or thin foam dressing at the skin/device interface(s)
      (2) High-flow nasal cannula (HFNC)/RAM/NC
         (a) Equipment: nasal cannulas
         (b) Prevention: silicone-based skin adhesive followed by a hydrocolloid. Top with a foam or hydroconductive dressing cut into a "T" shape
            i. Placed "T" upside down to protect the nasal septum and across the nasal base at the skin/device interface(s)
            ii. Tubing securement: silicone-based skin adhesive followed by a hydrocolloid, secured with a retention tape at the skin/device interface(s)

L. Debridement

Necrotic tissue is a barrier to healing, removal of this nonviable tissue is critical to wound bed preparation to promote and optimize wound healing. Debridement is a necessary part of the neonate's wound treatment. Nonviable tissue will delay wound healing and harbor bacteria. Debridement methods may be selective (targeting only areas of nonviable tissue) or nonselective (removing healthy tissue along with nonviable tissue) (11,29,30).

1. Indications
   a. When goal is to heal by optimization of a healthy wound bed
   b. Wound bed contains nonviable tissue, debris, or hypertrophied tissue that impairs contact inhibition of the epithelial cells
2. Contraindications
   a. When goal is maintenance or comfort/palliative
   b. Stable eschar on the heel
   c. Stable dry gangrene/dry ischemic limbs
   d. High risk for bleeding
   e. Malignant wounds

PI STAGE	DESCRIPTION
Stage 1 Pressure Injury-Lightly Pigmented 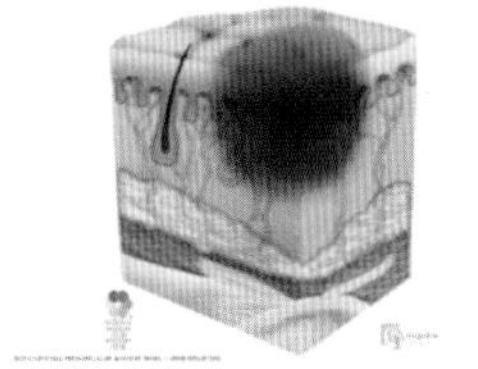	Intact skin with nonblanchable redness in a localized area, that persists 30 min after pressure relief. The area may be painful, firm, soft, warmer or cooler as compared to adjacent tissue.
Stage 2 Pressure Injury 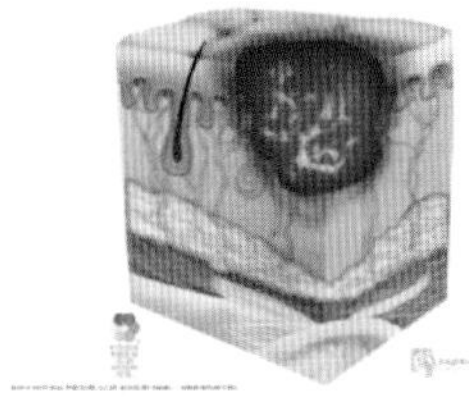	Partial-thickness loss of dermis. Presenting as a shallow open injury with a red pink wound bed, without slough. May also present as an intact or open/ruptured serum-filled or serosanginous-filled blister.
Stage 3 Pressure Injury 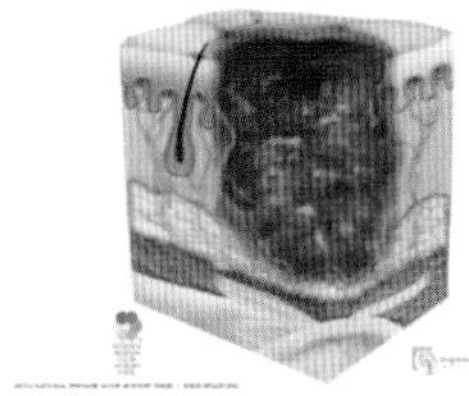	Full-thickness tissue loss. Subcutaneous fat may be visible, however bone, tendon, or muscles are not exposed. Sloughing may be present but does not obscure the depth of tissue loss. May include undermining or tunneling.
Stage 4 Pressure Injury 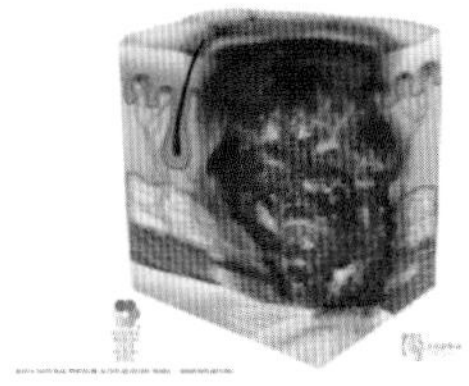	Full-thickness tissue loss with exposed bone, tendon, cartilage, or muscle. Sloughing or eschar may be present on some parts of the wound bed. There is often undermining or tunneling. Cartilage is considered bone.
Deep Tissue Pressure Injury 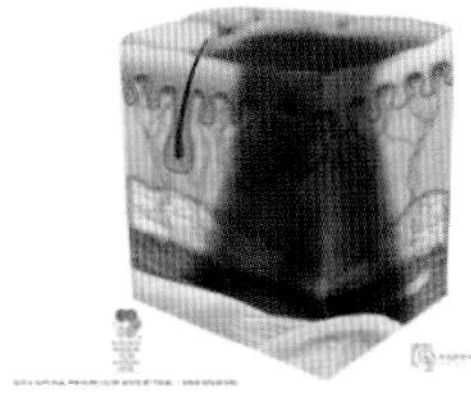	Purple or maroon localized area of discolored intact skin or blood-filled blister due to damage of underlying soft tissue from pressure and/or shearing.
Unstageable Pressure Injury-Slough and Eschar 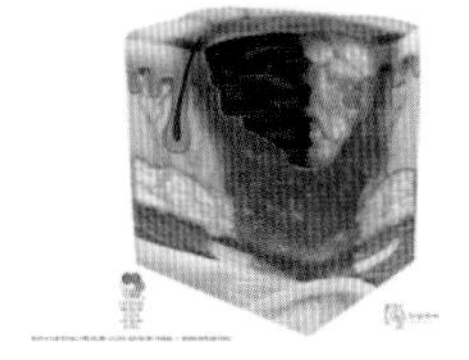	Full-thickness tissue loss in which the actual depth of the injury is completely obscured by slough (yellow, tan, gray, or brown) and/or eschar (tan, brown, or black) in the wound bed. Until enough slough or eschar is removed to expose the base of the wound, the true depth cannot be determined.
Mucous Membrane 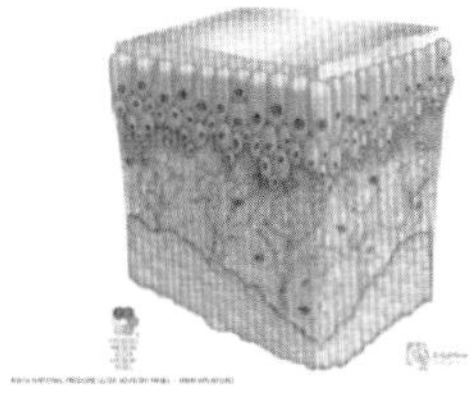	These PIs are found on mucous membranes with a history of a medical device in use at the location of the injury. Due to the anatomy of the tissue these injuries cannot be staged.

FIGURE 54.7 Pressure injury staging. (Adapted with permission of the National Pressure Ulcer Advisory Panel (NPUAP), 2016.)

3. Types of debridement (11,29,30)
   a. Noninstrumental
      (1) Autolytic: selective
         (a) Mechanism of action: use of the body's own enzymes (white blood cells) found in wound exudate
         (b) Appropriate for: slough, ideally noninfected wounds
         (c) Dressing: occlusive, moisture retentive
      (2) Enzymatic: selective
         (a) Mechanism of action: topical application of enzymes that digest denatured collagen
         (b) Appropriate for: slough and eschar (requires crosshatching), (non)infected wounds
         (c) Dressing: nonadherent plus secondary dressing
      (3) Mechanical: nonselective
         (a) Mechanism of action: mechanical force used
         (b) Appropriate for: nonadherent slough, infected wounds without visible granulation
         (c) Dressing: wet-to-dry, wound irrigation, or manual shearing to wound bed with gauze
   b. Instrumental
      (1) Conservative sharp: selective, removal of loosely adherent slough/necrotic tissue by scalpel, forceps, and/or scissors
         (a) Often used in conjunction with noninstrumental debridement
         (b) To be performed only by trained practitioner
         (c) Conservative sharp debridement
            i. Supplies
               (i) Clean gloves
               (ii) Sterile gloves
               (iii) Antiseptic solution
               (iv) Sterile saline
               (v) Sterile gauze
               (vi) Sterile scalpel, forceps, and/or scissors
               (vii) Appropriate topical treatment, if necessary
               (viii) Appropriate sterile dressing(s), if necessary
            ii. Procedure
               (i) Technique: aseptic
               (ii) Wash hands, don clean gloves
               (iii) Remove old dressing
               (iv) Remove gloves, wash hands, don sterile gloves
               (v) Cleanse the wound with antiseptic solution
               (vi) Allow to dry

        (vii) Using sterile instrument(s)
           1) Grasp nonviable tissue
           2) Lift away from wound base
           3) Carefully cut away small amounts of nonviable tissue, avoiding all vascular structures
      (viii) Cleanse with sterile saline
        (ix) Gently pat wound bed and periwound dry with new sterile gauze
        (x) Proceed to prescribed wound treatment plan
    (2) Surgical: nonselective, sterile removal of slough/necrosis by scalpel

M. Surgical Incisions

Surgical wounds heal by reepithelialization at the skin incisional level and surgical restoration of the underlying tissue layers below. Although healing times vary, most acute wounds heal within 4 to 6 weeks. The preterm neonate's skin presents integrity challenges due to immature skin structure (31).

1. Routine surgical incision care: leave the original postoperative dressing in place for 48 hours. This allows hemostasis to occur and protects from bacterial invasion
   a. First 48 hours: if the dressing becomes saturated, replaced with a new sterile dressing, using aseptic technique
      (1) Aseptic surgical incision dressing change, first 48 hours
         (a) Supplies
            i. Clean gloves
            ii. Sterile gloves
            iii. Sterile gauze
            iv. Cleaning solution
            v. Appropriate sterile dressing(s)
         (b) Procedure
            i. Technique: aseptic
            ii. Wash hands, don clean gloves
            iii. Remove old dressing
            iv. Remove gloves
            v. Wash hands, don sterile gloves
            vi. Clean incision with cleaning solution
            vii. Gently pat incision with sterile gauze until completely dry
            viii. Apply sterile dressing
   b. After 48 hours: the dressing may be removed, leaving the incision open to air. Cleanse daily, using aseptic technique, until the incision is healed
2. Sternotomy: leave the original postoperative dressing in place for 48 hours. This allows hemostasis to occur and protects from bacterial invasion

a. Routine care of the closed sternotomy
   (1) First 48 hours: if the dressing becomes saturated, replaced with a new sterile dressing, using aseptic technique
   (2) After 48 hours and extubated (**Fig. 54.8**): dressing may be removed, leaving incision open to air. Cleanse daily, using aseptic technique, until the incision is healed

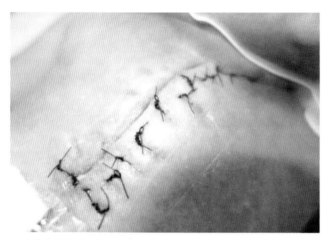

FIGURE 54.8 Healing sternotomy. (Copyright © 2018 Children's National Medical Center.)

   (a) Incisional protection
      i. Keep the neck clean and dry
      ii. Cover incision when there is an increased risk for soiling (e.g., suctioning, feeding, performing mouth care)
   (3) After 48 hours and intubated/tracheostomy: a dressing should remain in place. Cleanse daily, using aseptic technique, until the incision is healed, or the patient is extubated
b. Delayed sternal closure (DSC)
   (1) Following cardiac surgery, a DSC, also referred to as open sternotomy (OS), may be clinically necessary. These incisional sites are covered with a sterile mediastinal dressings (silicone/elastomer sheeting) attached to external skin edges, and covered with an occlusive dressing (32)
      (a) Follow organizational policy/procedures, typically only removed/changed by surgeon
      (b) Frequent dressing assessments for
         i. Occlusiveness
         ii. Fullness: concave, convex, bulging, flat
         iii. Drainage
   (2) Associated complications (32)
      (a) Infection: sternal, mediastinitis, sepsis
      (b) Bleeding
      (c) Tamponade: bulging dressings may be a sign of impending tamponade
      (d) Sternal instability

3. Surgical incision complications
   a. Hematoma and seromas
      (1) Definitions
         (a) Hematoma: a collection of clotted blood between the tissue layers
         (b) Seroma: a collection of serum between the tissue layers
      (2) Treatment
         (a) Fluid should reabsorb, if it fails to in a timely manner, a needle aspiration or drain may be necessary
   b. Incisional failure: incisional opening along the wound edges
      (1) Definitions
         (a) Partial dehiscence: superficial skin separation at the incision site. Skin edges are separated, deeper tissues remain intact
         (b) Full dehiscence: dehiscence to the fascia level
         (c) Evisceration: dehiscence extends past the fascia level, resulting in protrusion of abdominal organs
            i. Treatment: surgical emergency, notify appropriate surgical team
      (2) Treatment
         (a) Follow principles of moist wound healing
         (b) Refer to Wound Dressing Selection section
            i. Frequently used dressings include, but are not limited to alginates, hydrofibers, hydrogels, hydrocolloids, and foams
            ii. NPWT may be considered in select patients. Refer to NPWT section.
   c. Surgical site infections (SSI): range from localized infections involving superficial skin layers to more serious infections involving tissues under the skin, organs, or implanted material (33)
      (1) Identification: refer to NERDS/STONES section
         (a) Wound culture: refer to section on wound culture
      (2) Treatment: localized, systemic, or surgical. For localized management, refer to sections on wound cleaning and treatment and dressing selection

N. Congenital Anomalies With Skin Integrity Alterations

1. **Neural tube defects**
   Myelomeningocele (spina bifida) is the most common congenital neural tube defect. Corrective surgery is typically performed within the first 24 to 78 hours of life to avoid meningitis and other associated complications (34,35)

a. Preoperative care
   (1) Goal: protect sac from rupture and patient from infection
      (a) Prevention
         i. Prophylaxis with broad-spectrum antibiotics
         ii. Positioning: prone or slide lying alleviates pressure
         iii. Skin protection: apply protective hydrocolloid dressings to bony prominences and utilize gel pads/fluidized positioners
      (b) Exposed sac protection
         i. Immediately cover the sac in a sterile protective dressing. Use of sterile saline soaked sterile gauze dressing is an ideal dressing choice. Plastic wrap over the gauze dressing assists in maintaining a moist environment
            (i) Use of sterile saline soaked sterile gauze dressing is an ideal dressing choice. Plastic wrap over the gauze dressing assists in maintaining a moist environment
            (ii) Protection from fecal contamination is essential. A cut-to-fit flap that directs stool away from the exposed sac, further decreasing risk of infection
      (c) Other considerations
         i. Latex free environment, neonates are at high risk for developing a latex allergy
         ii. All iodine containing products should be avoided; they cause further injury to the exposed tissue
b. Postoperative care
   (1) Goal: protect incision from damage and infection
      (a) Maintain prone/side-lying position until cleared by neurosurgery
      (b) Ensure dressing remains clean, dry, and intact. Continue to utilize the fecal containment device until incision is healed
      (c) Monitor for hydrocephalus
      (d) Maintain latex precautions

2. **Giant omphalocele**
   An abdominal wall defect, exceeding 5 to 6 cm in diameter, characterized by herniation of the abdominal viscera, to include parts of the liver through the base of the umbilical cord, and a covering of the peritoneum. When primary surgical closure is not feasible, treatment options include staged repair and conservative treatment with delayed surgical closure (26,36)
   a. Delayed surgical closure
      (1) Goal: decrease infection risk through promotion of eschar formation and epithelization of the sac

(2) Treatment: application of topical escharotic agents directly onto the sac. Initial cleansing and application of escharotic agent should be done using aseptic technique
   (a) Topical escharotic agents
      i. Certain toxicities are associated with several escharotic agents, and currently there is no standard treatment (27)
         (i) Povidone-iodine (PVP-I): thyroid dysfunction
         (ii) Silver sulfadiazine and silver nitrate: seizures, peripheral neuropathy, ocular pathology, nephrotic syndrome, elevated liver enzymes, leukopenia, argyria
         (iii) Alcohol: alcohol intoxication
      ii. Recent expert opinions suggest silver impregnated hydrofiber dressings for their antimicrobial properties and low silver associated toxicity
   (b) Dressing changes should be completed
      i. Every 3 days, or more frequently for significant drainage in the first several weeks
      ii. Every 5 to 7 days as drainage slows
   (c) Omphalocele sac changes
      i. Evolves through various toughening and thickening stages
      ii. Membrane may appear yellow/green/grey and the hydrofiber dressing will liquefy the slough to reveal the new epithelized tissue (37)
(3) Promotion of omphalocele epithelization
   (a) Supplies:
      i. Clean gloves
      ii. Cleansing solution
      iii. Sterile water
      iv. Scissors
      v. Escharotic agent: silver impregnated hydrofiber dressing
      vi. Nonadherent dressing
      vii. Securement warp (e.g., Kling, ACE bandage)
   (b) Procedure
      i. Technique: clean
      ii. Wash hands and apply clean gloves
      iii. Remove soiled dressings
      iv. Wash hands and apply clean gloves
      v. Cut silver impregnated hydrofiber dressing into small strips
      vi. Lightly moisten the hydrofiber strips and apply them over the open areas of the omphalocele (areas that are epithelized do not require further treatment)
      vii. Cover with nonadherent dressing
      viii. Utilize securement wrap to hold dressing in place

3. Aplasia cutis congenita

Aplasia cutis congenita (ACC) is a rare congenital disease characterized by local absence of epidermis, dermis, and occasionally, subcutaneous tissue or bone that usually involves the scalp vertex. ACC lesions can occur on any body surface, although localized scalp lesions form the most frequent pattern, accounting for over 70%, with complete aplasia involving bone defects occurring in approximately 20% of the case (**Fig. 54.9**) (38)

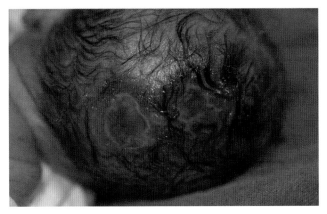

FIGURE 54.9 Aplasia cutis congenita full thickness with exposed dura.

   a. Treatment: approach to treatment for ACC is controversial. It is based upon size, depth, and location, of the defect and involvement of scalp veins (39–42)

     (1) Conservative treatment

       (a) Type of defect(s): scalp (<1 cm in diameter with intact dura, no sagittal sinus involvement, no large vascular malformation), large scalp without bone involvement, large nonscalp

       (b) Treatment requires preservation of a moist wound environment that prevents desiccation, promotes epithelialization, and minimizes risk of infection (**Fig. 54.5**)

         i. Petrolatum gauze, nonadhering dressings, and emollients

         ii. Use of topical antimicrobials or antimicrobial dressings only if signs of infection are present

     (2) Surgical

       (a) Type of defect(s): large defects involving the scalp and skull with exposed sagittal sinus or brain tissue, and exposed vessel (40)

         i. Urgent surgical treatment is indicated for exposed sagittal sinus or large vessel

       (b) Treatment: options include primary closure, flaps, skin or bone grafts

         i. It is of the utmost importance to keep the wound moist and covered at all times to avoid the risk of desiccation, resulting in dura rupture and fatal hemorrhage (40)

4. Epidermolysis bullosa

Epidermolysis bullosa (EB) refers to a diverse group of inherited skin fragility disorders (**Figs. 54.10 and 54.11**) (43,44). Neonates with EB can have skin fragility at birth, or develop blistering of the skin within the neonatal period. Development of acute and chronic wounds that cause pain, joint contractures, fusion of fingers/toes, and premature death related to secondary infection and squamous cell carcinoma from chronic wounds is possible. In severe cases, blistering can occur internally within the gastrointestinal tract and other mucosal membranes. Skin may blister or sheer in response to minimal friction or trauma, and the extent of skin layer and mucosal membrane involvement is determined by the subtype of EB and severity of disease (44,45)

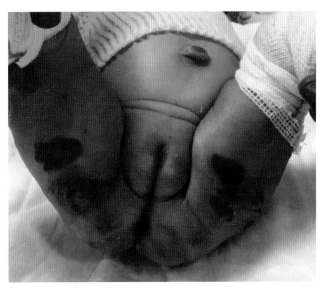

FIGURE 54.10 Epidermolysis bullosa. (Copyright © 2018 Children's National Medical Center.)

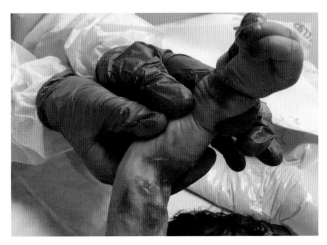

FIGURE 54.11 Epidermolysis bullosa. (Copyright © 2018 Children's National Medical Center.)

a. Treatment

(1) Premedication: recommended prior to all dressing changes

(2) Cleansing: sterile normal saline or approved antimicrobial cleanser

(3) Blister management: blisters occur following friction and minor trauma

    (a) Intact blisters require lancing with a sterile needle, as they are not self-limiting and will expand rapidly leading to epidermal separation

        i. Parallel lancing creating an entry and exit hole (44)

        ii. Puncturing allows for further drainage, while keeping the roof of the blister intact, serving as a protective covering

(4) Dressings

    (a) Dressing removal: sterile normal saline soaks are beneficial for dressings that have become dried to exudate prior to removal

    (b) Moist wound healing principles should be utilized

    (c) Cover all open areas with nonadherent dressings prior to wrapping

    (d) Intact skin under wrapping should be coated with an emollient for added protection from friction (44)

    (e) Small studies and expert opinion support the use of specialized nonadherent dressings that minimize skin trauma and promote wound healing in the neonate with EB (16). Dressing options include, but are not limited to

        i. Contact layer: soft silicone mesh

            (i) Increased risk of hypergranulation in junctional EB and blistering in EBS-DM

        ii. Impregnated gauze: petroleum or hydrogel

            (i) Cover with a nonadherent dressing

            (ii) Secure with a secondary dressing

        iii. Absorption: hydrofiber, soft silicone foam

        iv. Protection: soft silicone foam

        v. Critical colonization/infection: polymeric membrane

        vi. Secondary dressings: gauze wrap, tubular netting, tubular bandage, soft silicone tape

b. Integumentary considerations

(1) Infection prevention

    (a) Scratching: prevent by placing mittens or nonadherent dressings over the hands. Topical emollients may also help relieve itching by adding moisture to the skin

(2) Medical equipment

    (a) Medical devices: avoid the use of medical devices and tapes when possible. If necessary, use a contact layer (silicone mesh) or protective (soft silicone foam) dressing under medical devices

    (b) Incubators: do not use unless medically necessary. Heat and moisture exacerbate blistering

(3) Clothing: loose fitting and made of a soft material such as cotton

(4) Diapers: remove elastic components that cause additional friction. Line diaper edges with a nonadherent dressing

    (a) Utilize barrier cream to the perineum with each diaper change to avoid further friction in this area

O. Ischemic Injuries

Irreversible tissue damage can be caused by thrombotic and inflammatory responses as early as 3 hours after an extreme ischemic event. The extent of the injury depends on the duration of the ischemic event and level of damage to collateral vessels. The extent of injury can present as patchy or specific to one localized area, frequently occurring in the distal aspect of the involved extremity. Once hemodynamics have stabilized, the extent of the reperfusion injury is noted. The full extent of the tissue damage is often seen days later following the ischemic event, initially presenting as discoloration of the skin, but can progress to nonviable tissue (**Fig. 54.12**).

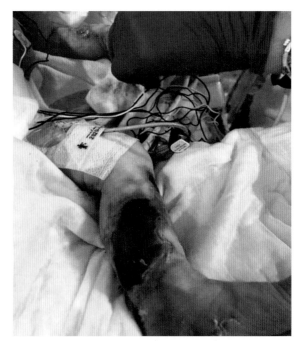

FIGURE 54.12 Ischemic injury. (Copyright © 2018 Children's National Medical Center.)

Management goals include: preserve viable tissue, prevent infection, and debride nonviable tissue.

1. Viable tissue preservation
   a. Principles of moist wound healing (refer to moist wound healing section)
   b. Prevention of infection
2. Nonviable debridement methods
   a. Adherent: autolytic, enzymatic, surgical
   b. Nonadherent: autolytic, enzymatic, mechanical, conservative sharp, surgical
3. Promotion of reperfusion
   a. Patient position: neutral alignment with nondependent/elevated extremities
   b. Methods: heel warmers, nitroglycerine paste
   c. Indications: improve perfusion to distal extremities, localized etiology
   d. Contraindications: hemodynamic instability, gangrene

References

1. Meszes A, Talosi G, Mader K, et al. Lesions requiring wound management in a central tertiary neonatal intensive care unit. *W J Pediatr.* 2017;13(2):165–172.
2. Sardesai SR, Kornacka MK, Walas W, et al. Iatrogenic skin injury in the neonatal intensive care unit. *J Matern Fetal Neonatal Med.* 2011;24(2):197–203.
3. Scheans P. Neonatal pressure ulcer prevention. *Neonatal Netw.* 2015;34(2):126–132.
4. Hoath SB, Mauro T. Fetal skin development. In: Eichenfield LF, Frieden IJ, Mathes EF, Zaenglein AL eds. *Neonatal and Infant Dermatology.* 3rd ed. London, New York, Oxford, Philadelphia, St Louis, Sydney, Toronto: Elsevier Saunders; 2015:1–13.
5. Dolack M, Huffines B, Stikes R, et al. Updated neonatal skin risk assessment scale (NSRAS). *Ky Nurse.* 2013;61(4):6.
6. Lund CH, Osborne JW. Validity and reliability of the neonatal skin condition score. *J Obstet Gynecol Neonatal Nurs.* 33(3):320–327.
7. Rogers VR. Wound management in neonates, infants, children, and adolescents. In: Browne NT, McComiskey CA, Flanigan LM, Pieper P eds. *Nursing Care of the Pediatric Surgical Patient.* 2nd ed. Sudbury, MA: Jones and Barlett Publishers; 2007:167–181.
8. Thames Valley Neonatal ODN Quality Care Group. Guideline framework for neonatal wound care. Thames Valley & Wessex Neonatal Operational Delivery Network. 2012. https://www.networks.nhs.uk/nhs-networks/thames-valley-wessex-neonatal-network/documents/guidelines/Wound%20Guideline.pdf
9. Bingham D, Pettit J, Thape JM, et al. *Neonatal Skin Care, Third Edition. Evidenced Based Clinical Practice Guideline.* Washington, DC: Association of Women's Health, Obstetric and Neonatal Nurses; 2013.
10. Lund C, Singh C. Skin and wound care for neonatal and pediatric populations. In: Doughty DB, McNichol LL eds. *Wound, Ostomy, and Continence Nurses Society Core Curriculum Wound Management.* Philadelphia, PA, Baltimore, New York, London, Buenos Aires, Hong Kong, Sydney, Tokyo: Wolters Kluwer; 2016:198–218.
11. Doughty DB, McNichol LL. *Core Curriculum Wound Management.* Philadelphia, PA: Wolters Kluwer; 2016.
12. Sibbald G, Woo K, Ayello E. Increased bacterial burden and infection: NERDS and STONES. *Wounds UK.* 2007;3(2):25–46.
13. Spear M. Best techniques for obtaining wound cultures. *Plast Surg Nurs.* 2012;32(1):34–36.
14. Levine NS, Lindberg RB, Mason AD Jr, et al. The quantitative swab culture and smear: a quick, simple method for determining the number of viable aerobic bacteria on open wounds. *J Trauma.* 1976;16(2):89–94.
15. Kuller JM. Infant skin care products what are the issues? *Adv Neonatal Care.* 2016;16(Suppl 5S):S3–S12.
16. King A, Stellar JJ, Blevins A, et al. Dressings and products in pediatric wound care. *Adv Wound Care (New Rochelle).* 2014;3(4):324–334.
17. Upadhyayula S, Kambalapali M, Harrison CJ. Safety of anti-infective agents for skin preparation in premature infants. *Arch Dis Child.* 2007;92(7):646–647.
18. Boswell N, Waker CL. Comparing 2 adhesives methods on skin integrity in the high-risk neonate. *Adv Neonatal Care.* 2016;16(6):449–454
19. U.S. Food & Drug Administration. Guidance for industry and FDA staff – class II special controls guidance document: non-powered suction apparatus device intended for negative pressure wound therapy (NPWT). 2010. https://www.fda.gov/medicaldevices/deviceregulationandguidance/guidancedocuments/ucm233275.htm
20. Baharestani MM. Use of negative pressure wound therapy in the treatment of neonatal and pediatric wounds: a retrospective examination of clinical outcomes. *Ostomy Wound Manage.* 2007;53(6):75–85.
21. Aldridge B, Ladd AP, Kepple J, et al. Negative pressure wound therapy for initial management of giant omphalocele. *Am J Surg.* 2016;211(3):605–609.
22. Baharestani M, Amjad I, Bookout K, et al. V.A.C. therapy in the management of paediatric wounds: clinical review and experience. *Int Wound J.* 2009;6(Suppl 1):1–26.
23. Blume-Peytavi U, Hauser M, Lunnemann L, et al. Prevention of diaper dermatitis in infants—literature review. *Pediatr Dermatol.* 2014;31(4):413–429.
24. Esser M. Diaper dermatitis what do we do next? *Adv Neonatal Care.* 2016;16(5S):S21–S25.
25. National Pressure Ulcer Advisory Panel. NPUAP pressure injury stages. 2017. http://www.npuap.org/resources/educational-and-clinical-resources/npuap-pressure-injury-stages/
26. Lee SL, Beyer TD, Kim SS, et al. Initial nonoperative management and delayed closure for treatment of giant omphaloceles. *J Pediatr Surg.*2006;41(11):1846–1849.
27. Pittman J. Medical device related pressure injuries. 2018. https://www.npuap.org/wp-content/uploads/2018/09/Medical-Device-Related-Pressure-Injury-Webinar.-Sept-2018-Handouts.pdf
28. Imbulana DI, Manley BJ, Dawson JA, et al. Nasal injury in preterm infants receiving non-invasive respiratory support: a systematic review. *Arch Dis Child Fetal Neonatal Ed.* 2018;103:F29–F35.
29. Sound West Regional Wound Care Program. Wound debridement guide. 2015. http://www.swrwoundcareprogram.ca/Uploads/ContentDocuments/DebridementGuideline.pdf

30. Acelity. *V.A.C. Therapy Clinical Guidelines a Reference Source for Clinicians*. San Antonio, TX: Acelity; 2015.

31. Knoerleim K, McKenney WM, Mullaney DM, et al. The surgical neonate. In: Browne NT, McComiskey CA, Flanigan LM, & Pieper P eds. *Nursing care of the pediatric surgical patient* 2nd ed. Sandbury, MA: Jones and Barlett Publishers; 2007:167–181.

32. Pye S, McDonnell M. Nursing considerations for children undergoing delayed sternal closure after surgery for congenital heart disease. *Crit Care Nurse*. 2010;30(3):50–61.

33. Center for Disease Control. Surgical site infections (SSI). 2017. https://www.cdc.gov/hai/ssi/ssi.html

34. Dias M. Neurosurgical management of myelomeningocele (spina bifida). *Pediatr Rev*. 2005;26(2):50–60.

35. McLone D, Bowman R. Overview of the management of myelomeningocele (spina bifida). *UpToDate*. 2018. https://www.uptodate.com/contents/overview-of-the-management-of-myelomeningocele-spina-bifida

36. Bauman B, Stephens D, Gershone H, et al. Management of giant omphaloceles: a systematic review of methods of staged surgical closure vs. nonoperative delayed closure. *J Pediatr Surg*. 2016;51(10):1725–1730.

37. Oquendo M, Agrawal V, Reyna R, et al. Silver-impregnated hydrofiber dressing followed by delayed surgical closure for management of infants born with giant omphaloceles. *J Pediatr Surg*. 2015;50(10):1668–1672.

38. Alexandros B, Dimitrios G, Elias A, et al. Aplasia cutis congenita: two case reports and discussion of the literature. *Surg Neurol Int*. 2017;8:273.

39. Gupta D. Aplasia cutis congenita. *UpToDate*. 2018. http://www.uptodate.com/contents/aplasia-cutis-congenita/print

40. Alexandros B, Dimitrios G, Elias A, et al. Aplasia cutis congenita: two case reports and discussion of the literature. *Surg Neurol Int*. 2017;8:273.

41. Wollina U, Chokoeva A, Verma SH, et al. Aplasia cutis congenita type I—a case series. *Georgian Med News*. 2017;3(264):7–11.

42. Cherubino M, Maggiulli F, Dibartolo R, et al. Treatment of multiple wounds of aplasia cutis congenita on the lower limb: a case report. *J Wound Care*. 2016;25(12):760–762.

43. Kirkorian AY, Weitz NA, Tlougan B, et al. Evaluation of wound care options in patients with recessive dystrophic epidermolys bullosa: a costly necessity. *Pediatr Dermatol*. 2013;31(1):33–37.

44. Denyer J, Pillay E. *Best Practice Guidelines for Skin and Wound Care in Epidermolysis Bullosa*. International Consensus. DEBRA; 2012.

45. Fine J, Bruckner-Tuderman L, Eady RA, et al. Inherited epidermolysis bullosa: updated recommendations on diagnosis and classification. *J Am Acad Dermatol*. 2014;70(6):1103–1126.

Phototherapy

Suhasini Kaushal and Jayashree Ramasethu

Phototherapy is the most common therapeutic intervention used for the treatment of unconjugated hyperbilirubinemia in neonates. The aim of phototherapy is to reduce serum bilirubin levels to decrease the risk of acute bilirubin encephalopathy and the chronic sequel of bilirubin toxicity, kernicterus (1).

Phototherapy causes isomerization of the bilirubin molecule (bilirubin IX-α, Z,Z configuration) to polar, water-soluble photoproducts (conformational photoisomers Z,E and E,Z bilirubin, and structural photoisomers E,Z and E,E lumibilirubin). These photoisomers can be excreted in bile and urine without the need for conjugation or further metabolism (2,3). Photo-oxidation plays a smaller role in the excretion of bilirubin.

A. Indications

1. Clinically significant hyperbilirubinemia. Indications to start phototherapy in babies with unconjugated hyperbilirubinemia vary depending on gestational age, birth-weight, age in hours, presence of hemolysis, and other risk factors such as acidosis and sepsis (1,4).
2. The total serum bilirubin (TSB) level must be considered when making the decision to commence treatment, as there is significant variability in laboratory measurement of direct bilirubin levels (1).
3. The American Academy of Pediatrics has published clinical practice guidelines for phototherapy in newborn infants at 35 weeks' or more gestation (**Fig. 55.1**) (1).

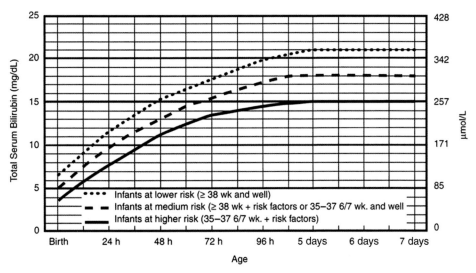

- Use total bilirubin. Do not subtract direct reacting or conjugated bilirubin.
- Risk factors = isoimmune hemolytic disease, G6PD deficiency, asphyxia, significant lethargy, temperature instability, sepsis, acidosis, or albumin <3.0 g/dL (if measured)
- For well infants 35–37 6/7 wk can adjust TSB levels for intervention around the medium risk line. It is an option to intervene at lower TSB levels for infants closer to 35 wks and at higher TSB levels for those closer to 37 6/7 wk.
- It is an option to provide conventional phototherapy in hospital or at home at TSB levels 2–3 mg/dL (35–50 mmol/L) below those shown but home phototherapy should not be used in any infant with risk factors.

FIGURE 55.1 Guidelines for phototherapy in hospitalized infants of 35 or more weeks' gestation. (Reprinted with permission from American Academy of Pediatrics Subcommittee on Hyperbilirubinemia. Management of hyperbilirubinemia in the newborn infant 35 or more weeks of gestation. *Pediatrics.* 2004;114(1):297–316. Erratum: *Pediatrics.* 2004;114(4):1138. Copyright © 2004 by the AAP.)

4. Guidelines for phototherapy for preterm infants <35 weeks' gestation have been proposed, but are much more variable and highly individualized (see Table 49.1 (5–7).
5. In extremely low–birth-weight (ELBW) infants, aggressive early phototherapy reduces peak bilirubin levels and rates of neurodevelopmental disability, but has been associated with higher mortality (8).

B. Contraindications

1. Congenital porphyria or a family history of porphyria is an absolute contraindication to the use of phototherapy. Severe purpuric bullous eruptions have been described in neonates with congenital erythropoietic porphyria treated with phototherapy (9).
2. Concomitant use of drugs or agents that are photosensitizers (10).
3. Concurrent therapy with metalloporphyrin heme oxygenase inhibitors has been reported to result in mild transient erythema (11).
4. Although infants with cholestatic jaundice may develop the "bronze baby syndrome" when exposed to phototherapy (see H), the presence of direct hyperbilirubinemia is not considered to be a contraindication (1). However, because the products of phototherapy are excreted in the bile, the presence of cholestasis may decrease the effectiveness of phototherapy.

C. Equipment

Terminology

It is important to be familiar with specific terminology to understand the functioning of the equipment available for phototherapy (2,12).

1. *Spectral qualities* of the delivered light (wavelength range and peak). Bilirubin absorbs visible light within the wavelength range of 400 to 500 nm, with peak absorption at 460 to 490 nm considered to be the most effective (2,3,13). *Note:* Phototherapy is not ultraviolet (UV) light (wavelength 10 to 400 nm).
2. *Irradiance* (intensity of light), expressed as watts per square centimeter (W/cm^2), refers to the number of photons received per square centimeter of exposed body surface area.
3. *Spectral irradiance* is irradiance that is quantitated within the effective wavelength range for efficacy and is expressed as $\mu W/cm^2/nm$. This is measured by various commercially available radiometers. Specific radiometers are generally recommended for each phototherapy system, because measurements of irradiance may vary depending on the radiometer and the light source (1,2,12).

Devices

Phototherapy equipment may be freestanding, attached to a radiant warmer, wall-mounted, suspended from the ceiling, or fiberoptic systems. These in turn may contain various light sources to deliver the phototherapy. The clinician is, therefore, faced with a vast array of equipment to choose from and must be aware of advantages and disadvantages of each type.

1. Gallium nitride light-emitting diodes (LEDs)
   a. These systems are semiconductor phototherapy devices capable of delivering high spectral irradiance levels of >200 $\mu W/cm^2/nm$ with very little generation of heat within a very narrow emission spectrum in the blue range (460 to 485 nm), with low infrared emission and no UV emission (2,12,13).
   b. LEDs have a longer lifetime (>20,000 hours) and have become cost effective for use in phototherapy devices.
2. Fluorescent tubes
   a. "Special blue" tubes, such as F20T12/BB, provide more irradiance in the blue spectrum than other tubes and are the most effective fluorescent light source (2). "Special blue F20T12/BB" tubes provide much greater irradiance than regular blue tubes, labeled F20T12/B. The flickering glare of the blue light has been reported to cause giddiness, nausea, and temporary blurring of vision in nursing personnel (12). One way to overcome this has been to use cool white light in conjunction with the special blue, but this combination can decrease efficacy by as much as 50%, depending on the proportion of cool white light used (14).
   b. Daylight lamps, like cool white lamps, have a wider wavelength spectrum and are less effective than blue light (15).
   c. Turquoise (peak irradiance 490 nm) and blue-green lights have also been used for phototherapy (16,17).
3. Fiberoptic systems
   a. UV-filtered light from a tungsten–halogen bulb enters a fiberoptic cable and is emitted from the sides and end of fiberoptic fibers inside a plastic pad.
   b. The pad emits insignificant levels of heat, so it can be placed in direct contact with the infant to deliver up to 35 $\mu W/cm^2/nm$ of spectral irradiance, mainly in the blue–green range (18).
   c. The orientation of the fiberoptic fibers determines the uniformity of emission and is unique to each of the commercially available devices.
   d. The main advantage of these systems is that, while receiving phototherapy, the infant can be held and/or nursed, thereby minimizing infant–parent separation. In addition, covering the infant's eyes is not necessary, decreasing parental anxiety.

e. The disadvantage of the fiberoptic pads is that they cover a relatively small surface area and, therefore, have less efficacy compared to overhead sources. They should not be used as the sole means of providing phototherapy in an infant with significant hyperbilirubinemia (1,12,14,18).

f. These devices are often used as an adjunct to conventional overhead application of phototherapy to provide "double" phototherapy (circumferential phototherapy), which has greater efficacy because greater body surface area is exposed to the light (12,18).

4. Halogen lamps
   a. Halogen spotlight systems utilize single or multiple metal halide lamps as the light source and can provide high irradiance over a small surface area (>20 μW/cm²/nm).
   b. These units can generate considerable heat, with the potential of causing thermal skin injury; therefore, they must not be in close proximity to the patient.
   c. The variable positioning with respect to the distance from the infant as well as heterogeneity of the irradiance can lead to unreliable dosing and unpredictable clinical responses. In addition, they are more expensive than fluorescent bulbs (2).

5. Filtered sunlight
   a. The largest burden of significant hyperbilirubinemia is in resource-poor countries.
   b. Innovative film canopies to filter sunlight and provide phototherapy have been developed and are being studied (19,20). The film canopies, Air Blue 80 and Gila Titanium filter out UV light while allowing passage of blue therapeutic light in the 400 to 520 range, maintaining an irradiance of 8 to 10 μW/cm²/nm. Further work needs to be done before these are widely adopted.

D. Technique (Conventional Phototherapy)

Conventional Phototherapy

Standard phototherapy is defined as the delivery of spectral irradiance of 10 μW/cm²/nm in the 430- to 490-nm band at the surface of the infant's body.

Intensive phototherapy is defined as the use of blue-green light in the 430- to 490-nm band delivered at 30 μW/cm²/nm or higher to the greatest possible body surface area in the infant (1,3,12,13).

1. Position the phototherapy unit over the infant to obtain desired irradiance (10 to 40 μW/cm²/nm).
2. Check irradiance (21)
   a. Measure irradiance below the center of the lights at the level of the infant's skin, using specific radiometers.
   b. Ideally, irradiance should be measured at several sites under the area illuminated by the phototherapy unit and the measurements averaged.
   c. Keep the photo radiometer calibrated and perform periodic checks of phototherapy units to make sure that adequate irradiance is being delivered.
   d. Using ordinary photometric or colorimetric light meters or relying on visual estimations of brightness is inappropriate.
3. The distance of the light from the infant has a significant effect on the intensity of phototherapy. Lights should be positioned as close to the infant as possible to achieve maximal intensity. Fluorescent tubes may be brought within approximately 10 cm of term infants without causing overheating, but halogen spot phototherapy lamps should not be positioned closer to the infant than recommended by the manufacturer, because of the risk of burns.
4. If increased irradiance is required, add additional units (22) or place a fiberoptic phototherapy pad under the infant (18). Additional surface area may be exposed to phototherapy by lining the sides of the bassinet with aluminum foil or a white cloth.
5. Due to the concerns for increased mortality in the ELBW premature infants, start with lower irradiance in preterm infants, and increase irradiance or surface area exposed based on rate of drop of TSB (23).
6. Maintain an intact acrylic/safety glass shield over phototherapy light bulbs to block UV radiation and to protect the infant from accidental bulb breakage.
7. Provide ventilation to the phototherapy unit to prevent overheating light bulbs.
8. Maintain cleanliness and electrical safety.

Fiberoptic Phototherapy

Fiberoptic phototherapy can be used as the sole source of phototherapy or as an adjunct to conventional treatment (18).

1. Insert the panel into disposable cover so that it is flat and directed toward the infant.
2. Place the covered panel around the infant's back or chest and secure in position. The phototherapy blanket/pad must be positioned directly next to the infant's skin to be effective. Avoid constriction and skin irritation under the infant's arms if the panel is wrapped around the infant.
3. Discard disposable covers after each treatment and when soiled.
4. Use eye patches and smallest fitting diapers if there is any direct exposure to lights in panel or if used with conventional phototherapy for double-sided effect.

5. Ensure stability and adequate ventilation of the illuminator unit by placing it on a secure surface.
6. Connect the fiberoptic panel to illuminator.
7. Keep the fiberoptic panel and illuminator clean and dry.
8. Allow the lamp to cool for 10 to 20 minutes before moving the illuminator. Do not place sharp or heavy objects on the panel or cable.

Care of the Infant Receiving Phototherapy

1. Monitor temperature, particularly of infants in an incubator, who may develop hyperthermia.
2. Monitor intake, output, and weight. Fluid supplementation may be necessary secondary to increased insensible losses and frequent stooling. Encourage breastfeeding. Healthy term breastfed infants may be supplemented with milk-based formula if maternal milk supply is inadequate (1). Milk feeding may inhibit the enterohepatic circulation of bilirubin (1).

   Intravenous (IV) fluids are rarely required. There is no evidence that IV fluid supplementation improves outcomes as compared to oral supplementation (24).
3. Use eye protection in the form of eye patches for infants receiving overhead phototherapy.
4. Maximize skin exposure to phototherapy source by using the smallest possible diapers as well as keeping blanket rolls from blocking light.
5. Avoid fully occlusive dressings, bandages, topical skin ointments, and plastic in direct contact with the infant's skin, to prevent burns.
6. Remove plastic heat shields and wraps that decrease irradiance delivered to the skin (25).
7. If in use, shield the oxygen saturation monitor probe from the phototherapy light.
8. Encourage parents to continue feeding, caring for, and visiting their infant.

E. Home Phototherapy

Home phototherapy decreases costs of hospitalization and eliminates separation of mother and infant. It is safe and effective for selected infants (26). Home phototherapy should be used only in infants whose bilirubin levels are in the "optional phototherapy" range (see **Fig. 55.1**).

1. Make arrangements to measure the infant's serum bilirubin every 12 to 24 hours, depending on the previous concentration and rate of rise. The infant should be examined daily by a visiting nurse or at an office.
2. The supervising physician should be in contact with the family daily during the period of treatment.
3. The infant should be hospitalized if he or she shows signs of illness, if the rate of rise in bilirubin level is rapid, or if TSB concentration exceeds 18 mg/dL.

F. Efficacy of Phototherapy

The conversion of bilirubin to water-soluble photoisomers occurs very quickly, with 20% to 30% of TB being converted to 4Z,15E bilirubin within seconds, but this is a reversible reaction (2). The clinical impact of effective phototherapy should be evident within 4 to 6 hours of initiation, with a decrease of more than 2 mg/dL (34 μmol/L) in TSB concentration (13). The clinical response depends on the rates of bilirubin production, tissue deposition and elimination, and photochemical reactions of bilirubin. The therapeutic efficacy of phototherapy depends on several factors (2,3).

1. Exposed body surface area: The rate of decline in bilirubin levels is directly proportional to the surface area of the skin exposed.
2. Distance of the infant from the light source: Phototherapy is more effective if the light source is placed closer to the infant.
3. Skin thickness and pigmentation as well as hemoglobin levels.
4. TSB at initiation of phototherapy.
5. Duration of exposure to phototherapy.

G. Discontinuation of Phototherapy and Follow-Up

1. There is no single standard bilirubin level for discontinuing phototherapy. The TSB level that determines the discontinuation of phototherapy depends on the gestational age of the infant, the postnatal age and total bilirubin level at which phototherapy was initiated, rate of fall of bilirubin level, and the etiology of the unconjugated hyperbilirubinemia (1,27).
2. If TSB does not fall steadily following intensive phototherapy, or is moving closer to level for exchange transfusion or the TSB/albumin ratio exceeds levels recommended, consider exchange transfusion (1).
3. In infants ≥35 weeks GA, when TSB level is <13 to 14 mg/dL (239 μmol/L), phototherapy can be discontinued (1).
4. Based on the etiology of the unconjugated hyperbilirubinemia, rebound TSB may be measured 12 to 24 hours later.
5. For infants who are readmitted to the hospital (usually for TSB levels of 18 mg/dL or higher), phototherapy may be discontinued when the serum bilirubin level falls below 13 to 14 mg/dL.
6. For infants who are readmitted with hyperbilirubinemia and then discharged, significant rebound is uncommon, but may still occur. The likelihood of rebound is much higher in premature infants, neonates with positive direct antiglobulin (Coombs) test, and in infants requiring phototherapy in <72 hours after birth,

and these risk factors should be taken into account when planning follow-up after phototherapy (27). Generally, a follow-up bilirubin measurement within 24 hours after discharge is recommended (1).

H. Complications of Phototherapy

Although phototherapy has been "used in millions of infants for more than 30 years, and reports of significant toxicity are exceptionally rare" (1), there are rare severe complications and increasing data that phototherapy is not always benign.

1. Separation of mother and infant and interference with bonding. This may be ameliorated by allowing infants to come out of the lights very few hours to bond with parents and breastfeed once bilirubin levels begin to fall on phototherapy (1).
2. Diarrhea or loose stools.
3. Dehydration secondary to insensible water loss, specifically with exclusively breastfed infants. Halogen and tungsten lamps contribute; insensible water loss is minimized with use of LED lights.
4. Although there is a risk of potential retinal damage from light exposure, adverse effects have not been reported in neonates because eye patches are used routinely (28).
5. "Bronze baby syndrome" occurs in some infants with cholestatic jaundice who are exposed to phototherapy due to accumulation in the skin and serum of porphyrins. The bronzing disappears in most infants within 2 months (29).
6. Rare complications of purpuric eruptions due to transient porphyrinemia have been described in infants with severe cholestasis who receive phototherapy (30).
7. Skin changes ranging from minor erythema, increased pigmentation, and skin burns (halogen/tungsten lamps), to rare and more severe blistering and photosensitivity in infants with porphyria and hemolytic disease. Concerns about an increase in the number of melanocytic nevi have not been substantiated (31).
8. Concerns for increased incidence of patent ductus arteriosus (PDA) and reopening of PDA in infants treated with phototherapy continue. There are ongoing trials of the role of chest shielding during phototherapy to prevent PDA (32).
9. Increased mortality has been noted in ELBW infants following intensive phototherapy. Cycled and intermittent phototherapy as opposed to continuous phototherapy is now being investigated as an alternative safer method (23).
10. Association with childhood cancer and phototherapy: An association was noted between receipt of phototherapy and an increased risk of myeloid leukemia, kidney cancer, and "other cancers" in the California Late Impact of Phototherapy Study (CLIPS) (33). The Late Impact of Getting Hyperbilirubinemia or Phototherapy (LIGHT) study (34) showed that although crude incidence ratios were elevated for myeloid leukemia, liver, and kidney cancers, the associations were no longer significant when adjusted with the propensity score. The actual number of cases were small and it is unclear if the associations discovered by analysis of big data sets denote causality (35). Nevertheless, since blue light has been associated with DNA damage, it would be prudent to weigh the risks versus the benefits in every case, and to use phototherapy only for appropriate indications.

References

1. American Academy of Pediatrics Subcommittee on Hyperbilirubinemia. Management of hyperbilirubinemia in the newborn infant 35 or more weeks of gestation. *Pediatrics.* 2004;114:297.
2. Lamola AA. A pharmacologic view of phototherapy. *Clin Perinatol.* 2016;43:259–276.
3. Ebbessen F, Hansen TWR, Maisels MJ. Update on phototherapy in jaundiced neonates. *Curr Pediatr Review.* 2017;13:176–180.
4. Watchko JF, Jeffrey Maisels M. Enduring controversies in the management of hyperbilirubinemia in preterm neonates. *Semin Fetal Neonatal Med.* 2010;15:136–140.
5. van Imhoff DE, Dijk PH, Hulzebos CV, et al. Uniform treatment thresholds for hyperbilirubinemia in preterm infants: background and synopsis of a national guideline. *Early Hum Dev.* 2011;87:521–525.
6. Maisels MJ, Watchko JF, Bhutani VK, et al. An approach to the management of hyperbilirubinemia in the preterm infant less than 35 weeks of gestation. *J Perinatol.* 2012;32: 660–664.
7. Morioka I. Hyperbilirubinemia in preterm infants in Japan: new treatment criteria. *Pediatr Int.* 2018;60:684–690.
8. Tyson JE, Pedroza C, Langer J, et al. Does aggressive phototherapy increase mortality while decreasing profound impairment among the smallest and sickest newborns? *J Perinatol.* 2012;32:677–684.
9. Baran M, Eliaçık K, Kurt I, et al. Bullous skin lesions in a jaundiced infant after phototherapy: a case of congenital erythropoietic porphyria. *Turk J Pediatr.* 2013;55:218–221.
10. Kearns GL, Williams BJ, Timmons OD. Fluorescein phototoxicity in a premature infant. *J Pediatr.* 1985;107:796–798.
11. Bhutani VK, Poland R, Meloy LD, et al. Clinical trial of tin mesoporphyrin to prevent neonatal hyperbilirubinemia. *J Perinatol.* 2016;36:533–539.
12. Bhutani VK; The Committee on Fetus and Newborn. Phototherapy to prevent severe neonatal hyperbilirubinemia in the newborn infant 35 or more weeks of gestation. *Pediatrics.* 2011;128:e1046–e1052.
13. Hansen TW. Biology of bilirubin photoisomers. *Clin Perinatol.* 2016;43(2):277–290.
14. Sarici SU, Alpay F, Unay B, et al. Comparison of the efficacy of conventional special blue light phototherapy and fiberoptic phototherapy in the management of neonatal hyperbilirubinemia. *Acta Paediatr.* 1999;88:1249–1253.
15. De Carvalho M, De Carvalho D, Trzmielina S, et al. Intensified phototherapy using daylight fluorescent lamps. *Acta Pediatr.* 1999;88:768–771.

16. Ebbesen F, Madsen P, Støvring S, et al. Therapeutic effect of turquoise versus blue light with equal irradiance in preterm infants with jaundice. *Acta Paediatr.* 2007;96:837–841.

17. Seidman DS, Moise J, Ergaz Z. A prospective randomised controlled study of phototherapy using blue and blue-green light emitting devices and conventional halogen quartz phototherapy. *J Perinatol.* 2003;23:123.

18. Tan KL. Comparison of the efficacy of fiberoptic and conventional phototherapy for neonatal hyperbilirubinemia. *J Pediatr.* 1994;125:607–612.

19. Slusher TM, Olusanya BO, Vreman HJ, et al. A randomized trial of phototherapy with filtered sunlight in African neonates. *N Engl J Med.* 2015;373:1115–1124.

20. Slusher TM, Vreman HJ, Brearley AM, et al. Filtered sunlight versus intensive electric powered phototherapy in moderate-to-severe neonatal hyperbilirubinaemia: a randomized controlled non-inferiority trial. *Lancet Glob Health.* 2018;6:e1122–e1131.

21. Borden AR, Satrom KM, Wratkowski P, et al. Variation in the phototherapy practices and irradiance of devices in a major metropolitan area. *Neonatology.* 2018;113:269–274.

22. Donneborg ML, Vandborg PK, Hansen BM, et al. Double versus single intensive phototherapy with LEDs in treatment of neonatal hyperbilirubinemia. *J Perinatol.* 2018;38:154–158.

23. Stevenson DK, Wong RJ, Arnold CC, et al. Phototherapy and the risk of photo-oxidative injury in extremely low birth weight infants. *Clin Perinatol.* 2016;43:291–295.

24. Lai NM, Ahmad Kamar A, Choo YM, et al. Fluid supplementation for neonatal unconjugated hyperbilirubinaemia. *Cochrane Database Syst Rev.* 2017;8:CD011891.

25. Karsdon J, Schothorst AA, Ruys JH, et al. Plastic blankets and heat shields decrease transmission of phototherapy light. *Acta Paediatr Scand.* 1986;75:555–557.

26. Walls M, Wright A, Fowlie P, et al. Home phototherapy in the United Kingdom. *Arch Dis Child Fetal Neonatal Ed.* 2004;89:F282.

27. Chang PW, Kuzniewicz MW, McCulloch CE, et al. A clinical prediction rule for rebound hyperbilirubinemia following inpatient phototherapy. *Pediatrics.* 2017;139:e20162896.

28. Hunter JJ, Morgan JL, Merigan WH, et al. The susceptibility of the retina to photochemical damage from visible light. *Prog Retin Eye Res.* 2012;31:28–42.

29. Rubaltelli FF, Da Riol R, D'Amore ESG, et al. The bronze baby syndrome: evidence of increased tissue concentration of copper porphyrins. *Acta Pediatr.* 1996;85:381–384.

30. Karg E, Kovács L, Ignácz F, et al. Phototherapy-induced blistering reaction and eruptive melanocytic nevi in a child with transient neonatal porphyrinemia. *Pediatr Dermatol.* 2018;35:e272–e275.

31. Lai YC, Yew YW. Neonatal blue light phototherapy and melanocytic nevus count in children: a systematic review and meta-analysis of observational studies. *Pediatr Dermatol.* 2016;33(1):62–68.

32. Bhola K, Foster JP, Osborn DA. Chest shielding for prevention of a haemodynamically significant patent ductus arteriosus in preterm infants receiving phototherapy. *Cochrane Database Syst Rev.* 2015;(11):CD009816.

33. Wickremasinghe AC, Kuzniewicz MW, Grimes BA, et al. Neonatal phototherapy and infantile cancer. *Pediatrics.* 2016;137:e20151353.

34. Newman TB, Wickremasinghe AC, Walsh EM, et al. Retrospective cohort study of phototherapy and childhood cancer in northern California. *Pediatrics.* 2016;137: e20151354.

35. Frazier AL, Krailo M, Poynter J. Can big data shed light on the origins of pediatric cancer? *Pediatrics.* 2016;137: e20160983.

56

Intraosseous Infusions

Mary E. Revenis and Lamia Soghier

A. Indications

1. Emergency intravenous access in hospital or during prehospital transport (1) when other venous access is not readily available; to restore intravascular volume so that peripheral venous access becomes possible. In delivery room resuscitation simulation settings, intraosseous access can be established more quickly than umbilical venous catheterization (2,3). See **Table 56.1**

TABLE 56.1 Types of Intraosseous Infusates

1. Fluids
    a. Normal saline
    b. Crystalloids
    c. Glucose (12)
    d. Ringer's lactate (10)

2. Blood and blood products

3. Medications
    a. Anesthetic agents (13,14)
    b. Antibiotics
    c. Atropine (10)
    d. Calcium gluconate
    e. Dexamethasone (10)
    f. Diazepam (10)
    g. Diazoxide (10); phenytoin (15)
    h. Dobutamine (11)
    i. Dopamine (11,12,16)
    j. Ephedrine (17)
    k. Epinephrine (17)
    l. Heparin (10)
    m. Insulin
    n. Isoproterenol (16)
    o. Lidocaine
    p. Morphine
    q. Sodium bicarbonate (dilute if possible)
    r. Adenosine (18)

4. Contrast material (19)

for categories of fluid and medications that have been infused (4–9).

B. Contraindications (6,8,9)

1. Bone without cortical integrity (fracture, previous penetration): Extravasation of infusate
2. Sternal site: Potential damage to heart and lungs (20)
3. Overlying soft tissue infection or burn
4. Osteogenesis imperfecta
5. Obliterative diseases of marrow such as osteopetrosis

C. Equipment (Fig. 56.1)

Sterile

1. Surgical gloves
2. Antiseptic swabs
3. Gauze squares
4. Aperture drape
5. 1% lidocaine in 1-mL syringe with 25-gauge needle
6. Needle, in order of preference (4–6,21)
    a. Bone marrow or intraosseous needle (18-gauge) (stylet and adjustable depth indicator preferred)
    b. Short spinal needle with stylet (18- or 20-gauge)
    c. Short hypodermic needle (18- or 20-gauge) (13)
    d. Butterfly needle (16- to 19-gauge) (22)
7. 5-mL syringe on a three-way stopcock and IV extension set with clamp
8. Intravenous infusion set and intravenous fluid
9. 5-mL syringes with saline flush solution

Optional

Intraosseous needle placement device (intended for use at the proximal tibial location). Devices approved for newborns are the battery-operated driver EZ-IO PD (Pediatric) (Vidacare,

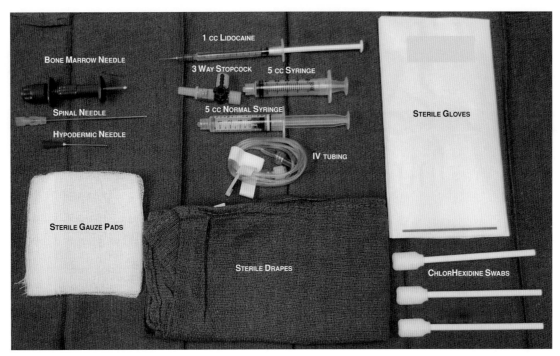

FIGURE 56.1 Sterile equipment necessary for intraosseous line placement.

San Antonio, TX, USA) (approved for 3 kg or larger), and the spring-activated (pediatric) B.I.G. Bone Injection Gun (WaisMed, Houston, TX, USA). There are company-provided reports of use in delivery rooms and intensive care nurseries. Published information on use of these devices in small premature infants is scarce. There is limited information on the incidence of success or complications when using these devices, as compared with manual insertion of the intraosseous needle (23).

Nonsterile

1. Small sand bag or rolled towel to aid in stabilizing limb
2. Tape
3. Armboard
4. Disposable plastic cup

D. Precautions

1. Limit use to emergency vascular access, when peripheral or central venous access is not feasible.
2. Avoid inserting needle through infected skin or subcutaneous tissue.
3. Stabilize limb with counterpressure, with sand bag or towel roll directly opposite proposed site of penetration, to avoid bone fracture.
4. If hand is also used to stabilize limb, do not position hand directly opposite puncture site, to avoid inadvertent puncture of hand by the intraosseous needle

if it goes through the limb. This is true regardless of whether a sand bag or towel is used. Limit needle size to decrease risk of bone fracture.
5. Administer drugs in the usual doses for intravenous administration; however, when possible, dilute hypertonic or strongly alkaline solutions prior to infusion, to reduce risk of bone marrow damage (5).
6. Discontinue intraosseous infusion as soon as alternative venous access is established, ideally within hours, to reduce risk of osteomyelitis or needle displacement. Complication rates may increase beyond 24 hours.

E. Technique (▶ Video 56.1: Intraosseous Infusion)

The proximal tibia is the site most commonly used in neonates due to ease of access, positioning for insertion, rapid determination of landmarks, and needle immobilization. Alternate sites can be used if the proximal tibia site is contraindicated.

Proximal Tibia (Fig. 56.2) (4–6,24)

1. Position patient supine.
2. Place sand bag or towel roll behind knee to provide countersupport behind puncture site.
3. Clean proximal tibia with antiseptic solution.
4. Put on sterile gloves.
5. Apply aperture drape.
6. If appropriate, inject lidocaine into skin, soft tissue, and periosteum (25,26).

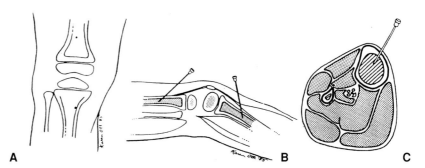

FIGURE 56.2 A: Anterior view. **B:** Sagittal section. **C:** Cross-section through tibia. (Reprinted with permission from Hodge D. Intraosseous infusions: A review. *Pediatr Emerg Care.* 1985;1(4):215.)

7. Determine penetration depth of needle: Rarely more than 1 cm in infants or 0.5 cm in small premature infants.
   a. For needle or bone needle injection device with adjustable depth indicator, adjust sheath to allow desired penetration.
   b. For needle without an adjustable depth indicator, hold the needle in the dominant hand with blunt end supported by the palm and the index finger approximately 1 cm from the bevel of the needle, to avoid pushing it past this mark.
8. Palpate tibial tuberosity with index finger **(Fig. 56.3)**.

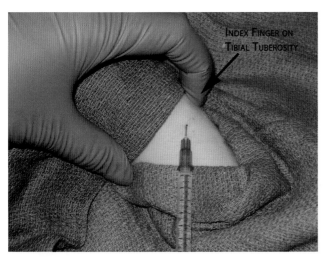

FIGURE 56.3 Palpation of tibial tuberosity with index finger.

9. Hold the thigh and knee above and lateral to the insertion site with the palm of the nondominant hand. Wrap fingers and thumb around, but not behind, the knee to stabilize the proximal tibia.
10. Insert needle on the flat, anteromedial surface of the tibia, 1 to 2 cm below and 1 cm medial to the tibial tuberosity. If the tibial tuberosity is not palpable, estimate penetration site 15 to 20 mm distal to the patella and medial along the flat aspect of the tibia.
11. Direct needle at a 90-degree angle (24).
12. Advance needle.
    a. For manual insertion, advance needle using firm pressure with a twisting motion until there is a

sudden, slight decrease in resistance, indicating puncture of the cortex. Avoid a rocking motion to minimize the risk of bone splintering or creating too large an opening.
    b. If an automatic spring-activated intraosseous needle injection device is used, turn the device to the "0" line to insert 0.5 cm. Hold the cylinder against the puncture site at a 90-degree angle with one hand. Release the safety latch on the cylinder with the other hand. Depress the cylinder, as with a syringe, without the use of force.
    c. If a battery-operated driver with attached needle is utilized, hold the driver in the dominant hand. Position the needle against the puncture site at a 90-degree angle. Depress the trigger to activate the driver. Do not force the driver, but apply gentle, steady pressure, allowing the driver to insert the needle. Stop when there is a sudden decrease in resistance.
13. Do not advance the needle beyond cortical puncture.
14. Remove the stylet.
15. Confirm the position of the needle in the marrow cavity.
    a. Needle should stand without support in larger patients, but should never be left unsupported **(Fig. 56.4)**.

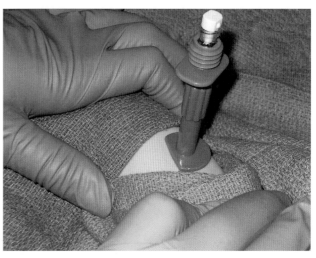

FIGURE 56.4 Intraosseous needle in place should stand without support.

b. Securely attach a 5-mL syringe and attempt to aspirate blood or marrow. Aspiration is not always successful when using an 18- or 20-gauge needle.

   If bone marrow is aspirated, it can be analyzed for blood chemistry values, partial pressure of arterial carbon dioxide, pH, hemoglobin level (27–29), type and cross-match, or cultured (28).

c. Attach syringe of saline flush solution and infuse 2 to 3 mL slowly, while palpating the tissue adjacent to the insertion site and beneath the extremity to detect extravasation. There should be only mild resistance to fluid infusion.

16. If marrow cannot be aspirated and significant resistance to fluid infusion is met:

a. The hollow bore needle may be obstructed by small bone plugs.

   (1) Reintroduce the stylet, or

   (2) Introduce a smaller-gauge needle through the original needle.

   (3) Attach syringe of saline flush and flush 2 to 3 mL of fluid.

b. The bevel of the needle may not have penetrated the cortex.

   (1) Redetermine estimated depth needed.

   (2) Advance.

   (3) Flush with saline.

c. The bevel of the needle may be lodged against the opposite cortex.

   (1) Withdraw needle slightly.

   (2) Flush with saline.

17. Observe the site for extravasation of fluid, indicating that:

a. The placement is too superficial, or

b. The bone has been penetrated completely.

c. If extravasation occurs, withdraw needle and select a different bone.

18. When needle position is confirmed:

a. Attach syringe and infuse medications or fluid directly into the needle or via an IV extension set with clamp. Clear medications with saline flush.

b. For continuous infusion, attach a standard intravenous infusion set with an infusion pump to the intraosseous needle and administer at the same rate as for IV infusion (5).

19. Secure intraosseous needle and maintain a clean infusion site while the needle is in place.

a. Tape the flanges of the needle to the skin to prevent dislodgement. If a needle safety latch is provided, attach the latch and then apply tape.

b. If desired, cover the exposed end of the needle with a disposable cup, taping the cover down. Cutting off the bottom of the cup will aid in visualization of the site for monitoring.

20. Secure intravenous tubing with tape to the leg.

21. Secure the leg to the armboard.

22. Obtain radiograph to confirm position of needle and to rule out fracture.

23. Monitor frequently for fluid extravasation.

24. Discontinue intraosseous infusion as soon as alternative intravenous access is achieved.

   In an infant with hypotension/hypovolemia, infusion via the interosseous route can restore peripheral perfusion to a point at which venous access is possible in well under 30 minutes.

a. Remove needle gently, with slight rotation motion if needed.

b. Apply a sterile dressing over the puncture site.

c. Apply pressure to the dressing for 5 minutes.

d. Monitor the puncture site for 48 hours for cellulitis or drainage.

Distal Tibia (Fig. 56.5) (5,21,24)

1. Position patient supine.

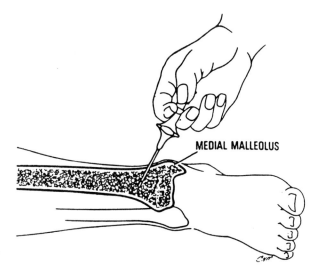

FIGURE 56.5 Intraosseous infusion into the distal tibia. (From Spivey WH. Intraosseous infusions. *J Pediatr*. 1987;111(5):639–643. Copyright © 1987 Elsevier. With permission.)

2. Prepare site and needle as for proximal tibia.

3. Insert needle in the medial surface of the distal tibia just proximal to the medial malleolus.

4. Direct needle cephalad away from the joint space.

5. Proceed as for proximal tibia.

Distal Femur (Fig. 56.2) (4)

1. Position patient supine.

2. Place sand bag or towel roll behind knee.

3. Prepare site and needle as for proximal tibia.

4. Insert needle 1 to 3 cm above the external condyles in the anterior midline.

5. Direct needle cephalad at an angle of 10 to 15 degrees.
6. Proceed as for proximal tibia.

F. Complications (4,7,30,31)

1. Fracture of bone (32)
2. Complete penetration of bone (10)
3. Osteomyelitis (30,31)
4. Periostitis
5. Subcutaneous abscess
6. Cellulitis
7. Sepsis
8. Extravasation of fluid from the puncture site
9. Subperiosteal or subcutaneous infiltration or hematoma
10. Compartment syndrome (33)
11. Subcutaneous sloughing
12. Death (reported only with sternal bone site) (20)
13. Amputation of limb (34)
14. Theoretical (as yet unreported) (35,36)
    a. Embolization of bone fragments or fat
    b. Damage to bone marrow
    c. Damage to growth plate

References

1. Sommer A, Weis M, Deanovic D, et al. Intraosseous infusion in the pediatric emergency medical service. Analysis of emergency medical missions 1990–2009. *Der Anaesthesia.* 2011;60:125–131.
2. Rajani AK, Chitkara R, Oehlert J, et al. Comparison of umbilical venous and intraosseous access during simulated neonatal resuscitation. *Pediatrics.* 2011;128:e954–e958.
3. Schwindt EM, Hoffmann F, Deindl P, et al. Duration to establish an emergency vascular access and how to accelerate it: a simulation based study performed in real-life neonatal resuscitation rooms. *Pediatr Crit Care Med.* 2018;19(5):468–476.
4. Fiser DH. Intraosseous infusion. *N Engl J Med.* 1990;322:1579–1581.
5. Spivey WH. Intraosseous infusions. *J Pediatr.* 1987;111:639–643.
6. De Boers S, Russell T, Seaver M, et al. Infant intraosseous infusion. *Neonatal Netw.* 2008;27:25–32
7. Ellemunter H, Simma B, Trawoger R, et al. Intraosseous lines in preterm and full term neonates. *Arch Dis Child Fetal Neonatal Ed.* 1999;80:F74–F75.
8. Engle WA. Intraosseous access for administration of medications in neonates. *Clin Perinatol.* 2006;33:161–168
9. deCaen A. Venous access in the critically ill child; When the peripheral intravenous fails! *Pediatr Emerg Care.* 2007;23:422–424.
10. Valdes MM. Intraosseous administration in emergencies. *Lancet.* 1977;1:1235–1236.
11. Berg RA. Emergency infusion of catecholamines into bone marrow. *Am J Dis Child.* 1984;138:810–811.
12. Neish SR, Macon MG, Moore JW, et al. Intraosseous infusion of hypertonic glucose and dopamine. *Am J Dis Child.* 1988;142:878–880.
13. Hamed RK, Hartmans S, Gausche-Hill M. Anesthesia through an intraosseous line using an 18-gauge intravenous needle for emergency pediatric surgery. *J Clin Anesth.* 2013;25:447–451.
14. Neuhaus D, Weiss M, Engelhardt T, et al. Semi-elective intraosseous infusion after failed intravenous access in pediatric anesthesia. *Paediatr Anaesth.* 2010;20:168–171.
15. Walsh-Kelly CM, Berens RJ, Glaeser PW, et al. Intraosseous infusion of phenytoin. *Am J Emerg Med.* 1986;4:523–524.
16. Bilello JF, O'Hair KC, Kirby WC, et al. Intraosseous infusion of dobutamine and isoproterenol. *Am J Dis Child.* 1991;145:165–167.
17. Shoor PM, Berrynill RE, Benumof JL. Intraosseous infusion: pressure-flow relationship and pharmacokinetics. *J Trauma.* 1979;19:772–774.
18. Helleman K, Kirpalani A, Lim R. A novel method of intraosseous infusion of adenosine for the treatment of supraventricular tachycardia in an infant. *Pediatr Emer Care.* 2017;33:47–48.
19. Cambray EJ, Donaldson JS, Shore RM. Intraosseous contrast infusion: efficacy and associated findings. *Pediatr Radiol.* 1997;27:892–893.
20. Turkel H. Deaths following sternal puncture. *JAMA.* 1954;156:992.
21. Iserson K, Criss E. Intraosseous infusions: a usable technique. *Am J Emerg Med.* 1986;4:540–542.
22. Lake W, Emmerson AJ. Use of a butterfly as an intraosseous needle in an oedematous preterm infant. *Arch Dis Child Fetal, Neonata Ed.* 2003;88:F409.
23. Geritse BM, Scheffer GJ, Draaisma JM. Prehospital intraosseous access with the bone injection gun by a helicopter transported emergency medical team. *J Trauma.* 2009;66:1739–1741.
24. Boon JM, Gorry DL, Meiring JH. Finding an ideal site for intraosseous infusion of the tibia: an anatomical study. *Clin Anat.* 2003;16:15–18.
25. Mofenson HC, Tascone A, Caraccio TR. Guidelines for intraosseous infusions. *J Emerg Med.* 1988;6:143–146.
26. Neuhaus D. Intraosseous infusion in elective and emergency pediatric anesthesia: when should we use it? *Curr Opin Anaesthesiol.* 2014;27:282–287.
27. Johnson L, Kissoon N, Fiallos M, et al. Use of intraosseous blood to assess blood chemistries and hemoglobin during cardiopulmonary resuscitation with drug infusions. *Crit Care Med.* 1999;27:1147–1152.
28. Orlowski JP, Porembka DT, Gallagher JM, et al. The bone marrow as a source of laboratory studies. *Ann Emerg Med.* 1989;18:1348–1351.
29. Miller LJ, Philbeck TE, Montez D, et al. A new study of intraosseous blood for laboratory analysis. *Arch Pathol Lab Med.* 2010;134:1253–1260.
30. Rosetti V, Thompson B, Miller J, et al. Intraosseous infusion: an alternative route of pediatric intravascular access. *Ann Emerg Med.* 1985;14:885–888.

31. Hallas P, Brabrand M, Folkestad L. Complication with intraosseous access: Scandinavian users' experience. *West J Emerg Med*. 2013;14:440–443.

32. La Fleche FR, Slepin MJ, Vargas J, et al. Iatrogenic bilateral tibial fractures after intraosseous infusion attempts in a 3-month-old infant. *Ann Emerg Med*. 1989;18:1099–1101.

33. Vidal R, Kissoon N, Gayle M. Compartment syndrome following intraosseous infusion. *Pediatrics*. 1993;91:1201–1202.

34. Suominen PK, Nurmi E, Lauerma K. Intraosseous access in neonates and infants: risk of severe complications—a case report. *Acta Anaesthesiol Scand*. 2015;59:1389–1393.

35. Pediatric Forum. Emergency bone marrow infusions. *Am J Dis Child*. 1985;139:438–439.

36. Fiser RT, Walker WM, Seibert JJ, et al. Tibial length following intraosseous infusion: a prospective, radiographic analysis. *Pediatr Emerg Care*. 1997;13:186–188.

CHAPTER

57

Tapping a Ventricular Reservoir

Lara M. Leijser and Linda S. de Vries

A. Introduction

The subcutaneous ventricular access device or ventricular reservoir **(Fig. 57.1)** is used to drain cerebrospinal fluid (CSF) from the ventricular system in preterm infants with posthemorrhagic ventricular dilatation (PHVD) and occasionally in term infants with obstructive hydrocephalus following intracranial hemorrhage or aqueduct stenosis (1–7). The ventricular reservoir is inserted in preterm infants who are too small and/or unstable to have a ventriculoperitoneal (VP) shunt inserted and it may abrogate or delay the need for a VP shunt in some infants. It also allows drainage and clearing of CSF which may be bloody and have a high protein content, particularly in the early posthemorrhagic phase, thereby decreasing the risk of blockage when a VP shunt is inserted (2,3,6–8). A ventricular reservoir is preferably not placed within the first postnatal week because of the risk of rebleeding.

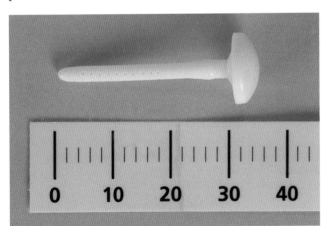

FIGURE 57.1 Ventricular reservoir: lateral view.

Insertion of a ventricular reservoir under ultrasound guidance is recommended. The reservoir is usually tapped immediately following insertion, by the neurosurgeon, to ensure proper placement. Subsequently, initially daily taps are performed in the neonatal intensive care unit (NICU),

aiming to remove enough CSF to prevent further ventriculomegaly and preferably reduce ventricular size, maintain normal head growth, and reduce pressure on the surrounding periventricular white matter (2,6,7,9).

B. Indications for Tapping the Reservoir

Based on Ultrasound Measurements

Ultrasound (or radiologic) evidence of progressive ventriculomegaly, based on progressive ventricular measurements from serial cranial ultrasonography, such as the ventricular index and anterior horn width (10–12).

Based on Clinical Symptoms

1. Rapidly increasing head circumference, more than 1.5 to 2 cm/wk (9).
2. Clinical signs of raised intracranial pressure (ICP), such as a full or tense anterior fontanelle, separation of the sutures, apnea and bradycardia, poor feeding, or vomiting.

C. Contraindications

1. Low circulating blood volume
2. Cellulitis or abrasion over the reservoir site
3. Sunken fontanelle or overlapping sutures
4. Severe coagulopathy or low platelet count
5. Active sepsis or meningitis

D. Equipment

Other than the cap and mask, all equipment is sterile.
1. Sterile gloves and gown, mask
2. Sterile dressing tray table

459

3. Sterile drape with hole; in case the hole is too large to maintain sterility or not present, a small hole can be cut in the drape using sterile scissors

4. Gauze swabs with chlorhexidine in 70% alcohol solution (in the United States chlorhexidine is not recommended in infants <2 months of age, but is still used in selected cases; 10% povidone-iodine is an alternative)

5. Port-a-cath or butterfly needle 24 gauge × 25 mm

6. Connector flexible tube of 10 cm with luer lock at both ends

7. Syringe of 10 or 20 mL

8. Three tubes with caps for CSF collection and sampling

9. Adhesive bandage

E. Precautions

1. Use strict aseptic technique

2. Maintain continuous cardiorespiratory monitoring during the procedure

3. Connect port-a-cath or butterfly needle to a 10-cm connector and syringe

4. Do not use local anesthetic

5. Do not place intravenous lines on the same side of the scalp

6. Always try to use a fresh site for insertion of the needle for each puncture to avoid leakage from one central puncture site

7. Insert needle just far enough into the reservoir to obtain CSF; inserting the needle too deep may damage the reservoir base

F. Technique

1. Infant should preferably be asleep and otherwise gently restrained and comfortable, preferably with the head turned to the side without the reservoir.

2. Palpate reservoir and locate puncture site. Clean skin over the reservoir with a radius of at least 5 cm of the surrounding skin using chlorhexidine in 70% alcohol or povidone-iodine solution for 30 to 60 seconds. Use light but firm contact.

3. Let dry in air for 1 to 2 minutes.

4. Prepare as for major procedure. Put on mask. Wash hands thoroughly. Put on gown and sterile gloves.

5. Clean reservoir area two times with antiseptic. Allow antiseptic to dry.

6. Position sterile drape to maintain a sterile field while maintaining patient visibility.

7. Insert needle at an angle of 30 to 45 degrees through the skin and at 90 degrees into the reservoir bladder as in Figure 57.2

8. Slowly aspirate the appropriate amount of CSF, at a maximum rate of 1 mL/min or a maximum procedure time of 15 to 20 minutes (**Fig. 57.2**). Remove no more

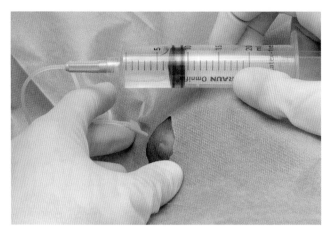

FIGURE 57.2 Tapping a ventricular reservoir.

than 10 to 15 mL/kg per tap. Some authors advocate letting the CSF drain spontaneously, rather than aspirating, in order to reduce fresh bleeding into the ventricles (13). This may however increase the risk of infection.

9. Remove needle and hold firm pressure for 2 minutes, until CSF leakage stops. Place adhesive bandage over puncture site.

10. Remove the restraints if used.

11. Collect CSF sample for bacterial culture, cell count, glucose, and protein at least twice per week (the frequency of testing CSF varies among institutions from daily to weekly).

12. Check urine sodium and potassium levels twice per week. Supplement sodium if required to maintain urine sodium >20 mmol/L.

13. Supplement collected CSF (initially 10 to 20 mL/kg per day) by increasing the intake of total fluid per kg per day.

G. Successful Tap

1. In case the indication for ventricular tapping is based on ultrasound measures of ventricular size, the ventricular measurements should have reduced at the end of the procedure. In this case, none of the findings below apply as the fontanel is hardly ever full and the sutures never widened.

2. In case the indication for reservoir tapping is based on the onset of clinical symptoms, the following points apply:

   a. At the end of the procedure, the anterior fontanelle should be soft and flat (not sunken), the cranial bones approximated well at the sutures, and the signs of raised ICP alleviated.

   b. If sufficient volume is removed, the fontanelle may be full 24 hours later.

3. If the fontanelle remains flat and signs of raised ICP do not reappear, or ventricular measurements from ultrasound decrease, the interval for tapping may

TABLE 57.1 Complications of Ventricular Reservoir Drainage

PROBLEM (INCIDENCE)	WHAT TO DO
Hyponatremia (20–60%)	Monitor serum electrolytes every other day and supplement sodium intake
Hypoproteinemia (15%)	Ensure adequate protein intake. Monitor serum albumin weekly
Infection (0–8%)	A combination of intravenous and intrareservoir antibiotics may rarely be successful. Removal of the reservoir is usually necessary and recommended
Subgaleal CSF collection (0–9%)	Percutaneous aspiration of fluid using a different needle at the same time as the reservoir is tapped. Tap larger volume of CSF from the reservoir or increase frequency of taps to reduce pressure
CSF leaks through incision (0–3%)	Increase frequency of reservoir taps
Ventricular access device occlusion (0–10%)	Replace reservoir
Trapped contralateral ventricle (6%)	Consider placing second reservoir if no stabilization or decrease in PHVD
Fresh bleeding into the ventricle or subarachnoid space (0–40%)	Prevent by using 24-gauge needle, aspirate slowly or let CSF drain spontaneously rather than aspirating. Do not remove more than 10–15 mL/kg during one procedure
Bradycardia, pallor, hypotension (rare)	Stop or reduce rate of aspiration. Infuse 10–15 mL/kg of normal saline IV bolus. Remove a smaller volume at a slower rate at next tap
Skin breakdown over reservoir (rare)	Avoid abraded skin when tapping the reservoir. Avoid excoriating skin while prepping site

be lengthened to every other day or less and/or the amount of CSF removed at each tap reduced.

H. Follow-Up

1. Assess ventricular measurements with initially daily cranial ultrasonography, clinical response to taps, and daily head circumference.
2. Interval between taps may range from twice a day to once every 2 to 3 days.
3. In case of persistent or progressive PHVD, taps should be continued until the infant weighs 2 to 2.5 kg and is a suitable candidate for VP shunt placement, and protein levels are <1.5 g/L and erythrocyte count is <100/mm^3 in CSF.

I. Complications

See **Table 57.1** (4,9,13,14).

References

1. McComb JG, Ramos AD, Platzker AC, et al. Management of hydrocephalus secondary to intraventricular hemorrhage in the preterm infant with a subcutaneous ventricular catheter reservoir. *Neurosurgery.* 1983;13:295–300.
2. Limbrick DD Jr, Mathur A, Johnston JM. Neurosurgical treatment of progressive posthemorrhagic ventricular dilation in preterm infants: a 10 year single institution study. *J Neurosurg Pediatr.* 2010;6:224–230.
3. Willis B, Javalkar V, Vannemreddy P, et al. Ventricular reservoir and ventriculoperitoneal shunts for premature infants with posthemorrhagic hydrocephalus: an institutional experience. *J Neurosurg Pediatr.* 2009;3:94–100.
4. Peretta P, Ragazzi P, Carlino CF, et al. The role of the Ommaya reservoir and endoscopic third ventriculostomy in the management of post-hemorrhagic hydrocephalus of prematurity. *Childs Nerv Syst.* 2007;23:765–771.
5. Brouwer AJ, Groenendaal F, Koopman C, et al. Intracranial hemorrhage in full term newborns: a hospital based cohort study. *Neuroradiology.* 2010;52:567–576.
6. Leijser LM, Miller SP, van Wezel-Meijler G, et al. Posthemorrhagic ventricular dilatation in preterm infants: When best to intervene? *Neurology.* 2018;90(8):e698–e706.
7. de Vries LS, Groenendaal F, Liem KD, et al. Treatment thresholds for intervention in posthaemorrhagic ventricular dilation: a randomised controlled trial. *Arch Dis Child Fetal Neonatal Ed.* 2019;104(1):F70–F75.
8. Wellons JC, Shannon CN, Kulkarni AV, et al. A multicenter retrospective comparison of conversion from temporary to permanent cerebrospinal fluid diversion in very low birth weight infants with posthemorrhagic hydrocephalus. *J Neurosurg Pediatr.* 2009;4:50–55.

9. Whitelaw A, Evans D, Carter M, et al. Randomized clinical trial of prevention of hydrocephalus after intraventricular hemorrhage in preterm infants: brain-washing versus tapping fluid. *Pediatrics.* 2007;119:e1071–e1078.

10. Levene MI, Starte DR. A longitudinal study of post-haemorrhagic ventricular dilatation in the newborn. *Arch Dis Child.* 1981;56:905–910.

11. Davies MW, Swaminathan M, Chuang SL, et al. Reference ranges for the linear dimensions of the intracranial ventricles in preterm neonates. *Arch Dis Child Fetal Neonatol Ed.* 2001;82:F219–F223.

12. Brouwer MJ, de Vries LS, Groenendaal F, et al. New reference values for the neonatal cerebral ventricles. *Radiology.* 2012;262:224–233.

13. Moghal NE, Quinn MW, Levene MI, et al. Intraventricular hemorrhage after aspiration of ventricular reservoirs. *Arch Dis Child.* 1992;67:448–449.

14. Kormanik K, Praca J, Gorton HJL, et al. Repeated tapping of ventricular reservoir in preterm infants with post-hemorrhagic ventricular dilatation does not increase the risk of reservoir infection. *J Perinatol.* 2010;30: 218–221.

58

Treatment of Retinopathy of Prematurity

William F. Deegan III

A. Introduction

Retinopathy of prematurity (ROP), a disorder of developing retinal blood vessels in the preterm infant, may lead to poor visual acuity or blindness. Screening and timely treatment improve visual outcomes.

B. Screening for ROP

Guidelines for screening preterm infants for ROP are published and updated regularly (1–3). Recommendations for screening in the United States are (1):

WHO:

1. Infants with a birth weight of <1,500 g or a gestational age of 30 weeks or less (as defined by the attending neonatologist).
2. Selected infants with a birth weight between 1,500 and 2,000 g or gestational age of more than 30 weeks with an unstable clinical course, including those requiring cardiopulmonary support and who are believed by their attending pediatrician or neonatologist to be a high risk.

WHEN: The timing of the first examination varies with gestational age.

1. The initial examination for infants born between 22 and 27 weeks' gestational age is at 31 weeks' postconceptional age (gestational age at birth plus chronologic age).
2. Infants born later than 27 weeks should be screened initially 4 weeks after birth.
3. Follow-up examinations depend on the retinal findings as classified by the International Classification of ROP

(4). **Tables 58.1** and **58.2** have been adapted from the joint policy statement of the American Academies of Pediatrics and Ophthalmology, and the American Association for Pediatric Ophthalmology and Strabismus (1).

4. Babies whose clinical condition deteriorates should be followed closely (i.e., weekly), as rapid progression and reactivation are possible.

BY WHOM:

1. It is imperative that babies are screened by ophthalmologists who are facile with binocular indirect ophthalmoscopy with scleral depression; who are comfortable with the examination of premature infants; who have experience with the various presentations and diagnosis of ROP. If residents or fellows are involved in the screenings, attending physicians must always be present and verify the examination findings. The examinations are done at the bedside with the assistance of the baby's nurse.
2. Telemedicine screening with wide-field imaging has been shown to have excellent sensitivity and specificity in some centers (5).

C. Classification of ROP (4)

1. Location: Three zones based on concentric circles, centered on the optic disc **(Fig. 58.1)**
   a. Zone I: Circle whose center is the optic disc and whose radius is twice the distance from the optic disc to the center of the macula (the fovea)
   b. Zone II: Circle whose radius extends from the optic disc to the nasal ora serrata and is peripheral to Zone I
   c. Zone III: Temporal crescent of retina anterior to Zone II

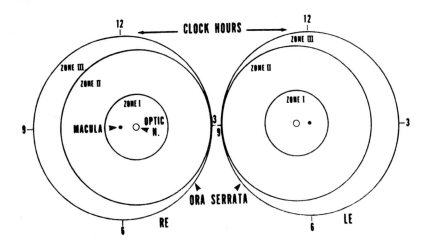

FIGURE 58.1 Scheme of retina of right eye (RE) and left eye (LE), showing zone borders and clock hours employed to describe location and extent of retinopathy of prematurity. (Reprinted with permission from An International classification of retinopathy of prematurity. The Committee for the Classification of Retinopathy of Prematurity. *Arch Ophthalmol.* 1984;102(8):1130–1134. Copyright © 1984 American Medical Association. All rights reserved.)

2. Extent of disease: The retina is divided into 12 equal segments, or clock hours. The extent of retinopathy specifies the number of clock hours involved.
3. Staging the disease (**Table 58.1**, **Figs. 58.2** and **58.3**) (4,10)
4. Additional signs indicating severity of active ROP
   a. "Plus" disease: Dilation and tortuosity of native retinal vessels in at least two quadrants of the eye. This is seen best in the posterior pole. A "+" symbol is added to the ROP stage number to designate the presence.
   b. "Preplus" disease: More arterial tortuosity and more venous dilation than normal, but insufficient for diagnosis of "plus" disease; may progress to frank "plus" disease.

   c. Aggressive posterior ROP: (**Table 58.3**). This is an uncommon, severe form of ROP, characterized by posterior location, prominent plus disease, out of proportion to peripheral findings, and usually in all four quadrants) and rapid progression.
5. Additional features
   a. Iris vascular engorgement (**Fig. 58.3**) and pupillary rigidity (manifested by poor dilation after mydriatic instillation) are harbingers of active, advanced ROP (6).
   b. Corneal and lenticular opacity may be present in the eyes of any premature infant regardless of the presence of ROP (7).

TABLE 58.1 **Stages of Retinopathy of Prematurity**

Stage 1	Demarcation line	A flat white line in the plane of the retina, separating avascular retina anteriorly from vascularized retina posteriorly
Stage 2	Ridge	Elevated primitive fibrovascular tissue extending out of the plane of the retina and separating the vascularized and avascular retina
Stage 3	Extraretinal fibrovascular proliferation	Neovascularization extending from the ridge into the vitreous. This tissue may cause the ridge to appear ragged or "fuzzy" (Fig. 52.2)
Stage 4	Partial retinal detachment	A separation of the retina from the underlying choroid. Traction by the vitreous, through the presence of neovascular tissue, pulls the retina away from its underlying attachments. The intervening (subretinal) space fills with a proteinaceous fluid Stage 4A: Detachment spares the macula Stage 4B: Involves the macula
Stage 5	Total retinal detachment	Retinal tissue becomes inextricably bound to reactive vitreous and is pulled by the vitreous into the retrolental space (hence the older term, retrolental fibroplasia)

From An International Committee for the Classification of Retinopathy of Prematurity. The international classification of retinopathy of prematurity revisited. *Arch Ophthalmol.* 2005;123:991–999.

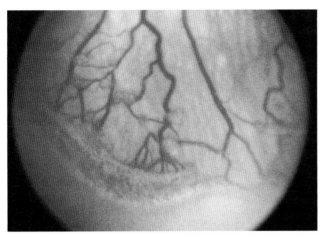

FIGURE 58.2 Dilated, tortuous vessels end in vascular shunts at a thickened ridge of fibrovascular tissue. Avascular retina lies anterior to the ridge.

TABLE 58.2 Follow-Up Examination Schedule

FINDINGS	FOLLOW-UP
Stage 1–2 in Zone I Stage 3 in Zone II	1 wk or less
Immature retina (no ROP) in Zone I Stage 2 in Zone II Regressing ROP in Zone I	1–2 wk
Stage 1 in Zone II Regressing ROP in Zone I	2 wk
Immature retina (no ROP) in Zone II Regressing or Stage 1–2 in Zone III	2–3 wk

Derived from Section on Ophthalmology American Academy of Pediatrics, American Academy of Ophthalmology, American Association for Pediatric Ophthalmology and Strabismus. Screening examination of premature infants for retinopathy of prematurity. *Pediatrics*. 2006;117:572–576. Erratum: *Pediatrics*. 2006;118:1324.

D. Laser Treatment of ROP (8,9)

Currently, most eyes with Zone I ROP (Stage 3, plus disease, or both) are treated with intravitreal anti-vascular endothelial growth factor (anti-VEGF) agents (discussed below). Laser treatment of Zone II and III disease remains the recommended primary modality in eyes with clear media and type 1/threshold ROP disease. Ablation of the avascular portion of the retina decreases the production of angiogenic growth factors and reduces the risk of retinal detachment. Laser photocoagulation, which has replaced cryotherapy, delivered via an indirect ophthalmoscope through a dilated pupil, can precisely ablate the targeted tissue and improve structural and functional outcomes. Laser treatment requires sedation, which can lead to cardiopulmonary complications and the need for emergent or elective intubation.

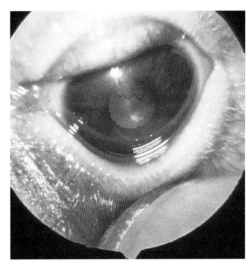

FIGURE 58.3 Dilation and tortuosity of iris vessels may be seen in severe threshold retinopathy of prematurity.

1. **Indications for laser treatment (Table 58.3)**
   Early treatment for ROP study guidelines (10,11):
   a. Peripheral retinal ablation should be considered for any eye with type 1 ROP.
   b. Consider close monitoring (weekly examinations) as opposed to retinal ablation for any eye with type 2 ROP. Regression of ROP can occur in about 50% of these patients without treatment (10); treatment should be considered if progression to type 1 status occurs.
   c. Treatment is recommended within 72 hours of detection of a stage of ROP requiring ablative therapy, when possible, in order to minimize the risk of retinal detachment.

2. **Contraindications**
   a. Stage 4 to 5 ROP, in which case laser may be done (intraoperatively) in conjunction with incisional surgery (vitrectomy) (12)
   b. Vitreous hemorrhage sufficient to obscure a view of the retina; these eyes are typically treated with intravitreal anti-VEGF injection(s)
   c. Instability of medical condition sufficient to make the stress of sedation and laser inadvisable
   d. Lethal medical illness

TABLE 58.3 Indications for the Treatment of ROP

Type 1 ROP	Zone I: Any stage of ROP with plus disease Zone I: Stage 3 ROP with or without plus disease Zone II: Stage 2 or 3 ROP with plus disease
Type 2 ROP	Zone I: Stage 1 or 2 ROP without plus disease Zone II: Stage 3 ROP without plus disease

From Early Treatment for Retinopathy of Prematurity Cooperative Group. Revised indications for the treatment of retinopathy of prematurity: Results of the early treatment for retinopathy of prematurity randomized trial. *Arch Ophthalmol*. 2003;121:1684–1694.

3. **Personnel**
   a. Ophthalmologist
      (1) Determines the need for treatment and discusses the findings and risks of treatment (i.e., obtains consent) with the parent(s)
      (2) Administers topical anesthetic to the eyes
      (3) Ensures that all personnel present at the treatment are wearing laser-safety goggles
      (4) Performs the laser
      (5) Watches for and treats ocular complications that may arise during and after the procedure
      (6) Follows the baby postoperatively until ROP is resolved
   b. Neonatology fellow, attending neonatologist, or pediatric anesthesiologist
      (1) Administers systemic sedative agents (midazolam, morphine, fentanyl, ketamine, or a combination)
      (2) Monitors patient for and treats any systemic complications that develop during or after treatment
      (3) Provides information to the ophthalmologist regarding the patient's overall condition throughout the procedure
   c. Assistant to the ophthalmologist
      (1) Helps with laser and instruments
      (2) Records the treatment parameters used during treatment
   d. Neonatal nurse
      (1) Instills dilating drops several times in the hour preceding treatment
      (2) Immobilizes the patient during treatment

4. **Equipment**
   a. Cardiorespiratory, blood pressure, and pulse oximeter
   b. Appropriate respiratory support (ventilator, laryngoscope and endotracheal tubes, face mask, self-inflating resuscitation bag, suction, and oxygen source)
   c. Emergency medications (atropine, epinephrine, calcium)
      Note: Precalculation of weight-appropriate doses is helpful
   d. Topical ocular anesthetic (e.g., tetracaine, proparacaine)
   e. Cycloplegic/mydriatic eye drops: Cyclomydril (Alcon Laboratories, Fort Worth, Texas) (cyclopentolate hydrochloride 0.2% and phenylephrine hydrochloride 1%) or 0.5% cyclopentolate and 1% or 2.5% phenylephrine
   f. Calcium alginate-tipped nasopharyngeal applicators or Flynn depressor (**Fig. 58.4**), for scleral depression
   g. Balanced salt solution for rewetting cornea during procedure

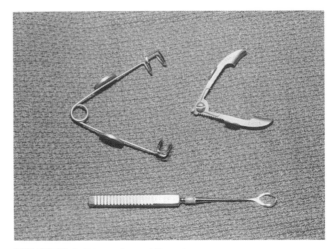

FIGURE 58.4 Lid speculae and Flynn depressor.

   h. Neonatal eyelid speculum (**Fig. 58.4**)
   i. 28- and 20-diopter lenses
   j. Portable argon or diode laser (9) with indirect (headlamp) delivery system
   k. Appropriate laser safety goggles

5. **Precautions and complications (Table 58.4)**
   a. Ensure that laser is fully functional.
   b. If the infant is at high risk for an adverse event that would terminate treatment prematurely, treat the more advanced eye first (assuming both have threshold ROP).
   c. Discontinue feedings at least 4 hours before the procedure, or empty the stomach with an orogastric tube.
   d. Establish IV access for infusions of medications and IV fluids.
   e. Observe oxygen saturation monitor carefully, and adjust administered oxygen appropriately.
   f. Stabilize the infant: Correct electrolyte imbalances, platelet deficiency, etc.
   g. Use only 1% phenylephrine if there is a history of hypertension.
   h. Wipe off any excess drops spilling onto the skin to avoid transcutaneous absorption (skin vessel blanching occurs with phenylephrine).

6. **Technique**
   a. General preparation
      (1) Instill mydriatic eyedrops (per orders from ophthalmologist) into both eyes multiple times in the hour prior to procedure. Maximal dilation is critical for optimum laser, and the pupils tend to constrict with the application of the laser; therefore, several (three or four) instillations of drops are required, especially in eyes with neovascularization/vascular engorgement of the iris. To properly check dilation, a bright light is shined directly into the eye; any movement of the pupil indicates inadequate dilation.

TABLE 58.4 Complications of Laser for Retinopathy

COMPLICATION	TREATMENT/ACTION
Systemic: Intra- and Immediately Postoperative	
Bradycardia	Interrupt treatment Assess airway, oxygen delivery Atropine 0.1 mg IV
Hypoxia/cyanosis	Evaluate airway Administer supplemental oxygen
Apnea	Evaluate airway Gentle stimulation Administer supplemental oxygen Provide positive pressure ventilation (self-inflating resuscitation bag or T piece face mask)
Tachycardia	Assess pain control Administer additional analgesic Monitor blood pressure and perfusion
Hypertension	Assess pain control Administer additional analgesic If moderate, observe If severe, consider hydralazine 0.1 mg/kg IV
Arrhythmia	Manage as appropriate for arrhythmia
Seizure (mechanism uncertain: possible anticholinergic effect)	Supportive care Antiseizure medication
Ocular: Intraoperative	
Closure of central artery	Relieve pressure on globe (stop scleral depression)
Corneal clouding/abrasion	Rinse with balanced salt solution/saline Interrupt treatment
Retinal/vitreous/choroidal hemorrhage	Gentle pressure on globe (until arterial pulsations visible) Avoid lasering blood May have to terminate treatment or switch to intravitreal bevacizumab if extensive
Ocular: Postoperative	
Conjunctival hemorrhage	Observation
Conjunctival laceration	Antibiotic ointment t.i.d. for 3–4 days
Corneal abrasion	Antibiotic ointment t.i.d. for 3–4 days Follow with slit lamp exam with fluorescein
Hyphema	Topical cycloplegic and steroids Follow intraocular pressure closely Consider washout if high pressure, no resolution in 7–10 days
Retinal/vitreous/choroidal hemorrhage	Close follow-up
Ocular: Late	
Amblyopia, strabismus, myopia	Pediatric ophthalmology assessment 3–4 mo after treatment(s). Educate parents prior to discharge regarding need for regular ophthalmology follow-up

t.i.d., three times per day.

(2) Transport the patient to surgical suite or designated procedure room in the nursery.

(3) Ensure monitors are attached and functioning.

b. Immobilize infant: Swaddle in a clean towel or blanket to immobilize arms and legs.

c. Ensure that the IV tubing is accessible.

d. Administer IV sedation. Instill local/topical anesthesia (e.g., tetracaine, proparacaine) during and again shortly after the sedation is given.

e. Distribute laser safety goggles and dim overhead lights.

f. Retract lids.

g. Perform laser: Cover the avascular retina with confluent gray–white burns (**Fig. 58.5**).

7. **Postoperative care**

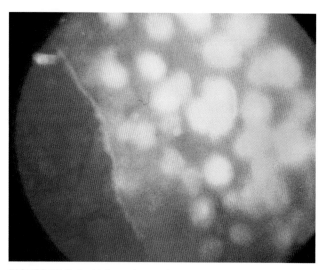

FIGURE 58.5 Freshly lasered avascular retina.

a. Apply antibiotic–steroid preparation (e.g., tobramycin–dexamethasone) to treated eye(s) three to four times daily for 3 days.

b. Monitor the patient with a cardiorespiratory monitor for 24 to 72 hours.

c. Perform a dilated retinal examination 1 to 2 weeks after treatment.

d. If opaque media are present at the time of laser, or if the pupil does not dilate adequately, complete treatment of the avascular retina may be impossible, and "skip areas" may be visible in the weeks after treatment. Supplemental laser treatment of these areas should be considered if there is not marked resolution of the adjacent plus disease and/or neovascularization. In the setting of persistence of plus disease or active neovascularization after complete laser ablation of the avascular retina in all quadrants, anti-VEGF treatment is warranted

e. Follow the infant every 1 to 2 weeks until the ROP resolves completely. If at the time of discharge ROP is still present, ensure that the parents and the physicians responsible for the care of the infant after discharge are aware of the extreme importance of maintaining a regular schedule of outpatient examinations.

f. Once the ROP has resolved completely, the baby should be seen by a pediatric ophthalmologist within 1 to 2 months to assess vision, ocular alignment and motility, refractive status, etc.

g. Long-term follow-up over several years is necessary. See outcomes and postdischarge follow-up below.

E. Intravitreal Injection for ROP

1. **Background.** Since the efficacy of anti-VEGF drug bevacizumab (Avastin; Genentech) for use in ROP has been reported (13,14), this treatment regimen has blossomed. Initial reports showed good results for eyes with Zone I disease. Given its relative ease of use compared with laser, and the lack of consensus on anti-VEGF agents (also ranibizumab/Lucentis; Genentech) in the premature infant (15,16), its use for Zone II disease has become widespread. It does provide an excellent first-line agent in any eye with ROP that develops opaque media, especially vitreous hemorrhage (a strong indication of active neovascularization/disease progression). It has the advantage over laser of requiring minimal to no sedation, eliminating those attendant risks.

   Like laser, anti-VEGF drugs halt disease progression by causing involution of active neovascular tissue. Intravitreal injections of anti-VEGF agents have been used to treat wet (neovascular) age-related macular degeneration (AMD), proliferative diabetic retinopathy, neovascular glaucoma, and other retinal vascular diseases.

2. **Precautions**

a. The major concern with bevacizumab in premature infants with ROP is systemic absorption and its effect on the developing infant. Bevacizumab is absorbed systemically after intravitreal injection. The risks of systemic effects on developing neonates have not been established (17).

b. The optimal and safe dose of bevacizumab in ROP has not been determined; the initially chosen (and most commonly employed) dose (0.625 mg) is extrapolated from that used in adults with ocular neovascular disease (1.25 mg), and may represent a severalfold increase in drug delivered/body weight over adults. Some studies with lower and "ultra-low" doses (0.16 mg) have shown efficacy (18).

c. No protocol for near- and long-term monitoring of bevacizumab in neonates has been developed.

d. The informed consent process for the use of intravitreal bevacizumab for ROP must reflect the uncertain status of the treatment, the off-label use of the drug, and the lack of long-term results, including the possibility of unknown systemic side effects.

e. Unlike laser, intravitreal injection is an INVASIVE procedure with the attendant risk of infection (endophthalmitis), cataract, retinal tear and detachment, and occlusion of the central retinal artery (due to a sudden rise in intraocular pressure) (see **Table 58.5**).

TABLE 58.5 Ocular Complications of Intravitreal Injection

COMPLICATION	TREATMENT
Immediate	
Closure of central retinal artery	Paracentesis (withdrawal of fluid from anterior chamber with needle)
Conjunctival hemorrhage	Observation
Vitreous hemorrhage	Observation and reevaluation (with ultrasonography if hemorrhage obscures view of retina) in 3–5 days
Within Days/Wks	
Infection/endophthalmitis	Prompt treatment with intravitreal antibiotics (vancomycin and ceftazidime)
Vitreous hemorrhage	As above
Retinal detachment	Incisional surgery (vitrectomy)
Retinal tear	Immediate laser or cryotherapy retinopexy
Within Wks/Mo/Yrs	
Reappearance of neovascularization/ reactivation of ROP	Close follow-up with low threshold for treatment, typically laser

f. The efficacy of anti-VEGF agents in ROP can be pyrrhic in nature as there have been multiple reports of reactivation of ROP and poor outcomes (retinal detachment) months or even *years* later (19–21). Close and extended follow-up (much more frequently than is typically seen in babies treated with laser) is mandatory.

3. Indications
  a. Threshold ROP in posterior Zone I disease. An early report showed benefit over laser in posterior (Zone I) disease (13).
  b. In unstable infants in whom laser may be contraindicated. Intravitreal injection does not require systemic sedation/anesthesia; in this regard, the procedure may be preferable to laser in unstable infants.
  c. In eyes with known or suspected ROP that develop a media opacity (inability to visualize the retina with indirect ophthalmoscopy), especially a vitreous hemorrhage or extensive preretinal hemorrhage.
  d. In eyes that have had an incomplete response to laser (14,17).
4. Contraindications
  a. Infection in or around the eyes
  b. Lethal medical illness
  c. Failure of consensus between parent(s), treating physicians, and hospital personnel about the uncertain nature of intravitreal bevacizumab in ROP and the risks of intravitreal injection (inability to obtain informed consent)
5. Personnel
  a. Ophthalmologist
    (1) Determines the need for treatment
    (2) Participates in informed consent process; unlike laser this should be the responsibility of the treating ophthalmologist, who discusses the ocular issues, and the neonatologist, who addresses the possible systemic effects of the drug
    (3) Administers topical anesthetic
    (4) Preps the lids, lashes, and conjunctivae with sterile 5% Betadine
    (5) Places the sterile lid speculum and performs the injection
    (6) Performs indirect ophthalmoscopy after the injection(s); if the central retinal artery is compromised, immediately performs a paracentesis, lowering the IOP
    (7) Instills antibiotic (e.g., ciprofloxacin 0.3%) drop and/or ointment to the treated eyes
    (8) Follows the baby for ocular complications and resolution of ROP
  b. Neonatologist
    (1) Provides information about the status of the infants to the treating ophthalmologist
    (2) Participates in the informed consent process
    (3) Monitors infant for systemic complications during and after treatment
  c. Nurse/assistant at bedside
    (1) Helps prepare the baby for injection (i.e., swaddles the baby)
    (2) Helps prepare the instruments at the bedside

6. **Equipment**
   a. Topical anesthetic
   b. Sterile lid speculum (one per eye)
   c. Caliper (one per eye)
   d. Sterile cotton-tipped applicators (CTA)
   e. Sterile gloves
   f. Topical 5% Betadine
   g. Topical antibiotic drops (ciprofloxacin 0.3%) and/or ointment
   h. Sterile syringe of bevacizumab (0.625 mg in 0.025 mL) with 30-gauge needle (one per eye)
7. **Complications (Table 58.2)**
   a. The most worrisome risk is postinjection infection (endophthalmitis). Babies with active or recent ocular surface or lid infections (e.g., conjunctivitis) should not have intravitreal injection
   b. Other serious ocular complications are ruled out by indirect ophthalmoscopy immediately after the injection (see sections 2e and 5a6, above)
   c. The risk of adverse systemic side effects (bradycardia, oxygen desaturation) is mitigated by the absence of systemic sedation/anesthesia, and the rapid nature of the procedure. However, it is reasonable to follow those precautions listed for laser treatment in F4.
8. **Technique**
   a. The baby's eyes are dilated according to the standard dilation protocol.
   b. Sterile towels are placed around the baby's head.
   c. Topical anesthetics are instilled.
   d. The lids, lashes, and conjunctiva are prepped with 5% Betadine.
   e. Wire lid speculum is placed.
   f. The caliper is used to mark a spot on the sclera 1.5 to 2.0 mm posterior to the limbus in the inferotemporal quadrant.
   g. A Betadine-soaked CTA is gently pressed over the mark and excess Betadine is allowed to collect in the inferior fornix.
   h. The injection is given.
   i. A topical antibiotic drop (ciprofloxacin 0.3%) is given.
   j. The ophthalmologist performs binocular indirect ophthalmoscopy.
   k. Dexamethasone/polymyxin B/dexamethasone ointment may be instilled.
9. **Postinjection Care/concerns**
   a. Topical antibiotic drops should be instilled three to four times a day for 3 days.
   b. Portable slit-lamp examination should be performed 48 to 72 hours postinjection.
   c. Any signs of infection (lid edema and erythema, conjunctival injection, clouding of the cornea and/or anterior chamber) should be reported immediately to the treating ophthalmologist.
   d. Examination by treating ophthalmologist in 1 week.

F. Postdischarge Care

A critical component of treatment of ROP is postdischarge care.

1. No baby with any ROP, or who has regressed ROP after treatment, should leave the neonatal intensive care unit (NICU) without a scheduled follow-up examination (1,22).
2. It is imperative that infants who develop any stage of ROP, especially those with prethreshold stage 3 or those who have received treatment, are seen within 1 to 2 weeks of discharge, or as directed by the ophthalmologist involved in the baby's care.
3. A careful, reproducible tracking system for arranging follow-up should be established by every NICU. A member of the staff of each NICU should be responsible for maintaining and periodically auditing this system (22,23).
4. Verbal and written instructions for follow-up should be given to the parents. Parents should be given a discharge form indicating their baby's *scheduled* follow-up among their discharge instructions. The importance of scheduled follow-up should be prominently stated on the form.
5. The possibility of reactivation of quiescent or "resolved" ROP in eyes treated with intravitreal anti-VEGF agents should be well documented and explicitly discussed with the parent(s), the ophthalmologist assuming the baby's outpatient care, and the pediatrician (see 2f above).

G. Outcome

1. Early treatment for type 1 high-risk prethreshold ROP has been shown to improve retinal structural outcome and visual acuity outcomes at 6 years of age (11).
2. Favorable outcome with vision of 20/40 or better was noted in 35% of treated eyes.
3. However, 65% of eyes receiving early treatment develop visual acuity worse than 20/40.
4. Unfavorable outcome despite treatment: Visual acuity 20/200 in 15%; blindness or low vision in 9%.
5. The outcome for eyes with Zone I disease, although poor, has improved with laser and intravitreal anti-VEGF agents.
6. Treated eyes carry a risk of retinal dystopia, myopia, and subsequent strabismus and amblyopia (11,24). To minimize the effect of refractive errors and strabismus, careful follow-up by a pediatric ophthalmologist is mandatory.
7. Reactivation of quiescent ROP in eyes treated with anti-VEGF agents (20) is a new phenomenon and may necessitate repeat treatments long after the baby has been discharged from the NICU.

8. Premature infants are at risk for intracranial pathologies that may limit visual function. Pediatric ophthalmologists, neurologists, and others involved in the care of former preemies should be in frequent contact in order to address the often complex and changing visual deficits present in these children.

References

1. Fierson WM; American Academy of Pediatrics Section on Ophthalmology, American Academy of Ophthalmology, American Association for Pediatric Ophthalmology and Strabismus, American Association of Certified Orthoptists. Screening examinations of premature infants for retinopathy of prematurity. *Pediatrics*. 2013;131:189–195.
2. Wilkinson AR, Haines L, Head K, et al. UK retinopathy of prematurity guidelines. *Early Hum Dev*. 2008;84:71–74.
3. Jefferies AL; Canadian Paediatric Society, Fetus and Newborn Committee. Retinopathy of prematurity: an update on screening and management. *Paediatr Child Health*. 2016;21(2):101–108.
4. An International Committee for the Classification of Retinopathy of Prematurity. The international classification of retinopathy of prematurity revisited. *Arch Ophthalmol*. 2005;123:991–999.
5. Silva RA, Murakami Y, Lad EM, et al. Stanford University network for diagnosis of retinopathy of prematurity (SUNDROP): 36 month experience with telemedicine screening. *Ophthalmic Surg Lasers Imaging*. 2011;42:12–19.
6. Kivlin JD, Biglan AW, Gordon RA, et al. Early retinal vessel development and iris vessel dilatation as factors in retinopathy of prematurity. Cryotherapy for retinopathy of prematurity (CRYO-ROP) cooperative group. *Arch Ophthalmol*. 1996;114:150–154.
7. Marcus I, Salchow DJ, Stoessel KM, et al. An ROP screening dilemma: hereditary cataracts developing in a premature infant after birth. *J Pediatr Ophthalmol Strabismus*. 2012;14:49;e1–e4.
8. Simpson JL, Melia M, Yang MB. Current role of cryotherapy in retinopathy of prematurity. A report by the American Academy of Ophthalmology. *Ophthalmology*. 2012;119:873–877.
9. Houston SK, Wykoff CC, Berrocal AM, et al. Laser treatment for retinopathy of prematurity. *Lasers Med Sci*. 2013;28(2):683–692.
10. Early Treatment for Retinopathy of Prematurity Cooperative Group. Revised indications for the treatment of retinopathy of prematurity: results of the early treatment for retinopathy of prematurity randomized trial. *Arch Ophthalmol*. 2003;121:1684–1694.
11. Early Treatment for Retinopathy of Prematurity Cooperative Group. Final visual acuity results in the early treatment for retinopathy of prematurity study. *Arch Ophthalmol*. 2010;128:663–671.
12. Klufas MA, Patel SN, Chan RV. Surgical management of retinopathy of prematurity. *Dev Ophthalmol*. 2014;54:223–233.
13. Mintz-Hittner HA, Kennedy KA, Chuang AZ, et al. Efficacy of intravitreal bevacizumab for stage 3+ retinopathy of prematurity. *N Engl J Med*. 2011;364:603–615.
14. Hwang CK, Hubbard GB, Hutchinson AK, et al. Outcomes after intravitreal bevacizumab versus laser photocoagulation: a 5-year retrospective analysis. *Ophthalmology*. 2015;122:1008–1015.
15. Sankar MJ, Sankar J, Chandra P. Anti-vascular endothelial growth factor (VEGF) drugs for treatment of retinopathy of prematurity. *Cochrane Database Syst Rev*. 2018;1:CD009734.
16. Tolentino M. Systemic and ocular safety of intravitreal anti-VEGF therapies for ocular neovascular disease. *Surv Ophthalmol*. 2011;56:95–113.
17. Morin J, Luu TM, Superstein R, et al. Neurodevelopmental outcomes following bevacizumab injections for retinopathy of prematurity. *Pediatrics*. 2016;137(4):pii: e20153218.
18. Hillier RJ, Connor AJ, Shafiq AE. Ultra-low-dose intravitreal bevacizumab for the treatment of retinopathy of prematurity: a case series. *Br J Ophthalmol*. 2018;102:260–264.
19. Snyder LL, Garcia-Gonzalez JM, Shapiro MJ, et al. Very late reactivation of retinopathy of prematurity after monotherapy with intravitreal bevacizumab. *Ophthal Surg Lasers and Imaging Retina*. 2016;47:280–283.
20. Lim LS, Mitchell P, Wong TY. Bevacizumab for retinopathy of prematurity. *N Engl J Med*. 2011;364:2360.
21. Yonekawa Y, Wu WC, Nitulescu CE, et al. Progressive retinal detachment in infants with retinopathy of prematurity treated with intravitreal bevacizumab or ranibizumab. *Retina*. 2018;38(6):1079–1083.
22. Day S, Menke AM, Abbott RL. Retinopathy of prematurity malpractice claims: the ophthalmic mutual insurance company experience. *Arch Ophthalmol*. 2009;127:794–798.
23. Moshfeghi DM. Top five legal pitfalls in retinopathy of prematurity. *Curr Opin Ophthalmol*. 2018;29(3):206–209.
24. Davitt BV, Quinn GE, Wallace DK, et al. Astigmatism progression in the early treatment for retinopathy study to 6 years of age. *Ophthalmology*. 2011;118:2326–2329.

Renal Replacement Therapy

Kara Short, Daryl Ingram, Vincent Mortellaro, Traci Henderson, and David Askenazi

Acute Renal Replacement Therapy

The two most common types of acute renal replacement therapy used in the neonatal population when management of electrolytes and/or fluid balance by less invasive means fails are peritoneal dialysis (PD) and continuous renal replacement therapy (CRRT). Variables to be considered when deciding between these modalities include:

- ability to gain access (vascular for CRRT and peritoneal catheter for PD)
- degree of fluid overload and/or electrolyte instability
- goals of therapy
- intoxication of a drug that can only be removed adequately by CRRT or hemodialysis (HD)
- degree of uremia
- condition of the abdomen, and
- availability of resources/center experience (1).

Indications

1. In general, like any procedure, RRT is indicated when the potential benefits outweigh the potential risks of not performing the procedure. RRT should begin when one or more vital functions of the kidney are failing and that result is likely to impede vital organ function. The clinician should not wait for complete kidney failure to initiate RRT. This is analogous to intubation for respiratory support. One would not wait for complete respiratory failure to intubate, but would intubate a patient when impending respiratory failure is likely.
2. Specifically, RRT is indicated when conservative management has failed to adequately control any of the following conditions (2,3):
   a. Hypervolemia
   b. Hyperkalemia
   c. Hyponatremia
   d. Refractory metabolic acidosis
   e. Hyperphosphatemia
   f. Inability to provide necessary blood products, drugs, and/or nutrition without progressive fluid overload
   g. Toxicity of certain medications
   h. Inborn errors of metabolism (4,5)

Contraindications

Although not a true contraindication, PD for severe hyperammonemia does not provide adequate ammonia clearance. Thus, either high-dose CRRT or HD followed by CRRT is the modality of choice (6,7). In the event that no HD or CRRT is available, starting PD while arranging transport to a medical center with HD and/or CRRT capabilities can be life saving (8). Contraindications to PD include any abdominal wall defects (omphalocele, gastroschisis), diaphragmatic or abdominal wall disruptions, perforated bowel due to necrotizing enterocolitis or other causes, acute abdomen, and/or recent surgery that disrupts the integrity of the peritoneum (9,10). In babies with imminent or current intracranial hemorrhage, PD may be preferred as this procedure does not require anticoagulation (6).

Acute Peritoneal Dialysis

For a comprehensive discussion on guidelines for PD during AKI, the International Society of Peritoneal Dialysis provides specific, comprehensive guidelines which are beyond the scope of this chapter (9). For this chapter, we will discuss the issues pertinent to neonates. In neonates, acute PD is frequently preferred over intermittent HD and CRRT because it is technically easier to perform. Peritoneal surface area per kilogram of bodyweight is relatively larger in newborns and children than in adults. Therefore, PD usually allows adequate clearance and removal of excess fluid. In addition, PD avoids the need for anticoagulation and maintenance of adequate vascular access, which are required for the other methods (11).

A. Equipment

(Figs. 59.1 and 59.2)

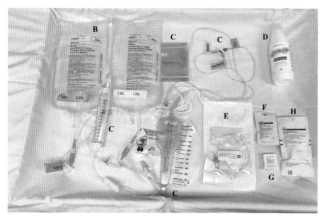

FIGURE 59.1 A: IV pole (Fig. 59.2). **B:** Dianeal Peritoneal Dialysis Solution (Baxter, Deerfield, Illinois). **C:** Dialy-Nate Set with luer connections: Peritoneal Dialysis set for Neonates (Utah Medical Products, Inc. www.utahmed.com.), which includes a 150-mL inline burette set, a 3-way stopcock, coiled tubing, and a drainage bag. **D:** ExSept Plus, skin-exit site wound cleanser; electrolytically produced 0.114% sodium hypochlorite (Courtesy of Angelini Pharma). **E:** Effluent Sample Bag (Baxter, Deerfield, Illinois). **F:** MiniCap with Povidone-Iodine Solution (Baxter, Deerfield, Illinois). **G:** Beta-Cap Clamp. **H:** FlexiCap Disconnect Cap with Povidone-Iodine Solution (Baxter, Deerfield, Illinois).

Sterile

1. Masks, drapes, gowns, and gloves
2. Chlorhexidine, povidone-iodine, or center-approved disinfectant scrub
3. 1% lidocaine without epinephrine
4. 3-mL syringe with 25-gauge needle
5. IV cutdown tray with no. 11 surgical blade
6. 3-0 Prolene sutures (either as part of cutdown tray or separately)
7. 22-gauge angiocatheter or a femoral catheter with guidewire
8. A temporary catheter such as a 14-gauge angiocatheter or one of the commercially available temporary dialysis catheters (e.g., a Trocath [Trocath Peritoneal Dialysis Center, Kendall McGaw Laboratories, Sabana Grande, Puerto Rico])
9. Dialysis solution (1.5%, 2.5%, or 4.25%)
   a. Other concentrations can be made by manual mixing of standard solutions once the system is set up

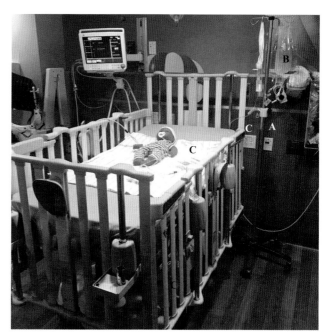

FIGURE 59.2 An assembled peritoneal dialysis circuit illustrates an IV pole (**A**) with Dianeal (**B**) attached to a Dialy-Nate Set (**C**). The patient line of the Dialy-Nate Set is attached to a Tenckhoff catheter exiting from the abdominal cavity of a doll, and the drain line of the Dialy-Nate Set has a bag at the end (located at the base of the crib).

10. Heparin
11. In-line burette set
12. Ultra-Set continuous ambulatory peritoneal dialysis (CAPD) Disposable Disconnect Y-Set or Dialy-Nate Set (Utah Medical Products, Midvale, Utah) made for patients <10 kg or fill volumes <150 mL
13. MiniCap Extended Life PD Transfer Set with Twist Clamp (Baxter, Deerfield, Illinois)
14. Medicap with Povidone-Iodine Solution
15. FlexiCap Disconnect Cap with Povidone-Iodine Solution

Nonsterile

1. Waterproof tape.
2. Baby weighing scale with low resolution (e.g., Medela, which has a resolution of 2 g from 0 to 6,000 g) or a hanging scale.
3. HomeChoice Automated PD System (minimum fill volume 150 mL) or any other reliable fluid warmer, such as the Gay-Mar Blanketrol and heating blanket. An alternative approach is to utilize a pediatric cycler set. Experience in using this equipment is necessary. We recommend a commercially available cycler that provides a minimum fill volume of 50 mL with 10-mL increments.

B. Preprocedure Care

1. Obtain informed consent.
2. Check bodyweight and abdominal girth.
3. Check for infection at the insertion site.
4. Decompress the stomach.
5. Catheterize the bladder.
6. Place preweighed diaper under the patient.

   Before assembly of system, wash hands and put on a mask. All connections should be made using sterile technique. Universal precautions should be observed (see Chapter 6). Keep all tubing clamped. See **Figure 59.2** for connections.
7. Prepare irrigation fluids per type of PD catheter.
8. Dwell volume for infusion = 10 to 15 mL/kg.
   a. Temporary catheter: Add 500 U of heparin to each 1 L of the dialysis solution. Start with 1.5% dialysate.
   b. Tunneled Tenckhoff catheter Quinton Pediatric Tenckhoff Neonatal 31-cm catheter (Kendall Healthcare, Mansfield, Massachusetts). Add 250-U heparin to each 1 L of sodium chloride 0.9% solution. Add 200-mg/L cefazolin and 8-mg/L gentamicin to sodium chloride 0.9% solution. If patient is allergic to either of those antibiotics, use vancomycin 20 mg/L.
9. Warm a liter bag of dialysate (Dianeal or other), or a larger bag if 1-L dialysate is not available, by resting it on the heating surface of the HomeChoice Automated PD System (Baxter, Deerfield, IL). You may also warm the tubing system with the Gay-Mar warmer and can hang bags as they are. The temperature can be set between 35°C and 37°C. For a newborn, keep the temperature at 37°C (in older pediatric patients, the temperature is usually set to 36°C, and occasionally to 35°C if the environmental temperature is high).
10. Spike the Dialy-Nate Set (Utah Medical Products, Midvale, Utah) into the dialysate (Dianeal or other).
11. Prime the circuit in a sterile fashion, clamp, and cap the end of the transfer set.
12. Connect the short-arm end of the Dialy-Nate Set to the twist clamp end of a MiniCap Extended Life PD Transfer Set with Twist Clamp (Baxter, Deerfield, Illinois). After surgical placement of the PD catheter, a sterile drainage bag is generally connected to the catheter. As PD is initiated, the Dialy-Nate Set is attached and the drainage bag discarded by a trained dialysis nurse.

C. Placement of a PD Catheter

The ideal technique is surgical insertion of a permanent PD catheter, which can be placed by an experienced surgeon in the neonatal intensive care unit (12). Catheters placed to exit the skin in a caudal direction carry a lower risk of peritonitis. The catheter is tunneled from the peritoneum to an exit site on the skin, which usually works well and leaks infrequently.

1. Monitor vital signs.
2. Sedate/anesthetize infant in supine position.
3. Scrub using sterile surgical procedure.
4. Prepare the skin of the abdomen (see Chapter 6).
5. Drape to expose the entire abdomen.
6. Elevate the umbilicus with two Addison graspers and incise the umbilicus with a no. 11 blade to enter into the peritoneal cavity.
7. Place a 5-mm Step trocar into the peritoneum and gain pneumoperitoneum with insufflation set based on the child's size; insert a 5- or 4-mm 30° laparoscope.
8. On the left side of the abdomen at the lateral rectus muscle border use a no. 11 blade to incise the abdominal wall with a 2-cm incision; perform a 1-cm incision mirrored on the right side of the abdomen.
9. Use a hemostat to dilate the incision on the left, then with a laparoscopic grasper in the right side incision; feed the Tenckhoff catheter through the dilated left incision into the abdomen making sure the distal cuff is below the abdominal wall fascia but still extraperitoneal.
10. Use the right-sided grasper to place the catheter into the pelvis behind the bladder/uterus and in the pouch of Douglas.
11. Most catheters have a colored strip for orientation; take note if the strip is anterior or posterior for the intra-abdominal catheter as maintaining this orientation for the tunneled portion will keep the catheter from flipping out of the pelvis.
12. Remove the right-sided grasper; from the left side, use a hemostat to create a curved subcutaneous tunnel that will accept the proximal cuff; the tract will extend from the incision medially arching over the umbilicus.
13. In the right-sided incision, close abdominal wall fascia with a 3-0 Vicryl suture. Then pass a curved tendon grasper through the subcutaneous tissues medially arching over the top of the umbilicus, through the previously created left-sided tunnel and out the left-sided incision.
14. Orient the catheter with the strip in the proper position and then pull the catheter to the right-sided incision with the tendon grasper. Use a hemostat to assist the proximal cuff into subcutaneous tunnel and into proper position.
15. A correctly placed catheter will have a gentle curve from one side of the abdomen to the other over top of the umbilicus with no kinking. The proximal cuff will be situated in the subcutaneous tissues of the left side of the abdomen while the distal cuff will be located in the subfascial plane outside of the peritoneal lining. The colored strip on the catheter will be in the same orientation through its course to prevent any catheter twist that

could result in obstruction or flipping of the catheter outside of the pelvis. The catheter course should have at least 1 cm of subcutaneous distance between its course and the umbilical stalk. If a gastrostomy tube is present, the catheter will need a similar buffer of soft tissue.

16. Close the left-sided incision with running subcuticular 4-0 Monocryl suture. Remove the trocar from the umbilicus; close the umbilical fascia with 2-0 or 0 Vicryl depending on the child's size. Close umbilical skin incision with a 4-0 Monocryl.

17. Place catheter metal fittings on the catheter and fasten them. Attach the connection tubing and test the catheter with saline. Saline should freely and quickly flow through the catheter into the abdomen and should drain as promptly.

18. If there are any flow issues, the catheter should be reevaluated along its length for any kinking, and if necessary a trocar placed back into the abdomen to assess any intra-abdominal kinking, malpositioning, or clogging.

19. If the omentum readily surrounds, obstructs, or gives suspicion of causing issue in the future, an omentectomy is indicated. This may be performed laparoscopically before placement of the catheter using the right-sided grasper and an energy device in the left-sided incision.

20. Once the catheter has been confirmed to have perfect function, dress the left side incision and the umbilicus with skin glue. Apply a dressing over the catheter with Bactroban cream, dry 2 × 2 gauze, and a Tegaderm. Place an antibiotic lock and Betadine cap over the catheter.

If surgical insertion of a permanent catheter is not possible, an alternative approach is to utilize an angiocatheter or a temporary PD catheter for no longer than a few days to minimize infection risk. Note that surgically inserted catheters are associated with fewer acute complications (13).

a. Monitor vital signs.
b. Restrain infant in supine position.
c. Scrub as for a major surgical procedure.
d. Prepare the skin of the abdomen (see Chapter 5).
e. Drape to expose the insertion site. The choice of insertion site is influenced by the preference of the physician and/or the presence of postoperative wounds, abdominal wall infection, or organomegaly. A location one-third the distance from the umbilicus to the symphysis pubis in the midline or a site lateral to the rectus sheath in either of the lower quadrants is preferred.
f. Infuse approximately 0.5 mL of lidocaine around the insertion point.
g. Select either a 14-gauge angiocatheter or a temporary dialysis catheter.
h. If you elect to use a 14-gauge angiocatheter:
   (1) Insert the angiocatheter at the insertion site.
   (2) Remove the stylet.
   (3) Infuse approximately 20 mL of normal saline to confirm a free flow. Clamp.
   (4) Proceed to step 10.
i. If using a soft and flexible temporary catheter, such as a Cook catheter (Cook Critical Care, Bloomington, Indiana), follow the manufacturer's instructions. Then proceed to step 10.
j. Test patency.
   (1) Unclamp. May observe flow of a few drops of saline. Connect the free end of the transfer set to the catheter.
   (2) Allow approximately 30 mL of dialysis solution to enter peritoneal cavity by gravity.
   (3) Clamp the short arm of the Y-Set (inflow).
   (4) Unclamp the long arm of the Y-Set (outflow).
   (5) Repeat steps a through d several times.
   (6) Secure the temporary catheter with a purse-string suture and tape if inflow and outflow occur readily.

D. Management

1. Establish a cycle time. This is usually about 60 minutes and consists of a fill by gravity, dwell time of 45 minutes, and drain by gravity. For ease of performing and charting manual PD, it is recommended that fill time be a 10-minute period, dwell a 40-minute period, and drain by gravity a 10-minute period.

2. Establish a dialysis fill volume per pass. Starting volume is usually 10 mL/kg. For continuous PD, volume will stay at 10 mL/kg. For shorter dialysis length, volume will be slowly increased as patient tolerates. It is important to note that for temporary catheters, fill volumes are not to exceed 10 mL/kg. For higher volumes and/or less cycles, a tunneled catheter is recommended.

3. Clamp the long arm of the Y-Set (outflow line).

4. Unclamp the inflow line.

5. Allow the dialysate to flow in as quickly as possible by gravity.

6. Vital signs can be monitored per unit standards or every hour, whichever is more frequent.

7. Clamp the inflow line.

8. Allow the fluid to dwell.

9. Unclamp the outflow when dwell time is completed.

10. Allow 10 minutes for draining.

11. If there are issues with drain or fill time, it may be acceptable to give additional time; however, should the catheter seem to be obstructed, an intervention may be needed (**Table 59.2**).

12. Clamp the outflow line.

13. Repeat the cycle.

14. If the goal is to perform intermittent PD, the usual goal will be 40 mL/kg dwells × 10–12 hourly cycles

per day. Dwell volume can be slowly increased by 10 to 20 mL every few days until the desired volume is achieved.

15. If not on 24-hour continuous cycles, a final dwell volume of 20 mL/kg (or ½ of the cycle dwell volume) is recommended. The next intermittent cycle should begin with a drain time of 10 minutes.

16. Add 500 U of heparin/L of dialysate, until dialysate effluent return is clear, with no evidence of cloudiness.

17. Add 3 mEq/L of potassium (K) if serum K level is ≤4 mEq/L.

E. Monitoring

1. Maintain hourly PD flow sheet.
   a. Volume in
   b. Volume out
   c. Net/hr (+/−)
   d. Net over the course of dialysis (+/−)
   e. Intakes (enteral, parenteral)
   f. Outputs (urine, gastric, insensible water loss, etc.)

2. Establish a desired fluid balance. Increase dextrose cocentration slowly if negative balance is required. Reassess the state of hydration frequently.

3. Measure serum glucose and potassium every 4 hours for the first 24 hours or until stable, then twice a day. Obtain other serum electrolyte levels twice daily. Check blood urea nitrogen, serum creatinine, serum calcium, serum phosphorus, and serum magnesium once a day.

4. Evaluation of the fluid should be done every shift—if the fluid appears cloudy, assessment for peritonitis (cell count and culture) should be performed.

5. Recognize that some drug dosages may need adjustments (**Table 59.1**) (14).

TABLE 59.1 Antimicrobial Dosing Recommendations for Renal Dysfunction in Patients

ANTIBIOTIC	CrCl <10 mL/min AND HEMODIALYSIS/PD^a ≤40 kg	CRRT ≤40 kg	PERITONEAL DIALYSIS
Acyclovir (IV)	5 mg/kg q24h—schedule after dialysis	5–10 mg/kg/dose q12h	5 mg/kg/dose q24h; no supplemental dose needed
Ambisome IV	3–5 mg/kg q24h—schedule after HD	3–5 mg/kg q24h	Poorly dialyzed—no adjustment recommended
Amikacin IV	10 mg/kg ×1 dose—random level prior to next HD treatment	10 mg/kg ×1 dose random level 24 hr	5 mg/kg ×1 dose, then base dosing on levels
Amphotericin B IV	0.75–1 mg/kg q24h—schedule after HD	0.75–1 mg/kg q24h	
Ampicillin IV	50 mg/kg/dose q12h	200 mg/kg/day divided q8h	50 mg/kg q12h
Bactrim (TMP/SMZ) IV	Not recommended. If needed 5 mg/kg/24 hr	5 mg/kg q12h	Use is not recommended
Cefepime IV	50 mg/kg/q24h	50 mg/kg/dose q8h (max 2 g/dose)	50 mg/kg/dose q24h
Fluconazole IV/PO	6 mg/kg/dose every other day after dialysis	6 mg/kg/dose q24h (max 400 mg)	Administer 50% of recommended dose q48h
Ganciclovir (induction) IV	1.25 mg/kg post HD	2.5 mg/kg q24h	IV 1.25 mg/kg dose 3× wk
Ganciclovir (maintenance) IV	0.625 mg/kg post HD	1.25 mg/kg q24h	IV 0.625 mg/kg/dose 3× wk
Gentamicin IV	One-time dose after dialysis, random level next day	One-time dose with 12h level	2.5 mg/kg ×1 dose, then based on levels
Meropenem IV	20 mg/kg/dose q24h—schedule after dialysis	40 mg/kg/dose q8h (2 g max)	20 mg/kg/dose q24h

TABLE 59.1   Antimicrobial Dosing Recommendations for Renal Dysfunction in Patients (*Continued*)

ANTIBIOTIC	CrCl <10 mL/min AND HEMODIALYSIS/PD[a] ≤40 kg	CRRT ≤40 kg	PERITONEAL DIALYSIS
Metronidazole IV/PO	4 mg/kg/dose q6h (extensively removed)	No adjustment needed	4 mg/kg/dose q6h
Micafungin IV	No adjustment needed	No adjustment needed	No adjustment needed
Nafcillin IV	No adjustment needed	No adjustment needed	No adjustment needed
Piperacillin/tazobactam IV	50 mg/kg/dose q12h	75 mg/kg/dose q8h	75 mg piperacillin/kg/dose q12h
Tobramycin IV	One-time dose after dialysis, random level next day	One-time dose with 12h level	2.5 mg/kg ×1 dose then based on levels
Vancomycin IV	15 mg/kg ×1 dose—random level next day or prior to next HD treatment	One-time dose with 12h level	15 mg/kg ×1 dose, then based on levels
Voriconazole (IV)			Not recommended
Voriconazole (PO)			Poorly dialyzed; no dosage adjustment necessary. Due to accumulation of the intravenous vehicle (cyclodextrin), the manufacturer recommends the use of oral voriconazole in these patients unless an assessment of risk: benefit justifies the use of IV voriconazole

Reviewed and edited April 2019.

[a]Dosing for PD is not always the same; please use your best clinical judgment.

Lexicomp (2019). Lexicomp Online; Aronoff GR, Bennett WM, Berns JS, et al. *Drug Prescribing in Renal Failure: Dosing Guidelines for Adults and Children.* 5th ed. Philadelphia, PA: American College of Physicians; 2007.

F. Complications

See **Table 59.2**.

Continuous Renal Replacement Therapy

CRRT has become a popular modality for dialysis in the neonatal population. With the development of smaller filters, it has become possible to use CRRT on neonates when they require it. Several circuits have been either adapted or designed specifically for use in neonates. This area of investigation and clinical use is exciting and we anticipate that CRRT for infants will be greatly enhanced with the use of these safer devices (12,14,15). Use of CRRT should be limited to regional centers and performed by those with the required expertise. CRRT is performed using a double-lumen catheter or two single-lumen catheters. **Table 59.3** provides the types of catheter sizes. Placement of these catheters depends on location of access, size of the vessel, and estimated duration of therapy (cuffed catheters are preferred if the estimated duration of the CRRT will be for at least 2 weeks). Blood from the patient is removed from one side of the catheter and run through a hemofilter composed of many fine capillaries of highly water-permeable membranes, located within a cylindrical case. The blood is pumped through the machine and returned to the patient on the other side of the vascular catheter.

CRRT can provide clearance of waste products and electrolyte balance by using the principles of dialysis, convection, or both. When dialysis is used, small molecules

TABLE 59.2 Complications of Peritoneal Dialysis

PROBLEM (RISK)	WHAT TO DO
Perforation of bladder, bowel, or major vessels (3–7%)	Surgical consultation
Puncture-site bleeding (3–15%)	Apply pressure gently Purse-string suture
Blood-stained dialysis maintained after several cycles	Check hematocrit frequently. Continue heparin. Rule out major vessel bleeding
Leakage from exit site (2–20%)	Reduce dwell volume until leakage stops. Stop dialysis
Extravasation of dialysate into the anterior abdominal wall	Replace with new catheter
More than 10% of solution retained in each of several consecutive cycles (outflow obstruction) (15–30%)	Reposition infant gently Reposition catheter by rotation and slight retraction. *Do not advance.* Remove if unchanged. Replace with new catheter
Two-way obstruction (3–20%)	Irrigate catheter with small amount of dialysate or saline aseptically. Never aspirate from a PD catheter with a syringe. Doing so can pull and entrap the omentum into the catheter space Reposition Remove if unchanged
Dislodgment of catheter (3%)	Replace with new catheter
Hydrothorax (0–10%)	Reposition infant, head and chest above level of abdomen. Decrease dwell volume
Hyperglycemia (10–60%)	Avoid high concentrations of dialysate unless outflow is inadequate Low dose of insulin if needed
Lactic acidosis	Use bicarbonate dialysate[a]
Hyponatremia	Reduce fluid intake. Aim to increase outflow if secondary to fluid overload
Hypernatremia	Increase fluid intake if secondary to excessive ultrafiltrate
Exit site infection (4–30%)	Systemic antibiotics
Peritonitis (0.5–30%)	Several rapid flushing exchanges Blood culture. Systemic vancomycin plus ceftazidime or an aminoglycoside For fungal peritonitis, systemic therapy is needed and catheter should be removed
Hernia (inguinal or umbilical) (2–13%)	Possible need for future repair
Small-bowel herniation and gangrene at catheter-exit site (one case report)	Surgical consultation
Removal of therapeutic drugs	See **Table 59.1**

[a]1.5% bicarbonate dialysis solution: 140 mEq/L Na, 110 mEq/L Cl, 30 mEq/L HCO_3, 15 g of glucose; add sterile water to 1,000 mL.

Data from Kohli HS, Barkataky A, Kumar RS, et al. Peritoneal dialysis for acute renal failure in infants: A comparison of three types of peritoneal access. *Ren Fail*. 1997;19:165–170; Kohli HS, Bhalla D, Sud K, et al. Acute peritoneal dialysis in neonates: Comparison of two types of peritoneal access. *Pediatr Nephrol*. 1999;13:241–244; Matthews DE, West KW, Rescorla FJ, et al. Peritoneal dialysis in the first 60 days of life. *J Pediatr Surg*. 1990;25:110–115; Wong KK, Lan LC, Lin SC, et al. Small bowel herniation and gangrene from peritoneal dialysis catheter exit site. *Pediatr Nephrol*. 2003;18:301–302.

TABLE 59.3 Available Vascular Catheters Commonly Used in Pediatric Patients

WEIGHT	CUFFED (TUNNELED)	UNCUFFED (UNTUNNELED)
<4 kg	■ Bard 6 Fr × 50 cm (POWERLINE)	■ Bard 6 Fr × 50 cm (PowerHohn) ■ Gambro 6 Fr × 15 cm ■ Medcomp 7 Fr × 7 cm ■ Medcomp 7 Fr × 10 cm
4–10 kg	■ Medcomp 8 Fr × 18 cm ■ Or as above for <4 kg	■ Medcomp 8 Fr × 12 cm ■ Mahurkar 8.5 Fr × 11 cm ■ (or as above for <4 kg)

General guidelines to choosing a dialysis catheter:
1. Cuffed catheters should be placed when the expected time for use is >2 wks; uncuffed for those expected to need access for <2 wks
2. Place the largest-diameter catheter with the shortest length that will be unlikely to cause harm to patient

cross the tiny holes in the filters across a concentration gradient and this procedure is referred to as continuous veno-venous hemodialysis (CVVHD). When only convective clearance is used, small and middle-sized molecules are "dragged" across through filtration, and fluids that do not contain such toxins are "replaced", either before or after the filter. This procedure is referred to as continuous veno-venous hemofiltration (CVVH). When both diffusion and convection are used, the procedure is referred to as continuous veno-venous hemodiafiltration (CVVHDF). Convective clearance has the advantage of being able to remove "middle-sized molecules," which has some theoretical benefit in rhabdomyolysis, sepsis, and intoxications of drugs that are "middle-sized molecules." However, most centers choose one or another based on availability. Ultrafiltration of fluid beyond what is being given (nutrition, blood products, medications, anticoagulation, and

replacement fluid for convective clearance) allows for removal of excess fluid from the patient. See **Figure 59.3**.

Prescription

Prescription components include type of fluids used for prime (blood, saline, or albumin), blood flow rate, type/mode/rate of fluids for clearance (the amount of fluids drives the dose of clearance), net ultrafiltration rate, and anticoagulation.

The type of fluid used to prime the machine is important for neonates.

1. **Saline prime:** chosen when the circuit volume is <10% of the patient's total blood volume and the patient is stable. Currently most circuits are not designed for neonates, because the circuit volume is >10% of a neonate's blood volume.
2. **Albumin prime:** chosen when the circuit volume is 10% to 15% of the patient's total blood volume.
3. **Blood prime:** chosen when the circuit volume is >15% of the patient's blood volume or for any patients not stable enough for a saline or albumin prime. It is important to note that packed red blood cells (pRBCs) are acidic, hyperkalemic, hemoconcentrated, and have a very low ionized calcium. Most programs have interventions in place to counteract acidosis, hyperkalemia, and to dilute the PRBCs, creating a more physiologic product as it is introduced to the patient (16).

There are two widely used types of anticoagulation for CRRT. A registry from 14 centers in the United States showed equal circuit survival with either anticoagulation choice, which was higher than circuits that did not have any anticoagulation. Patients who had heparin had more bleeding (14).

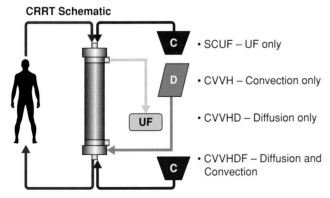

CRRT Schematic

- SCUF – UF only
- CVVH – Convection only
- CVVHD – Diffusion only
- CVVHDF – Diffusion and Convection

FIGURE 59.3 Terminology and types of clearance for the modes of continuous renal replacement therapy (CRRT). SCUF, slow continuous ultrafiltration (no convection nor diffusion); CVVH, continuous veno-venous hemofiltration (convection only); CVVHD, continuous veno-venous hemodialysis (diffusion only); CVVHDF, continuous veno-venous hemodiafiltration (both convection and diffusion).

a. **Systemic heparin:** Heparin is infused into the patient through the CRRT machine or through another type of vascular access and titrated to achieve the desired effect with the lowest dose. Anticoagulation labs (either PTT, anti-Xa, or ACT) are followed every 2 to 6 hours and heparin drip is adjusted for desired effect. It should be noted that anti-Xa labs are not commonly used in the neonatal population as anti-Xa levels can be affected by hemolysis and hyperbilirubinemia, which affect the color of the blood and the way the machine reads the result.

b. **Regional citrate:** Citrate and calcium can be used to anticoagulate the circuit. Citrate is given at the access line of the patient which will cause the ionized calcium in the circuit to become very low (desired range = 0.25 to 0.4), which prevents coagulation. Either calcium chloride or calcium gluconate infusions are given to the patient (either on the return line or via a separate central line) to achieve normal patient–ionized calcium levels (1.1 to 1.3 mmol/L). Patient, and circuit, ionized calcium labs are measured every 2 to 6 hours to monitor for therapeutic dosing. The biggest risk of citrate anticoagulation is citrate accumulation. Patients who have liver dysfunction, immature livers, or are receiving high blood flow or high clearance rates are at risk for systemic hypocalcemia.

Equipment

1. HD **access**: double-lumen or two single-lumen large-gauge centrally placed catheters.
   a. It is important to note one may have a tunneled or nontunneled line depending on length of HD needed. Generally, in the acute setting, a nontunneled catheter is placed initially.
   b. See **Table 59.3** for list of vascular catheters.
2. **Machine:** use machine available at your center
3. Heater post circuit to warm the blood before it returns to the patient
4. **Circuit:** many types with different volume choices
5. Masks, gloves, chucks, gauze
6. Sodium hypochlorite disinfectant suitable for catheters or similar
7. **Syringes:** 3 and 10 mL
8. 4 1-L bags of normal saline for priming the circuit
9. 1 Y-connector
10. Supply bag of C-clamp (if needed), Y-connector, blood spike, 100-mL NS bag used for putting the machine into recirculation if needed
11. Dialysate
12. Blood for prime if patient meets parameters (see Prescription)

Preprocedure Care

1. Obtain informed consent.
2. Obtain venous access. The largest catheter able to be placed is recommended for optimal blood flow. See **Table 59.3.**
3. Check bodyweight, vital signs, venous blood gas, pre-CRRT anticoagulation lab (see procedure), and renal function panel.
4. Monitor for infection at venous access site.

Procedure

1. Set up machine per hospital protocol.
2. Assess patency of the catheter.
3. Set up CRRT anticoagulation.
4. Connect patient to the machine.
5. Start with low blood flows to confirm patient tolerance. Ramp blood flow slowly until at goal.
6. Confirm stability of patient via vital signs.
7. Document fluid removal goals in chart.

Management

1. **Fluid removal**
   a. In general, fluid should be removed fast enough to wean the ventilator (for cases of fluid overload) without causing hypotension. Removing up to 5% of bodyweight net per day is a generous rate of removal if there is high intravascular volume. Rates should be adjusted based on patient condition and how the patient tolerates different rates.
   b. Clarification should be made with medical team to count/not count fluid boluses needed for cardiac instability and blood products.

Monitoring

1. Intake/output
2. Daily weight
3. Electrolytes q day and PRN
4. CBC q day and PRN
5. Vital signs every hour or per unit protocol, whichever is more frequent

Complications

See **Table 59.4**.

TABLE 59.4 Complications of Continuous Renal Replacement Therapy

PROBLEM (RISK)	WHAT TO DO
Bleeding	Check anticoagulation labs. Consider decreasing or stopping anticoagulation.
Vascath-site bleeding	Surgical intervention.
Line infection	Systemic antibiotics. Consider replacing line.
Electrolyte imbalances	Modify dialysate. Monitor electrolytes more frequently until stable.
Blood loss if circuit clots	Obtain CBC. Give red blood cells as needed.
Hypotension	Decrease fluid removal. Consider giving a fluid bolus. We recommend no more than 10 mL/kg.
Hypertension	Consider increasing fluid removal rate.
Hypothermia	Check the warmer used to warm the return tubing. Consider adding a Bair Hugger.
Dislodgment of catheter	Replace with new catheter.
Removal of therapeutic drugs	See **Table 59.1**.

References

1. Kaddourah A, Goldstein SL. Renal replacement therapy in neonates. *Clin Perinatol.* 2014;41(3):517–527.
2. Selewski DT, Charlton JR, Jetton JG, et al. Neonatal acute kidney injury. *Pediatrics.* 2015;136(2):e463–e473.
3. Moghal NE, Embleton ND. Management of acute renal failure in the newborn. *Semin Fetal Neonatal Med.* 2006;11(3):207–213.
4. Batshaw ML, Brusilow SW. Treatment of hyperammonemic coma caused by inborn errors of urea synthesis. *J Pediatr.* 1980;97(6):893–900.
5. Gortner L, Leupold D, Pohlandt F, et al. Peritoneal dialysis in the treatment of metabolic crises caused by inherited disorders of organic and amino acid metabolism. *Acta Paediatr Scand.* 1989;78(5):706–711.
6. Daschner M, Schaefer F. Emergency dialysis in neonatal metabolic crises. *Adv Ren Replace Ther.* 2002;9(1):63–69.
7. Arbeiter AK, Kranz B, Wingen AM, et al. Continuous venovenous haemodialysis (CVVHD) and continuous peritoneal dialysis (CPD) in the acute management of 21 children with inborn errors of metabolism. *Nephrol Dial Transplant.* 2010;25(4):1257–1265.
8. Picca S, Dionisi-Vici C, Bartuli A, et al. Short-term survival of hyperammonemic neonates treated with dialysis. *Pediatr Nephrol.* 2015;30(5):839–847.
9. Cullis B, Abdelraheem M, Abrahams G, et al. Peritoneal dialysis for acute kidney injury. *Perit Dial Int.* 2014;34(5):494–517.
10. Mattoo TK, Ahmad GS. Peritoneal dialysis in neonates after major abdominal surgery. *Am J Nephrol.* 1994;14(1):6–8.
11. Chan KL, Ip P, Chiu CS, et al. Peritoneal dialysis after surgery for congenital heart disease in infants and young children. *Ann Thorac Surg.* 2003;76(5):1443–1449.
12. Askenazi D, Ingram D, White S, et al. Smaller circuits for smaller patients: improving renal support therapy with Aquadex. *Pediatr Nephrol.* 2016;31(5):853–860.
13. Bridges BC, Askenazi DJ, Smith J, et al. Pediatric renal replacement therapy in the intensive care unit. *Blood Purif.* 2012;34(2):138–148.
14. Rodieux F, Wilbaux M, van den Anker JN, et al. Effect of kidney function on drug kinetics and dosing in neonates, infants, and children. *Clin Pharmacokinet.* 2015;54(12):1183–1204.
15. Ronnholm KA, Holmberg C. Peritoneal dialysis in infants. *Pediatr Nephrol.* 2006;21(6):751–756.
16. Fleming GM, Askenazi DJ, Bridges BC, et al. A multicenter international survey of renal supportive therapy during ECMO: The kidney intervention during extracorporeal membrane oxygenation (KIDMO) group. *ASAIO J.* 2012;58(4):407–414.

CHAPTER

60

Neonatal Hearing Screening

Catherine Demirel

A. Purpose

1. To identify hearing loss in the neonatal period in order to provide early intervention so that delay in speech and language development may be minimized.
2. To support accurate reporting by state of incidence of congenital hearing loss.

B. Background

1. The prevalence of congenital hearing loss in newborns is 1.4 (range 0 to 4.6) per 1,000 infants screened with 97% of newborns screened in the United States (1).
2. The risk of hearing loss can increase substantially when infants are exposed to certain perinatal risk factors (e.g., cytomegalovirus) or have medical conditions requiring certain interventions (e.g., extracorporeal membrane oxygenation) in intensive care nurseries (**Table 60.1**).
3. Delaying diagnosis of hearing loss can lead to significant problems in language and speech acquisition (2).

C. Indications

1. **Every newborn** should receive a hearing screen before discharge from the hospital (3,4).
   a. Currently, 47 states and the District of Columbia have passed legislation mandating universal newborn hearing screening for every infant regardless of background and risk factors (5).
   b. Every U.S. state and territory has established an Early Hearing Detection and Intervention (EHDI) program to help ensure infants receive hearing screening and intervention services (6).
   c. The Centers for Disease Control and Prevention's EHDI program recommends that infants identified by a failed hearing screen be referred for a comprehensive

audiology evaluation *as soon as possible and always before 3 months of age* (7).

2. Infants who meet **high-risk criteria** for acquiring hearing loss warrant immediate hearing screening, followed

TABLE 60.1 High Risk Criteria Associated With Hearing Loss in Childhood

- Illness or condition that requires admission of 5 days or longer to NICU
- Exposure to any of the following treatments regardless of NICU duration of stay
  - Extracorporeal membrane oxygenation
  - Ventilator
  - Ototoxic medication
  - Loop diuretics
  - Hyperbilirubinemia requiring exchange transfusion
- Stigmata or other findings associated with a syndrome known to include sensorineural or permanent conductive hearing loss
- Family history of permanent childhood sensorineural hearing loss
- Craniofacial anomalies, including those with morphologic abnormalities of the pinna and ear canal and temporal bone anomalies
- In utero infection, such as cytomegalovirus, herpes, toxoplasmosis, or rubella
- Parental or caregiver concern regarding hearing, speech, language, and developmental delay
- Postnatal infections associated with sensorineural hearing loss, including bacterial meningitis
- Syndromes associated with progressive hearing loss, such as neurofibromatosis, osteopetrosis, and Usher syndrome
- Neurodegenerative disorders, such as Hunter syndrome, or sensory motor neuropathies, such as Friedreich ataxia and Charcot–Marie–Tooth syndrome
- Head trauma
- Chemotherapy

Derived from American Academy of Pediatrics, Joint Committee on Infant Hearing. Year 2007 position statement: Principles and guidelines for early hearing detection and intervention programs. *Pediatrics.* 2007;120:898.

by ongoing monitoring. Table 60.1 lists factors known to be associated with permanent congenital, late-onset, or progressive hearing loss in childhood. *Even if they have passed their initial hearing screen,* it is critical that infants with any of these risk factors be referred to audiology after discharge so that they may continue to be monitored during the early years of language acquisition and development (5).

D. Types of Hearing Loss

1. Conductive: resulting from impaired sound transmission through ear canal, tympanic membrane, and middle ear.
2. Sensorineural: due to cochlear or retrocochlear disorder.
3. Mixed: has both conductive and sensorineural components.
4. Auditory neuropathy spectrum disorder (ANSD): resulting from normal or near normal cochlear hair cell function and absent or abnormal auditory nerve function (8).

E. Types of Hearing Screen

1. Otoacoustic emissions (OAE): A noninvasive screening tool that measures sounds generated by a functioning cochlea. A probe containing a miniature microphone delivers a sound stimulus, either click or tone, into the ear canal and records the cochlear response that travels from the cochlea back into the ear canal. This assembly is coupled to a computer for analysis of the sound in the ear canal and for processing of the otoacoustic emission. Results may be automatically analyzed and interpreted as either "pass" or "refer" for each ear. **Figure 60.1** shows an infant undergoing OAE screening. This screening tool evaluates the peripheral auditory system extending to cochlear function.

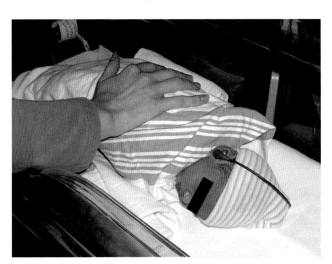

FIGURE 60.1 An infant undergoing OAE screening.

2. Automated auditory brainstem response (AABR): A noninvasive screening tool that records auditory brainstem responses (ABR) and compares them to a template representing typical results in neonates. Occlusive earphones cover the ears and emit sound stimuli into the ear canal. Electrodes are placed on the head and nape of neck to detect electrical activity from the auditory nerve and brainstem in response to the sound stimuli. A computer registers samples of the electrical activity over a fixed period of time. The averaged responses are then compared to a normal newborn template to determine if the result is a "pass" or a "refer" for each ear. **Figure 60.2** shows an infant undergoing AABR screening. In addition to assessing middle ear and cochlear activity, this test evaluates the function of the auditory nerve and auditory brainstem.

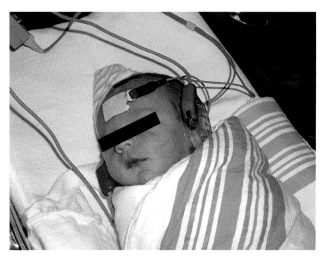

FIGURE 60.2 An infant undergoing AABR screening.

3. ABR also referred to as brainstem auditory evoked response (BAER): Not typically used as the initial hearing screen tool, BAER is a diagnostic test used to predict type and severity of hearing loss. BAER testing is conducted after a failed screening measurement. ABRs are determined in each ear for both click and tone stimuli. These sounds are presented by air (earphone) as well as bone conduction. Severity of hearing loss is expressed in decibels and described as conductive, sensorineural, or mixed.

F. Techniques

1. Both OAE and AABR screening systems can be automated: An individual only needs to be appropriately trained to set up and apply the equipment. A computer processes the incoming information and gives a readout of the result, usually as "pass" or "refer."

2. Care should be taken to attempt screening in a relatively quiet environment, as well as ensuring that the infant is resting comfortably and the ear canals are free from obvious debris, to avoid false "refer" result.

G. Specific Protocols

1. For infants admitted to **neonatal intensive care unit (NICU) for more than 5 days:** the Joint Committee on Infant Hearing recommends AABR technology as the only appropriate screening technique for use in the NICU (5). This specific population is at high risk for having ANSD which is detected by AABR but not by OAE (10,11). Immediate and direct referral should be made to an audiologist if an infant does not pass AABR in the NICU.
2. For well-nursery infants: Although OAE is more often used than AABR, both methods are widely used in many hospitals, as there is no standardization of newborn hearing screening protocols for well infants. Some hospital programs screen neonatal hearing with OAE first. If infant does not pass OAE, AABR will be used to rescreen. There are advantages and disadvantages to using OAE as the first newborn hearing screen (Section H). Infants who do not pass AABR should not be rescreened by OAE and "passed," because such infants are presumed to be at risk of having ANSD (5).
3. For infants **readmitted** to hospitals: A repeat hearing screen is recommended for infants *<1 month old,* who were readmitted to hospital, if the medical condition is associated with increased risk of hearing loss (e.g., meningitis or significant hyperbilirubinemia) (5).
4. The following timeline is a goal objective in Healthy People 2020 (5,9,11)
   a. By 1 month old: All newborns to have hearing screened
   b. By 3 months old: Those that do not pass initial screening need to have a comprehensive evaluation by an audiologist.
   c. By 6 months old: Infants with confirmed hearing loss should receive appropriate interventions.

H. Limitations

1. Infant hearing screening can be compromised by environmental noise (such as a busy intensive care unit) or infant movement. OAE screening, more so than AABR, is particularly affected by vernix occluding the ear canal, or middle ear pathology such as effusion (12).
2. OAE screening, although less time-consuming to set up and conduct, has a higher "refer" (fail) rate than AABR. The refer rates for OAE screening alone are reported to be between 5.8% and 6.5%, with refer rates using AABR screening around 3.2% (13,14). False-positive rates are reported to be approximately 2.5% to 8% in some newborn hearing screening programs (15). In particular, infants who are <48 hours old are more likely to have a "refer" result if screened with OAE, as the presence of vernix and debris in the ear canal can be a significant factor (16).
3. Some infants who pass newborn screening will later demonstrate permanent hearing loss. Although this loss may reflect delayed hearing loss, both ABR and OAE screening technology will miss some hearing loss (mild or isolated frequency losses) (5).

I. Contraindications

1. Patient has significantly atretic or total lack of external ear canal: Refer directly to pediatric audiologist.
2. Although it is certainly fair to rescreen an infant who has potentially failed screening because of excessive background noise, vernix in ear canal, etc., multiple rescreening attempts in hopes of eventually obtaining a "pass" should not be completed as they can contribute to delayed identification of congenital hearing loss. Newborns who fail the initial screening can be rescreened *once* before hospital discharge or in an outpatient setting, but not both. If the newborn fails the second screening in one or both ears, the newborn is referred for to an audiologist for outpatient diagnostic testing (17).

J. Special Circumstances

1. *Hearing parents whose infant does not pass a hearing screening:* Parents are often quite concerned to learn their infant has not passed a hearing screening. The result can be especially stress-provoking for parents whose infant may have spent a good deal of time in a NICU and may be facing additional medical concerns upon discharge. It is extremely important to remember that *a failed hearing screening is not a definitive diagnosis of hearing loss.* It is an important indicator that the infant needs immediate referral to an audiologist for further detailed evaluation, which may or may not result in a formal diagnosis of hearing loss.
2. *Deaf parents whose infant does not pass a hearing screen:* Deaf parents, especially culturally deaf individuals who use American Sign Language and identify strongly with being members of the deaf community, are often thrilled to find out that their infant may have hearing loss. This is a cultural identification. These parents are rejoicing in the fact that their infant is like them and will have a cultural place of significance in

their social world. This is often in direct opposition to the traditional medical perspective on hearing loss. The parental reaction can be frankly surprising for involved health care professionals. It is very important to realize *that these infants of culturally deaf parents are not facing the immediate crisis* of delayed language development referred to earlier. American Sign Language is a well-researched, intact language that is immediately accessible to an infant of deaf parents (16,18, 19). Although it is still extremely important to establish audiologic follow-up for these infants of deaf parents who fail a hearing screen, it is also critical to respect the potential cultural implication for such families. These parents may be celebrating in a manner very similar to hearing parents who are happy that their infant has passed the hearing screening.

K. Complications

OAE and AABR are considered to be noninvasive and safe procedures. Like any procedure that involves the application of electrode pads, mild superficial skin abrasions could possibly occur with the removal of the electrode pads after AABR testing.

References

1. Gaffney M, Eichwald J, Gaffney C, et al. Early hearing detection and intervention among infants—Hearing screening and follow-up survey, United States, 2005–2006 and 2009–2010. Centers for Disease Control and Prevention (CDC). Available at https://www.cdc.gov/
2. Ching TYC, Dillon H, Button L, et al. Age at intervention for permanent hearing loss and 5-year language outcomes. *Pediatrics*. 2017;140(3):pii: e20164274.
3. U.S. Department of Health & Human Services. Detecting Hearing loss in infants and young children. *NIH*, 2000. Available at https://www.nidcd.nih.gov/
4. American Academy of Pediatrics, Joint Committee on Infant Hearing. Year 2007 position statement: Principles and guidelines for early hearing detection and intervention programs. *Pediatrics*. 2007;120:898–921.
5. American Speech-Language-Hearing Association. State trends in hearing screening. Available at https://www.asha.org/
6. National Center for Hearing Assessment and Management Utah State University. State EHDI information. Available at http://www.infanthearing.org/
7. Centers for Disease Control and Prevention (CDC). Hearing loss in children: Recommendations and guidelines. Available at http://www.cdc.gov/
8. Xoinis K, Weirather Y, Mavoori H, et al. Extremely low birth weight infants are at high risk for auditory neuropathy. *J Perinatol*. 2007;27:718–723.
9. Norrix LW, Velenovsky DS. Auditory neuropathy spectrum disorder: a review. *J Speech Lang Hear Res*. 2014;57(4):1564–1576.
10. US Department of Health and Human Services, Office of Disease Prevention and Health Promotion. Healthy People 2020 topics and objectives: Hearing and other sensory or communication disorders. July 18, 2011. Available at http://healthypeople.gov/
11. Delaney A. Newborn hearing screening. *eMedicine*. 2016. Available at http://www.emedicine.com/
12. Vohr B, Oh W, Stewart EJ, et al. Comparison of costs and referral rates of 3 universal newborn hearing screening protocols. *J Pediatr*. 2001;139:238–244.
13. Clarke P, Iqbal M, Mitchell S. A comparison of transient-evoked otoacoustic emissions and automated auditory brainstem responses for pre-discharge neonatal hearing screening. *Int J Audiol*. 2003;42:443–447.
14. Lin H, Shu M, Lee K, et al. Comparison of hearing screening programs between one step with transient evoked otoacoustic emissions (TEOAE) and two steps with TEOAE and automated auditory brainstem response (AABR). *Laryngoscope*. 2005;115:1957–1962.
15. Clements C, Davis S. Minimizing false-positives in universal newborn hearing screenings: a simple solution. *Pediatrics*. 2001;107:(3):e29.
16. Nussbaum D, Waddy-Smith B, Doyle J. Students who are deaf and hard of hearing and use sign language: considerations and strategies for developing spoken language and literacy skills. *Semin Speech Lang*. 2012;33(4):310–321.
17. American Speech-Language-Hearing Association. Expert panel recommendations on newborn hearing screening. Available at http://www.asha.org. 2013.
18. Stokoe WC. Sign language structure. *Ann Rev Anthropol*. 1980;9:365–390.
19. Stokoe W. *A Dictionary of American Sign Language on Linguistic Principles*. Washington, DC: Gallaudet Press; 1965.

CHAPTER

61

Management of Natal and Neonatal Teeth

Priyanshi Ritwik, Kimberly K. Patterson, and Robert J. Musselman

Introduction

The occurrence of teeth in the oral cavity at birth or within the first 30 days of life is uncommon. Such teeth have been called natal and neonatal teeth, respectively. This distinction, however, is artificial and not relevant to clinical decision making. Relevant clinical inferences can be made by further describing these teeth as mature or immature based on the quality of dental tissue and degree of dental development (1). Hebling et al. (2) classified natal teeth into four clinical categories **(Table 61.1) (Figs. 61.1** to **61.3).**

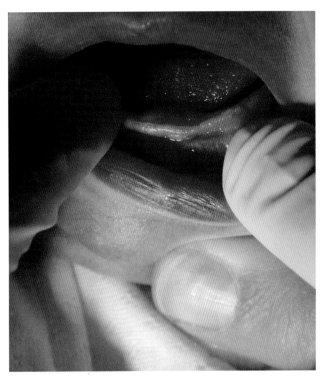

FIGURE 61.1 Normal (edentulous) alveolar ridge in neonate.

TABLE 61.1 Hebling Classification of Natal Teeth

1. Shell-shaped crown poorly fixed to the alveolus by gingival tissue with absence of a root
2. Solid crown poorly fixed to the alveolus by gingival tissue with little or no root
3. Eruption of the incisal margin of the crown through the gingival tissue
4. Edema of gingival tissue with an unerupted but palpable tooth

The reported incidence of natal and neonatal teeth varies from 1 in 2,000 to 3,500 (3). Overall, natal teeth occur more frequently than neonatal teeth at a 3:1 ratio (4). However, in a study of 18,155 infants, the reported incidence of natal and neonatal teeth was 1:716 (5). Most (85%) of natal and neonatal teeth are mandibular incisors (6,7), but natal teeth may also occur in the posterior regions of the alveolar process **(Figs. 61.4** and **61.5)** (3,8–10). Most (95%) of natal and

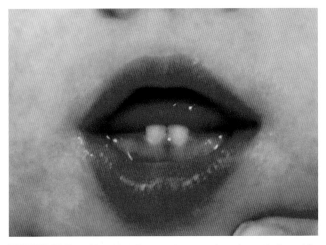

FIGURE 61.2 Hebling classification #3 neonatal tooth; not indicated for extraction.

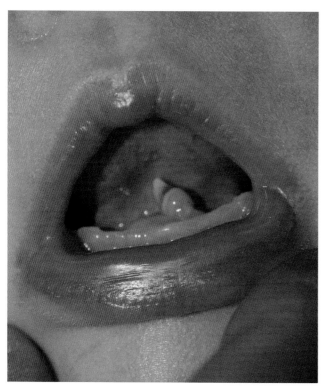

FIGURE 61.3 Hebling classification #2 natal tooth; this tooth was extracted.

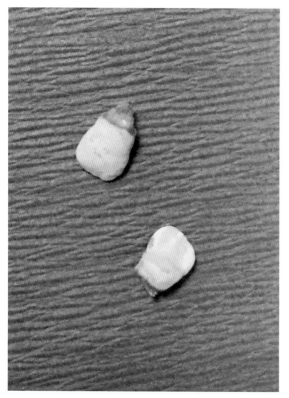

FIGURE 61.4 Hebling classification #1 mandibular natal teeth extracted by emergency room physician.

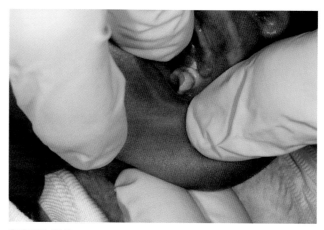

FIGURE 61.5 Maxillary posterior natal tooth in 9-day-old infant, Hebling classification #1 indicated for extraction, emphasizing evaluation of the posterior oral cavity in newborns. (Image courtesy Dr. Benjamin Hanks.)

neonatal teeth are part of the normal complement of the deciduous dentition (11,12); this indicates that supernumerary natal and neonatal teeth are rare. Hence, natal and neonatal teeth should be retained if possible. In certain instances, such teeth may need to be removed (see C).

Natal and neonatal teeth have been reported in preterm infants (13,14). The incidence of natal and neonatal teeth is higher in infants born with cleft lip and/or palate (15,16). The reported incidence ranges from 2% to 7%, with a higher incidence in cases of bilateral cleft lip and palate (15). In cases with unilateral cleft lip and palate, the natal/neonatal teeth are usually found to be present on the side of the cleft (15). This is important to identify, since the presence of natal/neonatal teeth in the cleft site will require modifications in the presurgical treatment. One study also noted the presence of natal/ neonatal teeth in the mandible, not in the site of the cleft, emphasizing the evaluation of maxillary as well as mandibular arches in infants born with cleft lip and palate. An example of a natal tooth in the site of the cleft is illustrated in **Figure 61.6**.

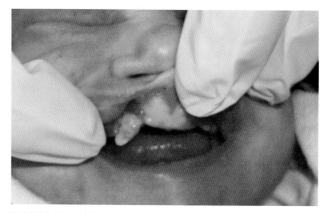

FIGURE 61.6 Hebling classification #2 natal tooth; indicated for extraction. The natal tooth was present at the site of alveolar cleft in this 3-day-old girl. This tooth was extracted with topical anesthetic.

A. Etiology

1. Superficial positioning of the primary tooth germ (12)
2. Infection and malnutrition (12)
3. Febrile illness (12)
4. Maternal exposure to toxins (polychlorinated bisphenol, polychlorinated dibenzofuran, polychlorinated dibenzo-*p*-dioxin) (17)
5. Syndrome/medical condition (**Table 61.2**) (12)

TABLE 61.2 **Conditions Associated With Higher Incidence of Natal/Neonatal Teeth**

Ellis–van Creveld syndrome
Hallermann–Streiff syndrome
Craniofacial synostosis
Multiple steatocystoma
Congenital pachyonychia
Sotos syndrome
Cleft palate
Pierre Robin anomalad

B. Clinical Presentation

There is variability in the clinical presentation of natal and neonatal teeth. Although some have normal crown shape and color and are held firmly in the alveolar process, others present as discolored microdonts with hypermobility, a feature common to the immature type of natal/neonatal teeth. The management of the patient depends on the clinical presentation.

C. Clinical Assessment

Clinical assessment should include an assessment of the tooth, oral soft tissues, and the systemic disposition of the patient.

1. Dental assessment
   a. Mobility: Tooth mobility greater than 1 mm is usually an indication for the extraction to prevent aspiration during feeding or natural tongue/lip movement.
   b. Color and shape of tooth: Discoloration and abnormal morphology indicate an immature natal/neonatal tooth, which usually will require removal.
   c. Root formation: A mobile tooth is likely to be lacking in root structure and is prone to spontaneous early exfoliation, with the risk of aspiration.
2. Soft tissue assessment
   a. Ventral surface of the tongue: Riga–Fede disease is the term given to an ulcerative granuloma formed on the ventral surface of the tongue. It results from irritation of the tongue by the sharp margins of

mandibular natal/neonatal teeth during feeding. Riga–Fede disease may appear severe, but it is a reactive and benign lesion. Excision biopsy is rarely required and the lesion regresses after conservative treatment has been rendered (18).
   b. Natal and neonatal teeth should be differentiated from cystic lesions such as Bohn nodules (gingival cysts of the newborn, located on the hard plate or alveolar ridges) and Epstein pearls (palatal cysts of the newborn, found along the midline), by both palpation and location in the infant's mouth. Bohn nodules and Epstein pearls are firm and have a smooth, rounded surface. There will usually be several nodules/pearls visible. Each of these entities will spontaneously resorb, and thus no treatment is required.
   c. Gingival tissue: Soft tissue around the natal/neonatal tooth should be examined for presence of inflammation or granulomatous lesion, caused by irritation by the sharp cervical margins of an immature tooth.
3. General assessment
   The problem-focused evaluation should be for any interference with feeding and the possibility of trauma to the ventral surface of the tongue, degree of mobility and maturity of the dental tissue. **Table 61.2** lists systemic conditions associated with higher incidence of natal/neonatal teeth.
4. **Indications for extractions:**
   a. Hypermobility of natal and neonatal tooth
   b. Discoloration or dysmorphology of the visible tooth crown
   c. Gingival irritation from natal and neonatal tooth

D. Precautions

1. The initial question in management of natal teeth is whether extraction is indicated. Indiscriminate extraction of natal/neonatal teeth is discouraged (19). Treatment should be individualized to each tooth and to each infant.
2. Should extraction be indicated, it must be confirmed that the patient has received the appropriate dose of vitamin K at birth (12). Current literature supports the extraction of mobile natal tooth at 10 days or later after birth to ensure establishment of appropriate intestinal flora to produce vitamin K, essential for the production of prothrombin by the liver, unless there is significant risk of aspiration (6,11), at which time sooner extraction may be warranted using additional precautions.
3. A detailed family history should be obtained, to rule out inherited coagulopathy.
4. Following the extraction, the socket should be curetted to remove odontogenic tissue (see F).
5. Long-term care: Whether the patient receives conservative restorative treatment or extraction, the parents should be encouraged to maintain regular dental appointments with a pediatric dentist. This referral supports monitoring

of the tooth for function and mobility or the residual extraction site for proper healing and providing parental guidance in oral hygiene practices for their infant.

E. Technique

Nonextraction Case

If the tooth is firmly anchored in the gingival tissues and appears of normal color and shape, extraction is not indicated.

1. Should the mother complain of discomfort while breast-feeding, the use of a breast pump and bottle feeding of expressed breast milk should be encouraged.
2. If the patient presents with Riga–Fede disease, a pediatric dentist should be consulted. The sharp margins of the tooth can be altered using photopolymerized dental composite restorative resin or glass ionomer cement to create a smooth contour. This results in spontaneous resolution of the tongue lesion (20,21).
3. Pain relief and faster healing may be accomplished by carefully applying triamcinolone acetonide (22).
4. If it is determined that extraction is not warranted, the parents must receive guidance on infant oral health. The tooth/teeth should be brushed gently with a soft-bristled toothbrush and a smear of fluoridated toothpaste in the morning and at night after the last feeding. The infant should not be put to sleep in a crib with a feeding bottle containing formula, milk, or juice.

Extraction Case

Preprocedure recommendations include:

1. Verification of vitamin K supplementation at birth
2. At least 10 days of age unless excess mobility results in risk of aspiration
3. Evaluation for heart disease, anemia, G6PD and NADH reductase deficiencies (23).
   a. **Equipment**
      (1) 2- × 2-in gauze piece
      (2) Cotton-tipped applicator
      (3) Topical anesthetic lidocaine 2% gel is the local anesthetic of choice. Topical oral anesthetic agents containing benzocaine should be avoided due to the risk of methemoglobinemia (24)
      (4) Blunt-nosed sterile surgical scissors and small surgical curette
   b. **Technique**
      (1) After drying the gingiva around the tooth with gauze, use a cotton-tipped applicator to apply a smear of topical anesthetic to the soft tissue attachment encircling the tooth.
      (2) Hold the tooth between thumb and index finger in gauze square and gently remove the tooth by rotational movement, with the tooth secure within the gauze square (**Figs. 61.7** to **61.9**).

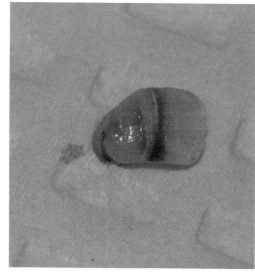

FIGURE 61.7 The natal tooth that was removed by grasping the tooth with gloved fingers, holding the tooth with a 2- × 2-in gauze square.

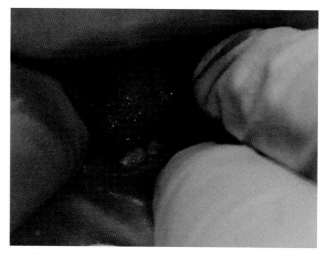

FIGURE 61.8 Healing of extraction site in 12 hours after extraction of two mandibular natal teeth.

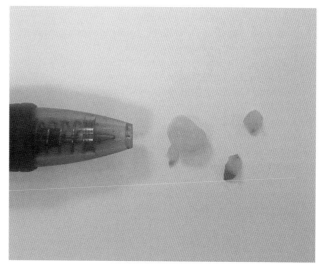

FIGURE 61.9 Extracted tooth fragments and soft tissue juxtaposed to ball point pen tip for size reference. (Image courtesy Dr. Benjamin Hanks.)

(3) Blunt-nosed scissors can be used to cut the connecting tissue if it is very fibrous or tenacious.

(4) If a small surgical curette is available, the extraction site should be gently curetted to remove residual odontogenic tissue.

If in the medical professional's clinical judgment, the tooth cannot be removed by the above technique, then the infant needs to be referred to a pediatric dentist for evaluation and possible extraction.

F. Complications of Extraction

1. Tissue tags comprising dental papilla and/or Hertwig epithelial root sheath remain in the extraction socket (25). These tissues may continue to form dental hard tissues, that is, dentin and root structure (25,26). These aberrant dental hard tissues may interfere with the normal eruption of adjacent primary teeth (25).

2. There has been one published report of difficulty in achieving hemostasis using localized pressure after the extraction of a natal tooth. This patient received microfibrillar collagen hemostat over the extraction site (3).

3. The development of postextraction pyogenic granuloma (27) and hamartoma (28) has been reported.

4. In 9% of patients with natal/neonatal teeth associated with alveolar cleft, a second tooth-like structure may develop later. This emphasizes the necessity to maintain regular dental evaluations and examinations for these patients following conservative or surgical management of natal or neonatal teeth.

References

1. Spouge JD, Feasby WH. Erupted teeth in the newborn. *Oral Surg Oral Med Oral Pathol.* 1966;22:198–208.
2. Hebling J, Zuanon ACC, Vianna DR. Dente natal—a case of natal teeth. *Odontol Clin.* 1997;7:37–40.
3. Brandt SK, Shapiro SD, Kittle PE. Immature primary molars in the newborn. *Pediatr Dent.* 1983;5:210–213.
4. Haberland C, Persing J. Neonatal teeth in a 6-week-old baby with bilateral cleft lip and palate: case report and review of the literature. *Oral Surg Oral Med Oral Pathol Oral Radiol Endod.* 2010;110:e20–e21.
5. Kates GA, Needleman HL, Holmes LB. Natal and neonatal teeth: a clinical study. *J Am Dent Assoc.* 1984;109:441–443.
6. American Academy of Pediatric Dentistry. Guideline on management considerations for pediatric oral surgery and oral pathology. *Pediatr Dent.* 2016;38(6):315–324.
7. Badenhoff J, Gorlin RJ. Natal and neonatal teeth: Folklore and fact. *Pediatrics.* 1963;32:1087–1093.
8. Friend GW, Mincer HH, Carruth KR, et al. Natal primary molar: case report. *Pediatr Dent.* 1991;13:173–175.
9. Masatomi Y, Abe K, Ooshima T. Unusual multiple natal teeth: case report. *Pediatr Dent.* 1991;13:170–172.
10. Kumar A, Grewal H, Verma M. Posterior natal teeth. *J Indian Soc Pedod Prev Dent.* 2011;29:68–70.
11. Leung AK, Robson WL. Natal teeth: a review. *J Natl Med Assoc.* 2006;98(2):226–228.
12. Cunha RF, Boer FA, Torriani DD, et al. Natal and neonatal teeth: review of the literature. *Pediatr Dent.* 2001;23:158–162.
13. Dahake PT, Shelke AU, Kale YJ, et al. Natal teeth in premature dizygotic twin girls. *BMJ Case Rep.* 2015;2015. doi:10.1136/bcr-2015-211930.
14. Cizmeci MN, Kanburoglu MK, Uzun FK, et al. Neonatal tooth in a preterm infant. *Eur J Pediatr.* 2013;172(2):279.
15. Yilmaz RB, Cakan DG, Mesgarzadeh N. Prevalence and management of natal/neonatal teeth in cleft lip and palate patients. *Eur J Dent.* 2016;10(1):54–58.
16. Kadam M, Kadam D, Bhandary S, et al. Natal and neonatal teeth among cleft lip and palate infants. *Natl J Maxillofac Surg.* 2013;4(1):73–76.
17. Alaluusua S, Kiviranta H, Leppaniemi A, et al. Natal and neonatal teeth in relation to environmental toxicants. *Pediatr Res.* 2002;52:652–655.
18. Hong P. Riga-Fede disease: traumatic lingual ulceration in an infant. *J Pediatr.* 2015;167:204.
19. Watt J. Needless extractions. *Br Dent J.* 2004;197:170.
20. Slayton R. Treatment alternatives for sublingual traumatic ulceration (Riga-Fede disease). *Pediatr Dent.* 2000;22:413–414.
21. Volpato LE, Simoles CA, Simoles F, et al. Riga-Fede disease associated with natal teeth: two different approaches in the same case. *Case Rep Dent.* 2015;2015:234961.
22. Seminario AL, Ivancakova R. Natal and neonatal teeth. *Acta Med (Hradec Kralove).* 2004;47:229–233.
23. Bayat A, Kosinski RW. Methemoglobinemia in a newborn: a case report. *Pediatr Dent.* 2011;33:252–254.
24. U.S. Food and Drug Administration. FDA Drug Safety Communication: reports of a rare, but serious and potentially fatal adverse effect with the use of over-the-counter (OTC) benzocaine gels and liquids applied to the gums or mouth. http://www.fda.gov/Drugs/DrugSafety/ucm250024.htm. Accessed July 1, 2011.
25. Nedley MP, Stanley RT, Cohen DM. Extraction of natal teeth can leave odontogenic remnants. *Pediatr Dent.* 1995;17:457.
26. Kim SH, Cho YA, Kim MS, et al. Complication after extraction of natal teeth with continued growth of dental papilla. *Pediatr Dent.* 2016;38:137–142.
27. Muench MG, Layton S, Wright JM. Pyogenic granuloma associated with a natal tooth: case report. *Pediatr Dent.* 1992;14:265–267.
28. Oliveira LB, Tamay TK, Wanderley MT, et al. Gingival fibrous hamartoma associated with natal teeth. *J Clin Pediatr Dent.* 2005;29:249–252.

Reducing the Dislocated Newborn Nasal Septum

Christine M. Clark, Kelly A. Scriven, and Earl H. Harley, Jr.

A. Background

Transient nasal deformations can occur secondary to fetal compression in utero or during delivery, and they typically resolve within the first several days of life without intervention (**Fig. 62.1**). In some cases, fetal compression during delivery can be sufficient to result in true dislocation of the nasal septum (**Fig. 62.2**). The incidence of true nasal septal dislocations is estimated to range from 0.6% to 4%, and correction within the first 3 to 4 days of life for severe septal dislocations with nasal obstruction is suggested to ensure the best possible long-term outcomes; however, observation with serial examinations can be considered in less severe cases without obstruction (1–7).

Physical examination of the newborn can distinguish between transient compression deformity and true dislocation. In order to make this distinction, gentle pressure should be applied to the nasal tip. If the septum moves from the midline at the base, dislocation should be suspected, as the compressed septum will not demonstrate this mobility. Additionally, application of gentle pressure will restore normal nasal anatomy in cases of compression deformity; however, this is not observed with true septal dislocations. Nasal endoscopy can also be performed to differentiate between the two.

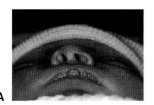 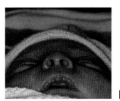

A   **B**

FIGURE 62.1 Nasal compression without septal deviation. **A:** Shortly after birth, the nose is asymmetrical from simple compression with an angled septum at rest. **B:** The septum assumes its normal angle. (From Fletcher MA. *Physical Diagnosis in Neonatology*. Philadelphia, PA: Lippincott-Raven; 1998:211.)

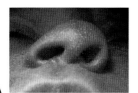 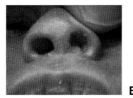

A   **B**

FIGURE 62.2 A: At rest, it is difficult to distinguish a true deviation. **B:** Attempts to restore normal anatomy are unsuccessful as the septum remains deviated at the base. (From Fletcher MA. *Physical Diagnosis in Neonatology*. Philadelphia, PA: Lippincott-Raven; 1998:211.)

B. Indications

1. Severe septal dislocation with presence of nasal obstruction.
2. To prevent difficulty with breathing and feeding, and to avoid epistaxis, malocclusion, and nasal obstruction.
3. Reduction in the newborn period may obviate the need for future surgery.

C. Contraindications

1. Concomitant nasal or midline congenital anomalies necessitating more extensive management
2. Posterior septal dislocation as determined by rhinoscopy
3. Small nasal cavity unfavorable to instrumentation with septal forceps

D. Equipment

1. Modified Walsham septum forceps or other septal forceps of appropriate size **(Fig. 62.3)**

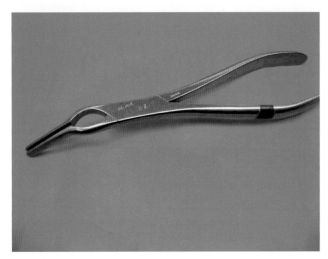

FIGURE 62.3 Walsham septum forceps.

E. Preprocedural Considerations

1. **The dislocated nasal septum should be reduced within the first 3 to 4 days of life.**
2. A thorough otolaryngologic evaluation for refractory dislocations and/or concomitant facial anomalies should be performed.
3. Placement of an oral airway or large-bore nasogastric tube to separate the tongue from the palate and facilitate oral respiration should be considered, as many newborns are obligate nasal breathers.

F. Technique

1. First, ensure that the infant's head is adequately restrained.
2. Carefully advance the septal forceps past the columella and into the nares along the anterior aspect of the cartilaginous septum. The forceps should be advanced to a depth of approximately 0.5 to 1.0 cm and should not be passed beyond the inferior aspect of the middle turbinate. Advancement should always be gentle and not forced **(Fig. 62.4)**.
3. The forceps should be carefully closed onto the septum. In order to move the septum into alignment with the nasal groove on the vomer, pressure should be directed on the lower edges of the forceps blades toward the midline. The forceps may need to be directed slightly upward to lift the inferior aspect of

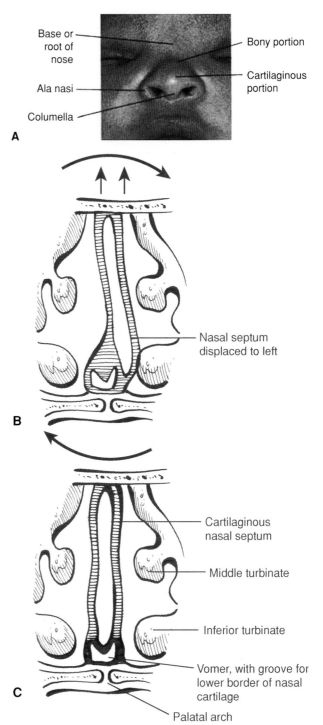

FIGURE 62.4 A: Landmarks of nasal anatomy. **B:** The cartilaginous nasal septum displaced to the left from the ridge on the vomer. *Large arrows* indicate the direction of turn of the forceps blades needed to replace the septum into the groove; *small arrows* indicate the concurrent upward pull. **C:** The septum postreplacement. (A: From Fletcher MA. *Physical Diagnosis in Neonatology.* Philadelphia, PA: Lippincott-Raven; 1998:211.)

the septum over the vomer and into the spinal groove **(Fig. 62.4B,C)**.

4. Reexamine the nasal septum to ensure adequate reduction.

G. Complications

1. Epistaxis
2. Injury to the septum and/or adjacent nasal structures
3. Injury to the skull base leading to cerebrospinal fluid (CSF) leak (extremely uncommon complication)
4. Persistent septal dislocation

References

1. Kawalski H, Spiewak P. How septum deformations in newborns occur. *Int J Pediatr Otorhinolaryngol.* 1998;44(1):23–30.
2. Podoshin L, Gertner R, Fradis M, et al. Incidence and treatment of deviation of the nasal septum in newborns. *Ear Nose Throat J.* 1991;70:485.
3. Tasca I, Compradretti GC. Immediate correction of nasal septal dislocation in newborns: long-term results. *Am J Rhinol.* 2004;18(1):47–51.
4. Cashman EC, Farrell T, Shandilya M. Nasal birth trauma: a review of appropriate treatment. *Int J Otolaryngol.* 2010; 2010:752974.
5. Hughes CA, Harley EH, Milmoe G, et al. Birth trauma in the head and neck. *Arch Otolaryngol Head Neck Surg.* 1999;125(2): 193–199.
6. Harugop AS, Mudhol RS, Hajare PS, et al. Prevalence of nasal septal deviation in new-borns and its precipitating factors: a cross-sectional study. *Indian J Otolaryngol Head Neck Surg.* 2012;64(3):248–251.
7. Jeppesen F, Windfeld I. Dislocation of the nasal septal cartilage in the newborn. Aetiology, spontaneous course and treatment. *Acta Obstet Gynecol Scand.* 1972;51:5–15.

CHAPTER

63

Lingual Frenotomy

Kelly A. Scriven and Earl H. Harley, Jr.

A. Definitions

1. **Lingual frenulum**—a fold of mucosa connecting the midline of the inferior surface of the tongue to the floor of the mouth (1). Generally thin, membranous, and avascular in the newborn (**Fig. 63.1**).

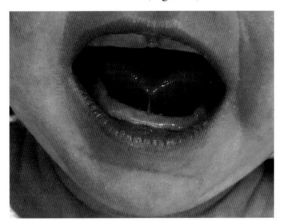

FIGURE 63.1 Newborn with significant anterior type 1 ankyloglossia. Note heart-shaped tongue, inability to raise tongue tip toward roof of mouth. (Photo courtesy of Earl Harley, MD.)

2. **Ankyloglossia (tongue tie)**—a congenital oral abnormality, characterized by an abnormally short, thick, and/or tight lingual frenulum (1). "Ankyloglossia" derives from the Greek *ankylos*—crooked, and *glossa*—tongue.
   (a) Many different variations of tongue tie with differing degrees of severity, location, and clinical significance.
   (b) May restrict mobility of the tongue tip and cause breastfeeding difficulties for the infant, as well as maternal complications such as sore nipples and mastitis.
   (c) Tongue tie has a genetic predisposition with increased incidence in first born males with a male to female ratio of 2.6:1 (2,3).
   (d) Incidence of ankyloglossia in infants has been estimated between 0.1% and 12.1% (4).

3. **Anterior tongue tie**—anterior position of the lingual frenulum, usually very thin and membranous, with resultant restricted tongue movement (up to 94% of tongue ties) (1).
   (a) Generally readily apparent on physical examination.
   (b) Can also be divided into type 1 (tongue is tethered to the floor of the mouth anteriorly, creating a heart-shaped tongue, **Fig. 63.1**) and type 2 (the tongue is proximally tethered with restricted tongue elevation, **Fig. 63.2**) (3).

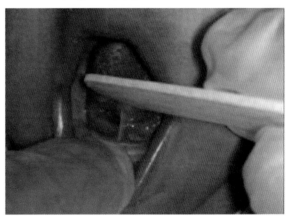

FIGURE 63.2 Newborn with type 2 ankyloglossia. (Photo courtesy of Earl Harley, MD.)

4. **Posterior tongue tie**—more subtle, and thus more difficult to diagnose, as anterior tongue tip usually has free movement; however, overall tongue movement may be restricted.
   (a) If not visible, can be palpated with gloved finger as "bump" or thick band at the ventral surface of the tongue.
   (b) Can also be subdivided into type 3 (tongue appears normal, but mobility limited by a short fibrous band halfway to the tip of the tongue) and type 4 (limited tongue mobility in the setting of a fibrous limitation at the most posterior aspect of the frenulum) (2,3).

5. **Lingual frenotomy (tongue clipping)**—a minor surgical procedure, appropriate for treatment of significant ankyloglossia in infants.
   a. "Frenotomy" involves isolation of the frenulum, which is cut with sharp instruments down to the base of muscle.
   b. Can be accomplished at the bedside in the neonatal intensive care unit or postpartum unit, or in an outpatient clinic setting by a trained physician (4).
6. **Frenuloplasty, frenulectomy, or frenectomy**—more complicated surgical procedures in which the lingual frenulum is excised, incorporating flap elevation or Z-plasty techniques.
   a. Reserved for older children, adults, or infants with a complicated lingual frenulum, such as a thickened frenulum containing genioglossus muscle or a "complete" ankyloglossia in which tongue is fused to the floor of the mouth. Performed in the operating room, by an otolaryngologist or oral surgeon, under conscious sedation or general anesthesia.
   b. Other techniques involve cautery with the use of carbon dioxide, erbium:YAG, or Nd:YAG lasers, requiring a trained laser professional (4–6).

B. Purpose

1. *Lingual frenotomy:* performed when the presence of ankyloglossia restricts or impedes an infant's ability to successfully latch.
   a. Most common in breastfeeding infants.
   b. Occasionally required in infants using an artificial teat (7).
2. Other problems related to ankyloglossia that may manifest in older children and adults, for which prophylactic frenotomy in infancy (when procedure is relatively simple and safe) should be considered:
   a. *Mechanical problems:* gingival recession, malocclusion, dental problems, difficulty cleaning the oral vestibule, difficulty playing an instrument, difficulty consuming ice cream.
   b. Articulation errors in speech (8,9).

C. Background

1. There is much controversy surrounding ankyloglossia regarding:
   a. *Definitions:* range from vague descriptions of a tongue that functions with a less than normal range of activity to specific description of a frenulum that is short, thick, muscular, or fibrotic (2–4,7,8)
   b. Clinical significance
      (1) Prior to the introduction and widespread use of breast milk substitutes in the early 20th century, breastfeeding was necessary for survival.

(a) Release of tongue tie was commonly performed by the midwife at delivery (2).
(b) Tongue tie does not generally pose a problem for the more passive process of bottle feeding.
(c) With a decrease in breastfeeding rates, frenotomy became unnecessary for infant feeding.
(d) However, more recent research about the benefits of breastfeeding on both mothers and infants began to emerge in the 1980s and 1990s. These benefits have led to more targeted attempts to resolve breastfeeding problems in infants, such as ankyloglossia (2,4,7).
   c. Need for surgical intervention
      (1) Some infants with tongue tie can breastfeed successfully with no surgical intervention (1,4). Nonsurgical interventions include nipple shields, changes in positioning, and tongue stretching exercises.
      (2) Each breastfeeding dyad is a unique combination of many factors, including the infant's intraoral structures, adequacy of suckling, and the size, shape, and elasticity of maternal nipples.
      (3) An emerging body of literature suggests that, for those mother–baby dyads who are experiencing difficulty breastfeeding associated with the presence of tongue tie, frenotomy is a safe, effective, and immediate means of providing relief of symptoms and supporting breastfeeding.
   d. Timing of surgical intervention
      (1) Controversy exists regarding when exactly frenotomy should be performed, and in what setting.
      (2) Historically, frenotomy was performed at birth; however, more recently the procedure has been performed safely in children as old as 5 years of age.
      (3) Emerging literature suggests frenotomy to be more effective in the 1st week of life (*Section K*).

D. Indications

1. In the neonate, presence of ankyloglossia, usually in a breastfeeding infant, causing one or more of the following:
   a. Maternal nipple trauma, pain, nipple/breast infection
   b. Poor latch
   c. Ineffective suckling, continuous suckling
   d. Weight loss, poor infant weight gain, failure to thrive
   e. Early weaning
      (1) An analysis of online breastfeeding forums showed that mothers experienced frustration

from providers' overlooking or missing the diagnosis of ankyloglossia. Similarly, they noted both physical and subjective improvement after frenotomy (2,7,8).

E. Contraindications

1. Presence of genioglossus muscle or vascular tissue in the frenulum, with no thin membranous tissue for incision. Refer to appropriate surgeon for consideration for frenuloplasty.
2. Known bleeding disorder (e.g., hemophilia). Refer to otolaryngologist for repair in the operating room.

F. Limitations

1. If the difficulty with breastfeeding was not caused by the tongue tie, release of the tongue tie will not result in improvement. Infants with multifactorial causes of difficulty feeding may derive little benefit from the procedure (4).
2. Even when tongue tie is the cause, attention must be paid to latch and suckling after release to ensure the best outcome.
   a. Postfrenotomy, it is not unusual for a period of suck training, by an appropriately trained lactation specialist, to be required to correct abnormal tongue movements.
   b. Follow-up with a trained lactation specialist is extremely important for breastfeeding success.

G. Equipment

Sterile

1. Iris or tenotomy scissors
2. Grooved retractor (optional—see below) **(Fig. 63.3)**

3. Gloves
4. Gauze pads
5. 24% oral sucrose (optional)
6. Topical anesthetic gel for oral use (optional—see below)
7. Cotton swab
8. Topical Neo-Synephrine, Gelfoam, or silver nitrate sticks (optional—see below)

Nonsterile

1. Blanket or towel for swaddling

H. Precautions

1. Ensure, by careful examination of the frenulum, that there is no vascular or muscular tissue in the field of incision. Transillumination may be used to enhance visualization.
2. Avoid submandibular duct orifices lateral to the frenulum.

I. Technique (1,2,4,10)

1. Obtain informed consent including risks of no benefit and bleeding (see Chapter 3).
2. Firmly swaddle the infant in a blanket or towel.
3. Infant is held in a firm, upright position by parent or assistant, with assistant holding the infants head to prevent lateral motion.
4. Stand on right side of infant if right handed, or directly in front of the infant.
5. Visualize the frenulum by positioning light source to the left of the infant, allowing essentially transillumination of the frenulum.
6. Retraction can be performed by several methods. One involves placement of two gloved fingers of the left hand

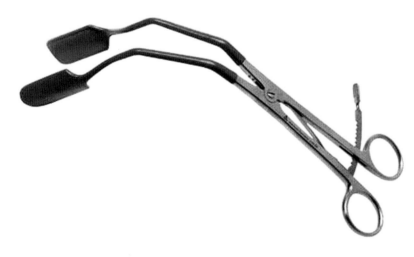

FIGURE 63.3 Grooved retractor used to raise tongue. Iris scissors make incision. (Photo provided courtesy of CooperSurgical, Inc.)

below the tongue, on either side of the midline. Alternatively, a grooved retractor or two cotton-tipped applicators can be used to push the tongue up toward the roof of the mouth, exposing the frenulum. When retracted, inspect the frenulum for any vascular or muscular structures. Identify the submandibular ducts, located on the floor of the mouth, and avoid disruption.

7. Utilization of local anesthesia (optional).
   a. With no anesthesia, there is minimal, brief discomfort because the frenulum is poorly innervated.
   b. Topical anesthetic gel can be applied to the frenulum with a cotton swab.

8. Divide the membranous frenulum with sterile iris or tenotomy scissors.
   a. *For anterior tongue tie*
      (1) Begin at the free border and proceed posteriorly, taking care to stay close to the ventral surface of the tongue and away from the floor of mouth. This avoids injury to the submandibular and sublingual salivary ducts.
      (2) In most cases, a single cut will free the tongue sufficiently.
      (3) Occasionally, two to three small, sequential cuts (1 to 3 mm) are required.
      (4) Each subsequent cut allows improved retraction and visualization for the next cut.
      (5) The posterior limit of dissection is the genioglossus muscle and the vascular bundle. At this point, the tongue is freed and can extend past lower alveolar ridge and lips and elevate to the roof of the mouth, which is crucial for breastfeeding.
      (6) Observe and palpate for posterior tongue tie, which may have been obscured by anterior tongue tie. If present, the next step may be required.
   b. *For posterior tongue tie*
      Should be performed only by practitioners with experience in treating posterior tongue tie, given proximity to genioglossus muscle and neurovascular bundle. Damage to muscular structures can cause postoperative pain, and disruption of neurovascular bundle can cause bleeding.
      (1) Visualize and palpate the sublingual area and ventral surface of the tongue. A membranous small band may or may not be visible.
      (2) Diagnosis is made by palpation. With the index finger nail down push the midline posteriorly. A posterior tongue tie will feel like a vertical tight band under the mucous membrane.
      (3) Clip in center of band with iris scissors as narrowly as possible until diamond shape opens **(Fig. 63.4)**.

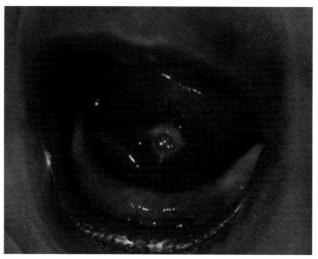

FIGURE 63.4 Completed frenotomy of posterior tongue tie with open diamond evident. (Photograph courtesy of Kimberlie Furness.)

      (4) Palpate edges of the "diamond." There can be taut edges laterally, which may need a clip of another millimeter until no longer taut and "diamond" is wide open.

9. Control any bleeding (usually minimal) with direct pressure applied with a sterile gauze pad. There is generally more bleeding with posterior frenulum clipping. If excessive bleeding (more than 3 to 5 mL):
   a. Continue to apply pressure. The steps below are rarely required.
   b. Apply topical Neo-Synephrine or oxymetazoline as vasoconstrictor on cotton swab, *or*
   c. Apply small piece of Gelfoam soaked in Neo-Synephrine *or*
   d. Dab with silver nitrate stick

10. Inform mother that breastfeeding may resume immediately. This helps stop bleeding and comforts the infant. Mothers frequently note an immediate and dramatic improvement in breastfeeding, with reduced discomfort, improved latch, stronger suckling, and absence of the clicking sounds frequently produced by the tongue-tied infant while breastfeeding. Occasionally, continued suck training with a lactation consultant is required. Encourage the mother to breastfeed exclusively when possible, as more passive bottle feeding may discourage the infant from breastfeeding.

11. Antibiotic therapy is not required.

12. Postoperatively, a white fibrin clot will form. Reassure parents that this is not a sign of infection.

13. Arrange follow-up in 1 to 2 weeks to check healing and reassess the infant's weight gain and latch.

14. Instruct the mother to consult her pediatrician immediately for weight loss, inability to feed, fevers, or other concerns.

15. Instruct the mother to perform massage at the surgical site two to three times per day in the healing stage to prevent postoperative scarring.

J. Complications (1,2,4,11,12)

1. Extremely rare when performed by a practitioner familiar and comfortable with the procedure.
    a. Excessive bleeding virtually never occurs unless deep lingual arteries and/or veins are severed. There have been rare case reports of postoperative hemorrhage resulting in hypovolemic shock.
    b. *Infection:* extremely rare.
    c. *Damage to tongue:* extremely rare, could be due to continued dissection beyond the genioglossus muscle, or continued dissection beyond the open "diamond" in posterior tongue tie.
    d. *Damage to submandibular ducts:* extremely rare, can be avoided by performing frenotomy as close to the ventral tongue as possible.
    e. Recurrent ankyloglossia due to excessive scarring.
        (1) Most common complication.
        (2) Often due to not performing tongue exercises and massage postoperatively.
        (3) Typically this is less severe than the original presentation of ankyloglossia, and is amenable to revision surgery.
    f. Glossoptosis (tongue collapse posteriorly) due to excessive tongue mobility. Generally only a concern in infants with underlying glossoptosis (such as from Pierre Robin sequence).

K. Outcomes (2–4,7–9,13–17)

1. Though frenotomy has been performed for centuries, outcomes data on the subject have been limited in the past decade.
2. Frenotomy appears to effectively decrease breastfeeding difficulties by decreasing compression of the nipple from the tongue and leading to a better latch, more effective feeding, and decreased maternal pain.
    a. Studies to date have shown significant improved scores in infant breastfeeding assessments after frenotomy has been performed.
    b. In one study, mothers strongly believed frenotomy benefited their child's ability to breastfeed, and were more inclined to continue breastfeeding. Mothers noted decreased pain and discomfort with breastfeeding after the procedure.
3. Additionally, mothers have noted increased benefit when frenotomy is performed in the 1st week of life in some series, compared to those performed later.
4. Other benefits to frenotomy noted in the literature include earlier introduction of solid foods, improved speech, and improved oral hygiene and ability to eat foods such as ice cream. Further studies are needed to evaluate the long-term effects of frenotomy.

References

1. Hong P, Lago D, Seargeant J, et al. Defining ankyloglossia: a case series of anterior and posterior tongue ties. *Int J Pediatr Otorhinolaryngol.* 2010;74:1003.
2. Steehler MW, Steehler MK, Harley EH. A retrospective review of frenotomy in neonates and infants with feeding difficulties. *Int J Pediatr Otorhinolaryngol.* 2012;76:1236–1240.
3. Coryllos E, Genna CW, Salloum AC. Congenital tongue-tie and its impact on breastfeeding. *American Academy of Pediatrics Newsletter (Summer).* 2004;1–6.
4. Walsh J, Tunkel D. Diagnosis and treatment of ankyloglossia in newborns and infants: a review. *JAMA Otolaryngol Head Neck Surg.* 2017;143(10):1032–1039.
5. Choi YS, Lim JS, Han KT, et al. Ankyloglossia correction: Z-plasty combined with genioglossus myotomy. *J Craniofac Surg.* 2011;22(6):2238–2240.
6. Chiniforush N, Ghadimi S, Yarahmadi N, et al. Treatment of ankyloglossia with carbon dioxide (CO2) laser in a pediatric patient. *J Lasers Med Sci.* 2013;4(1):53–55.
7. Srinivasan A, Dobrich C, Mitnick H, et al. Ankyloglossia in breastfeeding infants: the effect of frenotomy on maternal nipple pain and latch. *Breastfeed Med.* 2006;1(4):216–224.
8. Walls A, Pierce M, Wang H, et al. Parental perception of speech and tongue mobility in three year olds after neonatal frenotomy. *Int J Pediatr Otorhinolaryngol.* 2014;78:128–131.
9. Vaz AC, Bai PM. Lingual frenulum and malocclusion: an overlooked tissue or a minor issue. *Indian J Dent Res.* 2015; 26(5):488–492.
10. Buryk M, Bloom D, Shope T. Efficacy of neonatal release of ankyloglossia: a randomized trial. *Pediatrics.* 2011;128:280–288.
11. Tracy LF, Gomez G, Overton LJ, et al. Hypovolemic shock after labial and lingual frenulectomy: a report of two cases. *Int J Pediatr Otorhinolaryngol.* 2017;100:223–224.
12. Genther DJ, Skinner ML, Bailey PJ, et al. Airway obstruction after lingual frenulectomy in two infants with Pierre-Robin Sequence. *Int J Pediatr Otorhinolaryngol.* 2015;79(9):1592–1594.
13. Kumar RK, Nayana Prabha PC, Kumar C, et al. Ankyloglossia in Infancy: an Indian Experience. *Indian Pediatr.* 2017;54(2): 125–127.
14. Wong K, Patel P, Cohen MB, et al. Breastfeeding infants with ankyloglossia: insight into mothers' experiences. *Breastfeed Med.* 2017;12:86–90.
15. Geddes DT, Langton DB, Gollow I, et al. Frenulotomy for breastfeeding infants with ankyloglossia: effect on milk removal and sucking mechanism as imaged by ultrasound. *Pediatrics.* 2008;122:188–194.
16. O'Callahan C, Macary S, Clemente S. The effects of office-based frenotomy for anterior and posterior ankyloglossia on breastfeeding. *Int J Pediatr Otorhinolaryngol.* 2013;77:827–832.
17. Ricke LA, Baker NJ, Maldon-Kay DJ, et al. Newborn tongue-tie: prevalence and effect on breastfeeding. *J Am Board Fam Pract.* 2005;18:1–7.

A

Appendix

Chapter 2
Checklists for Selected Procedures

The following checklists are provided to complement the chapters. They may be used for training purposes or to ensure quality and consistency in performing procedures.

SUPRAPUBIC BLADDER TAP CHECKLIST	
STEPS OF PROCEDURE	**COMMENTS**
1.	No contraindications—voided <1 hr ago, dehydration, distended belly, uncorrected bleeding problem	
2.	Time out—right patient, right procedure, consent Application of local anesthetic cream	
3.	Check equipment ☐ Mask/sterile gloves ☐ Small sterile gauze ☐ Antiseptic swab sticks × 3 (povidone iodine) ☐ Clean water ☐ Sterile towel or aperture drape ☐ Small adhesive bandage ☐ 3 mL syringe ☐ Transillumination light or portable ultrasound (optional) ☐ 22-gauge × 1.5-in needle or butterfly needle ☐ Sterile specimen bottle with cap	
4.	Have assistant restrain infant in supine frog leg position	
5.	Locate landmarks: palpate top of pubic bone, percuss bladder Use transilluminator or portable ultrasound to check if bladder is full	
6.	Wear mask; "scrub" hands, wear sterile gloves	
7.	Clean suprapubic area and area over pubic bone with antiseptic swabs × 3 and air dry for 30 sec	
8.	Place sterile drapes over baby's thighs and below suprapubic area	
9.	Attach needle to syringe; palpate symphysis pubis	
10.	Insert needle 1–2 cm above symphysis pubis in midline Maintain needle perpendicular to surface or slightly caudad	
11.	Advance needle 2–3 cm—aspirate gently as needle is advanced; stop advancing needle when urine enters syringe Collect urine sample and withdraw needle	
12.	Do not advance needle more than 3 cm Do not redirect needle in different directions "looking for" urine	
13.	Apply pressure over puncture site with sterile gauze to stop any bleeding Wipe off antiseptic with clean water, and apply small adhesive bandage	
14.	Remove needle and transfer urine specimen into sterile container for urine culture and other tests	

LUMBAR PUNCTURE CHECKLIST	
STEPS OF PROCEDURE	**COMMENTS**
1.	Time out—right patient/right procedure/consent No contraindications? Application of local anesthetic cream	
2.	Check equipment ☐ Cap/mask/gown/sterile gloves ☐ LP kit OR ☐ Cup with iodophor antiseptic solution or antiseptic swab sticks ☐ Sterile towels or aperture drape ☐ Local anesthetic/pain medication ☐ Spinal needle 22-gauge × 1.5-in—two needles ☐ Specimen tubes with caps × 3 ☐ Small adhesive bandage ☐ Pain medication (fentanyl for ventilated infant; local 1% lidocaine injection for nonventilated infant; oral sucrose if appropriate)	
3.	Cardiorespiratory monitor and pulse oximeter	
4.	Have assistant restrain infant in lateral decubitus or sitting position with spine flexed; avoid flexion of the neck	
5.	Locate landmarks: Interspace L4–5 just below or interspace L3–4 just above imaginary line between iliac crests (*Note: Spinal cord termination between T12 to L3 is achieved only at 2 mo post term. Between 25 and 40 wks, the cord termination gradually ascends from L4 to L2. Use L4–5 interspace for preterm infants to avoid cord penetration.*)	
6.	Wear cap and mask (gown optional) "Scrub" hands, wear sterile gloves	
7.	Clean lumbar area with antiseptic × 3 times and air dry for 30 sec	
8.	Sterile drapes: Large flat drape under baby; fenestrated drape over the back	
9.	Local anesthetic injection (or IV fentanyl in ventilated baby) if local anesthetic cream was not applied prior to procedure	
10.	Insert spinal needle in L4–5 interspace in midline; aim slightly cephalad. Depth of 1–1.5 cm in term infant; less in preterm infant	
11.	Feel for "pop"—change in resistance as needle passes through ligamentum flavum and dura (may not be felt in small infants)	
12.	Remove stylet frequently to check for fluid Always replace stylet before advancing needle	
13.	Collect CSF—allow to flow passively into three sterile tubes	
14.	Replace stylet before removing needle	
15.	Place adhesive bandage over puncture site Clean off iodophor from skin with sterile water	

ENDOTRACHEAL INTUBATION CHECKLIST		
ENDOTRACHEAL TUBE DIAMETER FOR PATIENT WEIGHT AND GESTATIONAL AGE		
TUBE SIZE (mm)	WEIGHT (g)	GESTATIONAL AGE (wks)
2.5	<1,000	<28
3.0	1,000–2,000	28–34
3.5	2,000–3,000	34–38
4.0	>3,000	>38

	STEPS OF PROCEDURE	COMMENTS
1.	Time out	
2.	Check equipment ☐ Sterile gloves ☐ 10-Fr suction catheter and suction device ☐ Endotracheal tube of appropriate diameter ☐ Endotracheal tube stylet ☐ Pediatric laryngoscope: Miller blade 1 (term), 0 (preterm), 00 (extreme preterm) ☐ Adhesive tape ☐ Resuscitation bag and mask or T—piece resuscitator ☐ Oxygen source ☐ End-tidal CO_2 detector ☐ Stethoscope ☐ CR monitor and pulse oximeter	
3.	Position infant with head in midline and the neck slightly extended (sniff position)	
4.	Clear oropharynx with gentle suctioning	
5.	Turn on laryngoscope light; hold laryngoscope with LEFT hand with blade directed toward patient	
6.	Open infant's mouth and depress tongue toward the left with right forefinger. Stabilize infants head with remaining fingers of right hand. (*Do not use laryngoscope blade to open the mouth*)	
7.	Under direct visualization, insert laryngoscope blade, sliding over the tongue until the tip of the blade is in the vallecula	
8.	Lift the laryngoscope handle to elevate the epiglottis and visualize the vocal cords (Avoid rocking motion)	
9.	Assistant may apply cricoid pressure to help visualize the vocal cords (optional)	
10.	Insert endotracheal tube through the vocal cords to predetermined length (Length of insertion [cm] = Weight in kg + 6)	
11.	Confirm endotracheal tube position in trachea by end-tidal CO_2 detector and auscultation	
12.	Ensure appropriate position of endotracheal tube; secure with adhesive tape; attach to mechanical ventilator device	
13.	Cut off excessive tube length	

UMBILICAL CATHETER PLACEMENT CHECKLIST	
STEPS OF PROCEDURE	**COMMENTS**
1. Time out (consent as per institutional policy)	
2. Check equipment ☐ Mask/cap/sterile gown/sterile gloves ☐ Measuring tape ☐ Sterile drapes ☐ Antiseptic solution/swabsticks ☐ Umbilical catheter kit ☐ Sterile drapes ☐ Heparinized saline (1 unit heparin/mL saline) ☐ Soft restraints for infant	
3. Wash hands, immobilize baby using soft restraints	
4. Measure or calculate length of insertion for UAC and UVC	
5. Wear hat and mask "Scrub hands" and wear sterile gown and gloves	
6. Open equipment tray maintaining sterility	
7. Prepare catheter(s) in sterile field: ☐ Select appropriate sized catheter(s) ☐ Attach stopcocks ☐ Flush catheters with heparinized saline removing all air bubbles ☐ Keep syringes attached to stopcocks/catheters	
8. Hold cord clamp or distal end of umbilical cord with hemostat (or have assistant hold)	
9. Clean umbilical cord and surrounding skin with antiseptic solution × 3 times	
10. Place sterile drapes around cord	
11. Place umbilical tape at base of cord with a loose knot	
12. Cut umbilical cord about 1 cm above skin surface with sharp scalpel blade	
13. Identify two umbilical arteries and one umbilical vein	
14. Stabilize umbilical cord with hemostats or with gauze	
15. Use iris forceps to dilate umbilical artery slightly	
16. Using small forceps insert catheters into umbilical artery and umbilical vein to predetermined depths	
17. Check for blood return and flush with small volume of heparinized saline	
18. Suture catheters in place using silk and needle holder	
19. Clean off povidone iodine (if used) with sterile water	
20. Tape catheters securely to abdomen	
21. Check position of catheters with x-ray or ultrasound scan	
22. Connect appropriate tubing—transducer for UAC and fluids for UVC	

Note: Break in sterile technique or letting air get into the UAC/ UVC are major errors.

NEEDLE THORACENTESIS CHECKLIST	
EMERGENCY EVACUATION OF AIR LEAKS	
STEPS OF PROCEDURE	COMMENTS
1. Time out—right patient, correct side, right procedure	
2. Check equipment ☐ Cap/mask/sterile gown/sterile gloves ☐ Antiseptic solution ☐ Sterile drapes ☐ 18–20-gauge angiocatheter ☐ IV extension tubing ☐ Three-way stopcock ☐ 10 and 20 mL syringes ☐ Petrolatum gauze	
3. Position infant: supine	
4. Skin prep: Clean hemithorax with antiseptic solution Sterile drapes	
5. Locate landmarks: 2nd intercostal space in midclavicular line OR 4th/5th intercostal space in anterior axillary line (avoid areola of breast)	
6. Connect 3-way stopcock to IV extension tubing Connect syringe to 3-way stopcock	
7. Insert angiocatheter at superior edge of rib at 45 degree angle chest wall, directed cephalad	
8. As angiocatheter enters pleural space, decrease angle to 15 degrees with chest wall Slide cannula in while removing stylet	
9. Attach IV extension tubing to angiocatheter, open stopcock and evacuate air with syringe	
10. Continue evacuating air as patient's condition warrants (Prepare for chest tube placement if required)	
11. Remove cannula and cover insertion site with petrolatum gauze and small dressing after procedure	

PICC (PERIPHERALLY INSERTED CENTRAL CATHETER) CHECKLIST	
STEPS OF PROCEDURE	**COMMENTS**
1.	Consent Time out—right patient/right procedure	
2.	Check equipment ☐ Mask/hat/sterile gown/two pairs of sterile gloves ☐ Antiseptic swabs chlorhexidine or povidone iodine ☐ Cardiorespiratory monitor/pulse oximeter PICC tray or procedure tray with components for PICC ☐ Extra sterile introducer needle ☐ Heparinized saline (1 unit heparin/mL of saline) 5–10 mL ☐ 3 mL syringe ☐ Sterile tourniquet (optional) ☐ Large sterile drape ☐ Tape measure ☐ Local anesthetic cream/pain medication (IV fentanyl) ☐ Steristrips/transparent dressing	
3.	Wash hands	
4.	Select appropriate vein (veins) for placement of PICC Apply local anesthetic cream on insertion site (optional) Measure distance from insertion site to right atrium in centimeters	
5.	Position infant appropriately; swaddle infant if possible, leaving limb for cannulation exposed	
6.	Wear hat and mask Wash hands again as for sterile procedure Wear sterile gown and gloves	
7.	Prepare catheter Cut catheter if required, based on the measurements obtained earlier Attach 3 mL syringe and flush catheter through with heparinized saline	
8.	Have assistant provide IV fentanyl for pain relief/sedation	
9.	Paint insertion site and limb with antiseptic swabs × 3 Allow to air dry for 1 min	
10.	Cover limb/baby with large sterile drape leaving insertion site exposed	
11.	Place sterile tourniquet (optional) Cannulate vein with introducer needle	
12.	Thread catheter through introducer needle to appropriate distance	
13.	Remove introducer needle and "break/peel" it away	
14.	Check markings to confirm depth of insertion of catheter Place small piece of steristrip to secure catheter in place at insertion site	
15.	X-ray confirmation of appropriate position of tip of catheter Upper extremity CXR: catheter tip at SVC/RA junction Lower extremity: Abdominal x-rays—AP and cross-table lateral to confirm catheter is in IVC and not in spinal venous complex	
16.	Dressing: Coil excess catheter into small loops and secure with steristrips and sterile transparent dressing	
17.	Remove excess povidone iodine from skin with sterile water	
18.	Start continuous infusion of fluids through catheter	

B

Appendix
Chapter 7

TABLE B.1 **Neonatal Pain Scales**

SCALE	ASSESSMENT PARAMETERS	AGE LEVEL (GA)	PAIN STIMULUS	RELIABILITY DATA[a]	SCORING/ THERAPEUTIC THRESHOLD	CLINICAL UTILITY
Behavioral Indicators of Infant Pain (BIIP)	■ Behavioral (Combines sleep/wake states, five facial actions and two hand actions)	24–32 wks	Procedural—acute pain	Inter-rater reliability 0.8–0.92	0–10 Intervention suggested for pain score ≥5	■ Assesses the two developmentally relevant hand movements shown to be indicators of pain/stress in preterm infants
Crying Oxygen requirement Vital signs Expression Resting Signaling distress (COVERS) Neonatal Pain Scale	■ Behavioral ■ Physiologic (Assesses crying, oxygen requirement, vital signs, expression, resting and signaling distress)	27–40 wks	Procedural—acute pain	Inter-rater reliability of >0.84 in preterm neonates and >0.95 in term neonates	0–18 Intervention suggested for pain score >7	■ Not for use in paralyzed neonates. ■ Criteria used for scoring applicable to a wider range of infants (e.g., visible crying in the intubated neonate as a behavioral response, looks at a change in need of oxygen) ■ Multidimensional scale[b]
Crying, oxygenation, vital signs, facial expression, and sleeplessness (CRIES)	■ Behavioral ■ Physiologic (Assesses crying, facial expression, sleeplessness, requires oxygen to stay at >95 % saturation, increased vital signs)	32–60 wks	Postoperative—prolonged pain	Inter-rater reliability >0.72	0–10 Intervention suggested for pain score >4	■ Easy to use ■ Limited usefulness in measuring pain in the intubated, paralyzed, or extremely premature infant. ■ Multidimensional scale
Douleur Aiguë du Nouveau-né (DAN)	■ Behavioral (Assesses facial expression, limb movements, vocal expression)	24–41 wks and up to 3 mo	Procedural—acute pain	Inter-rater reliability >0.92	0–10 Intervention suggested for pain score ≥3	■ Multidimensional scale

(continued)

TABLE B.1 Neonatal Pain Scales (*Continued*)

SCALE	ASSESSMENT PARAMETERS	AGE LEVEL (GA)	PAIN STIMULUS	RELIABILITY DATA[a]	SCORING/ THERAPEUTIC THRESHOLD	CLINICAL UTILITY
Echelle Douleur et inconfort du nouveau-né (Modified EDIN6)	■ Behavioral Assessment of 5 items: (1) facial expression (2) body movements (3) quality of sleep, (4) quality of contact with nurses (5) consolability (6) gestational age	25 wk to >37 wks	Pain in the NICU (basal or prolonged Pain)	Inter-rater reliability >0.82–0.86	0–15 Intervention suggested for pain score ≥7	■ Modified EDIN scale to account for pain expression in preterm infant —not solely discomfort ■ One-dimensional scale
EValuation ENfant DOuleur (EVENDOL)	■ Behavioral (Assesses vocal expression, facial movements, posture and interaction with environment)	Newborn to 7 yrs	Acute or prolonged	Inter-rater reliability >0.79–0.92	0–15 Intervention suggested for pain score >4	■ Designed for use in the Emergency Department ■ Simple, easy to use
Faceless Acute Neonatal Pain Scale (FANS)	■ Behavioral ■ Physiologic (Assesses HR change, desaturations, limb movements, vocal expression)	30–35 wks	Procedural	Inter-rater reliability >0.92	0–10 Intervention suggested for pain score >4	■ First scale to evaluate pain in preterm neonate when the face is not accessible ■ Simple and easy bedside pain scale ■ Limited to infants not intubated allowing assessment of vocal expressions ■ Multidimensional scale
Neonatal Facial Coding System (NFCS)	■ Behavioral (Assesses facial actions)	25 wks to term neonates	Procedural	Inter- and intrarater reliability >0.85	0–8 Intervention suggested for pain score >2	■ Established scale to assess pain in newborns and infants
Neonatal Infant Pain Scale (NIPS)	■ Behavioral (Assesses facial expression, crying, breathing patterns, arm and leg movements, arousal)	28–38 wks	Procedural	Inter-rater reliability >0.92–0.97	0–7 Intervention suggested for pain scores ≥4	■ Easy and fast to use ■ Adapted from CHEOPS scale ■ Multidimensional scale
Neonatal Pain, Agitation and Sedation Scale (NPASS)	■ Physiologic ■ Behavioral ■ Contextual (Assesses crying, irritability, facial expression, extremity tone, vital signs)	23–40 wks	Acute, sedation, postopera-tive, ventilated	Inter-rater reliability >0.85	0–10 pain 0–10 sedation Intervention suggested for pain scores >3	■ Combined pain and sedation scale ■ First neonatal combined pain and sedation scale; includes a premature pain assessment that adds to score based on GA

TABLE B.1 Neonatal Pain Scales (*Continued*)

SCALE	ASSESSMENT PARAMETERS	AGE LEVEL (GA)	PAIN STIMULUS	RELIABILITY DATA[a]	SCORING/ THERAPEUTIC THRESHOLD	CLINICAL UTILITY
Premature Infant Pain Profile (PIPP)	■ Physiologic ■ Behavioral ■ Contextual (Assesses Heart rate, oxygen saturation, facial actions)	Term and preterm neonates	Postoperative, Procedural	Inter- and intrarater reliability >0.93–0.96	0–21 Score ≥12 indicated moderate to severe pain	■ Not fast to use ■ Scoring of infant occurs 15 sec immediately before event and 30 sec immediately after event ■ Modified PIPP scale now developed for easier use ■ Limited use in the intubated, paralyzed, and extremely premature neonate
Scale for Use in the Newborn (SUN)	■ Behavioral ■ Physiologic (Assesses CNS state, breathing, movement, tone, facial expression, heart rate changes, and mean blood pressure changes)	Term and preterm neonates	Procedural Intubation — acute pain		0–28 Average baseline scores 10–14	■ Not an easy scale to use compared to NIPS

[a]Internal consistency considered as high when the coefficient is between 0.77 and 0.99.
[b]Combines behavioral, contextual, and physiologic information.
GA, gestational age.

TABLE B.2 Neonatal Sedation Scales

SCALE	ASSESSMENT PARAMETERS	AGE LEVEL (GA)	SEDATION	RELIABILITY DATA[a]	SCORING/THERAPEUTIC THRESHOLD	CLINICAL UTILITY
Neonatal Pain, Agitation, Sedation Scale (NPASS)	■ Physiologic ■ Behavioral ■ Contextual (Assesses crying, irritability, facial expression, extremity tone, vital signs)	23–40 wks	Acute, sedation, postoperative, ventilated	Inter-rater reliability >0.85	0–10 pain 0–10 sedation score between −2 and −5 on the sedation subscale indicates light sedation and a score between −6 and −10 indicates deep sedation	■ Combined pain and sedation scale ■ First neonatal combined pain and sedation scale; includes a premature pain assessment that adds to score based on GA
Modified COMFORT scale	■ Physiologic ■ Behavioral (Assesses alertness, calmness, movement, mean arterial pressure, heart rate, facial expression)	23–54 wks	Acute, sedation ventilated	Inter-rater reliability >0.8	7–35	■ Respiratory assessment is for mechanically ventilated patients ■ Less useful in distinguishing distress caused by pain vs. from delirium or drug withdrawal
State Behavioral Scale (SBS)	Seven dimension ratings: respiratory drive, response to ventilation, coughing, best response to stimulation, attentiveness to care provider, tolerance to care, consolability, movement after consoled	6 wks to 6 yrs[a]	Describing sedation/agitation levels in young intubated patients supported on mechanical ventilation	Inter-rater reliability >0.79	−3 to +2 −3 (unresponsive) −2 (responsive to noxious stimuli) −1 (responsive to gentle touch or voice) 0 (awake and able to calm) +1 (restless and difficult to calm) +2 (agitated)	■ Describing sedation/agitation levels in young intubated patients supported on mechanical ventilation ■ Excludes postop and patients on neuromuscular blockade

[a]Chronological age.

TABLE B.3 Neonatal Withdrawal Scales

SCALE	ASSESSMENT PARAMETERS	AGE LEVEL (CA)	WITHDRAWAL	RELIABILITY DATA[a]	SCORING/ THERAPEUTIC THRESHOLD	CLINICAL UTILITY
Finnegan Neonatal Abstinence Score (NAS) (1975) Finnegan Neonatal Abstinence Syndrome Scale (NASS)—Short Form (2013)	■ Physiologic ■ Behavioral	Newborn	Assessment of withdrawal symptoms in otherwise healthy neonates with prenatal drug exposure	Inter-rater reliability <0.62	0–62 Intervention for scores ≥8 in three consecutive assessments or scores >12 in two consecutive assessments 0–16 Intervention for score ≥8	■ Developed in 1975 for assessment of withdrawal symptoms in otherwise healthy neonates with prenatal drug exposure ■ Most widely used tool ■ Initial scale too long, complex for routine use ■ Recently modified
Lipsitz Neonatal Drug Withdrawal Scoring System	■ Physiologic ■ Behavioral (Assesses tremors, irritability, reflexes, stools, muscle tone, skin abrasions, respiratory rate, repetitive sneezing, yawning, forceful vomiting, and fever)	Newborn	Screen for newborn infants with prenatal exposure	Inter-rater reliability >0.77	0–20 Intervention for score ≥4	■ Only 11 items to score—less resource intensive ■ Four items of scale list yes/no outcome responses
Neonatal Narcotic Withdrawal Index	Consists of 6 signs of NAS plus an "other" category of 12 additional signs	Newborn	Screen for newborn infants with prenatal exposure	Inter-rater reliability >0.77	0–14 Intervention for score ≥5 on two evaluations in 24 hrs	■ Performed twice daily ■ Assesses a brief list of key withdrawal signs and symptoms
Neonatal Withdrawal Inventory (NWI)	An eight point checklist of seven NAS symptoms with a four point behavioral distress scale	Newborn	Screen for newborn infants with prenatal exposure	Inter-rater reliability >0.89	0–19 Intervention for first score >8	■ Simple and easy to use
Withdrawal Assessment Tool— version 1 (WAT-1)	■ Physiologic ■ Behavioral (Assesses previous 12 hr stools, vomiting and temperature, a 2 min pre stimulation observation, 1 min stimulus observation and post stimulus recovery)	2 wks to 18 yrs	Monitoring opioid and benzodiazepine withdrawal symptoms in pediatric patients	Inter-rater reliability >0.8	0–12 Score >3 indicates withdrawal	■ WAT-1 is better at detecting symptoms of opioid versus benzodiazepine withdrawal ■ Performed twice daily ■ Validated to evaluate iatrogenic withdrawal in a broader pediatric population

[a]CA, chronological age.

TABLE B.4 Sedative and Analgesic Agents Commonly Used in Neonates and Infants

THERAPEUTIC CLASS	MEDICATION	MECHANISM OF ACTION	METABOLISM	ROUTE OF ADMINISTRATION (NEONATES)	DOSE AND FREQUENCY	REVERSAL AGENT	COMMENTS
Nonopioid analgesic	Acetaminophen (paracetamol) (Tylenol) (Ofirmev)	Weak inhibitor of prostaglandin synthesis. Inhibits peripheral pain impulse generation via descending serotonergic pathways, L-arginine/nitric oxide pathway, cannabinoid system and redox mechanism[a]	**Hepatic:** Cytochrome P450 (CYP) enzymes; sulfate and glucuronide metabolites CYP2E1, 1A2, 3A4 metabolize small amount to hepatotoxic NAPQI "detoxified" by glutathione conjugation[b]	Oral, rectal, IV infusion 10-mg/mL IV dose FDA labeled for >2 yrs of age: 15 mg/kg q6h or 12.5 mg q4h *Limit: 75 mg/kg/day Infuse dose over 15 min*	*GA 28—32 wks:* **Oral:** 10–12 mg/kg/ dose q6–8h[c] **Rectal:** 20 mg/kg/dose q12h *Limit: 40 mg/kg/day* *GA 33–37 wk and term ≤10 days:* **Oral:** 10–15 mg/kg/ dose q6h **Rectal:** 30 mg/kg then 15 mg/kg/dose q8h *Limit: 60 mg/kg/d* *Term ≥10 days:* **Oral:** 10–15 mg/kg/ dose q4-6h **Rectal:** 30 mg/kg then 20 mg/kg/dose q6–8h *Limit: 75 mg/kg/day*	None: GI decontamination/ acetylcysteine for toxicity	Antipyretic, analgesic, very weak anti-inflammatory activity Inducers of CYP2E1, 1A2, 3A4: (phenobarbital, phenytoin, rifampin) alter metabolism; ↑hepatotoxicity Neonates: ↓ CYP activity; ↓ toxicity with ↑ serum concentrations (lower toxic metabolite) Additive analgesic effect with opioid (opioid sparing)[d] *Ineffective for acute procedural pain[e]* Rectal absorption slow and unreliable[c] IV form: OFIRMEV[g] 1,000 mg/100 mL *Single-use vial, 6 hrs expiration*

		Mechanism of Action	Dosage Forms	Dose	Interactions	Comments
Nonsteroidal anti-inflammatory drugs (NSAIDs) Arylpropionic	Ibuprofen	Inhibition of cyclooxygenase enzyme (COX-1 and COX-2 isoforms) thereby decreasing prostaglandin biosynthesis (PGI2)	**Hepatic:** Phase I and II enzyme biotransformation with urinary and biliary excretion. Metabolism primarily by CYP2C9 and CYP2C8 ↓ CYP2C9 activity in newborn, increasing over first year of life Polymorphisms CYP2C9 may cause ADRs Clearance ↑ after birth also affected by weight, age $t_{1/2}$: 24–30.5 hrs (newborn) vs. 2 hrs (adults)	IV, Oral tablets, solutions	**Oral:** 4–10 mg/kg/ dose q 6–8h as needed[i] *Limit:* 40 mg/kg/day **IV:** Ibuprofen lysine: 10 mg/kg then two doses: 5 mg/ kg at 24 and at 48 hrs "off label" for analgesia *No data regarding use for > 3 days*	None: Maintain hydration, avoid nephrotoxin use Discontinue anticoagulants, replace blood loss if needed, correct low platelets	*NSAIDS not recommended for routine analgesic use in neonate. Limited data on use of ibuprofen analgesia for infants <3 mo of age; monitor urine output, renal function* **NSAID precautions:** Use lowest effective dose for shortest duration possible May displace bilirubin. Caution in asthma, renal or hepatic insufficiency, bleeding disorders, GI disease (bleeding or ulcers), and with anticoagulants[i] Use of ≥1 NSAID not recommended All NSAIDs have potential adverse cardiovascular effects Oral solutions may contain benzoate: *"gasping syndrome"* in newborn IV: No data for analgesic dosing for newborns IV ibuprofen lysine (Neoprofen) is labeled for patent ductus arteriosus (PDA) closure *High incidence of renal and GI side effects reported with use of ibuprofen to treat PDA*
Heteroaryl acetic acid NSAIDs	Ketorolac	Inhibition of cyclooxygenase enzyme (COX-1 and COX-2 isoforms) thereby decreasing prostaglandin biosynthesis (PGI2)	**Hepatic:** Phase I and II enzyme biotransformation with urinary and biliary excretion Metabolism primarily by CYP2C9 and CYP2C8 ↓ CYP2C9 activity in newborn, increasing over first year of life	IV, IM, oral tablets	**IV:** 0.5 mg/kg/ dose q6–8h up to 3 days Infants >1 mo and children <2 yrs of age[i] **IM:** Avoid—painful, erratic absorption	None: Maintain hydration, avoid concomitant nephrotoxins Discontinue anticoagulants, replace blood loss if needed, and correct low platelets	Limited data in infants and children <2 yrs **Do NOT exceed 48–72 hrs treatment** FDA labeled for ≤5 d therapy: ↑ adverse effects and no data[i] Monitor: hematologic parameters (platelets, Hct, Hgb), clinical signs bleeding, fluid status, BUN/Scr, urine output during therapy **Follow NSAID precautions** Infants younger than 21 days and less than 37 wks CGA are at significantly increased risk for bleeding events[i]

(continued)

TABLE B.4 Sedative and Analgesic Agents Commonly Used in Neonates and Infants (Continued)

THERAPEUTIC CLASS	MEDICATION	MECHANISM OF ACTION	METABOLISM	ROUTE OF ADMINISTRATION (NEONATES)	DOSE AND FREQUENCY	REVERSAL AGENT	COMMENTS
Opioid agonists (μ) receptor	Morphine	Binds to Mu opiate receptors in CNS inhibiting ascending pain pathways; altering the perception of and response to pain; generalized CNS depression	**Hepatic:** Glucuronide conjugation to morphine-6-glucuronide (active) and morphine-3-glucuronide (inactive) Onset of action: 5 min (lower lipid solubility) Peak effect: 15 min Neonates: delayed maturation of CYP enzyme/conjugation resulting in a longer half-life, slower clearance, and longer elimination Half-life: Preterm neonates: 10–20 hrs Neonates: 4.5–13.3 hrs	Oral, rectal, IM, intranasal, IV, SC, epidural	**IV:** 0.05–0.1 mg/kg/dose q4–6h **Continuous infusion:** 0.01–0.03 mg/kg/hrs (10–30 mcg/kg/hr) **Intranasal:** 0.2 mg/kg/dose **Oral:** 0.3 mg/kg/dose q3–4h	**Naloxone:** Neonatal depression: 0.1 mg/kg/dose IV/IM/SC. May repeat q2–3 min minutes as needed Neonatal opiate intoxication: 0.1 mg/kg/dose IV	**Use preservative free (PF) formulations.** *Neonates are more susceptible to respiratory depression secondary to immature glucuronidation* [K] *Morphine-3-glucuronide—is the predominant metabolite in preterm neonates; responsible for analgesic antagonism and rapid tolerance.* **Morphine dosage increases may not increase analgesia yet result in respiratory depression.** Adult clearance values by 6 mo of age. Slower rates of dependence and withdrawal vs. fentanyl. May delay attainment of full enteral feeding in the preterm neonate. Long-term AE on neurologic system in preterm infants remains unclear. **Analgesic effect on acute pain in preterm neonates remains controversial** Morphine considered safer than midazolam for neonates requiring sedation. *May require exceeding maximum dose in opioid tolerance with close monitoring.* Dosing interval is inversely related to corrected gestational age.

| Synthetic opioid agonists | Fentanyl | Binds with stereospecific receptors at many sites within CNS, ↑s pain threshold, alters pain reception, inhibits ascending pain pathways | **Hepatic:** CYP3A4 oxidative N dealkylation to norfentanyl (>90%) and inactive metabolites ↑ lipid solubility: Onset of action: 3 min Duration: 30 min Clearance 70% of adult values in term neonates, ↑s rapidly at birth | Intranasal, IV | IV: Pain/sedation: 0.5–4 mcg/kg/dose slow IV q2–4h **Intranasal:** 1.5–2 mcg/kg/dose **Continuous IV:** 0.5–2 mcg/kg/h and titrate | **Naloxone:** Neonatal depression: 0.1 mg/kg/dose May repeat q2–3 min as needed Neonatal opiate intoxication: 0.1 mg/kg/dose IV Neuromuscular blocking agent (prevents chest wall rigidity)[m] | Infusion of IV fentanyl can lead to chest wall rigidity[m] Infuse slowly over 3–5 min Less histamine release than morphine; more suitable for neonates with chronic lung disease (CLD) ↓s pulmonary vascular resistance— may be useful in persistent pulmonary hypertension (PPHN) Induces rapid tolerance and withdrawal vs. morphine (3–5 days fentanyl vs. 2 wks morphine) Monitor for CYP3A4 drug interactions: e.g., inhibitors fluconazole, macrolide antibiotics. Consult reference/clinical pharmacist for updated information |
| | Methadone | Binds to opiate receptors in CNS. These mu-receptors inhibit ascending pain pathways, which alter perception and response to pain. Causes generalized CNS depression Desensitizes δ-opioid receptors, antagonizes NMDA receptors involved in pain sensitization[n] | **Hepatic:** CYP3A4/ CYP2D6 N-demethylated to an active metabolites Onset of action: 20 min IV, 30–60 min Oral (slow) Prolonged elimination half-life (15–55 hrs) Half-life: ↑ variability when used for analgesia in neonates: (3.8–62 hrs)[j,n] | Oral (liquid, tablets), IV, IM, SC | Neonatal abstinence syndrome: 0.05–0.2 mg/kg/ dose q12–24h[n] | **Naloxone** Neonatal depression: 0.1 mg/kg/dose IV/ IM/SC May repeat q2–3 min as needed Neonatal opiate intoxication: 0.1 mg/kg/dose IV | Difficult to titrate doses due to prolonged half-life *Oral solutions may contain propylene glycol or benzyl alcohol "gasping syndrome" in neonates* Some references consider equipotent with morphine Varies with age, disease state, and previous opioid exposure Use caution as incomplete cross-tolerance may occur with methadone and other opioids Long-term effects of NMDA-receptor antagonism in the neonate is unknown High oral bioavailability, low cost, minimal SE once optimal dose is achieved Many drug interactions with CYP3A4, CYP2D6 substrates in the NICU (fluconazole, zidovudine, macrolides, phenobarbital, etc.). Consult updated drug interaction databases |

(continued)

TABLE B.4 Sedative and Analgesic Agents Commonly Used in Neonates and Infants (*Continued*)

THERAPEUTIC CLASS	MEDICATION	MECHANISM OF ACTION	METABOLISM	ROUTE OF ADMINISTRATION (NEONATES)	DOSE AND FREQUENCY	REVERSAL AGENT	COMMENTS
α-adrenergic agonist analgesics	Clonidine	Stimulates alpha-2-adrenoreceptors in locus ceruleus, ↓s presynaptic calcium, inhibits NE release from sympathetic nerve endings reducing sympathetic outflow (useful in managing opioid withdrawal—activates K$^+$ channel via G inhibitory protein as opioids)	**Hepatic:** Primarily hydroxylation, via CYP2D6 **Onset of action:** Oral: 30–60 min	Oral, IV	**Oral:** 1 mcg/kg/dose q4–6h Maximum: 6 mcg/kg/dose **IV infusion:** 0.5 mcg/kg/hr increasing to maximum: 3 mcg/kg/hr	**None:** Discontinue Infusion/dose, support respiration, cardiac function, correct BP	Attenuates adrenergic hyperactivity; somatic and autonomic signs of withdrawal Consider as adjunct for infants with persistent and severe signs of withdrawal (i.e., long-term continuous opioid/benzodiazepine IV infusions)^l *Hold doses for SBP <50 mm Hg or HR <100 bpm* *Do not confuse with clonazepam (Klonopin)* Used for treating opioid induced myoclonus in neonates
	Dexmedetomidine	Hypnotic, analgesic, sympatholytic ↓ sympathetic response to pain; Selectively stimulates dorsal horn of spinal cord α₂-adrenergic receptors; produces sedation via α₁-effects in locus ceruleus, preserving spontaneous ventilation ↑ intraoperative hemodynamic stability	**Hepatic:** Primarily by CYP2A6 then N-glucuronidation and N-methylation Clearance in newborn ≈30% of adult, ↑ to adults rates by 12 mo of age^{n,o}	IV, IM (preservative-free solution) 100 mcg/mL (2 mL)	**IV:** 0.1–0.5 mcg/kg loading dose over 10–20 min Continuous: 0.1–0.3 mcg/kg/hr. Titrate to desired level of sedation Max: 1.5 mcg/kg/hr^p	Most adverse effects respond to discontinuing infusion or ↓ rate Treat bradycardia: atropine; hypotension: ↑ IVF or start vasopressor, hypertension during load dose: ↓ rate	Additive analgesic effect with ketamine, fentanyl, sevoflurane for surgical procedures Control of withdrawal with prolonged opioid use Sedation during mechanical ventilation Monitor pain scores; may cause significant ↓ body temperature^l Avoid abrupt discontinuation—rapid awakening, anxiety, "fighting" ventilator, and withdrawal ↓ dose in hepatic insufficiency Not labeled for use for <18 yrs Animal models suggest a potentially neuroprotective effect of dexmedetomidine

| General anesthetics | Ketamine | Direct action on cortex and limbic system to produce dissociative anesthesia. Blocks D-2 dopamine receptor. Noncompetitive agonist of NMDA No effect on pharyngeal or laryngeal reflexes[p] | **Hepatic:** N-dealkylation hydroxylation, glucuronide conjugation, dehydration of hydroxylated metabolites | IV | IV: 0.5–2 mg/kg Induction dose: 1–2 mg/kg **Continuous IV infusion** (sedation): 5–20 mcg/kg/min Titrate to desired level[p] | **None** Discontinue infusion, support respiration, cardiac function, emergence reactions (pediatrics < adults)[i,p] | Provides sedation, analgesia, amnesia. Sedation in mechanically ventilated neonates, especially during suctioning Caution in GERD: ↑ vomiting, will ↑ ICP Not adequate as sole anesthetic for surgical procedures of pharynx, larynx, and bronchial tree or visceral pain pathways Pre-medicate with IV atropine dose secondary to increased production of upper respiratory and salivary secretions *Limited neonatal use due to potential ↑ ICP and neurotoxicity[p,s]* Long-term effects unknown. Increase in neuronal apoptosis observed in neonatal animal studies The American College of Emergency Physicians (ACEP Green 2011) considers use of ketamine in infants aged <3 mo an absolute contraindication, due higher risk of airway complications |
| | Propofol | Alkylphenol sedative–hypnotic. Increases responsiveness of GABA receptor to GABA, potentiating glycine activity (mediates response to noxious stimuli) | **Hepatic:** Extensive metabolism via CYP, with glucuronide and sulfate conjugation | IV | IV: 200–300 mcg/kg/min initial dose[q,r] Usual dose range: 125–150 mcg/kg/min *Effective, safe dose range for neonates needs further study* | **None** Discontinue infusion, support respiration, cardiac function, correct acid-base status | Limited data for use in neonates Advantages: Rapid onset, short t₁/₂ SE: Pain at injection site, hypotension, apnea Generics: Contain benzyl alcohol, sodium benzoate *No analgesic properties/assess sedative effect* ↓ doses when giving with opioids[q,r] Monitor lipids, metabolic status during infusion Significant decrease in mean arterial pressure reported in preterm neonates[q,r] Restrict use to trained personal |

(continued)

TABLE B.4 Sedative and Analgesic Agents Commonly Used in Neonates and Infants (*Continued*)

THERAPEUTIC CLASS	MEDICATION	MECHANISM OF ACTION	METABOLISM	ROUTE OF ADMINISTRATION (NEONATES)	DOSE AND FREQUENCY	REVERSAL AGENT	COMMENTS
Benzodiazepines	Diazepam	Binds to GABA receptors in CNS decreasing excitability of neuronal cells[s]	**Hepatic:** CYP P450 oxidation and demethylation to active metabolites (oxazepam) **Half-life:** Diazepam Infants (40–50 hrs) Neonates (50–100 hrs)	IV, Oral	**IV:** 0.1–0.3 mg/kg dose over 3–5 min, maximum total dose of 2 mg **Oral:** 0.2–1 mg/kg q6–8h for NAS	Flumazenil 0.01 mg/kg IV (total dose 0.05 mg/kg)	Not first-line IV due to: benzoic acid, benzyl alcohol, sodium benzoate Extravasation may cause necrosis Benzodiazepine complications: myoclonic jerking, excessive sedation, respiratory depression
	Lorazepam	Binds to GABA receptors in CNS decreasing excitability of neuronal cells	**Hepatic:** Glucuronide conjugation to inactive metabolite: lorazepam glucuronide	IV, Oral	**IV/Oral:** 0.05–0.1 mg/kg q4–8h as needed **IV continuous infusion:** 0.05–0.1 mg/kg/hr Dilute with sterile water 1:1 prior to infusion	Flumazenil 0.01 mg/kg IV (total dose 0.05 mg/kg)	Risk of withdrawal (irritability, agitation, tremors, sleep problems) after long-term sedation with IV benzodiazepines[t] Slower BBB penetration vs. diazepam[i] Caution: Monitor for propylene glycol toxicity with continuous infusion Oral solutions contain propylene glycol +/− benzyl alcohol ("gasping syndrome") ↓ dose for hepatic dysfunction Incompatible with TPN
	Midazolam	Binds to GABA receptors in CNS decreasing excitability of neuronal cells	**Hepatic:** CYP-P450 hydroxylation followed by glucuronide conjugation, highly protein bound **Rapid onset:** 1–5 min IV <5 min intranasal **Peak sedative action:** <20 min	IV, Oral, intranasal	**IV (slow):** 0.05–0.15 mg/kg/ dose **Intranasal:** 0.1–0.3 mg/kg/dose **Oral:** 0.15–0.45 mg/kg/ dose **Continuous infusion:** 0.03–0.06 mg/kg/ hr = 0.5–1 mcg/ kg/min	Flumazenil 0.01 mg/kg IV (total dose 0.05 mg/kg)	*No analgesic effect.* Anxiolytic, sedative, muscle relaxant, anticonvulsant *Not recommended for continuous intravenous infusion in neonates* Caution in hepatic impairment Monitor for hypotension, respiratory depression, and seizure-like activity Decreases cerebral blood flow velocities Decrease dose in neonates with decreased cardiac output Data required on safety and efficacy of midazolam in neonates *Insufficient evidence to promote routine use of midazolam as sedative for neonates[s,t,u]* Reports of serious neurologic and hemodynamic effects, and of negative cerebral artery blood flow Midazolam induces apoptosis and is concentration dependent via activation of mitochondrial pathway in neonatal animal models[t,u]

Sucrose analgesia	Oral sucrose solution	Activation of endogenous opioid system through taste[o]	Oral	**Carbohydrate metabolism:** Undergoes gastric hydrolysis, utilized as a carbohydrate (3.94 kcal/g)	0.2–0.5 mL/kg Avoid >10 doses per 24 hrs, especially during first week of life and in preterm infants Limited data on safe maximum dose	**None** Adverse effects ≤1.5%: Choking, spitting-up, vomiting after dose	Use 12–24% sucrose or glucose 20–30% Administer 1–2 min prior to procedure Concentrated preparations are hyperosmolar (up to 1,000 mOsm/L). *Use with caution especially in preterm neonates* Long-term safety and neuro-developmental outcomes of repeated oral sucrose administration unknown. Higher number of sucrose doses associated with poorer motor development and attention/orientation scores at 36 and 40 wks postmenstrual age Coadministration of sucrose with nonnutritive sucking may be additive/synergistic Place on tip of tongue (location of opioid receptors) Reduces pain during venipunctures/heelsticks. Tolerance may develop with repeated doses Neonates of opioid-dependent mothers may not respond Synergistic effect with nonpharmacologic therapies such as facilitated tucking and skin-to-skin contact
Topical anesthetics	Lidocaine 1 mg with epinephrine	Blocks initiation and conduction of nerve impulses via ↓ sodium permeability	Subcutaneous (SC)	**Hepatic/dermal:** CYP-450 and small amount of dermal metabolism to monoethyl-glycinexylidide	**SC:** 2–5 mg/kg	**None** Mild swelling, bruising, and bleeding at site of injection. Systemic toxicity in neonate after inadvertent lidocaine intravascular injection during dorsal penile nerve block[v]	Available with epinephrine (vasoconstrictor) for select procedures (e.g., suture)[y] *Examine labels closely—avoid error* Consider adding sodium bicarbonate to buffer to ↓ pain or warming vial prior to injection to body temperature Use SC (without EPI) for ring or nerve blocks

(continued)

TABLE B.4 Sedative and Analgesic Agents Commonly Used in Neonates and Infants (Continued)

THERAPEUTIC CLASS	MEDICATION	MECHANISM OF ACTION	METABOLISM	ROUTE OF ADMINISTRATION (NEONATES)	DOSE AND FREQUENCY	REVERSAL AGENT	COMMENTS
	Lidocaine 4% liposomal cream	Blocks initiation and conduction of nerve impulses via ↓ sodium permeability	**Hepatic/dermal:** CYP-450 and small amount of dermal metabolism to monoethyl-glycinexylidide	Topical	Topical	Local skin reactions	Use in term infants for short term procedures **Avoid use in premature infants: contains benzyl alcohol** Avoid prolonged contact[v,w]
	Lidocaine 2.5%/ prilocaine 2.5% eutectic mixture cream	Blocks initiation and conduction of nerve impulses via ↓ sodium permeability	**Hepatic/dermal:** CYP-450 and small amount of dermal metabolism to monoethyl-glycinexylidide	Topical	**Topical:** 0.5–2 g under occlusive dressing 1 hr prior to procedure 2 g = Term infants 0.5 g = Preterm *Avoid applying over larger areas and for >2 hrs duration*	Local skin reactions Methemoglobinemia	Methemoglobinemia from prolonged contact/large amounts in young infants[w] Drugs predisposing to methemoglobinemia include: Sulfas, acetaminophen, benzocaine, nitrofurantoin, nitroglycerin, phenobarbital, phenytoin Has been used safely in preterm infants in small amounts once daily. Do not apply near or in open wounds. Avoid in severe hepatic disease. Caution in infants receiving class I antiarrhythmics.

[a]Wang C, Allegaert K, Tibboel D, et al. Population pharmacokinetics of paracetamol across the human age-range from (pre)term neonates, infants, children to adults. *J Clin Pharmacol.* 2014;54(6):619.

[b]Pacifici GM, Allegaert K. Clinical pharmacology of paracetamol in neonates: a review. *Curr Ther Res.* 2015;77:24.

[c]van Lingen RA, Deinum JT, Quak JM, et al. Pharmacokinetics and metabolism of rectally administered paracetamol in preterm neonates. *Arch Dis Child Fetal Neonatal Ed.* 1999;80(1)F59.

[d]Ceelie I, De Wildt SN, Van Dijk M, et al. Effect of intravenous paracetamol on postoperative morphine requirements in neonates and infants undergoing major noncardiac surgery: a randomized controlled trial. *JAMA.* 2013;309(2):149.

[e]Seifi F, Peirovifar A, Gharehbaghi MM. Comparing the efficacy of oral sucrose and acetaminophen in pain relief for ophthalmologic screening of retinopathy of prematurity. *Am J Med Sci Med.* 2013;1(2):24.

[f]Cook SF, Roberts JK, Samiee-Zafarghandy S, et al. Population pharmacokinetics of intravenous paracetamol (acetaminophen) in preterm and term neonates: model development and external evaluation. *Clin Pharmacokinet.* 2016;55(1):107–119.

[g]Ofirmev (acetaminophen). Injection package labeling. San Diego, CA: Cadence Pharmaceuticals, Inc.; revised November 2010.

[h]Reuters T. Red Book: Pharmacy's Fundamental Reference. Los Angeles, CA: PDR Network; 2018.

[i]Taketomo CK, Hodding JH, Kraus DM. Pediatric and Neonatal Dosage Handbook, 18th ed. Hudson, OH: Lexi-Comp; 2017.

[j]Aldrink JH, Ma M, Caniano DA, et al. Safety of ketorolac in surgical neonates and infants 0–3 months old. *J Pediatr Surg.* 2011;46(6):1081.

[k]Klimas R, Mikus G. Morphine-6-glucuronide is responsible for the analgesic effect after morphine administration: a quantitative review of morphine, morphine-6-glucuronide, and morphine-3-glucuronide. *Br J Anaesth.* 2014;113(6):935.

[l]Pacifici GM. Clinical pharmacology of fentanyl in preterm infants: a review. *Pediatr Neonatol.* 2015;56:143.

[m]Malik I, Wilks JA, Singh P, et al. Fentanyl-induced chest wall rigidity in the intensive care unit. *J Clin Anesth Pain Med.* 2015;2(1):1.

[n]Ward RM, Drover DR, Hammer GB, et al. The pharmacokinetics of methadone and its metabolites in neonates, infants and children. *Paediatr Anaesth.* 2014; 24(6):591.

[o]Estkowski LM, Morris JL, Sinclair EA. Characterization of dexmedetomidine dosing and safety in neonates and infants. *J Pediatr Pharmacol Ther.* 2015;20(2):112–118.

[p]Bhutta AT. Ketamine: a controversial drug for neonates. *Semin Perinatol.* 2007;31:303.

[q]Shah PS, Shah VS. Propofol for procedural sedation/anaesthesia in neonates. *Cochrane Database Syst Rev.* 2011;(3):CD007248.

[r]Merchaoui Z, Le Saché N, Julé L, et al. PO-0272 Evaluation of propofol for sedation in neonatal endotracheal intubation. *Arch Dis Child.* 2014:99:A334.

[s]Morriss FH, Jr, Saha S, Bell EF, et al. Eunice Kennedy Shriver National Institute of Child Health and Human Development Neonatal Research Network Surgery and neurodevelopmental outcome of very low-birth-weight infants. *JAMA Pediatr.* 2014;168:746.

[t]Hall W. Anesthesia and analgesia in the NICU. *Clin Perinatol.* 2012;39(1):239.

[u]Taddio A, Ohlsson A. Intravenous midazolam infusion for sedation of infants in the neonatal intensive care unit. *Cochrane Data Syst Rev.* 2012;6:CD002052.

[v]Tutag Lehr V, Taddio A. Practical approach to topical anesthetics in the neonate. *Semin Perinatol.* 2007;(5):323.

[w]Guay J. Methemoglobinemia related to local anesthetics; a summary of 242 episodes. *Anesth Analg.* 2009;108:837.

There are concerns about neurodevelopmental effects on the newborn brain. Chronic and early administration of opioids and benzodiazepines are discouraged in preterm infants on mechanical ventilation. Preclinical evidence suggest that early anesthetic exposure may lead to neuroapoptosis. Further evaluation is required. Use of these agents should be limited and assessed and reassessed over the course of treatment.

CGA, corrected gestational age.

C

Appendix

Chapter 37
Bedside Checklist for Each Infant While on b-CPAP

To Be Completed by Infant's Nurse Each Shift

Date: _____

CHECK POINTS	TIME	TIME	TIME
Blended air/oxygen supply is appropriate			
Flow meter at 5–7 L/min			
Humidifier water level is correct			
Excess rainout in the afferent tubing is drained			
Nasal prong size is correct			
Nasal prongs positioned correctly and not touching the septum			
Head cap fits snugly			
Corrugated tubing correctly placed			
Velcro moustache is correctly placed			
Septum is intact			
Neck roll is of correct size and position			
Head position is correct			
Preductal oxygen saturation probe			
Excess rainout in the efferent tube is drained			
Tape at 7 cm at base of bottle			
Sterile water (or acetic acid) level is at 0 cm			
Tubing securely fixed at 5 cm under water			
Gas bubbling in the bottle continuously			
Date circuit is due for a change (7 days max)			
Date CPAP prongs is due for a change (3 days max)			
Nurse Signature			

D

Appendix

Chapter 44

TABLE D.1 **Neonatal Surgical Tray**

QUANTITY	MANUFACTURER	CATALOG	INSTRUMENT NAME
			Forceps
2	Aesculap	OC020R	Iris Forceps Straight 4″
2	Aesculap	OC022R	Iris Forceps Curved Serrated 4″
2	Aesculap	BD511R	Adson Forceps with teeth 4¾″
2	Aesculap	FB400R	DeBakey Forceps 2 mm × 6″
			Clamps
2	Aesculap	BH104R	Hartmann Mosquito Clamp Straight 4″
2	Aesculap	BH105R	Mosquito Clamp Curved 4″
2	Aesculap	BH110R	Halsted Mosquito Clamp Straight 5″
2	Aesculap	BH111R	Halsted Mosquito Clamp Curved 5″
			Needle Holders
1	Aesculap	BM204R	Derf Needle Holder
1	Aesculap	BM218R	Crile Wood Needle Holder 6″
			Scissors
1	Aesculap	BC210R	Iris Scissors Straight 4⅜″
1	Aesculap	BC252R	Mayo Scissors Straight 6¾″
1	PW	35-2109	DeMartel Vascular Scissors 7¾″
			Retractors
1	Aesculap	BV010R	Alm Retractor 2¾″
1	Aesculap	BV011R	Alm Retractor 4″
2	Aesculap	OA338R	Blair Retractor Sharp 4-prongs × 5¾″
			Miscellaneous
4	Aesculap	BF431R	Towel Clip Small
1	Aesculap	MB603R	Eye Probe 5″
1	Aesculap	US063	Metal Iodine Cup 6 oz
12	Kendall	9132	Sponge Gauze 2″ × 2″
12	Kendall	9024	Sponge Gauze 4″ × 4″
6	MediAction	706-B	OR Blue Towel

TABLE D.1 Neonatal Surgical Tray (*Continued*)

QUANTITY	MANUFACTURER	CATALOG	INSTRUMENT NAME
			Add to Tray after Sterilization
1	BD Eclipse	305780	BD Eclipse Needle 1 mL 25-gauge × 5/8"
2	BD Eclipse	305062	Syringe Luer-Lok 5 mL BD Needle 18-gauge × 1.5"
1	BD Eclipse	371615	Disposable Scalpel Blade #15
1	BD Eclipse	371611	Disposable Scalpel Blade #11
1	Misc	0607	Connector Tubing Plastic 5 in 1
3	Misc	0610	Rubber Band # 16
1	Cardinal	U11 T	Umbilical Tape
1	Cardinal	683G	Black Silk Suture 4-0
1	Cardinal	682	Black Silk Suture 5-0

NB. These are the contents of the Neonatal Surgical Tray used at MedStar Georgetown University Hospital, Washington, DC. Descriptors are given for ordering but are subject to individual preference. Disposable, single-use, or plastic instruments from commercially prepared trays are suitable for many procedures.

TABLE D.2 Selected Sutures Appropriate for Common Neonatal Procedures

TYPE	RAW MATERIAL	TISSUE USE	ADVANTAGES	DISADVANTAGES
Vicryl or Dexon	Synthetic copolymers	Subcutaneous Fascia	Mild tissue reaction (2+) Low infectivity rate For absorbable suture or ligature Maintain knots	Cannot be used for approximation under stress 60% strength at 2 wks Safety in cardiovascular tissue not established Requires flat and square ties with extra throws
Silk	Braided protein filament from silk worm	Skin Fascia Securing chest tubes and catheters	Best knot holding Easiest to use Strong for size	High infectivity rate High tissue reaction
Nylon	Polyamide polymer Mono- or braided filament	Monofilament: skin closure and plastic surgery Braided: any tissue Securing chest tubes and catheters	Inert Least tissue reaction Lowest infectivity	Poor knot holding, requires at least six ties Not as easy to handle
Prolene	Polymer of propylene Monofilament	Skin Pull-out subcuticular	Inert Low tissue reaction (0–1+) Low infectivity Very strong for size Holds knot better than nylon	Remains encapsulated
Skin closure tape	Reinforced nylon filaments to back or porous paper tape	Skin superficial laceration or when subcuticular suture also used	Easy to place and remove Quick to apply No skin reactivity Least scarring No anesthetic required	Will not stick to wet or oily skin (wipe skin with alcohol first) Will not hold if wound is widely separated or under tension Cannot evert wound edges

E

Appendix

Chapters 48 and 49

TABLE E.1 **Blood Products**

WHOLE BLOOD PRODUCTS				
PRODUCT	SHELF LIFE	ADVANTAGES	DISADVANTAGES	COMMENTS
A. Whole blood Hct 38–44%	1. ACD/CPD/CP2D = 21 days 2. CPDA-1 = 35 days	1. Provides volume 2. Provides RBCs 3. Provides some coagulation factors	1. WBC, and platelets relatively nonfunctional unless fresh and unrefrigerated 2. Storage lesion defects (K^+) in plasma fraction	1. Used for exchange transfusion 2. PRBCs and FFP preferable for correction of massive blood loss
B. Reconstituted whole blood Hct variable	24 hrs	1. Allows preparation of whole blood from stored RBCs (packed or frozen) and FFP 2. Allows preparation of Group O cells with low-titer A and B antibody plasma	1. Time for preparation	1. Use for exchange transfusion 2. Hematocrit may be adjusted by formula 3. Provides replacement equivalent of fresh whole blood. 4. Formula for reconstitution: volume of plasma to add = volume PRBCs × (Hct PRBCs/Hct desired − 1).
C. Autologous fetal blood	1. Fresh heparinized <4 hrs 2. ACD/CPD/CP2D = 21 days 3. CPDA = 35 days 4. AS = 42 days	1. Potential immediate availability in delivery room or from blood bank	1. Risk of bacterial contamination 2. Difficult to obtain correct anticoagulant blood ratio 3. Requires anticipatory preparation for best procedural control 4. Complicated procedure to perform in DR and maintain sterility	1. Information on advantages of autologous blood is limited 2. Properly prepared and tested banked blood is a better choice if time permits 3. Developing countries exploring use 4. Competition for umbilical cord banking 5. Consider delaying cord clamping as alternative

TABLE E.1 Blood Products (*Continued*)

RED CELL PRODUCTS					
PRODUCTS	VOLUME (mL)	SHELF LIFE	ADVANTAGES	DISADVANTAGES	COMMENTS
A. PRBCs Hct 70–75% in CPDA-1 Hct 55–60% in additive solutions (AS)	1. CPDA-1 = 250 2. AS = 350	1. ACD/CPD/CP2D = 21 days 2. CPDA-1 = 35 days 3. AS = 42 days	1. Readily available 2. Easy to prepare	1. Accentuated storage lesion defects if unit is at end of shelf life 2. Less RBC mass/mL of transfused product, if PRBCs in additive solutions are used	1. Principal use for correction of anemia 2. With sterile connecting device, can remove aliquots for transfusion 3. If only AS products available, hard pack for massive transfusion or for exchange transfusion
B. Sedimented RBCs Hct 65–80% (variable)	Variable	As above	1. Does not require centrifugation 2. Contains less plasma than standard RBC units	1. Hct may not be as high as desired	An alternative to hard packing without centrifugation
C. Quad pack collection Hct 55–75%	Mother unit = 250–350 Each satellite unit ≤150	As above	1. Allows multiple transfusions to one infant 2. Volume of each quad adjustable	1. Outdate rates high unless NICU has a number of infants 2. Some wastage expected	Many neonatal units find this collection system valuable if they do not have sterile connecting equipment available.
D. Leukodepleted RBCs	CPDA-1 = 250 AS = 350	As above	1. WBC count $<1-5 \times 10^6$/product 2. Reduces risk of transmission of CMV	1. Prestorage LD preferred over bedside filters 2. Cannot LD a unit from sickle-trait donor 3. Leukodepletion failures occur	1. Indicated for prevention of febrile transfusion reactions and for leukocyte alloimmunization in older children, but these phenomena are rare in neonates 2. Does not prevent TA-GVHD
E. Irradiated PRBCs	1. CPDA-1 = 250 2. AS = 350	As above	1. Abrogates GVHD in susceptible infants	1. Storage limited to 28 days postirradiation or by original expiration date due to K^+ leak 2. Equipment not always available	1. Irradiation before issue preferable to long-term refrigerator storage postirradiation

(*continued*)

TABLE E.1 Blood Products (*Continued*)

RED CELL PRODUCTS					
PRODUCTS	VOLUME (mL)	SHELF LIFE	ADVANTAGES	DISADVANTAGES	COMMENTS
F. Washed RBCs	200	24 hrs	1. Removes 80% WBCs 2. Removes platelets, K^+, anticoagulant 3. Hct adjustable—less viscosity	1. Time required for preparation 2. Equipment not always available 3. Expires 24 hrs after washing as "open" system	1. Can wash portions of quad pack 2. May be combined with FFP for exchange transfusions. 3. Major indications include patients with hyperkalemia and T activation
G. Frozen deglycerolized RBCs	200	Frozen up to 10 yrs After thawing/deglycerolizing for 24 hrs unless stored using a closed system	1. Maintenance of 2, 3-DPG and ATP 2. Removes >80% WBCs	1. Higher cost than other preparations 2. Equipment not always available 3. Typically expires 24 hrs after washing (closed system may be 14 days)	1. RBCs frozen with glycerol, thawed, and deglycerolized by washing prior to transfusion, resuspended in 0.9% NaCl 2. Allows storage of rare types of blood

PLATELET PRODUCTS					
PRODUCTS	VOLUME (mL)	SHELF LIFE	ADVANTAGES	DISADVANTAGES	COMMENTS
A. Platelet concentrate (random donor platelet)	40–70	4 hrs to 5 days	Approximately 5.5×10^{10} platelets in 40–70 mL plasma	1. Contains some WBCs, few RBCs, and plasma 2. Rh D immunization possible	1. Use immediately on receipt from blood bank and never refrigerate 2. May be leukocyte reduced 3. Volume may be reduced by centrifugation for use when out of group or extreme volume restriction is necessary; changes expiration to 4 hrs
B. Single-donor apheresis platelets	250–300	5 days	1. $>3 \times 10^{11}$ platelets in 250–300 mL of plasma 2. Always LD with current collection equipment 3. If used over 5 days, can reduce donor exposures. 4. Repeated pheresis from some donor possible	1. Large volume; needs to be split or aliquoted into EUs	1. Allows selection of HLA- and HPA-compatible donors 2. 1 EU = 5.5×10^{10} platelets 3. Std dose = 1 EU/5–10 kg with minimum dose of one EU (volume reduction may be necessary for ELBW infants) 4. Platelet additive solutions (PAS) and pathogen reduction technologies being used in some centers

TABLE E.1 **Blood Products** (*Continued*)

PLASMA PRODUCTS					
PRODUCTS	VOLUME (mL)	SHELF LIFE	ADVANTAGES	DISADVANTAGES	COMMENTS
A. FFP	180–300	Frozen (−18°C) = 1 yr Thawed = 24 hrs	1. Contains plasma proteins, coagulation factors, anticoagulant proteins, complement, and albumin	1. 20–45 min thawing time 2. Not for volume expansion or fibrinogen replacement	1. Separated from WB within 6–8 hrs collection 2. Must be ABO compatible 3. Use blood filter 4. Confused with PF24, now more commonly available
B. Cryoprecipitate	12–20	Frozen (−18°C) = 1 yr Thawed = 6 hrs	1. Better source of fibrinogen and VWF than plasma products	1. Limited indications include F XIII and congenital/acquired fibrinogen deficiency	1. Must be ABO compatible 2. Use blood filter 3. Transfuse immediately after thaw 4. Dose = 1 U/5–10 kg
C. Albumin	5%	3 yrs at room temperature	1. Heat treated to reduce risk of infectious diseases 2. Requires no cross-match 3. Increases plasma oncotic pressure	1. Expensive 2. Does not provide coagulation factors	1. Five micron filter required 2. Na 130–160 mmol/L 3. Osmolarity ~330 mOsm/L 4. Isotonic
D. Albumin	25%	3 yrs at room temperature	1. Requires no cross-match 2. Increases plasma oncotic pressure with low volume	1. Expensive 2. Does not provide coagulation factors 3. Can produce pulmonary edema and cardiac failure	1. Five micron filter required 2. Na 130–160 mmol/L 3. Osmolarity ~330 mOsm/L 4. Hypertonic (high oncotic pressure)
E. Plasma frozen within 24 hrs (PF24)	180–300	1 yr if frozen; Thawed = 24 hrs	1. Contains plasma proteins, coagulation factors, anticoagulant proteins, complement, and albumin	1. May be less effective for FV, FVIII, and VWF replacement 2. Not indicated for volume expansion/fibrinogen replacement	1. Separated from WB and frozen with 24 hrs 2. Most commonly available from blood suppliers 3. Thawed plasma, released up to 5 days postthaw, may also be used but some decrement in clotting factors
F. Single source plasma	180–300		1. Contains plasma proteins, coagulation factors, anticoagulant proteins, complement, and albumin		1. From single-donor plasmapheresis 2. Can be aliquoted into small volumes and frozen for neonatal use
G. Recovered plasma	180–300		1. Contains plasma proteins, coagulation factors, anticoagulant proteins, complement, and albumin	1. May be less effective for FV, FVIII, and VWF replacement 2. Not indicated for volume expansion/fibrinogen replacement	1. Plasma recovered from WB without specialized time limit 2. Quality of factors/anticoagulant proteins not well studied

Index

Note: Page numbers followed by f refer to figure and t refer to table respectively.